Cancer Precursors

Springer
New York
Berlin
Heidelberg
Barcelona
Hong Kong
London
Milan
Paris
Singapore
Tokyo

Eduardo L. Franco, MPH, DrPH
Professor, Departments of Oncology and Epidemiology, and
Director, Division of Cancer Epidemiology, McGill University,
Montreal, Quebec, Canada

Thomas E. Rohan, MB, BS, PhD
Professor and Chairman, Department of Epidemiology and
Social Medicine, Albert Einstein College of Medicine, Bronx,
New York, USA

Editors

Cancer Precursors

Epidemiology, Detection, and Prevention

Foreword by Joseph F. Fraumeni, Jr., MD, MSc

With 50 Figures

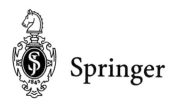

Springer

Eduardo L. Franco, MPH, DrPH
Professor
Departments of Oncology
 and Epidemiology
and
Director
Division of Cancer Epidemiology
McGill University
Montreal, Quebec H2W 1S6, Canada

Thomas E. Rohan, MB, BS, PhD
Professor and Chairman
Department of Epidemiology
 and Social Medicine
Albert Einstein College
 of Medicine
Bronx, NY 10461, USA

Cover illustration: For cover art, see Figure 15.1 on page 234.

Library of Congress Cataloging-in-Publication Data
Cancer precursors : epidemiology, detection, and prevention / editors, Eduardo L.
Franco, Thomas E. Rohan.
    p. ; cm
Includes bibliographical references and index.
ISBN 0-387-95188-1 (h/c : alk. paper)
1. Precancerous conditions.   I. Franco, Eduardo L.   II. Rohan, Thomas E.
[DNLM: 1. Precancerous Conditions–pathology. 2. Neoplasms—diagnosis. 3.
Neoplasms—prevention & control. QZ 204 C215 2001]
RC268.5.C328 2001
616.99′4–dc21   2001049595

Printed on acid-free paper.

Production coordinated by Chernow Editorial Services, Inc., and managed by Lesley
Poliner; manufacturing supervised by Jerome Basma.
Typeset by Best-set Typesetter Ltd., Hong Kong.
Printed and bound by Maple-Vail Book Manufacturing Group, York, PA.
Printed in the United States of America.

9 8 7 6 5 4 3 2 1

ISBN 0-387-95188-1   SPIN 10789389

Springer-Verlag   New York Berlin Heidelberg
A member of BertelsmannSpringer Science+Business Media GmbH

To Our Wives
Eliane and Rosa

Foreword

Dramatic advances in our understanding of cancer causation have come from epidemiologic and laboratory research, particularly over the past two decades. These developments have included a broadening interest in the critical events that take place during the early stages of the dynamic multistep process leading to invasive cancer. Increasingly, cancer epidemiologists are pursuing research into the origins and natural history of premalignant lesions, including intermediate or surrogate endpoints, a trend accelerated by the development of molecular technologies that are revolutionizing our understanding of the transformation of normal to malignant cells. There seems little doubt that this emerging knowledge will provide further insights not only into carcinogenic processes, but also into more sensitive methods of early detection and more effective means of prevention.

In this book, Drs. Franco and Rohan have succeeded in preparing a comprehensive, timely, and critical review of the substantial progress that has been made in our understanding of cancer precursors. They have enlisted experts in the field who have contributed authoritative chapters on the precursors to a wide variety of cancers, with emphasis on etiology and natural history, including the role of environmental and heritable factors that provoke normal cells to undergo malignant transformation. Epidemiologic data are linked whenever possible to molecular as well as classical cellular pathology, providing a fuller understanding of the causal events and mechanisms that initiate the carcinogenic process.

It is generally understood that preventing cancer is far preferable to treating it. While opportunities now exist for primary and secondary prevention of certain cancers, we are still limited by an incomplete understanding of causal factors and precursor lesions that hold the key to advances in cancer prevention. However, as a result of conceptual breakthroughs in our understanding of the fundamental mechanisms of cancer, there is growing optimism that the incorporation of molecular and genetic probes into epidemiologic and clinical approaches will more fully illuminate events on the causal pathway to cancer. By identifying and deploying sensitive biomarkers of carcinogenic exposure, susceptibility genes, and intermediate outcomes, it should be possible to more precisely define individuals at elevated risk of cancer, and to design and test novel approaches to diagnostic and preventive interventions.

This optimism is tempered, however, by the formidable challenges for epidemiologic and multidisciplinary research to identify, select, measure, validate, and integrate biomarkers that are predictive of cancer risk and amenable to preventive measures. While this book presents a wealth of information about cancer precursors, it also indicates the complexity of the task ahead for epidemiologists, as well as clinicians, molecular biologists, and other scientists, whose work on precursors may usher in new strategies to eliminate cancer before it develops and escapes control.

Joseph F. Fraumeni, Jr., MD, MSc
Director, Division of Cancer
Epidemiology and Genetics
National Cancer Institute
National Institutes of Health
Rockville, Maryland, USA

Preface

The purpose of this book is to bring together in one place reviews of the descriptive, analytical, and molecular epidemiological research on cancer precursors at specific anatomical locations, as well as a discussion of the methodological issues associated with the study of cancer precursors. We feel that such a book is particularly timely since the last few years have brought considerable progress in our understanding of the early natural history of cancer and of the etiology of precursor lesions. There have also been improvements in the means of detecting precursor lesions, either directly or via testing of surrogate biomarkers. While progress has perhaps been more rapid for cancer precursors at those anatomical sites which are more accessible and therefore more amenable to study, there is now a considerable body of knowledge bearing on the topic of precursor lesions at many sites.

The book is divided into five sections. Part I seeks to place subsequent chapters in context by providing brief overviews of the molecular basis of carcinogenesis and of the histological aspects of cancer precursors.

Part II addresses some of the issues related to the measurement, interpretation, and study of precursor lesions. Specifically, this section includes a chapter on the conceptual basis for studying precursor lesions, and on the practical aspects of obtaining, processing, and analyzing tissues containing either precancerous lesions or specimens enabling biomarkers of their presence to be detected. Intermediate markers (surrogate endpoints) have an increasingly important role to play in cancer research, and Part II also includes a chapter on the theoretical and practical problems involved in the use of surrogate endpoints in experimental and observational studies of cancer. The final chapter in this section discusses the assessment of epidemiologic relationships involving cancer precursors and the impact of measurement error on the study of such relationships.

The main section of the book, Part III, contains reviews of cancer precursors at the most important anatomical sites at which solid tumors occur. These reviews include discussion of the epidemiology of these lesions, and where appropriate, aspects of their detection and prevention. Somewhat inevitably, the authors have taken different approaches in responding to their task, given that there are considerable between-site differences in the current state of knowledge and that much of the information regarding risk factors for cancer precursors overlaps with that available for invasive cancers of the same organ site.

Part IV includes chapters on various aspects of the control of cancer precursors. A chapter on screening addresses issues concerning the role of secondary prevention of cancer precursors, with particular emphasis on screening for precursors of cervix and colorectal cancer, for which the relevant concepts are most developed. A chapter on chemoprevention discusses the use of precancerous lesions and early associated biomarkers as surrogate endpoints to characterize cancer chemopreventive efficacy. The third chapter of this section summarizes evidence-based policy recommendations from different national and international agencies on screening and prevention, with particular emphasis on cancer precursors.

Part V, the final section of the book, contains a brief chapter in which we attempt to peer into the future to anticipate how research on the etiology, detection, and prevention of cancer precursors might develop.

The book includes contributions by well-established scientists who work on topics related to the biology, epidemiology, and control of cancer precursors, and these scientists have written their chapters in the knowledge that the target audience encompasses a broad professional base, including basic cancer researchers, epidemiologists, oncologists, molecular biologists, pathologists, health policy professionals, and graduate students in cancer-related fields. We thank the contributors for their superb efforts to make their chapters accessible to such a wide audience. We also appreciate their patience and diligence in revising their chapter manuscripts in response to our editorial requests to meet the common style and content structure that we attempted to impose upon the contributions within each section.

Our task was simplified enormously by the wonderful editorial staff at Springer-Verlag who shepherded us through the entire publication process. In particular, we thank Laura Gillan, Carol Wang, and Cindy Chang for their excellent support and responsiveness to all of the issues that we raised during the production of the book. We also thank Eliane Duarte-Franco, Elvira Rocco Ickowicz, Nicolas Schlecht, Anita Koushik, Jason Parente, Javier Pintos, Marie-Claude Rousseau Sarah Mitchell-Weed, and Candida Pizzolongo, for their superb assistance with valuable discussions, locating references, and other tasks associated with the writing and editing of the book. J. Baron (author of the chapter on colorectal lesions) received helpful advice and photomicrographs from Jeremy Bass and Daniel Longnecker. Grants NCI CA54053, CA63933, and PHS 5M01-RR-00079 provided support for the work of J. Palefsky (chapter on anal lesions). The latter acknowledges the contributions of his collaborators in the UCSF anal neoplasia cohort study: Elizabeth Holly, Mary Ralston, Naomi Jay, Michael Berry, Maria Da Costa, and Teresa Darragh, and in the cost-effectiveness analysis study: Suzanne Goldie, Milton Weinstein, and Karen Kuntz. E. Franco's contributions were supported by a Distinguished Scientist Award from the Medical Research Council of Canada.

Finally, a short note on the history of this book. Over the last 11 years, the editors have collaborated closely on various projects on cancer epidemiology and prevention and on methodological issues related to error in the measurement of intermediate endpoints for cancer. The decision to jointly edit this book was taken about two years ago and was a natural consequence of this long-standing collaboration. Bringing this writing and editing project to bear fruit required more hours and exchanges of electronic mail messages and phone conversations than we care to count. The order of our names on the masthead reflects nothing other than a simple alphabetical listing. We both enjoyed producing this tome immensely, and we sincerely hope that the reader will find it a valuable resource.

Eduardo L. Franco   *Thomas E. Rohan*
MPH, DrPH   *MB, BS, PhD*
Montreal, Quebec   Bronx, New York

August 2001

Contents

Part III   Site-Specific Precancerous Conditions

Part IV   Control of Cancer Precursors

Contributors

John A. Baron, MD, MS, MSc
Departments of Medicine and Community and Family Medicine,
Dartmouth-Hitchcock Medical Center, Lebanon, NH 03756, USA

Neil Caporaso, MD
Pharmacogenetic Section, Genetic Epidemiology Branch, Division
of Cancer Epidemiology and Genetics, National Cancer Institute,
National Institutes of Health, Rockville, MD 20892, USA

Michael B. Cohen, MD
Department of Pathology, University of Iowa, Iowa City, IA 52242-
1087, USA

Carlos Cordon-Cardo, MD
Department of Pathology, Division of Molecular Biology, Memorial
Sloan-Kettering Cancer Center, New York, NY 10021, USA

Pelayo Correa, MD
Department of Pathology, Louisiana State University Health Sciences Center, New Orleans, LA 70112-1393, USA

Janet R. Daling, MD
Division of Public Health Sciences, Fred Hutchinson Cancer
Research Center, University of Washington, Seattle, WA 98109-1024,
USA

Alex Ferenczy, MD
Department of Pathology, Jewish General Hospital, Montreal,
Quebec H3T 1E2, Canada

Eduardo L. Franco, MPH, DR PH
Departments of Epidemiology and Oncology, Division of Cancer
Epidemiology, McGill University, Montreal, Quebec H2W 1S6,
Canada

Richard P. Gallagher, MD
Cancer Control Research Program, BC Cancer Agency, Vancouver, British Columbia V5Z 4E6, Canada

Michael Goggins, MD
Departments of Pathology, Oncology, and Medicine, Johns Hopkins Hospital, Baltimore, MD 21287, USA

Ralph H. Hruban, MD
Departments of Pathology and Oncology, Johns Hopkins Hospital, Baltimore, MD 21287, USA

Christine Iacobuzio-Donahue, MD, PhD
Department of Pathology, Johns Hopkins Hospital, Baltimore, MD 21287, USA

Rita A. Kandel, MD
Department of Pathology and Laboratory Medicine, Mount Sinai Hospital, Toronto, Ontario M5G 1X5, Canada

Gary J. Kelloff, MD
Division of Cancer Prevention, National Cancer Institute, National Institutes of Health, Bethesda, MD 20892, USA

Tim K. Lee, MSc, PhD
Cancer Control Research Program, BC Cancer Agency, Vancouver, British Columbia V5Z 4E6, Canada

Margaret M. Madeleine, MS, PhD
Department of Epidemiology, Program in Epidemiology, Fred Hutchinson Cancer Research Center, University of Washington, Seattle, WA 98109-1024, USA

Pamela M. Marcus, MS, PhD
Division of Cancer Prevention, National Cancer Institute, National Institutes of Health, Bethesda, MD 20895-7354, USA

James R. Marshall, PhD
Arizona Cancer Center, University of Arizona, Tucson, AZ 85724, USA

Anthony B. Miller, MB, ChB
Division of Clinical Epidemiology, Deutsches Krebforschungzen-trum, 69009 Heidelberg, Germany

Joel M. Palefsky, MD
Department of Laboratory Medicine, University of California, San Francisco, San Francisco, CA 94143, USA

Kamal S. Pohar, MD
Department of Urology, Memorial Sloan-Kettering Cancer Center, New York, NY 10021, USA

Thomas E. Rohan, MB, BS, PhD
Department of Epidemiology and Social Medicine, Albert Einstein College of Medicine, Bronx, NY 10461, USA

R. Sankaranarayanan, MD
Unit of Descriptive Epidemiology, International Agency for Research on Cancer, Lyon F-69372, France

Regina M. Santella, PhD
Division of Environmental Health Sciences, Mailman School of Public Health of Columbia University, New York, NY 10032, USA

Arthur Schatzkin, MD, DrPH
Nutritional Epidemiology Branch, National Cancer Institute, National Institutes of Health, Bethesda, MD 20892, USA

Joellen M. Schildkraut, PhD
Department of Community and Family Medicine, Cancer Prevention, Detection, and Control Research Program, Duke University Medical Center, Durham, NC 27710, USA

Morris Sherman, MB, BCh, PhD
Departments of Medicine and Pathology, University of Toronto, Toronto General Hospital, Toronto, Ontario M5G 2C4, Canada

Caroline C. Sigman, PhD
CCS Associates, Mountain View, CA 94043, USA

Thara Somanathan, MD
Department of Pathology, Regional Cancer Center, Trivandrum 695011, India

Hisham K. Tamimi, MD
Departments of Epidemiology and Obstetrics and Gynecology, Program in Epidemiology, Fred Hutchinson Cancer Research Center, University of Washington, Seattle, WA 98109-1024, USA

William D. Travis, MD
Department of Pulmonary and Mediastinal Pathology, Armed Forces Institute of Pathology, Washington, DC 20306-6000, USA

Thomas L. Vaughan, MD
Department of Epidemiology, Fred Hutchinson Cancer Research Center, University of Washington, Seattle, WA 98109-1024, USA

Jim Vaught, PhD
Division of Cancer Epidemiology and Genetics, Pharmacogenetic Section, Genetic Epidemiology Branch, National Cancer Institute, National Institutes of Health, Rockville, MD 20892, USA

Ian Wanless, MD
University of Toronto, Toronto General Hospital, Toronto, Ontario
M5G 2C4, Canada

David P. Wood, Jr., MD
Department of Urologic Oncology, Karmanos Cancer Institute,
Wayne State University, Harper Hospital, Detroit, MI, 48201, USA

Introduction

Thomas E. Rohan and Eduardo L. Franco

Cancer is generally considered to arise as a result of a multistep process involving changes in a number of genes following the initial clonal expansion of a mutated stem cell [1–4]. These genotypic changes are often accompanied by changes in tissue morphology, which result in progressively more severe cytologic and nuclear atypia. Writing many years ago, Foulds [5] stated that "lesions described as 'precancerous' are visible steps in a dynamic process of neoplasia; these lesions may or may not undergo progression to a more advanced stage of neoplasia." In this book, we use the term *cancer precursors* to refer to all lesions up to but not including invasive cancer. That is, essentially, we have adopted a morphological definition of cancer precursors, and we have included in our discussion carcinomas-*in-situ*, which are lesions with many of the morphological hallmarks of invasive cancer that do not extend below the basement membrane. Our focus is on precursors of epithelial malignancies because precursors of mesenchymal, hematopoietic, or lymphoid malignancies are not particularly well defined.

More than half a century ago, it was suggested that a useful definition of a cancer precursor is "a condition which may be associated with development of cancer" [6]. We concur with this definition, as have others before us [7]. However, this does not resolve the terminological difficulties and disagreement which surround such conditions. Indeed, the term *cancer precursors* is not one which is used universally. Other terms used to denote similar conditions

include *incipient neoplasia* [8] and *precancer* [9]. In contrast, the term *precancerous states* has been used to denote all conditions up to but not including carcinoma *in situ* [10], the latter being considered to represent preinvasive cancer rather than a precancerous lesion. These difficulties surrounding terminology highlight the need for improvements in and possibly alternative approaches to the definition of such lesions. Most importantly, the recognition that a given tissue abnormality is associated with cancer development does not necessarily imply that all cancers at that site will develop from such lesions, nor that any such abnormalities will acquire malignant characteristics. The plurality of histological abnormalities that are associated with the different types of endometrial cancer is a case in point.

Increasing attention is being devoted to the study of cancer precursors, as evidenced by the recent spate of books on various aspects of the topic [8,9,11]. As stated in one of those books, "Until now there has been such a heavy emphasis on cancer that we are only at a beginning in understanding precancer" [9]. In part, this might reflect the difficulty of defining the natural history of cancer development and of establishing, therefore, that a given lesion is a cancer precursor. Indeed, validation of cancer precursors as intermediate endpoints for cancer development is challenging, since tissue sampling necessarily interrupts or alters the course of the natural history of the neoplastic process. Furthermore, it is often difficult, if not impossible, to undertake the repeated tissue sampling

1

that would be required to study progression to more advanced precursor lesions (and, indeed, regression to earlier stages), although in some cases, alternative sampling techniques (e.g., Pap smears) might provide the possibility of doing so without encountering such problems; however, cytopathological and even histological examinations are prone to errors due to inadequate sampling of the affected tissue and/or to incorrect microscopic interpretation. Nevertheless, study of cancer precursors is important for several reasons. Firstly, elucidation of the etiology of precursors will provide insight into the etiology of the corresponding cancer, since if the precursor represents an intermediate stage in the causal pathway between exposure and the occurrence of invasive cancer, then etiological factors for the former must be a subset of those for the latter. Secondly, cancer precursors, if clearly defined, can provide targets for screening and hence early detection of those at increased risk of cancer, with obvious implications for the clinical management of individuals identified with such lesions. Thirdly, if etiological investigation of cancer precursors identifies potentially modifiable risk factors, it will provide opportunities for the primary prevention of both the precursors *per se* and of the corresponding cancer. And finally, study of the molecular and genetic changes occurring in cancer precursors can provide fundamental insight into the nature of the carcinogenic process.

As is revealed in the ensuing chapters, our knowledge of the etiology of cancer precursors varies considerably by anatomical site. In part, this might reflect the relative inaccessibility of a site to tissue sampling (e.g., pancreas) and hence the difficulty of detecting and diagnosing precursors at that site. For some cancers (e.g., ovarian), it might also be indicative of a relatively short premalignant phase which therefore eludes detection. Furthermore, for some anatomical sites, it might also reflect the fact that it is only relatively recently that we have identified putative precursors for the corresponding cancer, as is the case for prostatic intraepithelial neoplasia. Nevertheless, as indicated earlier, clues to the etiology of such con-

ditions come in part from knowledge of the etiology of the corresponding cancer, which is often easier to study.

Although screening is usually targeted at the detection of cancerous lesions at a relatively early stage, screening at some sites (in particular, the cervix and colon) does result in detection of a substantial proportion of cancer precursors. In principle, treatment or removal of such lesions will result in a reduction in the risk of subsequent invasive cancer. With the further development or improvement of screening modalities, it might be anticipated that detection of lesions at the earlier stages of carcinogenesis will increase. In some cases, this might pose diagnostic and therapeutic dilemmas, the former because of the need to establish that newly identified conditions (for example, at sites which were previously inaccessible) are indeed cancer precursors, and the latter because of concern over unnecessary treatment of lesions which might never have progressed. These issues might be resolved by conducting randomized trials to assess the effect of such screening and treatment modalities on cancer incidence and mortality.

To date, relatively few studies have been undertaken to test the effect of interventions on the risk of cancer precursors. However, with increasing recognition of the advantages that intermediate (or surrogate) endpoints offer for the study of preventive strategies, in terms of reductions in time, sample size, and cost, as compared to the corresponding requirements for trials involving cancer as an endpoint, one can anticipate a burgeoning of activity in this area. Indeed, cancer chemoprevention is a relatively new area of endeavor which has been described as involving the use of "agents that prevent cancer by either preventing or treating premalignant lesions" [12].

The advent of the genetic era has spawned many studies of the molecular changes that characterize histologically-defined cancer precursors [11]. Such studies might provide insight into the progressive accumulation of the fundamental molecular changes leading to carcinogenesis. In addition, the results of such studies might have clinical implications [13], since for those women who are identified as being at increased risk of progression to invasive cancer (on the basis of their status with respect to one or more molecular markers), close follow-up and perhaps early intervention might be warranted. Also, such studies might assist with the development and/or identification of chemopreventive agents that target cellular or molecular alterations in preinvasive epithelial carcinomatous tissue [12].

Although these factors are not a direct focus of this book, we note here that difficulty in defining the natural history of cancer development and of establishing that a lesion is a cancer precursor, and debate about the appropriate clinical management of cancer precursors, can have consequences that extend beyond the obvious scientific and public health aftereffects and into the legal arena. Increasingly, epidemiologists are being called upon to testify as to whether or not a given drug or putative environmental insult may have been linked etiologically to a possible precursor condition in individuals who subsequently developed cancer. This may place lay juries in the awkward position of having to decide whether a precursor condition was in the causal pathway of the plaintiff's cancer after hearing arguments that reflect a lack of consensus in the scientific community. One example of the controversy that can surround cancer precursors relates to the widespread use of hormonal replacement therapy, which began more than 30 years ago. The ensuing upsurge in endometrial cancer incidence fueled much of the scientific debate on whether endometrial hyperplasia is a true precursor lesion of endometrial cancer. The recent prevailing view is that it is not, and that atypical hyperplasia is a precursor (see Chapter 17). In relation to the clinical management of cancer precursors, medical malpractice cases have been built on whether or not a clinician acted sufficiently aggressively in treating a dysplastic lesion to prevent cervical cancer from occurring in a given patient, or on whether or not a cytopathology laboratory incorrectly reported a Pap test as negative.

Although we might be only at the beginning of the study of cancer precursors, it is clear that considerable headway has been made already. Our hope is that the ensuing chapters will provide a solid basis for practitioners and investigators wishing to learn more about these conditions or to undertake further research in this area.

References

1. Vogelstein B, Kinzler KW. The multistep nature of cancer. *Trends Genet* 1993; 9:138–41.
2. Nowell PC. The clonal evolution of tumor cell populations. *Science* 1976; 194:23–8.
3. Kern SE. Clonality: more than just a tumor-progression model. *J Natl Cancer Inst* 1993; 85:1020–1.
4. Boone CW, Henson DE, Kelloff GJ. Pathobiology of incipient neoplasia. In: Srivastava S, Henson DE, Gazdar A (eds) *Molecular pathology of early cancer*. Amsterdam: IOS Press, 1999, pp. 3–11.
5. Foulds L. The natural history of cancer. *J Chron Dis* 1958; 8:2–37.
6. Stout AP. *Human cancer*. Philadelphia: Lea and Febiger, 1932, p. 18.
7. Correa P. Morphology and natural history of cancer precursors. In: Schottenfeld D, Fraumeni JF Jr (eds) *Cancer epidemiology and prevention*, 2nd ed. New York: Oxford University Press, 1996, pp. 45–64.
8. Henson DE, Albores-Saavedra J. *Pathology of incipient neoplasia*, 2nd ed. Philadelphia: WB Saunders Company, 1993.
9. Pontén J (ed) *Precancer: biology, importance and possible prevention*. Cancer Surveys, Vol. 32. Cold Spring Harbor, NY: Cold Spring Harbor Laboratory Press, 1998.
10. Carter RL (ed) *Precancerous states*. London: Oxford University Press, 1984.
11. Srivastava S, Henson DE, Gazdar A. *Molecular pathology of early cancer*. Amsterdam: IOS Press, 1999.
12. Lippman SM, Lee JJ, Sabichi AL. Cancer chemoprevention: progress and promise. *J Natl Cancer Inst* 1998; 90:1514–28.
13. Ahrendt SA, Sidransky D. The potential of molecular screening. *Surg Oncol Clin North Am* 1999; 8:641–56.

Part I
Biological Basis of Carcinogenesis

1
Mechanisms and Biological Markers of Carcinogenesis

Regina M. Santella

Mechanisms of Carcinogenesis

Initiation

Cancer is a complex group of diseases with many causes, including chemical carcinogens, radiation, hormones, dietary factors, infectious agents and oxidative stress. Animal studies have provided the basis for our understanding of how these diverse agents result in the production of a malignant tumor. A model for the multistage process of carcinogenesis divides it into three stages: initiation, promotion, and progression [1–4]. Initiation is the irreversible interaction of a carcinogen with tissue DNA. This DNA damage is necessary but not sufficient for tumorigenesis since other events must also take place. It cannot be detected pathologically but produces cells that are precursors of the future tumor.

Chemical carcinogens can be divided into several categories. Direct-acting carcinogens have inherent reactivity, due to their electrophilic nature, and react with nucleophilic residues in cellular proteins and with nucleic acids (RNA and DNA) to form adducts, covalent products resulting from binding of the carcinogen [5–8]. Examples of direct-acting chemical carcinogens include epoxides, such as ethylene oxide, and cytotoxic chemotherapeutic agents, such as cyclophosphamide. Radiation, another example of a direct-acting agent, is known to induce nucleotide base damage, cross links, and DNA single- and double-strand breaks [9].

Most chemical carcinogens present in the environment, however, exist as procarcinogens (Figure 1.1) and are not active in their native form. Examples include polycyclic aromatic hydrocarbons (PAHs) (produced during the combustion of organic material and present in cigarette smoke, polluted air, and various foods), aromatic amines (also present in cigarette smoke and the diet as well as in certain occupational settings), and aflatoxin B_1 (a dietary carcinogen produced by a mold contaminant). Initiation by these agents is dependent upon their conversion to highly reactive electrophilic species (Figure 1.1). This process of metabolic activation of the procarcinogen to the "ultimate" carcinogen is carried out by a number of enzymes present in various human tissues [10,11]. The model PAH, benzo(a)pyrene (BP), for example, is not chemically reactive and does not bind to DNA. However, enzymes in the cytochrome P450 system, including CYP1A1, oxidatively metabolize BP and related PAHs to a variety of derivatives, including phenols and dihydrodiols. This process is part of the normal mechanism for conversion of xenobiotics to more water-soluble forms for excretion. Unfortunately, for PAH, highly reactive epoxides are one of the intermediates in this oxidative process. For BP, a specific diol epoxide has been identified as the critical reactive intermediate. This intermediate covalently binds DNA primarily at the N2 position of guanine, although adducts are also found on adenine. Adducts on RNA, and on proteins such as albumin, have also been

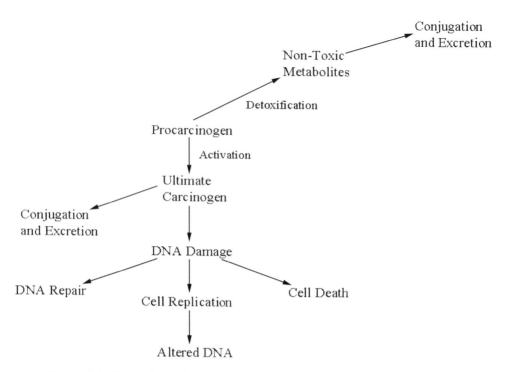

FIGURE 1.1. Metabolism of chemical carcinogens to DNA-reactive intermediates.

identified. Oxidative metabolism of exogenous chemicals such as BP also results in oxidative DNA damage, increasing the hazard of such exogenous chemicals. Further complicating the issue, many of the activation enzymes, such as CYP1A1, are inducible by PAH and other chemicals, enhancing the conversion of xenobiotics to toxic intermediates.

In addition to electrophilic intermediates, free radical derivatives of chemicals are implicated in carcinogenesis [5,12,13]. DNA damage also arises spontaneously from endogenous chemicals that arise during metabolism, oxidative stress, and chronic inflammation [14]. The types of damage produced include deaminations, alkylations, base loss, and oxidation. The level of these potentially mutagenic endogenous lesions is high, and they have been suggested to be major contributors to carcinogenesis and aging.

While chemical carcinogens are activated by a wide range of enzymes, there also exists a series of enzymes (phase II enzymes) that are involved in the detoxification of activated carcinogens, thus preventing their binding to DNA. These include epoxide hydrolase, N-acetyl transferases, glutathione S-transferases (GSTs), sulfotransferase, and glucuronide transferase [10]. The products of these reactions are generally more hydrophobic and thus more readily excreted. For example, the reactive diol epoxide of BP can be conjugated to glutathione and thus detoxified by both GST M1 and GST T1. However, in some relatively rare situations, phase II enzymes have also been shown to activate chemical carcinogens; GST activates 1,2-dihaloethanes [11].

Evidence that DNA is the critical target in carcinogenesis came from the increased incidence of cancer in individuals with genetic defects in DNA repair (e.g., xeroderma pigmentosa [15]). A relationship between the level of DNA adduct formation in animals and carcinogen potency has also been observed [16,17]. The association of particular mutations in specific genes (discussed later) with tumors provided additional evidence. But adducts also form in many tissues in which tumors do not arise. Guanine is the most common target, but modifications of all four bases of DNA have been reported [7,8]. The simple alkylating agents can methylate or ethylate any of the nitrogens or oxygens in the bases as well as the sugars and phosphate backbone.

Thus, different carcinogens can attack different sites on the DNA, and even a single carcinogen can form multiple types of adducts. The structures of many of these carcinogen–DNA adducts have been well characterized using physico-chemical methods; conformational changes induced by carcinogen binding have also been determined [12]. These chemical and physical alterations in the structure of DNA are responsible for errors which occur during DNA replication and cell division. Different adducts induce different types of mutations with varied efficiencies. For example, adducts that distort the double helix tend to induce frame-shift mutations, but those that lie outside the helix tend to produce transversion mutations [4,5,7].

Because of the importance of maintaining DNA's integrity, there are five evolutionarily conserved pathways for the repair of various types of DNA damage. Direct damage repair deals with damage such as alkylation of guanine (e.g., O^6-methylguanine) by removal of the alkyl group leaving the guanine intact. Base-excision repair generally repairs endogenous DNA damage such as 8-oxo-deoxyguanosine, an oxidized base. These types of damage tend to be more structurally subtle than those induced by exogenous chemicals. Nucleotide-excision repair is responsible for removal of bulky carcinogen adducts, such as those of BP, that distort the DNA structure. A number of genes are involved in this process, including helicases and endonucleases which respectively unwind the DNA and cut out a precisely defined section of the damaged DNA. Mismatch repair deals with replication errors that are missed by the proofreading functions of DNA polymerase. This pathway is important since loss of this function is found in sporadic as well as familial cancers. In hereditary non-polyposis colon carcer (HNPCC), germline mutations in genes involved in mismatch repair (*hMSH2*, *hMLH1*, *hPMS1* and *hPMS2*) are found. The last pathway repairs double-strand breaks. A number of detailed reviews on the various DNA repair pathways are available [18–22].

The cellular responses to DNA damage are complex and may result in repair of the damage, cell death by apoptosis, or continued cell proliferation (Figure 1.1). If modification of DNA by chemical carcinogens or by endogenous processes goes unrepaired before cell replication, an altered DNA sequence may result. These alterations can include base substitutions (either transitions of transversions), frame-shift mutations, deletions, recombination, chromosome translocation, and gene amplification.

Promotion

In contrast to tumor initiation, tumor promotion is a reversible process that facilitates the expression of the initiated cells and leads to the production of precursor lesions and benign tumors. A variety of chemicals have been shown to induce tumor promotion, including phenobarbital and the classic promoter isolated from croton oil, tetradecanoyl phorbol acetate (TPA). These agents do not directly interact with DNA, and their actions are reversible. The two-stage mouse skin carcinogenesis system has served as a model for understanding promotion and has demonstrated that treatment with promoting agents must follow that by initiators and must be long term in order for benign papillomas to arise [1]. Classic promoting agents interact with membrane-associated receptors, affect gene expression through alterations in signal transduction pathways, and interfere with gap-junctional intercellular communication. This concept may also apply to lung tumors since cigarette smoke contains both initiating agents and promoters. In addition to this classic mechanism of promotion, other agents promote the carcinogenic process by other means. For example, viral infection with hepatitis B virus (HBV) leads to liver cell death, inflammation, and liver regeneration, which over many years, leads to cirrhosis [23]. Human immunodeficiency virus (HIV) leads to immune suppression and promotion of cervical cancers initiated by human papillomavirus [24].

Progression

Progression is the process wherein benign tumors become malignant and further evolve with increasing malignancy. Accumulation of multiple genetic alterations, as briefly reviewed later, drives the progressive transformation of normal cells into highly malignant ones [3]. Studies on the age-dependent incidence of human cancers suggest that four to seven rate-limiting stochastic events are needed for a cell to become fully malignant [25]. Molecular analysis of cancers in various stages of progression have demonstrated that alterations in tumor suppressor genes and oncogenes accumulate during tumor progression and metastasis, and correlate with aggressiveness of the tumor [26]. A major characteristic of this stage of carcinogenesis is genomic instability. A genetic model was first constructed for colorectal carcinoma, since tumors in various stages of progression from small adenomas to large metastatic carcinomas could be readily obtained for analysis [27,28]. Similar models have been developed for other cancers including lung and prostate [29,30].

Oncogenes and Tumor Suppressor Genes

While DNA damage may occur throughout the genome, the critical cellular targets are oncogenes, also called proto oncogenes, and tumor suppressor genes [31–33] (Table 1.1). Many oncogenes code for components of signal transduction pathways that are involved in the control of normal growth and differentiation. Mutations in these genes distort the function of the associated proteins, resulting in abnormal growth control and differentiation. Signal transduction is a complex process involving many types of proteins including transmembrane growth factors (e.g., epidermal growth factor) and their receptors which have kinase activity. Protein phosphorylation by these kinases plays a central role in signal transduc-

TABLE 1.1. Examples of oncogenes and tumor suppressor genes.

Oncogenes	Function
ras, bcl-2	Membrane-associated G protein
myc, fos, jun	Nuclear transcription factor
sis, int-2	Growth factor
src, ret, erbB	Protein tyrosine kinase

Tumor suppressor genes	
hMLH1	Mismatch DNA repair
p53, WT	Transcription factor
RB	Transcriptional repressor

tion by changing the conformation of proteins and activating enzyme functions; phosphorylation also influences protein–protein interactions. *Ras* oncogenes were among the first oncogene products implicated in human cancers; at least one third of tumors contain mutated *Ras* genes. Proteins such as Ras become activated when they bind guanosine triphosphate (GTP) and inactivated when they hydrolyze GTP to guanosine diphosphate (GDP). In the activated state, Ras proteins switch on a cascade of other kinases, which in turn activate the transcription factors *Fos* and *Jun* committing the cell to DNA replication and division. Specific mutations in Ras result in the permanently activated state. Ras mutations in rodent tumors induced by chemical carcinogens have been well characterized and drive cell division [34]. Similar mutations are found in human lung, colon and pancreatic tumors [26,35,36].

While altered oncogenes result in enhanced cell proliferation, tumor suppressor genes block tumor growth. When they are inactivated, growth becomes constitutive, no longer subject to normal growth control. Several tumor suppressor genes have been identified and linked to heritable tumors. The first to be identified was the *RB* gene associated with retinoblastoma. Inactivation of this gene has also been associated with sarcomas, small cell lung carcinomas, and breast and bladder cancers [37]. Another example is the hereditary mutations which occur in the p53 tumor suppressor gene in Li-Fraumeni syndrome patients in whom cancers in multiple tissues are found [37]. P53 is also the most frequently mutated tumor suppressor gene in sporadic tumors. This may be related to its complex role in many central cellular processes, including gene transcription, DNA repair, cell cycling, genomic stability, chromosomal segregation, senescence, and apoptosis [38]. In addition, several oncogenic DNA viruses mediate their effects, in part, by targeting p53 protein for binding. Tumor suppressor genes are inactivated by "two hits", two successive genetic events which fully eliminate activity of both alleles of the gene. In familial cases, the first "hit" has already occurred in the germline of the patient, but in nonfamilial cases, one hit is a point mutation or small deletion, and the second hit is loss of heterozygosity (LOH). Mapping sites of LOH has been a major route by which new tumor suppressor genes have been identified. While several tumor suppressor genes, such as *p53* and *RB*, are found in both familial and sporadic cancers, others appear exclusively in familial cancers (e.g., *BRCA1*, *WT1*). Finally, epigenetic mechanisms, which do not involve alterations in DNA sequence, are also important in tumor suppressor gene inactivation through the process of DNA methylation. Extensive methylation of cytosine at CpGs in regulatory sequences such as promoters can turn off gene expression.

It is apparent that a given tumor can contain multiple types of mutations, and that there is considerable heterogeneity between tumors of the same histologic type, in terms of the types of mutations seen. However, a model has been suggested in which six essential alterations in the cell are required for malignant growth. These include: self-sufficiency in growth signals, insensitivity to growth-inhibitor (antigrowth) signals, evasion of programmed cell death (apoptosis), limitless replicative potential, sustained angiogenesis, and tissue invasion and metastasis [3]. It may be necessary in all types of tumors for these capabilities to be acquired, although the order in which they arise may vary, and the specific genes which are responsible for the acquisition of the particular capability may differ. The loss of genomic stability results in increased rates of mutations that drive the accumulation of the changes needed for tumor development. Loss of genomic stability is also responsible for tumor heterogeneity; that is, no two tumors are exactly alike, and no tumor is composed of genetically identical cells [39].

Biological Markers in Carcinogenesis

A variety of highly sensitive and specific laboratory procedures are now available for use as biomarkers to identify individuals exposed to particular chemical carcinogens, to determine individual risk for cancer development, to identify individuals with early-stage clinical disease, and also to use as intermediate endpoints in intervention studies. Figure 1.2 provides a schematic diagram of the sequence of events in the continuum from the initial exposure of an individual to a causative agent(s) to the eventual development of a fully malignant tumor. Several types of biomarkers make it possible to precisely monitor each of these events [40,41]. These biomarkers can be divided into specific categories: internal dose, biologically effective dose, early biologic effects (responses), and susceptibility. Biomarkers of internal dose take into account individual differences in absorption or bioaccumulation of the compound in question and indicate the actual level of the compound within the body and in specific tissues or compartments. Examples include measurement of cotinine in serum or urine, resulting from cigarette smoke exposure; measurement of 1-hydroxypyrene in urine from PAH exposure; measurement of aflatoxins in urine from dietary exposure; and measurement of organochlorines in serum from dietary exposure. These biomarkers occur early in the continuum from exposure to disease, and therefore, while they are good markers of exposure, they are generally not useful in the identification of risk or early stage disease.

Another major area of research has been the identification of genetic susceptibility factors specifically related to carcinogen metabolism

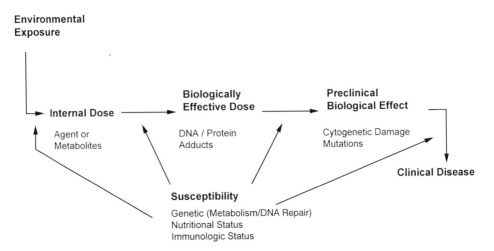

FIGURE 1.2. Biologic markers in chemical carcinogenesis.

and DNA repair. Phenotyping assays have been used in a number of studies to investigate relationships between enzyme activity and cancer risk. For example, a lack of activity of GST M1 has been associated with increased risk of lung cancer in a number of studies [reviewed in [42]]. Deletion of this gene can also be determined using polymerase chain reaction (PCR) methods, simplifying the investigation of the role of this enzyme. Similarly, single-nucleotide polymorphisms in a number of the phase I and II enzymes responsible for the activation and detoxification of chemical carcinogens have been identified [43]. These polymorphisms are frequently associated with altered enzyme level or function. Thus, a major area of research has been the determination of the frequency of specific polymorphisms in individuals with or without various cancers. A number of studies have demonstrated elevated risk for cancer development among carriers of specific alleles. While the increase in risk is often small (<2-fold) compared to that in carriers of germline mutations in specific tumor suppressor genes such as *p53* or *Rb*, the high prevalence of these alleles suggests that they are associated with a high attributable risk in the population. The recent discovery of polymorphisms in DNA repair genes have further expanded these studies. A number of published reviews summarize this area of research in detail [42–45].

Biomarkers of Biologically Effective Dose

These assays measure the amount of the compound that has actually reacted with DNA or with an established surrogate target, for example proteins in the blood. Assays for carcinogen–DNA adducts in the target tissue provide a more relevant marker than assays of the internal dose. This is because the former takes into account not only individual differences in absorption and distribution, but also differences in metabolism (activation versus detoxification) of the chemical and differences in the extent of repair of adducts. Unfortunately, for many studies in humans, DNA from the target tissue is not readily accessible, and thus surrogate tissues are often used (e.g., placenta, peripheral blood cells, buccal cells). The relationship between the types and levels of adducts in these more readily sampled sources and those in the target tissue have been established in some animal studies, but there are few similar studies in humans. A relationship between lung and blood DNA adducts has been observed [46,47]. The time frame of exposure, which can be monitored by measuring DNA adducts, is limited by cell turnover and DNA repair, and thus generally reflects recent exposure. Studies in former smokers have demonstrated that although lung tissue adducts are lost within several years of smoking cessation, blood adducts are lost within several months, and oral cell adducts within weeks [48–50].

Measurement of Carcinogen–DNA Adducts

Several highly sensitive and specific methods have been developed for detecting carcinogen–DNA adducts in humans, including physical methods such as fluorescence spectroscopy and gas-chromatography/mass-spectrometry (GC/MS), ^{32}P-postlabeling, immunoassays employing antisera to specific adducts, and combinations of these methods [reviewed in [12,51–53]]. These assays are highly sensitive (able to detect one adduct/10^7 to 10^9 nucleotides), but often require an appreciable amount of DNA (about 10–100 μg) and are fairly laborious. Immunoassays require the generation of antibodies, which frequently have cross-reactivity with structurally related adducts. However, the antibodies can be used for immunohistochemical detection of adducts in tissue biopsies or exfoliated cells. The ^{32}P-postlabeling method can detect multiple types of adducts resulting from exposure to complex mixtures; absolute quantitation is a problem, especially with poorly characterized adducts, since the efficiency and yield at each of the multiple steps cannot be easily determined. Other methods of adduct detection include high performance liquid chromatography with fluorescence (aflatoxin B$_1$ and BP) or electrochemical detection (oxidized bases), and GC/MS (alkylation adducts). These last two methods require the hydrolysis of DNA before analysis.

Carcinogen–DNA adducts have been detected and quantified in individuals exposed to carcinogens in various occupational or environmental settings. Increases in PAH–DNA have been found in foundry, aluminum-plant, and coke-oven workers' and in roofers, fire fighters, coal-tar–treated psoriasis patients, smokers, consumers of charbroiled foods, and subjects exposed to high levels of air pollution. These studies have generally observed consistent increases in DNA damage with increased exposure, but have also revealed large inter-individual differences in adduct levels, even in individuals with apparently comparable exposure. These differences are believed to be due to genetic differences in carcinogen metabolism and DNA repair, as well as differences in exposures to other substances (such as the intake of antioxidant vitamins), that may influence carcinogen metabolism.

Measurement of Carcinogen–Protein Adducts

Since the activated metabolites of several carcinogens can also form covalent adducts with proteins, assays of protein adducts have been used as a marker of carcinogen exposure and activation, thus serving as a convenient surrogate for DNA adducts [Reviewed in [12,52,54]]. Although proteins are not critical targets during carcinogenesis, the extent to which they are modified can be a useful biomarker of the biologically effective dose. Because of their abundance in blood, both hemoglobin (extracted from red blood cells) and serum albumin have been used for such assays. As with DNA adducts, protein adducts provide information on only relatively recent exposure, since the life span of the red blood cell is about four months, and the half life of serum albumin is about 21 days. However, protein adducts are not removed by any repair system. Therefore they may be a more sensitive marker of chronic exposure. All of the current assays for protein adducts require the isolation of the modified amino acid or the released carcinogen residues, which is followed by the analysis of these residues. GC/MS has been used to measure ethylene oxide-, 4-aminobiphenyl- and tobacco-specific nitrosamine-hemoglobin adducts resulting from occupational exposure or smoking [Reviewed in [12,54]]. Immunoassays have been used for quantitation of aflatoxin-albumin [52].

Adducts as Markers of Cancer Risk

While most of the studies on adducts have examined the relationship between exposure and adduct formation, a small number of studies have examined the relationship between adducts and cancer. Two types of studies have been carried out (Table 1.2): case-

TABLE 1.2. DNA and protein adducts in case-control and nested case-control studies (reference numbers in brackets).

Case-Control
PAH–DNA and lung cancer [46,55,56]
4-ABP–DNA and liver cancer [58]
Aflatoxin B$_1$–DNA and liver cancer [57]

Nested case-control
Aflatoxin B$_1$–guanine in urine and liver cancer [59,60]
Aflatoxin B$_1$–albumin in blood and liver cancer [61–63]
Aflatoxin metabolites in urine and liver cancer [64]

control studies, in which blood or tissue samples are collected from cases at the time of diagnosis; or nested case-control studies, in which samples are banked from healthy individuals, and cases are identified as the cohort is followed. The latter type of study is considered ideal since it eliminates the potential problem of the disease influencing the biomarker. In case-control studies, PAH–DNA adducts have been found to be elevated in white-blood-cell DNA of lung cancer cases compared to controls, adjusting for level of smoking [46,55,56], and aflatoxin- and 4-aminobiphenyl-DNA adducts have been found to be higher in liver tissue of hepatocellular carcinoma patients compared to tissue obtained from surgical controls [57,58]. In nested case-control studies, urinary aflatoxin-guanine adducts, aflatoxin metabolites, and albumin adducts have been found to be increased in liver cancer cases, and a synergistic interaction between chronic HBV infection and aflatoxin on liver cancer risk has also been observed [Reviewed in [52]].

Markers of Early Biologic Response

Cytogenetic Assays

These include assays for sister chromatid exchange (SCE), micronuclei (MN) and chromosomal aberrations (CAs). As with the adduct studies, these assays have been used most extensively for detection of exposure, but they are not chemical- or exposure-specific. CAs in peripheral lymphocytes have been used extensively as sensitive monitors of radiation exposure, but appear to be less sensitive for

detecting exposure to chemical carcinogens [Reviewed in [65]]. MN consist of small amounts of DNA in the cytoplasm which are not incorporated into daughter nuclei during mitosis because of chromosomal damage. MN are easy to score but reflect only a small proportion of the induced chromosome aberrations. A major advantage of assaying for MN is that this assay can also be carried out directly on exfoliated cells (such as oral mucosa cells) which can be sampled noninvasively. Assays for MN have been used to examine the toxic effects of cigarette smoking, and also the beneficial effects of β-carotene, in oral mucosal cells of betel-nut chewers [Reviewed in [66]]. SCEs in peripheral blood lymphocytes are considered a more sensitive, rapid and simple cytogenetic endpoint than CA for evaluation exposure to genotoxic agents. Increased levels of SCEs have been demonstrated as a result of exposure to cigarette smoke, certain occupational exposures, dietary factors, and certain drugs [Reviewed in [67]].

Cytogenetic assays have also been used in nested case-control studies to determine whether they are predictive of risk. Combined analyses of data from Nordic and Italian prospective cohort studies found that chromosomal aberrations were significant predictors of risk for all cancers and were independent of age at test, gender, and time since test; the relationship was not affected by the inclusion of occupational exposure level and smoking habit [68,69]. No association was found between MN or SCE and subsequent cancer incidence/mortality.

Acquired Gene Mutations in Oncogenes or Tumor Suppressor Genes

Numerous studies have investigated mutations in oncogenes and tumor-suppressor genes in tumors of both animals and humans. The *p53* tumor suppressor gene is probably the most extensively studied gene and is mutated in about 50% of various human tumors [reviewed in [70,71]]. This work has also demonstrated links between environmental exposures and specific mutational spectra present in the tumor. These links include a relationship between aflatoxin B1 exposure and codon 249 mutations in liver cancer, sunlight and mutations that are characteristic of those produced by UV-induced pyrimidine dimers in skin cancer, and G–T transversions, characteristic of bulky carcinogens, in cigarette smoke and lung cancer [72]. Similarly, studies of mouse skin, rat mammary tumors, and mouse liver tumors indicate that the types of base-substitution mutations seen in *ras* genes in these tumors depend on the specific carcinogen administered, and that these types of mutations often correlate with the type of DNA base modification and the mutational spectra of these chemicals in simpler systems [36].

While these studies have been very informative for understanding disease etiology, newer markers involving the use of blood, urine, and sputum to identify circulating tumor cells and DNA and oncogene and tumor suppressor gene proteins are more likely to be useful precursors to clinically detectable disease (Table 1.3). Blood levels of mutant oncogene and tumor suppressor gene proteins have been measured using Western blot and enzyme-linked immunosorbent assay (ELISA) technology. In one study, a subset of patients with mutations in the *p53* gene in their tumor carried mutant p53 protein in their serum [73]. However, in another study [74], p53 was only moderately increased in serum of lung cancer patients compared to controls. Thus, the relationship between tumor and serum assays requires further validation. In healthy workers with occupational exposure to vinyl chloride, a known liver carcinogen, mutant p53 protein was found more frequently in workers with higher exposure [75]. These results suggest that mutant p53 protein in serum might be an early indicator of risk. Antibodies to p53 protein have also been measured in about 30% of cases with cancer at various sites [reviewed in [76]]. Their presence in high-risk individuals such as exposed workers and smokers suggests that they may also be useful in the early detection of cancer. However, they are not site specific and may present problems in terms of accurate diagnosis.

A strong dose–response relationship between vinyl-chloride exposure and mutant ras p21 protein has also been observed [reviewed in [77]]. In a prospective study, p21 k-ras and p52 SIS were more frequently found in serum of subjects who went on to develop cancer, compared to healthy controls [78]. Plasma DNA has also been analyzed for mutations in *k-ras* [79]. In patients undergoing colonoscopy, 39% with mutations in plasma had neoplasms with *k-ras* mutation compared with 3% of patients without mutations. A major concern of this research is the meaning of positive assays in apparently healthy individuals. Studies have also been performed on *c-erbB-2* (*HER2/neu*) [Reviewed in [80]].

TABLE 1.3. Examples of biomarkers for early stage disease (reference numbers in brackets).

Proteins in Plasma/Serum
Mutant p53 and ras [74,75,77]
Overexpression of c-erbB-2 [80]
Antibodies to p53 [76]

DNA in Plasma/Serum
Mutant *ras* [79]
Mutant *p53* [90]

Exfoliated Cells
p53 Mutations [93,97]
Telomerase activity [84–86]
Loss of heterozygosity [91,92]
Microsatellite alterations [92,93]
mRNA in tumor cells in blood or urine [87–89]

Other Markers of Early Stage Disease

Telomerase contributes to the maintenance of telomere stability; its expression can be detected in 85 to 90% of primary cancer tissues [81]. Although it is not clear at what stage of cancer development telomerase is activated, measurement of telomerase activity may be useful for early diagnosis of cancer. Activity has been measured by the telomeric repeat amplification protocol (TRAP); an RNA component can be measured by in situ hybridization [82,83]. A study of exfoliated cells in urine from patients with bladder cancer found that measurement of telomerase activity was more sensitive in detecting the presence of cancer than standard cytologic examination [84]. However, a study in oral mucosa found activity in normal oral squamous epithelium, leukoplakia and carcinomas [85]. Similarly, a study of benign breast lesions (fibroadenoma and dysplasia) obtained by fine-needle aspiration found that 16% of samples were positive compared to 39% of carcinomas using strict criteria [86]. Further studies are necessary to determine the utility of this assay in detecting cancer precursors.

The detection of circulating tumor cells in blood, urine, and pleural effusions has been achieved using reverse transcriptase PCR (RT–PCR) methods to detect, for example, specific mRNAs including α-fetoprotein, a CD44 variant, and two tissue kallikrein family genes [87–89]. Loss of heterozygosity and microsatellite instability have also been used to identify tumor cells or tumor DNA in blood, exfoliated oral cells, and sputum [for example [90–92]]. The recent development of microarray technology should provide new ways to investigate early stage disease in apparently healthy individuals. Determination of the complex profiles of gene expression in precursor lesions and in tumors may also provide new insights into individual susceptibility and causative factors [for example [93–96]]. Advances in analyzing complex profiles of cellular proteins ("proteomics") should also provide similar insights.

Conclusion

Advances in basic research on the cellular and molecular mechanisms of carcinogenesis have contributed to our understanding of this complex multistage disease. This research has also led to the development of methods to monitor humans for early stages of disease. Studies on DNA and protein adducts have demonstrated associations of higher levels of adducts with disease status. However, these results have not been applicable to the individual; higher DNA adducts are not proof of higher risk. More-recent studies, identifying tumor cells or mutated DNA in biospecimens, hold promise for the early identification of

subjects with preclinical disease. Considerably more research will be necessary however, before these assays can be used for routine medical care.

References

1. Weinstein IB, Santella RM, Perera F. Molecular biology and molecular epidemiology of cancer. In: Greenwald P, Kramer BS, Weed DL (eds) *Cancer Prevention and Control*. Bethesda: Marcel-Dekker, 1995: 83–110.
2. Yuspa SH. Overview of carcinogenesis: past, present and future. *Carcinogenesis* 2000; 21: 341–5.
3. Hanahan D, Weinberg RA. The hallmarks of cancer. *Cell* 2000; 100:57–70.
4. Yuspa SH, Poirier MC. Chemical carcinogenesis: from animal models to molecular models in one decade. *Adv Cancer Res* 1988; 50:25–70.
5. Pitot III HC, Dragan Y. Chemical carcinogenesis; In: Klaassen CD (ed) *Casarett & Doull's Toxicology*. New York: McGraw-Hill, 1995, pp. 201–67.
6. Jeffrey AM. DNA modification by chemical carcinogens. *Pharmacol Ther* 1985; 28:237–72.
7. Grunberger D, Singer B. *Molecular Biology of Mutagens and Carcinogens*. New York, Plenum, 1983.
8. Dipple A. DNA adducts of chemical carcinogens. *Carcinogenesis* 1995; 16:437–41.
9. Little JB. Radiation carcinogenesis. *Carcinogenesis* 2000; 21:397–404.
10. Parkinson A. Biotransformation of xenobiotics; In: Klaassen CD (ed) *Casarett & Doul's Toxicology*. New York: McGraw-Hill, 1995, pp. 113–86.
11. Guengerich FP. Metabolism of chemical carcinogens. *Carcinogenesis* 2000; 21:345–51.
12. Poirier MC, Santella RM, Weston A. Carcinogen macromolecular adducts and their measurement. *Carcinogenesis* 2000; 21:353–60.
13. Lindahl T. Instability and decay of the primary structure of DNA. *Nature* 1993; 362:709–15.
14. Marnett LJ, Burcham PC. Endogenous DNA adducts: potential and paradox. *Crit Rev Toxicol* 1993; 6:771–85.
15. Kraemer KH, Lee MM, Scotto J. Xeroderma pigmentosum. Cutaneous, ocular, and neurologic abnormalities in 830 published cases. *Arch Dermatol* 1987; 123:241–50.
16. Lutz WK. Quantitative evaluation of DNA binding data for risk estimation and for classifi-

cation of direct and indirect carcinogens. *J Cancer Res Clin Oncol* 1986; 112:85–91.

17. Poirier MC, Beland FA. DNA adduct measurements and tumor incidence during chronic carcinogen exposure in animal models: Implications for DNA adduct-based human cancer risk assesment. *Crit Rev Toxicol* 1992; 5:749–55.

18. Friedberg EC. *DNA Repair*. New York: W. H. Freeman and Company, 1985.

19. Schmutte C, Fishel R. Genomic instability: first step to carcinogenesis. *Anticancer Res* 1999; 19: 4665–96.

20. Strauss BS. Frameshift mutation, microsatellites and mismatch repair. *Mutat Res* 1999; 437:195–203.

21. Lindahl T, Wood RD. Quality control by DNA repair. *Science* 1999; 286:1897–1905.

22. de Boer J, Hoeijmakeers JHJ. Nucleotide excision repair and human syndromes. *Carcinogenesis* 2000; 21:453–60.

23. Butel JS. Viral carcinogenesis: revelation of molecular mechanisms and etiology of human disease. *Carcinogenesis* 2000; 21:405–26.

24. Wright TC. Papillomavirus infection and neoplasia in women infected with human immunodeficiency virus; In: Franco E, Monsonego J (eds) *New developments in cervical cancer screening and prevention*. Oxford: Blackwell, 1997, pp. 131–46.

25. Renan MJ. How many mutations are required for tumorigenesis? Implications from human cancer data. *Mol Carcinog* 1993; 7:139–46.

26. Yokota J. Tumor progression and metastasis. *Carcinogenesis* 2000; 21:497–503.

27. Kinzler KW, Vogelstein B. Lessons from hereditary colorectal cancer. *Cell* 1996; 87:159–70.

28. Vogelstein B, Fearon ER, Hamilton SR, et al. Genetic alteration during colorectal-tumor development. *N Engl J Med* 1988; 319:525–32.

29. Shiseki M, Kohno T, Adachi J, et al. Comparative allelotype of early and advanced stage non-small cell lung carcinomas. *Genes Chromosom Cancer* 1996; 17:71–7.

30. Saric T, Brkanac Z, Troyer DA, et al. Genetic pattern of prostat cancer progression. *Int J Cancer* 1999; 81:219–24.

31. Bishop JM. Molecular themes in oncogenesis. *Cell* 1991; 25:235–48.

32. Fearon ER. Human cancer syndromes: clues to the origin and nature of cancer. *Science* 1997; 278:1049.

33. Haber D, Harlow E. Tumor suppressor genes: evolving definitions in the genomic age. *Nat Genet* 1990; 16:320–22.

34. Manques R, Pellicer A. Ras activation in experimental carcinogenesis. *Semin Cancer Biol* 1992; 3:229–39.

35. Bos JL. Ras oncogenes in human cancer: a review. *Cancer Res* 1989; 49:4682–9.

36. Balmain A, Harris CC. Carcinogenesis in mouse and human cells: parallels and paradoxes. *Carcinogenesis* 2000; 21:371–7.

37. Lindor NM, Greene MH, Mayo Cancer Family Program, et al. The concise handbook of family cancer syndromes. *J Natl Cancer Inst* 1998; 90:1039–71.

38. Harris CC. Structure and function of the p53 tumor suppressor gene: clues for rational cancer therapeutic strategies. *J Natl Cancer Inst* 1996; 88:1442–55.

39. Lengauer C, Kinzler KW, Vogelstein B. Genetic instabilities in human cancers. *Nature* 1998; 396:643–9.

40. Toniolo P, Boffeta P, Shuker DEG, et al. *Applications of biomarkers in cancer epidemiology*. Lyon: International Agency for Research on Cancer, 1997.

41. Perera FP. Molecular epidemiology: insights into cancer susceptibility, risk assessment, and prevention. *J Natl Cancer Inst* 1996; 88:496–509.

42. Houlston RS. Glutathione S-transferase M1 status and lung cancer risk: a meta-analysis. *Cancer Epidemiol Biomarkers Prev* 1999; 8:675–82.

43. Vineis P, Malats N, Lang M, et al. *Metabolic polymorphisms and susceptibility to cancer*. Lyon: International Agency for Reseach on Cancer, 1999.

44. Bartsch H, Nair U, Risch A, et al. Genetic polymorphism of CYP genes, alone or in combination, as a risk modifier of tobacco-related cancer. *Cancer Epidemiol Biomarkers Prev* 2000; 9:33–28.

45. d'Errico A, Taioli E, Chen X, et al. Genetic metabolic polymorphisms and the risk of cancer: a review of the literature. *Biomarkers* 1996; 1:149–73.

46. Tang DL, Santella RM, Blackwood MA, et al. A molecular epidemiological case-control study of lung cancer. *Cancer Epidemiol Biomarkers Prev* 1995; 4:341–6.

47. Wiencke JK, Thurston SW, Kelsey KT, et al. Early age at smoking initiation and tobacco carcinogen DNA damage in the lung. *J Natl Cancer Inst* 1999; 91:614–19.

48. Phillips DH, Schoket B, Hewer A, et al. Influence of cigarette smoking on the levels of DNA adducts in human bronchial epithelium and white blood cells. *Int J Cancer* 1990; 46:569–75.

49. Mooney LA, Santella RM, Covey L, et al. Decline of DNA damage and other biomarkers in peripheral blood following smoking cessation. *Cancer Epidemiol Biomarkers Prev* 1995; 4: 627–34.

50. Hsu TM, Zhang YJ, Santella RM. Immunoperoxidase quantitation of 4-aminobiphenyl- and polycyclic aromatic hydrocarbon–DNA adducts in exfoliated oral and urothelial cells of smokers and nonsmokers. *Cancer Epidemiol Biomarkers Prev* 1997; 6:193–9.

51. Schut HAJ, Shiverick KT. DNA adducts in humans as dosimeters of exposure to environmental, occupational, or dietary genotoxins. *FASEB J* 1992; 6:2942.

52. Santella RM. Immunologic methods for detection of carcinogen-DNA damage in humans. *Cancer Epidemiol Biomarkers Prev* 1999; 8: 733–9.

53. Beach AC, Gupta RC. Human biomonitoring and the ^{32}P-postlabeling assay. *Carcinogenesis* 1992; 13:1053–74.

54. Skipper PL, Tannenbaum SR. Protein adducts in the molecular dosimetry of chemical carcinogens. *Carcinogenesis* 1990; 11:507–18.

55. van Schooten FJ, Hillebrand MJX, vanLeeuwen FE, et al. Polycyclic aromatic hydrocarbon-DNA adducts in lung tissue from lung cancer patients. *Carcinogenesis* 1990; 11:1677–81.

56. Tang DL, Rundle A, Warburton D, et al. Associations between both genetic and environmental biomarkers and lung cancer: evidence of a greater risk of lung cancer in women smokers. *Carcinogenesis* 1998; 19:1949–54.

57. Lunn RM, Zhang YJ, Wang LY, et al. p53 Mutations, chronic hepatitis B virus infection, and aflatoxin exposure in hepatocellular carcinoma in Taiwan. *Cancer Res* 1997; 57:3471–7.

58. Wang LY, Chen CJ, Zhang YJ, et al. 4-Aminobiphenyl-DNA damage in liver tissue of hepatocellular carcinoma patients and controls. *Am J Epidemiol* 1998; 147:315–23.

59. Ross RK, Yuan JM, Yu MC, et al. Urinary aflatoxin biomarkers and risk of hepatocellular carcinoma. *Lancet* 1992; 339:943–6.

60. Qian GS, Ross RK, Yu MC, et al. A follow-up study of urinary markers of aflatoxin exposure and liver cancer risk in Shanghai, People's Republic of China. *Cancer Epidemiol Biomarkers Prev* 1994; 3:3–10.

61. Chen CJ, Yu MW, Liaw YF, et al. Chronic hepatitis B carriers with null genotypes of gluthione S-transferase M1 and T1 polymorphisms who are exposed to aflatoxin are at increased risk of hepatocellular carcinoma. *Am J Hum Genet* 1996; 59:128–34.

62. Chen CJ, Wang LY, Lu SN, et al. Elevated aflatoxin exposure and increased risk of hepatocellular carcinoma. *Hepatology* 1996; 24:38–42.

63. Pittelkow AR, Perry HO, Muller SA, et al. Skin cancer in patients with psoriasis treated with coal tar. *Arch Dermatol* 1981; 117:465–8.

64. Wang LY, Hatch M, Chen CJ, et al. Aflatoxin exposure and the risk of hepatocellular carcinoma in Taiwan. *Int J Cancer* 1996; 67:620–5.

65. Schwartz GG. Chromosome Aberrations, In: Hulka BS, Wilcosky TC, Griffith JD (eds) *Biological markers in epidemiology*. New York: Oxford University Press, 1990, pp. 173–95.

66. Vine MF. Micronuclei; In: Hulka BX, Wilcosky TC, Griffith JD (eds) *Biological markers in epidemiology*. New York: Oxford University Press, 1990, pp. 125–46.

67. Das BC. Factors that influence formation of sister chromatid exchanges in human blood lymphocytes. *Crit Rev Toxicol* 1988; 19:43–84.

68. Hagmar L, Bonassi S, Stromberg U, et al. Chromosomal aberrations in lymphocytes predict human cancer: a report from the European Study Group on Cytogenetic Biomakers and Health (ESCH). *Cancer Res* 1998; 58:4117–21.

69. Bonassi S, Hagmar L, Stromberg U, et al. Chromosomal aberrations in lymphocytes predict human cancer independently of exposure to carcinogens. *Cancer Res* 2000; 60:1619–25.

70. Lakin ND, Jackson SP. Regulation of p53 in response to DNA damage. *Oncogene* 1999; 18:7644–55.

71. Ashcroft M, Vousden KH. Regulation of p53 stability. *Oncogene* 1999; 18:7637–43.

72. Hollstein M, Hergenhahn M, Yang Q, et al. New approaches to understanding p53 gene tumor mutation spectra [see comments]. *Mutat Res* 1999; 431:199–209.

73. Husgafvel-Pursiainen K, Kannio A, Oksa P, et al. Mutations, tissue accumulations, and serum levels of p53 in patients with occupational cancers from asbestos and silica exposure. *Environ Mol Mutagen* 1997; 30:224–30.

74. Hemminki K, Palmgren J, Korhonen P, et al. Serum epidermal growth factor receptor and p53 as predictors of lung cancer risk in the ATBC study. *Biomarkers* 1999; 4:72–84.

75. Smith SJ, Li Y, Whitley R, et al. Molecular epidemiology of p53 protein mutations in workers exposed to vinyl chloride. *Am J Epidemiol* 1998; 147:302–8.

76. Soussi T. p53 antibodies in the sera of patients with various types of cancer: a review. *Cancer Res* 2000; 60:1777–88.

77. Marion MJ. Critical genes as early warning signs: example of vinyl chloride. *Toxicol Let* 1998; 102–103:603–7.

78. Weissfeld JL, Larsen RD, Niman HL, et al. Oncogene-related serum proteins and cancer risk: a nested case-control study. *Am J Epidemiol* 1996; 144:723–7.

79. Kopreski MS, Benko FA, Borys DJ, et al. Somatic mutation screening: identification of individuals harboring K-ras mutations with the use of plasma DNA. *J Natl Cancer Inst* 2000; 92:918–23.

80. Meden H, Kuhn W. Overexpression of the oncogene *c-erbB-2* (*HER2/neu*) in ovarian cancer: a new prognostic factor. *Eur J Obstet Gynecol Reprod Biol* 1997; 71:173–9.

81. Kim NW, Piatyszek MA, Prowse KR, et al. Specific association of human telomerase activity with immortal cells and cancer. *Science* 1994; 266:2011–15.

82. Yashima K, Milchgrub S, Gollahon LS, et al. Telomerase enzyme activity and RNA expression during the multistage pathogenesis of breast carcinoma. *Clin Cancer Res* 1998; 4:229–34.

83. Yashima K, Litzky LA, Kaiser L, et al. Telomerase expression in respiratory epithelium during the multistage pathogenesis of lung carcinomas. *Cancer Res* 1997; 57:2373–7.

84. Kinoshita H, Ogawa O, Kakehi Y, et al. Detection of telomerase activity in exfoliated cells in urine from patients with bladder cancer. *J Natl Cancer Inst* 1997; 89:724–30.

85. Kannan S, Tahara H, Yokozaki H, et al. Telomerase activity in premalignant and malignant lesions of human oral mucosa. *Cancer Epidemiol Biomarkers Prev* 1997; 6:413–20.

86. Villa R, Zaffaroni N, Folini M, et al. Telomerase activity in benign and malignant breast lesions: a pilot prospective study on fine-needle aspirates. *J Natl Cancer Inst* 1998; 90:537–9.

87. Hautkappe AL, Lu M, Mueller H, et al. Detection of germ-cell tumor cells in the peripheral blood by nested reverse transcription-polymerase chain reaction for α-fetoprotein-messenger RNA and β human chorionic gonadotropin-messenger RNA. *Cancer Res* 2000; 60:3170–4.

88. Okamoto I, Morisaki T, Sasaki J, et al. Molecular detection of cancer cells by comptetitve reverse transcription-polymerase chain reaction analysis of specific CD44 variant RNAs. *J Natl Cancer Inst* 1998; 90:307–15.

89. Kawakami M, Okaneya T, Furihata K, et al. Detection of prostate cancer cells circulating in peripheral blood by reverse transcription-PCR for hKLK2. *Cancer Res* 1997; 57:4167–70.

90. Silva JM, Dominguez G, Garcia JM, et al. Presence of tumor DNA in plasma of breast cancer patients: clinicopathological correlations. *Cancer Res* 1999; 59:3251–6.

91. Rosin MP, Epstein JB, Berean K, et al. The use of exfoliative cell samples to map clonal genetic alterations in the oral epithelium of high-risk patients. *Cancer Res* 1997; 57:5258–60.

92. Wistuba II, Lam S, Behrens C. Molecular damage in the bronchial epithelium of current and former smokers. *J Natl Cancer Inst* 1997; 89:1366–73.

93. Ahrendt SA, Chow JT, Xu LH, et al. Molecular detection of tumor cells in bronchoalveolar lavage fluid from patients with early stage lung cancer. *J Natl Cancer Inst* 1999; 91:332–39.

94. Alizadeh AA, Eisen MB, Davis RE, et al. Distinct types of diffuse large B-cell lymphoma identified by gene expression profiling [see comments]. *Nature* 2000; 403:503–11.

95. Sgroi DC, Teng S, Robinson G, et al. In vivo gene expression profile analysis of human breast cancer progression. *Cancer Res* 1999; 59:5656–61.

96. Kaminski N, Allard JD, Pittet JF, et al. Global analysis of gene expression in pulmonary fibrosis reveals distinct programs regulating lung inflammation and fibrosis. *Proc Natl Acad Sci USA* 2000; 97:1778–83.

97. Sidransky D, Von Eschenbach A, Tsai YC, et al. Identification of p53 gene mutations in bladder cancers and urine samples. *Science* 1991; 252:706–9.

2
Morphology of Cancer Precursor Lesions

Michael B. Cohen

Our understanding of the development and progression of cancer has rapidly evolved over the last several decades. The earlier clinical recognition of disease, more accurate histopathologic classification, and the identification of molecular alterations that underlie some of these cancers have all contributed to this understanding. However, many gaps in our knowledge base remain. For example, we do not understand the sequential changes, either morphologic or molecular, that underlie early neoplastic progression for most cancers. This is illustrated in many of the subsequent chapters dealing with site-specific cancer precursors. More importantly, our ability to predict the biology of individual precursors is lacking. In part, this is due to our inability to recognize precursor lesions for cancers such as lymphoma, but it is also related to inadequate understanding of the known morphologic lesions that are thought to be precursors, for example prostatic intraepithelial neoplasia (see Chapter 20 on prostate). Despite this perceived pessimism, there is a bright future because newer methodologies are now available that lend themselves to better characterization of these precursor lesions. With this information in hand, our ability to predict, prevent, and alter the natural history of cancer is eminently feasible.

This chapter, written from a pathologist's perspective, aims to outline some of the hurdles that need to be overcome before reliable insight can be obtained into the problem of cancer precursors. Underlying all of this is the need for reproducible classification systems for these precursor lesions that are predicated on consensus terminology. For some cancers, this has been reasonably well established. None-the-less, the main aim of this chapter is to ensure that all investigators can communicate effectively with the pathologist when discussing issues pertinent to cancer precursor lesions [1,2].

Terminology Issues

One of the key issues affecting the critical analysis of the literature on cancer precursors is terminology. The terms cancer, tumor, and neoplasm are often used interchangeably, particularly in a clinical setting. However, they have distinct meanings and every effort should be made to use the terms correctly:

Cancer (L., Crab): any malignant neoplasm (tumor)

Tumor: a nonspecific term meaning lump or swelling; in current usage, however, a synonym for a neoplasm, including cancer

Neoplasm (G., neos. new, *plasma*, anything formed, a growth): a new growth; an aberrant proliferation of cells; may be benign or malignant

Additional terms that are often misused are highlighted in Table 2.1. In particular, there is often confusion between hyperplasia and hypertrophy; for example, benign prostatic hypertrophy (BPH) is more appropriately

TABLE 2.1. Neoplasia and related terms.

Neoplasia: a process of clonal expansion due to defects in the molecular controls that regulate cellular proliferation and/or cell death.

Hyperplasia: an increase in size of a tissue or organ due to an increase in the number of cells. It may be physiologic, compensatory or pathologic.

Hypertrophy: an increase in size of an organ or tissue due to increase in cell size (not number of cells), for example in skeletal muscle.

Hypoplasia: inadequate growth of an organ or tissue.

Aplasia: no growth of an organ or tissue.

Atrophy: a decrease in size of an organ or tissue due to disuse or inadequate nutrition.

Metaplasia: an adaptive substitution of one type of adult tissue for another type of adult tissue. Under stress a more vulnerable type of tissue is replaced by another type more capable of meeting stress.

Dysplasia: an abnormal cellular proliferation in which there is loss of normal architecture and orientation—associated with protracted chronic irritation and inflammation. This term is often used in the context of a preneoplastic (precursor) lesion. Related terms include "atypia", intraepithelial neoplasia/lesion.

Anaplasia: a loss of structural differentiation, typically seen in malignant neoplasms.

Desmoplasia: the formation and proliferation of connective tissue; frequently, prominent proliferation of connective tissue in the growth of tumors.

referred to as nodular hyperplasia. Finally, the term dysplasia is most synonymous with precursor or premalignant lesions such as those that form the basis of this discussion.

Classification of Neoplasms

The ultimate goal of histopathologic "tumor" classification is to predict the biologic behavior [3]. The ends of the spectrum of severity are termed "benign" and "malignant" (Table 2.2). In general these characteristics define clinical behavior, but there are exceptions. The hallmark of a malignant neoplasm is metastatic spread.

Neoplasms are classified by their tissue of origin (histogenesis). Histogenesis cannot be interpreted without knowledge of normal histology, development, and tissue renewal. Benign tumors are designated by attaching the suffix *oma* to the prefix designating the cell type from which the tumor arises (Table 2.3). The generalities outlined are just that; there are numerous exceptions. For example: adenoma (adeno: gland or related to glands) is either a benign epithelial neoplasm that produces a glandlike pattern or a benign epithelial neoplasm that is derived from glands, but does not necessarily produce a glandular pattern. Malignant tumors are classified essentially in the same way as benign tumors with certain additions (Table 2.3). For example, adenocarcinoma combines adenoma and carcinoma, and is a malignant neoplasm of epithelial cell origin with glandular differentiation. Besides adenocarcinoma, the common epithelial malignances are squamous-cell carcinoma and urothelial (transitional-cell) carcinoma. Less common carcinomas include undifferentiated (small or large cell) carcinomas. Carcinomas are by the far the most common type of malignant neoplasm. Neoplasms also arise in or are derived from mesenchymal tissues. In this case, their malignant counterparts are called sarcomas. The third major category of neoplasms consists of those of hematopoietic or lymphoid origin. As a general rule, benign forms of these diseases are not well recognized, either clinically or pathologically. The malignant forms are called leukemias and lymphomas. The latter is a characteristic deviation from the usual benign–malignant nomenclature, and therefore these cancers are often referred to as malignant lymphomas. There are also eponyms for certain neoplasms named after people that discovered, defined, or described them. Examples include: Kaposi's sarcoma, Wilms' tumor and Hodgkin's disease.

Though it is true that the behavior of an individual precursor lesion or a cancer is often quite unpredictable, nevertheless the natural

TABLE 2.2. Pathologic differential diagnosis of neoplasms.

		Benign	Malignant
Gross		Slow growth	Rapid growth
		Small	Large
		Well-circumscribed/encapsulated	Infiltrative
		Compress adjacent tissue	Invasive
		Absent	Necrosis
		Absent	Hemorrhage
		Absent	Metastasis
Microscopic			
Architectural		Well-circumscribed/encapsulated	Infiltrative
		Expansive growth	Invasive
		Close resemblance to normal	Destruction of normal architecture
		Well-differentiated	Poorly differentiated
		Cohesive	Discohesion
Cytologic		Absent	Pleomorphism (size & shape)
		Absent	↑ Nuclear–cytoplasmic ratio (N/C)
		Absent	Hyperchromasia
		Absent	Irregularly granular chromatin
		Absent	Prominent nucleoli, multiple nucleoli
		Absent	Tumor giant cells
		Absent	(Abnormal) mitoses

TABLE 2.3. Terminology of neoplasms.

			Malignant tumor	
Tissue	Normal cell	Benign tumor	General name	Specific name
Epithelial	Squamous	Papilloma	Carcinoma	Squamous
	Glandular	Adenoma		Adeno-
	Urothelial	Papilloma		Urothelial
Mesenchymal	Fibroblast	Fibroma	Sarcoma	Fibro-
	Osteocyte	Osteoma		Osteogenic-
	Chondrocyte	Chondroma		Chondro-
	Fat cell	Lipoma		Lipo-
	Endothelial	Hemangioma		Endothelio-
	Cell	Lymphangioma		Lymphangio-
	Skeletal muscle	Rhabdomyoma		Rhabdo-(striated)
	Smooth muscle	Leiomyoma		Leio-(smooth)
Hematopoietic	Lymphocyte	Benign Neoplasms for this group are not defined	Leukemia	Lymphocytic Leukemia
	Myelocyte			Myelogenous Leukemia
	Plasma Cell			Multiple myeloma

Simple Microscopic Algorithm*

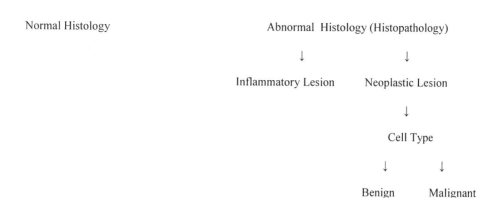

FIGURE 2.1. The pathologist's approach to microscopic evaluation. This algorithm does not neatly take into account precursor lesions, but most commonly would be applied at the stage when the distinction between benign and malignant neoplasms is rendered.

history of many specific types of neoplasms follows particular patterns which enable us to arrive at fairly accurate histopathologic classifications. To aid the nonpathologist, a simplified algorithm for the pathologist's approach to microscopic evaluation is shown in Figure 2.1.

Types of Malignant Neoplasms

Carcinomas are cancers that arise from epithelial precursor cells. These neoplasms usually spread via the lymphatics first to regional lymph nodes, and then later to more distant lymph nodes and, via the bloodstream, to other organs. The most common types are squamous cell carcinomas, urothelial cell carcinomas, and adenocarcinomas. The morphological pattern usually mimics that of the epithelial cell of origin. Sarcomas arise from stromal or mesenchymal components of organs. They may show varying degrees of differentiation, for example osteoid formation in osteogenic sarcomas. These neoplasms frequently metastasize via the bloodstream to distant sites. Hematopoietic neoplasms, including leukemias

and lymphomas, are malignant neoplasms of bone-marrow–derived cells. There are no well-recognized benign lesions for these cancers. They are typically found in the bone marrow and blood, and in the lymph nodes, respectively.

Malignant neoplasms may be derived from congenital rests, benign teratomas or malformations, from benign neoplasms, or from areas subjected to chronic irritation or inflammation in which cell injury necrosis, atrophy, and hyperplasia are seen in varying combinations [3]. The pre-malignant areas are often recognized by their dysplastic features, including irregular growth patterns and bizarre cytologic changes.

Biological and Clinical Behavior of Cancers

One of the fundamental distinctions in cancer is the separation between in situ and invasive disease. This is a crucial distinction that best applies to epithelial neoplasms, and separates, for example, adenocarcinoma in situ from adenocarcinomas. In situ carcinoma does not have the propensity to metastasize, since it is limited to the basement membrane. Once a tumor invades through the basement membrane, it may metastasize [3]. Precursor lesions are usually defined as lesions earlier than in situ disease, although in some instances, carcinoma-in-situ and minimally invasive cancer are included in the term "precursor lesion". For the former, (in situ disease), a compelling argument can be made for its inclusion; for the latter however, it cannot. Invasive cancer has the propensity to metastasize and cannot truly be viewed as a precursor lesion. In addition, there is often an attempt to grade the precursor lesions, as in the uterine cervix, with a numerical score or a qualitative term, similar to grading a cancer. In many instances however, this has been abandoned because of the lack of reproducibility amongst observers' scorings.

There are several factors that can affect the natural history of cancers. Histogenesis (tissue origin) is probably the most important factor in determining tumor behavior. The theory of histogenesis states that, in general, tumors derived from the same tissue will behave in a similar way, and tumors derived from different tissues will behave differently [3]. For example, there are three types of cancer that occur in the stomach: adenocarcinoma, derived from the lining glandular epithelium; lymphoma, derived from the lymphoid tissue of the stomach wall, and leiomyosarcoma, derived from the smooth muscle of the wall. They are similar in that they produce a mass, may ulcerate, and cause bleeding. They differ in their incidence, their tendency to metastasize, their response to different types of therapy, and their overall prognosis.

The theory of histogenesis also states that tumors derived from the same epithelium behave differently depending on the histological pattern of differentiation of the tumor. For example, squamous-cell carcinoma, adenocarcinoma and small cell carcinoma can each be derived from the bronchial epithelium. Small cell carcinoma differs from the others in its tendency to metastasize widely and early in its course. Pathologists base diagnoses and oncologists base therapy primarily on tumor histogenesis.

Tumor Grade or Degree of Differentiation

Grading of tumors is of fundamental importance in managing patients with cancer, as established by the American Joint Committee on Cancer (AJCC) [4]. It is a semiquantitative assessment of the extent to which a tumor resembles the normal tissue at that site. As a general rule, the more closely tumor cells resemble the normal tissue, the less malignant the behavior. Tumors are generally graded on a numerical scale, for example I, II, III, or well differentiated, moderately differentiated, and poorly differentiated. It is particularly interesting that there is an evolution in progress in this area. From the original four tier (I–IV) grading scheme introduced by Broder in the early part of the twentieth century we are moving towards a two tiered system: low and high grade [3]. Examples of this include the grading of tumors of the cervix as well as of the urinary bladder and colon [5,6].

Attempts have also been made to grade precursor lesions in a fashion similar to the grading of cancers. Perhaps the most notable example is the grading of cervical dysplasias (Table 2.4).

In the 1950s the concept of cervical dysplasia was established with a four-grade system. By the late 1960s, it became clear that the separation between severe dysplasia and carcinoma in situ was unreliable, and Richart developed the concept of cervical intraepithelial neoplasia (CIN), a three grade system [7]. In the late 1980s, the Bethesda System was established, which relied on a two grade system; this was modified slightly in the early 1990s and is due for revision in the spring of 2001 [8,9] (see Chapter 16 on the cervix). This evolution would

TABLE 2.4. Grading of cervical dysplasias.

Dysplasia	Cervical intraepithelial neoplasia	Squamous intraepithelial lesion
Mild	I	Low-grade
Moderate	II	High-grade
Severe	III	High-grade
Carcinoma-in-situ	III	High-grade

suggest that our ability to predict the natural history of a lesion needs refining and/or supplementation by ancillary techniques, such as prognostic markers, in order to be clinically useful.

Stage

The stages of tumor development correlate well with prognosis and direct therapy. *Stage* refers to the anatomic extent of the tumor at the time of presentation. As a rule, the higher the stage the poorer the prognosis. Components of tumor stage include: size, extent of invasion and penetration of anatomic boundaries by the primary tumor, presence and number of lymph nodes involved with metastatic spread, and presence of distant metastasis. This is the basis for the tumor-nodes-metastasis (TNM) classification adopted by the Union Internationale Contre le Cancer (UICC), the AJCC, and oncology subspecialty societies [4]. Staging does not apply to precursor lesions, since they are confined to the primary site.

Terminology of Precursor Lesions

Dysplasia may progress to a pattern of carcinoma-in-situ in which the cytologic features are those of a fully developed cancer, but the abnormal cells do not infiltrate below the basement membrane of the tissue. Once this infiltration occurs, the invasion of underlying lymphatics and blood may lead to widespread dissemination. This sequence is best demonstrated in the development of invasive squamous cell carcinoma of the cervix. In mesenchymal neoplasms, the transition from a benign to a malignant neoplasm is often reflected by an increase in the number of mitoses. Attempts have been made to try to quantify this, as in the case of smooth muscle neoplasms of the uterine corpus [2]. Although there has been some success in defining thresholds for the number of mitoses (and the degree of atypia), the use of such information in

attempting to predict the biology of particular borderline lesions (for example those that are neither clearly benign nor malignant) remains an inexact art.

Predicting the outcome (prognosis) in a particular case is the ultimate goal. While the degree of anaplasia (atypia), mitotic activity, and differentiation are helpful in predicting clinical outcome, better correlations are usually found with the depth of infiltration of a cancer and whether or not metastases are present. (For example, patients with carcinomas of the colon that are limited to the mucosa at the time of resection have a much better chance of being cured than those whose cancers have infiltrated through the muscle wall.) Similar efforts to predict the outcome of precursor lesions have been much less successful.

Recurrence and Progression

These important concepts generally apply to cancers. However, it is also reasonable to think in terms of the progression and recurrence of precursor lesions. Assuming the natural history is unaltered, precursor lesions may progress to an in situ carcinoma, and from there to invasive cancers and metastatic disease.

Carcinomas

Our ability to recognize precursor lesions for carcinomas has aided our attempts to better understand the underlying biology. Insights into this process have come from studies of many types of carcinomas. For example, as noted previously, the evolution of CIN I to metastatic disease is reasonably well defined from a morphologic perspective, although the molecular events remain to be fully elucidated. Clearly, human papillomavirus (HPV) is etiologically important, but the ability to predict disease progression in an individual patient remains the goal.

Perhaps, the most detailed studies of cancer development have come from the studies in the Vogelstein laboratory [10,11]. This large body of work has resulted in the elucidation of the

Normal → Hyperplasia → Early Adenoma → Late Adenoma → Adenocarcinoma → Metastasis

FIGURE 2.2. Development of colon cancer.

molecular events underlying the adenoma–carcinoma sequence for colorectal carcinomas where cancer is viewed as a multistage process (see Chapter 9). Using contemporary molecular biologic techniques and hereditary cancer syndromes, this group has been able to propose a model for the development and progression of colon cancer. Briefly, colon carcinogensis is thought to progress through a series of stages from normal to metastatic disease, with distinct molecular alterations underlying each step (Figure 2.2).

The results of these detailed studies form the framework for similar efforts on cancer in other locations. Two examples are the urinary bladder (urothelial carcinomas) (see Chapter 21) and the head and neck (squamous carcinomas) (see Chapter 6). The establishment of a correlation between morphologic and molecular alterations has been a significant advance in this field.

Hematopoietic Neoplasms

Although more common than soft tissue tumors, hematopoietic neoplasms are much less common than carcinomas [12,13]. This however, has not hindered our understanding of many of the fundamental molecular events that are critical to neoplastic progression amongst this group of tumors. In fact, our understanding of the molecular biologic alterations in lymphoid neoplasms is better than that for carcinomas. But the recognition of precursor lesions, including in situ lesions, remains poorly defined. Most hematopoietic cells, and lymphocytes in particular, have the ability to circulate throughout the body via the lymphatic and/or vascular systems. Therefore, the concept of precursor lesions is not applicable to these neoplasms. Certain diseases [such as autoimmune diseases (e.g., Hashimoto's thyroiditis), immunodeficiency syndromes (e.g., organ transplantation), and certain viral pathogens (e.g., HIV)] are known to confer an increased

risk of lymphoproliferative disorders [2]. It is expected that the application of molecular tools, such as gene rearrangements, will allow the recognition of select benign proliferations. Still, overall, our understanding of precursor lesions for hematopoietic neoplasms remains distinctly incomplete.

Soft Tissue Tumors (Mesenchymal Neoplasms)

Despite the relative abundance of mesenchymal tissues throughout the human body, the incidence of benign and, in particular, malignant neoplasms is very low [12,13]. There is a large array of mesenchymal cell types, and as a result, a large number of different soft tissue tumors. More importantly, precursor lesions have not been recognized for the vast majority of such tumors [2]. However, the malignant transformation of some benign soft tissue tumors, for example peripheral nerve sheath tumors (neurofibroma, Schwannoma), is well recognized. In addition, it is also well recognized that certain low-grade soft tissue tumors (liposarcoma for example) might progress to high-grade tumors. Lastly, the rarity of these neoplasms, with a few notable exceptions (one is Ewing's sarcoma), has hindered our understanding of the molecular events that underlie these neoplasms. Consequently, a fundamental understanding of the development and progression of soft tissue tumors from precursor lesions to metastatic disease is still in its infancy.

Prognostic Markers: A Word of Caution

A long-term goal is to be able to reproducibly recognize precursor lesions (or cancers at an early stage), predict their biology (presumably with ancillary studies), and institute therapy that would maximize clinical benefit while minimizing toxicity and cost to the individual patient. To this end there is a large body of literature that focuses on the utilization of prognostic and predictive markers. Unfortunately, the mainstays of prognostication and prediction remain pathologic observations: histopathologic tumor type, grade, and stage [14]. There are several issues, many of which are addressed throughout this book, that will need further refinement before this long-term goal can be achieved. Although pathology is viewed as the gold standard, the literature is replete with examples of the lack of inter- and intraobserver variability in pathological assessment, including the classification of precursor lesions. For example, Gleason, in utilizing the grading scheme for prostatic adenocarcinoma that he developed, had an intra-observer agreement of 50% for the same grade and an intra-observer agreement of 85% for deviations within one grade [15]. Hayes, among others, has tried to make some sense of these issues by developing the tumor marker utility grading system (TMUGS) [16,17]. A few key issues are worthy of specific mention. First, precursor lesions and cancers are heterogeneous both spatially and temporally. Thus, the application of specific prognostic markers may be of limited value due to sampling issues. Second, there is a redundancy of signaling pathways inside cells that may limit the applicability of select markers that focus on one pathway only. Third, variation in methodology and quality-control issues are well recognized concerns. As a result, it is difficult to analyze data from different laboratories together. In this regard also, the exclusion of noninformative cases is a real concern. Finally, data interpretation and statistical analysis have been far from uniform, and this has also contributed to the difficulty in reading the literature. Taken together, these are fundamental issues that need to be resolved before the goal of reproducibility in recognition, prediction, and treatment can be achieved.

Future Directions

The morphologic and molecular identification of precursor (premalignant) lesions is evolving, although our understanding is best concerning the carcinomas. The advent of molecular biologic tools will greatly enhance our further understanding of these lesions. Several new techniques will likely become fundamental in these ongoing studies. Three are worthy of special mention. The use of laser capture microdissection allows morphologic identification of these (putative) lesions and their isolation as a relatively pure population of cells [18–20]. These cells can then be analyzed at the molecular level (e.g., protein, mRNA or DNA) for alterations that might give insight into the development of these lesions and allow prediction of their biology (progression). This underscores a critical issue in much of the published literature: sampling. With variable success, attempts have been made in the past to microdissect out the cells of interest. Contamination with other cell types has confounded the reliable identification of prognostic/predictive markers. It is hoped that with more reliable microdissection methods more meaningful molecular information can be obtained.

A second inovative technique is the use of DNA microarrays that contain thousands of gene products that can be assayed with computer-based analytical tools [21]. In a paper by Golub, the separation of acute lymphocytic leukemia (ALL) from acute myelogenous leukemia (AML) was accomplished using such methodology [22]. Though, in the majority of cases, this distinction can be accomplished morphologically, especially in conjunction with phenotypic analysis, this is a proof of the principle that tumors may in the future be diagnosed by DNA microarrays and related methodology. Tumor classification using DNA microarrays is a goal at the National Cancer Institute. This has already been applied to other cancers such as breast carcinomas [23]. Ultimately, it is conceivable that molecular diagnosis of tumors will play an important role, although it seems unlikely that it will replace conventional histopathology. Rather, it seems that it will be useful in providing additional prognostic and predictive information. It is also likely that the diagnostic utility of protein-level information, for example that obtained by immunohistochemistry, will be enhanced, once the information from the larger DNA chip arrays have been refined and validated.

Perhaps the most intriguing is the use of this approach to study the natural history of tumors, such as that of melanoma [24].

The last technique, tissue microarray, may be particularly useful since it allows rapid screening of relatively large number of specimen samples [25,26].

Finally, some words of caution for the pathologist examining putative precursor lesions. It should be clear from this discussion that appropriate classification of precursor lesions is critical to enhance our understanding of their natural history. By and large, our knowledge is limited to epithelial lesions/carcinomas, but even for these, there remain significant gaps in our understanding. It is hoped that with an enhanced understanding, appropriate intervention will alter the biology of the disease. This would represent a fundamental evolution of medicine from a disease-based discipline to a preventive one. All this, however, is predicated on a fundamental understanding of the molecular epidemiology of precursor lesions. Overall, it is clear that molecular epidemiology has an exciting future, as shown throughout this book.

References

1. Ponten J. Cell biology of precancer. In: Ponten J (ed) *Precancer: biology, importance and possible prevention. Cancer Surv* 1998; 32:5–35.

2. Henson DE, Albores-Saavedra J. *Pathology of Incipient Neoplasia*, 3rd ed. Oxford: Oxford University Press, 2001.

3. Cotran RS, Kumar V, Collins T. Neoplasia. In: Cotran RS, Kumar V, Collins T (eds) *Robbins Pathologic Basis of Disease*, 6th ed. Philadelphia: WB Saunders Company, 1999, 260–327.

4. Fleming ID, Cooper JS, Henson DE, et al. (eds) *AJCC Cancer Staging Manual*, 5th ed. Philadelphia: Lippincott-Raven, 1997.

5. Compton CC, Fielding LP, Burgart LJ, et al. Prognostic factors in colorectal cancer. College of American Pathologists Consensus Statement 1999. *Arch Pathol Lab Med* 2000; 124:979–94.

6. Epstein JI, Amin MB, Reuter VE, et al. The World Health Organization/International Society of Urological Pathology consensus classification of urothelial (transitional cell) neoplasms of the urinary bladder. *Am J Surg Pathol* 1998; 22:1435–48.

7. Richart RM. Natural history of cervical intra-epithelial neoplasia. *Clin Obstet Gynecol* 1968; 5:748–84.

8. The 1988 Bethesda System for reporting cervical/vaginal cytologic diagnoses: developed and approved at the National Cancer Institute Workshop in Bethesda, Maryland, December 12–13, 1988. *Hum Pathol* 1990; 7:704–8.

9. The Bethesda System for reporting cervical/vaginal cytologic diagnoses: revised after the second National Cancer Institute Workshop, April 29–30, 1991. *Acta Cytol* 1993; 37:115–24.

10. Fearon ER, Vogelstein B. A genetic model for colorectal tumorigenesis. *Cell* 1990; 61:759–67.

11. Kinzler KW, Vogelstein B. Lessons from hereditary colorectal cancer. *Cell* 1996; 87:159–70.

12. Greenlee RT, Murray T, Bolden S, et al. *Cancer Statistics 2000*, CA Cancer J Clin 2000; 50:7–33.

13. Percy C (ed) Histology of cancer. Incidence and prognosis: SEER Population-Based Data, 1973–1987. *Cancer Suppl* 1995; 77:1–421.

14. Hammond MEH, Fitzgibbons PL, Compton CC, et al. College of American Pathologists Conference XXXV: solid tumor prognostic factors—which, how, and so what? summary document and recommendations for implementation. *Arch Pathol Lab Med* 2000; 124:958–65.

15. Gleason DF. Histologic grading of prostate cancer: a perspective. *Hum Pathol* 1992; 3:273–9.

16. Hayes DF, Bast RC, Desch CE, et al. Tumor marker utility grading scheme: a framework to evaluate clinical utility of tumor markers. *J Natl Cancer Inst* 1996; 88:1456–66.

17. Hayes DF, Trock B, Harris AL. Assessing the clinical impact of prognostic factors: when is "statistically significant" clinically useful? *Breast Cancer Res* 1998; 52:305–19.

18. Emmert-Buck MR, Bonner RF, Smith PD, et al. Laser capture microdissection. *Science* 1996; 274:998–1001.

19. Fend F, Raffeld M. Laser capture microdissection in pathology. *J Clin Pathol* 2000; 53:666–72.

20. Webb T. Laser capture microdissection comes into mainstream use. *J Natl Cancer Inst* 2000; 92:1710–11.

21. Perou CM, Brown PO, Botsetin D. Tumor classification using gene expression patterns from DNA microarrays. *Mol Med Today* 2000; 6:67–76.

22. Golub TR, Slonim DK, Tamayo P, et al. Molecular classification of cancer: class discovery and class prediction by gene expression monitoring. *Science* 1999; 286:531–7.

23. Perou CM, Jeffrey SS, van de Rijn M, et al. Distinctive gene expression patterns in human mammary epithelial cells and breast cancers. *Proc Natl Acad Sci USA* 1999; 96:9212–17.

24. Wang E, Marincola FM. A natural history of melanoma: serial gene expression analysis. *Immunol Today* 2000; 21:619–23.

25. Kononen J, Bubendorf L, Kallioniemi A, et al. Tissue microarrays for high-throughput molecular profiling of tumor specimens. *Nat Med* 1998; 4:844–7.

26. Camp RL, Charette LA, Rimm DL. Validation of tissue microarray technology in breast carcinoma. *Lab Invest* 2000; 80:1943–9.

Part II
Issues Related to Measurement and Interpretation of Cancer Precursors

3
Collection, Processing, and Analysis of Preneoplastic Specimens

Neil Caporaso and Jim Vaught

As the tools to explore the molecular basis for the cellular and tissue alterations that underlie neoplastic change and progression become more widely available and refined, there is increasing emphasis on the study of the earliest changes that characterize cancer. Molecular epidemiology uses biomarkers to complement traditional questionnaire approaches in determining the contribution of exposure and other factors to cancer. Preneoplastic tissue studies offer specific advantages with regard to investigations of cancer etiology and treatment. These include:

1. By definition, preneoplastic changes are not influenced by the clinical sequelae of cancer, and therefore studies of preneoplastic tissue and host factors (e.g., vitamin levels) are less biased than similar studies using neoplastic tissue. For example, weight loss due to cancer may result in host alterations that obscure more specific molecular changes that are intrinsic to the process of transformation.
2. The earliest and most specific changes that characterize cancer may be present.
3. Focus on changes in the tissue of interest permits study of gene expression and proteomics, which reveals patterns of changes specific to developing cancer.
4. Prospective studies of subjects with preneoplastic changes may shed light on the determinants of progression.
5. Genetic studies of tissue may reveal preneo-plastic alterations in tissue that lacks obvious histopathological features, thus refining and expanding the morphological definitions of preneoplasia.
6. Studies of preneoplastic lesions using biomarkers may represent a fertile area for combined clinical trials and etiological investigation.
7. Molecular characterization of these lesions (i.e., intermediate markers) may provide targets for intervention or monitoring. The former may be therapeutically useful, while the latter may help guide clinical decisions.
8. Clinical interventions on preneoplastic lesions are often less invasive and radical, have a higher probability of success, and generally involve the patient in the medical system at a stage where conventional treatment, if considered necessary, can take place at a time when it is likely to be most effective.

For these goals to be achieved, it is critical that biological specimens are obtained in a manner that is efficient, safe, and consistent with ethical guidelines; that preserves crucial marker characteristics; and that is optimal for subsequent processing, linkage with information, and long-term storage. This chapter describes issues relevant to the acquisition, processing, and storage of biological specimens that are integral to this study approach. Further details on the general approach [1] and implications of different study designs [2,3] can be found in the literature.

Molecular Epidemiology Paradigm

The general types of questions that can be addressed in studies of preneoplastic lesions can be categorized by considering a molecular epidemiological scheme (Figure 3.1). How do the molecular (somatic genetic changes, chromosomal alterations, protein or expression patterns, cell surface markers, etc.) features of preneoplastic lesions compare to:

1. Exposure. For example, what is the relation of cervical lesions to human papillomavirus (HPV), or of oral leukoplakia to alcohol and smoking? More broadly, how do extrinsic exposures as well as other host factors influence these lesions (i.e., gender, nutritional status, concurrent medical illness, etc.)?

2. Intermediate markers, including internal dose measures, such as macromolecular adducts, or markers of early biological effect, such as measures of cytogenetic damage. The former category reflects mostly exposure, and the latter reflects a combination of exposure, host factors, and accumulated "effects" that may border on the next stage, altered structure or function. So, for example, are DNA–carcinogen adducts related to preneoplastic bronchial lesions?

3. Inherited genetic factors. For example, are colon polyps related to the NAT2 or MTHFR genotypes?

4. Somatic genetic changes and other evidence of "altered structure or function." For example, are p53 lesions present in bronchial dysplasia?

5. Clinical outcome. For example, what findings in preneoplastic lesions predict benign or malignant outcomes?

6. Intervention. For example, what features of preneoplastic lesions predict a benign outcome or progression after specific therapeutic interventions? Are there certain molecular features associated with side effects?

Traditionally, each of these questions has been addressed by different study designs. Clinical trials are conducted to explore treatment issues, but epidemiological studies are conducted to examine etiological questions [1]. With progressive advances in molecular biology, the menu of possible investigations that can be conducted on biospecimens, and the efficiencies of using large cohort studies or clinical or screening trials to collect these materials, have become increasingly attractive. We consider first some broad principles relevant to many, if not most, studies that involve biospecimens and then address some aspects relevant to specific organ systems.

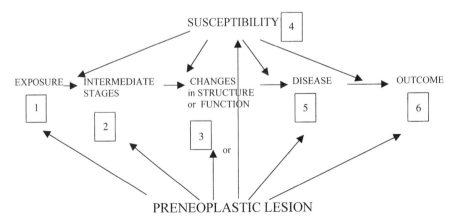

FIGURE 3.1. Types of questions that can be studied involving preneoplastic lesions (see text).

General Specimen Collection and Processing Considerations

Biomarkers for preneoplastic lesions are often measured in blood fractions including whole blood; serum or plasma; buffy coat (or lymphocytes); and red blood cells. Examples of analyses that may be conducted on such specimens include the measurement of serum prostate specific antigen (PSA), and genetic polymorphisms measured by polymerase-chain-reaction (PCR)–based methods in DNA extracted from blood or blood fractions.

For research projects involving the collection and processing of fresh blood, a research nurse or other appropriate personnel should verify that the study participant has been adequately informed about the study and has consented to participate. The nurse should inquire about medications or conditions that might exclude the participant from the collection, and about problems with previous blood donations. A blood pressure reading may also be appropriate. Procedures to prevent exposure of study personnel to HIV, hepatitis and other infectious agents (e.g., adherence to Universal Precautions practices, prior Hepatitis B vaccination) must be followed during the collection and handling of any biological specimens. All fresh or frozen specimens should be considered potentially infectious. Equipment and supplies should be organized ahead of time. For some projects it is necessary to ship blood collection kits to remote study sites. Procedures for collecting blood from donor subjects must be well established and documented, especially for remote sites. Experienced phlebotomists must be employed to avoid harmful side effects and the collection of suboptimal specimens. For studies of biomarkers of precancerous lesions, blood may be fractionated into plasma/serum, lymphocytes, monocytes, erythrocytes, granulocytes and platelets. If the blood fractions will not be used immediately, they may be separated into aliquots in small cryovials and stored in mechanical or liquid-nitrogen freezers.

For some studies it may be desirable to provide for an unlimited supply of DNA from blood specimens. Peripheral blood lymphocytes isolated from whole blood, or buffy coat samples collected from the fractionation of blood specimens, may be cryopreserved for the establishment of cell lines. In order to preserve the viability of lymphocytes, cryopreservation of specimens requires freezing using a controlled-rate freezing program and subsequent storage in the vapor phase of liquid nitrogen. Aliquots of cryopreserved lymphocytes may subsequently be removed from storage and transformed by Epstein–Barr virus (EBV) for the establishment of cell lines [4].

The following are additional important considerations when collecting and processing blood for study of precancerous biomarkers:

- Anticoagulant [4]: Determine whether anticoagulant is necessary for the intended laboratory analyses and use the appropriate evacuated tube system (i.e., vacutainer) containing either EDTA (ethylenediaminetetraacetic acid), heparin or acid–citrate–dextrose (ACD). Various anticoagulants have advantages and disadvantages that should be considered when used in specific laboratory applications.
- Stability: Consideration must be given to the stability of the biomarkers of interest under various conditions of collection and storage [5]. For some laboratory studies, it is necessary to process the sample immediately. However, many biomarkers are stable for long periods if the specimens are frozen and stored properly at −80°C or lower. For some laboratory applications, it is acceptable to store blood specimens as "spots" on specially designed blood-spot cards. Such samples are stable for long periods and are suitable for PCR-based biomarker assays.
- Secure Storage: Whether specimens are stored in mechanical or liquid-nitrogen freezers, quality-control (QC) procedures must be in place to maintain records concerning the proper operation and maintenance of the equipment. Emergency procedures must be in place in order to respond to unexpected equipment failures. Alarm systems and back-up generators are necessary components of biorepositories.

- Shipping: Shipping requirements vary according to the specimen type, shipping distance, and other factors. Blood that will be fractionated upon receipt at a laboratory should be shipped using cool packs that will limit temperature excursions and not result in freezing. Specimens that will be analyzed for unstable biomarkers will need to be shipped frozen with adequate dry ice to preserve their integrity. "Dry shippers" in which liquid nitrogen is absorbed into the walls of the shipping vessel are now used to ship specimens at temperatures of −100°C or lower. Very specific regulations govern the shipping of blood and other biological specimens within the United States and internationally. See the Appendix for additional information.

In addition to the site-specific tissue specimens described in this chapter and the general utility of blood fractions for many biomarker studies, it is often more convenient to meet a study's objectives through the collection of alternative biological specimens [4]. Some examples are:

- Urine, feces, sputum: These can be used to monitor metabolic disease processes, to measure exposure to xenobiotic agents, to conduct mutagenicity studies, to provide a source of DNA, and they can also be as a source of exfoliated cells.
- Buccal cells: These can be conveniently collected using a mouthwash protocol and used as a source of DNA for genotyping and other biomarker assays [6].
- Skin biopsies: Fibroblast lines can be established as a renewable source of consitutional DNA.
- Tissue biopsies: These can be bronchial brushings/washings, cervical cone biopsies, pleural/peritoneal fluid, bone marrow, or cerebrospinal fluid obtained in diagnostic or staging evaluations.
- Autopsy materials: These can provide a valuable source of tissue for many types of biomarker studies. However, special attention must be paid to assuring timely collection and processing due to the rapid deterioration of some tissues after death [7,8].
- Paraffin-embedded tissues: These are useful for many studies that require analysis of

tissue pathology with respect to precancerous conditions. Procedures have been developed for extraction and analysis of nucleic acids from paraffin tissue blocks, though the quality of the nucleic acids may be inferior to that purified from fresh specimens [8].

In collecting any of the tissue, blood, or other specimen types described in this chapter, it is necessary to establish a strict set of procedures that will result in specimens that are of optimal quality for the proposed studies. Such procedures form the basis of a QC program. The QC program must include standard operating procedures (SOPs) that define the specific forms and procedures for collecting, processing, storing, and shipping each specimen type necessary for the research program. In the QC program the specifics of collection, necessary forms, the stability of specimens, proper storage conditions, biohazard considerations, labeling and computerized inventory systems, and shipping details, are provided in sufficient detail for consistency to be maintained when new personnel are trained. Many of these considerations are described in the articles by Landi and Caporaso [4] and by Grizzle et al. [7]. The latter article describes the desirable characteristics of a program for collecting and processing biospecimens for a research program, based on the model developed for NCI's Cooperative Human Tissue Network (CHTN).

It is extremely important that the storage conditions for specimens be planned and established well before specimen collection begins. The intended length of time before specimens will be analyzed, and the stability of the analytes of interest, are major considerations in deciding whether to refrigerate, or freeze at −70°C, or in the vapor phase of liquid nitrogen (about −130°C). When in doubt, it is best to store tissues in the vapor phase of liquid nitrogen for maximum stability over an extended period. Liquid-nitrogen freezers have fewer maintenance problems than mechanical ultrafreezers with compressors and other moving parts. Modern liquid-nitrogen freezers have sophisticated electronic systems with automated filling mechanisms, temperature alarms, and nitrogen-level alarms.

Specimens may be stored in a variety of vessels using labeling systems specific for the study. However, there are some guidelines that must be followed to avoid problems in the long-term storage of specimens. Glass vials or vials with pop-up tops are generally not suitable as long-term storage vessels. Screw-cap cryovials specifically designed for long-term low-temperature storage are the storage vessels of choice.

Labeling systems also vary greatly in their stability when stored long-term in ultrafreezers, that is, at liquid-nitrogen temperatures. Some of the contacts listed in the internet sites in the Appendix, for example, those at the National Cancer Institute (NCI) and Centers for Disease Control (CDC) biorepositories, can advise researchers on the proper materials to use for storage of specimens. Bar-coding systems are now available for biorepository applications. Some of the codes, such as the two-dimensional data matrix system, can be used to store both numeric and textual information on the smallest cryovials. See the internet references included in the Appendix for more information and the names of vendors that provide a variety of bar-coding systems.

The security of the specimens is paramount in any biorepository. The repository's standard procedures should include plans for responding to severe weather and other disasters (floods, power failure, fire, security breaches, terrorism), including a plan to move the contents of the freezers to an alternative location if necessary. Alarm systems that alert security personnel whenever freezers exceed a preset temperature are a necessity. Generators that can reliably power the freezers and other critical equipment must be in place in the event of a power failure. An extra measure of security is provided by dividing replicates of specimens between two or more freezers to prevent loss of the entire sample in the event of freezer malfunction.

A specimen repository requires an adequate system for maintaining an accurate and current inventory of specimens. For smaller repositories with only a few freezers, such an inventory may consist of a small database with the freezer location, volume (or size), and condition of the specimen. For larger repositories containing millions of specimens, such as those maintained by the NCI and CDC, more sophisticated customized specimen inventory systems have been developed. At NCI, the primary system for maintaining an inventory of over 5 million specimens is the BSI-II, a web-based specimen inventory system. The BSI-II system is a key component in NCI's record keeping for repositories of biological specimens and for laboratory testing of these specimens. This system currently tracks specimens obtained from the participants in over 450 NCI epidemiological and genetic studies. The BSI-II maintains a complete description of each specimen vial as a full history from the date its information was first entered into the system. There are two basic types of data in the system: repository-specific data, and study-specific data. Repository-specific data consist of the sample identifier (ID), date received, freezer location, and specimen condition. Study-specific data include study ID, subject ID, sample ID, date of specimen collection, and other related information. When vials are removed from storage and sent to laboratories for analysis, or to other storage locations, the BSI-II maintains specimen tracking information. Many users access the BSI-II concurrently, including NCI investigators, repository staff, government contractors, and outside researchers.

Ethical Considerations

The collection of any specimens for research purposes requires strict adherence to institutional and federal regulations to protect the confidentiality of human subjects and to provide for their safety. In the United States, the Code of Federal Regulations (CFR, specifically 45 CFR 46) governs the protection of human subjects. The regulations are interpreted by local institutional review boards (IRBs), which review applications from investigators who intend to collect and use human tissues in their research programs. In addition, for many studies the IRBs require that investigators obtain approval from human subjects through informed-consent documents. The ethical implications of studies involving long-standing archives of paraffin-embedded tissue remain an area of intense discussion. See the discussion by Grizzle et al. [7] and the internet references in the Appendix for additional information.

Specific Malignancies

In this section, we provide several examples of standard methods of specimen collection and processing involving preneoplastic lesions of specific organs. Invasive neoplasia of the squamous epithelium occurs at a number of anatomical sites including the skin, oral cavity, esophagus, and cervix, and is normally preceded by several stages of intraepithelial evolution. Normal epithelium, via a process of genomic instability, goes through an initial stage of hyperplasia followed by several stages of preinvasive neoplasia, including mild, moderate, and severe dysplasias. The preneoplasias are denoted by different names for various organ sites, such as actinic keratosis in skin and dysplastic leukoplakia in the oral cavity. Generally the stages of preneoplasia take 1 to 15 years to develop into invasive neoplasia or carcinoma. Normal glandular epithelium, such as that found in the colon, breast, and prostate, undergoes a similar progression to hyperplasia and several stages of intraepithelial neoplasia or adenoma, before developing into invasive neoplasia or adenocarcinoma over a period of 5 to 20 years [9].

Cervix

Epidemiological studies have shown that human papillomavirus (HPV) is the central cause of cervical cancer, and the prevalence of HPV in cervical cancer has been shown to be close to 100% [10]. Screening for cervical cancer using cervical cytology has led to a significant decrease in incidence and mortality. In addition to standard Pap smears, cervical cell specimens can be collected in order to detect HPV types known to be associated with the more severe forms of cervical neoplasia. Studies are under way at the United States NCI and elsewhere to evaluate HPV testing for screening or as an adjunct to cytology.

Preneoplastic lesions of the cervix include cervical intraepithelial neoplasia grade 1 (CIN I), also known as mild dysplasia, CIN II, also known as moderate dysplasia, and CIN III, which includes severe dysplasia and carcinoma in situ (see Chapter 16 by Franco). The latter are precursors of invasive cervical cancer. A recently developed alternative classification system for cervical neoplasia is the Bethesda system: *ASCUS* is atypical squamous cells of undetermined significance; *LSIL* is low-grade squamous intraepithelial lesion; *HSIL* is high-grade squamous intraepithelial lesion. LSIL includes CIN 1 and HSIL includes CIN 2 and CIN 3. Abnormal cells that cannot be classified as low- or high-grade squamous intraepithelial lesions are described as ASCUS, which includes many of the minor abnormalities commonly designated "atypical" in the past [11].

Cervical cells can be collected by several clinical procedures that allow for analysis of potential preneoplastic conditions. The procedures include conventional Pap smears and newer technologies developed for automated processing of cervical cells and detection of HPV by PCR-based methodology.

For an ongoing study at the NCI [12], the following protocols were developed:

- Pap Smear: A Papette broom is used to collect a specimen that is smeared onto a slide for a conventional Pap smear evaluation. The slide is immediately fixed with a spray fixative or by immersion in 95% ethanol.
- ThinPrep: The Papette broom is rinsed in PreservCyt (CYTYC Corporation Boxborough, Massachusetts) for preparation of a ThinPrep and for HPV testing by Hybrid Capture Microplate analysis (Digene Corporation, Silver Spring, Maryland).
- Swab testing: A Dacron swab is used to collect a cervical cell specimen, which is placed into Specimen Transport Medium (STM, Digene Corporation, Silver Spring, Maryland) for HPV testing by PCR methodology.

The above specimens, including the Pap-smear slides, PreservCyt vials for ThinPrep, and

Hybrid Capture samples in STM, can be stored and transported at room temperature. Cervicovaginal specimens collected using the methods outlined above have been analyzed in a variety of studies of preneoplastic cervical disease. Fluorescent in situ hybridization (FISH) has been used to detect chromosomal changes in cells from archival cervical smears [13]. FISH allows for detection of specific chromosomal changes that may be useful in monitoring progression toward high-grade cervical dysplasia. Cells collected and fixed using PreservCyt are processed to prepare ThinPrep slides in an automated procedure developed by Cytyc Corporation. ThinPrep slides were developed in an effort to produce more representative cytologic preparations with fewer artifacts. Analysis of ThinPrep slides in comparison to standard PAP smears has shown ThinPrep slides to provide greater sensitivity in detecting preneoplastic cervical lesions [14].

Several methods are available to detect specific HPV types associated with increased cervical cancer risk. The Hybrid Capture system detects a variety of cancer-associated HPV types in cervical cell specimens prepared in STM [15]. More sensitive PCR-based methods have been developed to detect the high-risk HPV types, as well as the dozens of HPV types that are associated with lower risk of developing cervical neoplasia [16].

With the advent of laser-assisted microdissection, it is now possible to identify preneoplastic cells among specimens with mixtures of cells, including routine cervical smears. Analysis of selected microdissected cervical cells by comparative genomic hybridization has shown that it is possible to identify chromosomal aberrations in small numbers of cervical cells [17].

Prostate

High-grade prostatic intraepithelial neoplasia (PIN) is recognized as the most likely preinvasive stage of prostatic adenocarcinoma (see Chapter 20 by Marshall and Wood). PIN has a high predictive value as a marker for adenocarcinoma of the prostate [18]. Examination of biopsied tissue is the usual method of detection

of PIN as it is not distinctive by ultrasonography. PIN does not cause a consistent change in serum PSA concentration that can be reliably differentiated from cancer or benign prostatic hyperplasia. The prostate is organized into three major glandular regions that differ histologically and biologically: the central zone (about 25%), peripheral zone (70%) and the transitional zone (5–10%). The majority (about 70%) of prostatic carcinomas originate in the peripheral zone while about 25% occur in the transitional zone.

Depending on the nature of the analyses to be performed and the clinical setting, tissue may be collected from surgically resected prostate, from needle or core biopsies, and during transurethral resection of the prostate (TURP). Prostate tissue removed during radical prostatectomy is generally fixed in formalin (18 to 24 hours in formalin for each 3 cm of specimen) prior to further dissection for routine surgical pathology evaluation. Fresh prostate tissue may also be harvested from radical prostatectomy procedures for cytogenetic, molecular biology, and other laboratory studies [19]. Needle-biopsy specimens generally consist of tissue from the peripheral zone and seldom include the central zone or anterior portion of the transitional zone. Care must be taken in the processing of needle biopsies to ensure that there has been adequate tissue sampling for all lesions to be detected [20]. Labeling of needle-biopsy specimens should include the identifying location from which the biopsy was taken. At least two slides should be prepared from each needle biopsy block. Core biopsy has the advantage of including random samples of tissue from all prostate zones.

TURP was the major treatment modality for prostatic hyperplasia in the past. TURP specimens consist of tissue from the transitional zone, urethra, periurethral area, bladder neck and anterior fibromuscular stroma. As with other methods of prostate tissue sampling, TURP specimens must be collected and processed in a manner that allows for detection of all abnormal lesions. Based on the size of TURP specimens, algorithms have been recommended by the College of American Pathologists, that outline the number of tissue blocks and sections that will maximize the possibility of detecting PIN and prostatic carcinoma [21].

The processing of prostate specimens depends on the method of collection and the intended analysis. Since detection of PIN is based on examination of biopsied prostate tissue, the collection and processing of preneoplastic prostate lesions follows standard pathologic and histologic protocols. However, if prostate specimens are to be analyzed for hormones or other biomarkers of variable stability, fresh tissue from prostatectomy, cystoprostatectomy, or TURP, must be placed in labeled vials and flash-frozen within 10 minutes of resection to prevent degradation of the analytes of interest.

Another potential preneoplastic lesion in the prostate is atypical adenomatous hyperplasia (AAH) of the prostate. AAH is a small glandular proliferation that occurs most often in the transitional zone, where a subset of well-differentiated carcinomas also arise. A recent study used microdissected AAH lesions to study chromosomal alterations, suggesting an approach that may be useful in future studies of precursor lesions of prostate cancer [22]. Other studies, using techniques such as comparative genomic hybridization, have also implicated chromosomal alterations in the progression to prostate cancer. There is evidence that genes such as the androgen receptor gene, e-cadherin, and PTEN are involved in the development and progression of prostate cancer [23].

Skin

Dysplastic nevi (DN) are the preneoplastic lesions that have been demonstrated in multiple epidemiologic studies to be precursors of melanoma [24] (see Chapter 14 by Gallagher and Lee). DN are defined according to clinical criteria that include a macular component, irregular and indistinct borders, variable color, and diameter more than 5 mm. Histologic findings include basilar melanocytic hyperplasia of large epithelioid melanocytes with variable nuclear atypia, a patchy lymphocytic infiltrate,

concentric eosinophilic fibroplasia, and lamellar fibroplasia.

The Genetic Epidemiology Branch of NCI has engaged in long-term studies of families to evaluate the natural history of DN and melanoma in families predisposed to melanoma. The DN found in members of these families have been evaluated by nevus counts, photography, and biopsy of suspected lesions [25]. Biopsies are collected from normal and preneoplasic skin. Normal skin may be collected from study participants to provide a source of fibroblasts [26]. Alternatively, cryopreservation of lymphocytes obtained from peripheral blood may be conducted to obtain a renewable source of germline DNA. Skin fibroblast specimens are not frozen. The necessary supplies, including specific media, are mailed to the local physician along with a written protocol and a copy of the participant's signed informed consent. During the biopsy, the skin specimen is kept sterile, and the specimen is placed into a cryogenic vial with the media as soon as possible after it has been excised. Biopsied material left floating on top of the media may become contaminated or die, and therefore the tissue should be submerged in the media. The media are kept refrigerated before the surgery, and after collection, the specimen is refrigerated until it is shipped to a laboratory or biorepository. See the Appendix for information on shipment of biological specimens. At NCI these normal skin biopsies are sent to a laboratory for establishment of fibroblastic cell lines.

Preneoplastic skin or tumor tissue is collected in a manner similar to that for normal skin. The protocol for processing the biopsy material is as described for normal skin. Although most of a lesion is consumed for routine pathology, nevi or melanomas can be used to establish melanocyte cultures. The nevus cell cultures have limited lifespans but are very useful in establishing early changes in melanocytes. Melanomas, especially metastatic lesions, can provide long-term cell cultures for multiple laboratory investigations. Both nevi and melanomas can also be flash-frozen in the cryogenic vials and stored in a biorepository until needed for further laboratory investigation.

In addition to direct examination of skin biopsies, laboratory studies may be performed on lymphoblastoid cell lines established by EBV transformation of peripheral blood lymphocytes collected from members of melanoma-prone families. These studies of lymphoblastoid cell lines have shown that, using a shuttle vector plasmid, cell lines from significant numbers of patients with cutaneous melanoma or DN had elevated plasmid mutation frequencies [27].

Colorectum

The wide range of incidence rates around the world and observations from migrant studies suggest that environmental or lifestyle factors play an important role in colorectal carcinogenesis. Epidemiologic and laboratory studies strongly support the role of dietary factors in the development of colorectal adenomas and cancer. Adenomatous polyps are the precursors of colorectal cancers, though only a minority of polyps undergoes malignant transformation [28] (see chapter 9 by Baron). Molecular genetic studies suggest that the development of colorectal cancer is a multistep process resulting from the accumulation of oncogene activation and tumor suppressor gene inactivation [29]. Polymorphic genes may also play a role in colorectal carcinogenesis.

For NCI's Polyp Prevention Trial [30], polyps were collected during colonoscopy procedures. Polyps were removed by standard endoscopic procedures and retained for histologic examination. If a polyp was too small to remove in its entirety, a biopsy was obtained before cauterization. Ribbons were cut from three different levels of the central core, and slides were prepared from each of the three levels of paraffin-embedded tissue. For diminutive polyps (less than 5 mm in diameter), one ribbon was cut from one, two, or three different levels of the central core, depending on the judgment of the pathologist. For larger polypoid lesions (greater than 5 mm), the tissue was bisected through the stalk zone, and each half was embedded so that its full face was sectioned through the long axis. Three serial cuts were made from each half of the polyp, and six slides were prepared.

Colorectal polyps prepared in the manner described above can be examined by pathologists using the histologic classification outlined in the World Health Organization (WHO) Histologic Typing of Intestinal Tumors [31]. Lesions are classified as adenomas of tubular, villous, tubulovillous, or flat histological type. Dysplasias that occur in colorectal adenomas may be of low grade or high grade, the latter including severe dysplasia and carcinoma in situ. The WHO classification defines the specific characteristics of the dysplasias in terms of the atypia of glandular architecture and cytology. Complementing the detection of potentially preneoplastic colorectal adenomas by standard pathologic methods, archival colorectal tissues have been used to analyze surrogate biomarkers. In one such study, investigators used immunohistochemical methods to study *p53* protein expression in paraffin-embedded blocks from serrated adenomas [32]. Recent advances in nucleic acid purification and PCR technology have made it possible to study biomarkers in archival tissue. In a study of over 2,000 archival blocks of colorectal tissue, Slattery et al. [33] showed that DNA could be extracted and PCR-based genetic studies could be performed on over 85% of the specimens.

Proteomics-based approaches are now being used to study alterations in protein expression in preneoplastic colorectal lesions. In a study of both normal colonic mucosa and colon polyps, Melis and White [34] detected over seven hundred protein spots in two-dimensional gel analyses. They were able to show differential expression of over 50 proteins among the polyp specimens. They also used immunostaining, microsequencing, and mass spectrometry to further identify specific proteins.

As with other tissue types, paraffin-embedded tissue is ideal for histological characterization and immunohistochemical studies and can yield both germline and tumor (or precursor) lesions, albeit with some limitations. Frozen tissue is, however, superior for most genetic analyses (better quantity and quality of DNA, more suitable for cytogenetic analyses, etc.).

Oral

Leukoplakia is a clinical term for white lesions of the mucosa that represents a spectrum of histologic findings ranging from epithelial hyperplasia through dysplasia to carcinoma [35]. Certain histological types that are inflammatory in origin, for example lichen planus, may be excluded. The great majority of observed lesions are benign, but all carry a high risk of progression to carcinoma (see Chapter 6 by Sankaranarayanan and Somanathan). Simple excision does not influence the ultimate risk of malignancy [36]. Many studies involving histological characterization of the lesions involve a comparison of topical (bleomycin gel, fenretinoide, vitamin A) or systemic (e.g. 13-*cis*-retinoic acid, vitamin A) treatments. Simple punch biopsy of lesions is guided by toluidine blue application [37]. Recently, a computer-assisted method to analyze precancerous oral lesions using an oral brush biopsy has shown promising results in a multicenter trial with perfect sensitivity and 92.5% specificity in 945 patients [38]. Study questions will dictate the precise method and handling of specimens. Paraffin-embedded tissue biopsies are ideal for characterizing histological features and also for conducting many standard immunohistochemistry studies, but fresh frozen tissue is preferred for many types of genetic analysis that required DNA extraction.

Lung

Early efforts to effectively screen for lung cancer using chest radiographs and sputum cytology did not result in documented improvements in survival, but there is great hope that newer molecular tools will provide the means to intervene more effectively in this malignancy [39] (see Chapter 13 by Marcus and Travis). The large number of identified molecular lesions, the appreciation of the main etiologic agent (tobacco), the typically prolonged preclinical phase in lung cancer, and the general futility of the traditional modes of treatment of this cancer are strong incentives to pursue these avenues of research. The high frequency of both smoking (including former smokers who remain at high risk for some time after quitting) and lung cancer (which contributes to the mortality of 6% of Americans) is a further public health incentive [40].

There are many approaches used to obtain specimens from subjects at high risk for lung cancer. The first and most common approach involves lung tumor samples derived from formalin-fixed wax-embedded tumors (i.e., paraffin blocks). Often it is possible to identify preneoplastic changes in adjacent blocks, and microdissection can be used to obtain paired tumor and preneoplastic tissue. This method has been used to conduct loss-of-heterozygosity studies to localize tumor suppressor genes [41]. Another approach involves obtaining sputum samples. In the late 1960s, Saccomano proposed an early detection technique [42] based on the use of sputum cytology to evaluate cytomorphologic changes in exfoliated bronchial epithelium. A multicenter trial of sputum cytology as an early detection approach failed to reveal a survival benefit, and today sputum is used as a standard adjunct to the diagnosis of malignancy (albeit with low sensitivity), but it can also be used to characterize and grade premalignant lesions (i.e., dysplasia). It has been proposed that monoclonal antibodies (i.e., to difucosylated Lewis X epitope) may demonstrate changes indicative of malignancy a year or more prior to conventional diagnostic approaches [43]. The sensitivity of sputum-based approaches has been marginally improved by the addition of molecular markers (such as mutations in tumor supressor genes or oncogenes such as *p53* or *K-ras*) and the collection of bronchiolar alveolar lavage (BAL) samples [44]. Genetic alterations are observed in subjects with no evidence of lung cancer, but their significance remains unclear [45]. Automated image analysis of the DNA content of normal cell nuclei has been proposed as capable of improving the detection of abnormal nuclei characteristic of squamous cell carcinoma with morphologically normal appearing cells [46].

Flexible fiberoptic bronchoscopy is a standard approach to obtaining diagnostic and staging information in lung cancer, and more recently, this modality has been used to obtain tissue for the study of preneoplastic lesions [47]. Other methods used to diagnose lung cancer (transthoracic biopsy, mediastinoscopy, surgical procedures) can also provide appropriate samples. Autoflourescence bronchoscopy has been used to enhance the detection of both preneoplastic and neoplastic changes. Using LIFE (Light Induced Fluorescence Endoscopy, Life Imaging System, Vancouver, Canada) fluorescence bronchoscopy, lung cancer tissue fluoresces less than normal tissue, and this allows detection of preneoplastic lesions [48]. This technique can be performed on an ambulatory basis without profound anaesthesia, thus allowing the possibility that studies might be conducted on high-risk populations that lack specific findings suggestive of lung cancer. Sections of bronchial tissue (5 microns thick) are obtained via pinch forceps biopsy and/or bronchial brushings and stained with hemotoxylin-eosin to conduct histologic characterization of preneoplastic lesions [49,50]. Methods exist to conduct immunocytochemistry studies on either frozen sections or formalin-fixed tissues. Obtaining snap-frozen tissue from surgical or bronchoscopy biopsies is the best approach when RNA or protein extraction (Northern or Western blotting) is anticipated. New imaging techniques such as spiral Computerized Tomography (CT) have great potential for the sensitive noninvasive detection of early lesions and this approach is under investigation as a screening modality.

Appendix

Internet References

Additional information concerning many of the topics discussed in this chapter may be found on the internet.

NCI web site—including information on risks and causes of cancer:
ohsr.od.nih.gov/

Human subjects protection:
National Institutes of Health: *http:// ohsr.od.nih.gov/*
National Bioethics Advisory Commission: *http://bioethics.gov/cgi-bin/bioeth_counter.pl*

Specimen shipping information:
National Institutes of Health: *http:// www.nih.gov/od/ors/ds/shipping/index.html*
Saf-T-Pak Inc: *http://www.saftpak.com/*

Specimen resources:
NCI Cooperative Human Tissue Network: *http://www-chtn.ims.nci.nih.gov/*
Other NCI specimen resources: *http:// www-napbc.ims.nci.nih.gov/link.html*
International Agency for Research on Cancer: *http://www-dep.iarc.fr/direct/biolog.htm*
Coriell Cell Repositories: *http:// locus.umdnj.edu/ccr/*

Specimen inventory systems:
ASTRO system at CDC CASPIR repository: *http://www.cdc.gov/od/ads/caspir/*
NCI BSI-II System: *http://www. bsi2.ims.nci.nih.gov*

Repository equipment and supplies:
Freezers: *http://www.so-low.com/*
Cryovials and other supplies: *http:// www.nalgenunc.com/map/index.html*
Labels and bar codes: *http://www.adamsl.com/*
DNA extraction kits: *http://www.qiagen.com/ http://www.gentra.com/gentra2.html*

Laser capture microdissection:
http://dir.nichd.nih.gov/lcm/lcm.htm

References

1. Rothman N, Stewart WF, Schulte PA. Incorporating biomarkers into cancer epidemiology: a matrix of biomarker and study design categories. *Cancer Epidemiol Biomarkers Prev* 1995; 4: 301–11.
2. Caporaso N, Rothman N, Wacholder S. Case-control studies of common allele and environmental factors. *J Natl Cancer Inst* 1999; 26:25–31.
3. Langholz B, Rothman N, Wacholder S, et al. Cohort studies for characterizing measured genes. *J Natl Cancer Inst* 1999; 26:39–43.
4. Landi MT, Caporaso N. Sample collection, processing and storage. In: *Applications of biomarkers in cancer epidemiology*. IARC Scientific Publication No. 142. Lyon: International Agency for Research on Cancer, 1997, pp. 223–36.
5. Pero RW, Olsson A, Bryngelsson C, et al. Quality control program for storage of biologically banked blood specimens in the Malmo diet and cancer study. *Cancer Epidemiol Biomarkers Prev* 1998; 7:803–8.

6. Harty LC, Shields PG, Winn DM, et al. Self-collection of oral epithelial cell DNA under instruction from epidemiologic interviewers. *Am J Epidemiol* 2000; 151:199–205.

7. Grizzle WE, Aamodt R, Clausen K, et al. Providing human tissues for research. *Arch Pathol Med* 1998; 122:1065–76.

8. Pero RW, Olsson A, Bryngelsson C, et al. Feasibility and quality of biological banking of human normal and tumor tissue specimens as sources of DNA for the Malmo diet and cancer study. *Cancer Epidemiol Biomarkers Prev* 1998; 7: 809–12.

9. Boone CW, Kelloff GJ. Endpoint markers for clinical trials of chemopreventive agents derived from the properties of epithelial precancer (intraepithelial neoplasia) measured by computer-assisted image analysis. *Cancer Surv* 1998; 32:133–47.

10. Bosch FX, Manos MM, Munoz N, et al. Prevalence of human papillomavirus in cervical cancer: a worldwide perspective. International Biological Study on Cervical Cancer (IBSCC) study group. *J Natl Cancer Inst* 1995; 87:796–802.

11. Broder S. Rapid communication, from the National Institutes of Health. *JAMA* 1992; 287:1822.

12. *Alternatives in Women's Health Care (ALTS) Study Procedures Manual*, Rockville, MD: National Cancer Institute, Division of Cancer Epidemiology & Genetics, 1996.

13. Kurtycz D, Nunez M, Arts T, et al. Use of fluorescent in situ hybridization to detect aneuploidy in cervical dysplasia. *Diagn Cytopathol* 1996; 15:46–51.

14. Hutchinson M, Zahniser D, Sherman M, et al. Utility of liquid-based cytology for cervical carcinoma screening. *Cancer* 1999; 87:48–55.

15. Schiffman M, Kiviat NB, Burk RD, et al. Accuracy and interlaboratory reliability of human papillomavirus DNA testing by hybrid capture. *J Clin Microbiol* 1995; 33:544–50.

16. Hildesheim A, Schiffman M, Gravitt PE, et al. Persistence of type-specific human papillomavirus infection among cytologically normal women. *J Infect Dis* 1994; 169:235–40.

17. Aubele M, Zitzelsberger H, Schenck U, et al. Distinct cytogenetic alterations in squamous intraepithelial lesions of the cervix revealed by laser-assisted microdissection and comparative genomic hybridization. *Cancer Cytopathol* 1998; 84:375–9.

18. Bostwick D. Prostatic intraepithelial neoplasia is a risk factor for cancer. *Semin Urol Oncol* 1999; 17:187–98.

19. Bova G, Fox W, Epstein J. Methods of radical prostatectomy specimen processing: a novel technique for harvesting fresh prostate cancer tissue and review of processing techniques. *Mod Pathol* 1993; 6:201–7.

20. Renshaw A. Adequate tissue sampling of prostate core needle biopsies. *Am J Clin Pathol* 1997; 107:26–9.

21. Bane BL. The handling and reporting of prostate biopsies and radical prostatectomy specimens (personal communication).

22. Doll J, Zhu X, Furman J, et al. Genetic analysis of atypical adenomatous hyperplasia (adenosis). *Am J Pathol* 1999; 155:967–71.

23. Visakorpi T. Molecular genetics of prostate cancer. *Ann Chir Gynaecol* 1999; 88:11–16.

24. Albert LS, Rhodes AR, Sober AJ. Dysplastic melanocytic nevi and cutaneous melanoma: markers of increased melanoma risk for affected persons and blood relatives. *J Am Acad Dermatol* 1990; 22:69–75.

25. Novakovic B, Clark WH Jr, Fears TR, et al. Melanocytic nevi, dysplastic nevi, and malignant melanoma in children from melanoma-prone families. *J Am Acad Dermatol* 1995; 33:631–6.

26. NCI Division of Cancer Epidemiology & Genetics. *Specimen Collection Manual*, 1999.

27. Moriwaki S, Tarone R, Tucker M, et al. Hypermutability of UV-treated plasmids in dysplastic nevus/familial melanoma cell lines. *Cancer Res* 1997; 57:4637–41.

28. Tierney RP, Ballantyne GH, Modlin IM. The adenoma to carcinoma sequence. *Surg Gynecol Obstet* 1990; 171:81–94.

29. Kinzler KW, Vogelstein B. Lessons from hereditary colorectal cancer. *Cell* 1996; 87:159–70.

30. Schatzkin A, Lanza E, Freedman LS, et al. The polyp prevention trial I: rationale, design, recruitment, and baseline participant characteristics. *Cancer Epidemiol Biomarkers Prev* 1996; 5:375–83.

31. Sobin LH (ed) *WHO international histologic classification of tumours*. New York: Springer-Verlag, 1989.

32. Yao T, Kouzuki T, Kajiwara M, et al. "Serrated" adenoma of the colorectum, with reference to its gastric differentiation and its malignant potential. *J Pathol* 1999; 187:511–17.

33. Slattery M, Edwards S, Palmer L, et al. Use of archival tissue in epidemiologic studies: collection procedures and assessment of potential sources of bias. *Mutat Res Genomics* 2000; 432:7–14.

34. Melis R, White R. Characterization of colonic polyps by two-dimensional gel electrophoresis. *Electrophoresis* 1999; 20:1055–64.
35. Epstein JB, Gorsky M. *Topical application of vitamin A to oral leukoplakia. A clinical case series.* Vol. 86. American Cancer Society, 1999, pp. 921–7. Atlanta.
36. Schepman KP, van der Meij EH, Smeele LE, et al. Malignant transformation of oral leukoplakia: a follow-up study of a hospital-based population of 166 patients with oral leukoplakia from the Netherlands. *Oral Oncol* 1998; 34: 270–5.
37. Epstein JB, Scully C, Spinelli J. Toluidine blue and Lugol's iodine application in the assessment of oral malignant disease and lesions at risk of malignancy. *J Oral Pathol Med* 1992; 21; 160–3.
38. Sciubba JJ and the U.S. collaborative OralCDx Study Group. Improving detection of precancerous and cancerous oral lesions. Computer assisted analysis of oral brush biopsy. *J Am Dent Assoc* 1999; 130:1445–57.
39. Marcus PM, Bergstralh EJ, Fagerstrom RM, et al. Lung cancer mortality in the mayo lung project: impact of extended follow-up. *J Natl Cancer Inst* 2000; 92:1308–16.
40. Kubik A, Polak J. Lack of benefit from semi-annual screening for cancer of the lung: follow-up report of randomized controlled trial on population of high-risk males in Czechoslovakia. *Int J Cancer* 1990; 45:26–33.
41. Chung GTY, Sundaresan V, Hasleton P, et al. Sequential molecular genetic changes in lung cancer development. *Oncogene* 1995; 11:2591–8.
42. Saccomanno G, Saunders RP, Klein GM, et al. Cytology of the lung in reference to irritant, individual sensitivity and healing. *Acta Cytocol* 1970; 14:377–81.
43. Tockman MS, Cupta PK, Myers JD, et al. Sensitive and specific monoclonal antibody recognition of human lung cancer antigen on preserved sputum cells: a new approach to early lung cancer detection. *J Clin Oncol* 1988; 6; 1685–93.
44. Ahrendt AS, Chow L-HX, Yang SC, et al. Molecular detection of tumor cells in brochoalveolar lavage fluid from patients with early stage lung cancer. *J Natl Cancer Inst* 1999; 4:332–9.
45. Field JK, Liloglou T, Xinarianos G, et al. Genetic alterations in bronchial lavage as a potential marker for individuals with a high risk of developing lung cancer. *Cancer Res* 1990; 59:2690–5.
46. Payne PW, Sebo TJ, Doudkine A, et al. Sputum screening by quantitative microscopy: a reexamination of a portion of the National Cancer Institute cooperative early lung study. *Mayo Clin Proc* 1997; 72:697–704.
47. Franklin WA. Pathology of lung cancer. *J Thorac Imag* 2000; 15:3–12.
48. Vermylen P, Pierard P, Roufosse C, et al. Detection of bronchial preneoplastic lesions and early lung cancer with florescence bronchoscopy: a study about its ambulatory feasibility under local anaesthesis. *Lung Cancer* 1999; 25:161–8.
49. Barsky SH, Roth MD, Kleerup EC, et al. Histopathologic and molecular alterations in the bronchial epithelium in habitual smokers of marijuana, cocaine, and/or tobacco. *J Natl Cancer Inst* 1998; 90:1198–1204.
50. Wistuba II, Lam S, Behrens C, et al. Molecular damage in the bronchial epithelium of current and former smokers. *J Natl Cancer Inst* 1997; 89:1366–73.

4

Intermediate Markers in Cancer Research: Theoretical and Practical Issues in the Use of Surrogate Endpoints

Arthur Schatzkin

The existence of distinct precancerous lesions—the focus of this volume—certainly tells us a great deal about the developmental pathophysiology of invasive malignant disease. Such precursor lesions, particularly those that appear to be necessary stages on the path to frank malignancy, also present a potentially promising target for cancer research. The use of precancerous lesions as "surrogate endpoints" for invasive cancer has considerable biologic and logistical appeal and has engendered substantial interest in recent years. This chapter addresses theoretical and practical problems in using surrogate endpoints in experimental and observational studies of cancer.

Definition of Surrogate Endpoint

In an intervention study (clinical trial), a surrogate endpoint for incident cancer yields a valid test of the null hypothesis of no association between the intervention (treatment) and cancer [1]. In other words, the effect of an intervention on the surrogate is concordant with its effect on cancer incidence; for an observational epidemiologic study, the association of an exposure with the surrogate parallels its association with cancer incidence. ("Concordant" and "parallel" imply proportionality, whereby a large change in the surrogate endpoint implies a large change in cancer incidence, and a small change in the surrogate

means a small change in cancer incidence.) If a putative surrogate endpoint meets these conditions, it can be considered a "valid" surrogate for that cancer.

Attraction of Studies Using Surrogate Endpoints

The enthusiasm for surrogate endpoints derives from the relative rarity of cancer in the general population. The age-adjusted annual incidence rate of breast cancer among women in the United States, for example, is about 100 per 100,000, or 0.1%. The annual colorectal cancer incidence rate among men and women combined is around 50 per 100,000, or only 0.05%. Thus, although cancer is a leading cause of morbidity and mortality in developed countries, even our most common malignancies occur relatively infrequently.

The medical research implications of this simple fact are straightforward: intervention or prospective observational epidemiologic studies with incident cancer endpoints must be large, lengthy, and costly. Such studies must yield hundreds, or even thousands, of cancers to have adequate statistical power to detect a meaningful treatment effect (intervention study) or relative risk (epidemiologic investigation). The ongoing Women's Health Initiative, for example, requires several tens of thousands of participants to have adequate power to detect reasonable reductions in the incidence of breast and colorectal cancer [2]. (Even case-control studies today have become fairly costly, multiyear efforts.) Studies with surrogate endpoints are attractive because they are potentially smaller, shorter, and considerably less expensive than their counterparts with cancer endpoints.

Diversity of Potential Surrogate Endpoints for Cancer

There are a host of biologic phenomena—biomarkers in the most general sense—that could potentially serve as cancer surrogates. With the explosion in molecular and cell biology, this list is only growing. Potential surrogate biomarkers can be categorized as follows:

1. *Alterations in the microscopic or gross characteristics of tissues.* Such "pre-neoplastic" or frankly neoplastic changes are obvious candidates for surrogate endpoints. Examples include cervical intraepithelial neoplasia (for squamous cell carcinoma of the cervix) [3]; colorectal adenomatous polyps (as surrogates for colorectal cancer) [4]; bronchial metaplasia (a possible preneoplastic state for lung cancer) [5]; and dysplastic changes in the esophagus (for esophageal cancer) [6].
2. *Imaging techniques for detecting histologic change.* Examples include mammographic parenchymal patterns as a surrogate for breast carcinogenesis [7], and ovarian ultrasound abnormalities in ovarian cancer [8].
3. *Cellular phenomena.* Surrogates in this category include several assays of epithelial cell proliferation, including tritiated thymidine or bromodeoxyuridine incorporation into DNA, proliferating cell nuclear antigen (PCNA), and Ki67 [9]. These assays have been extensively used in studies of intestinal mucosa, but have been used in other epithelial tissues as well. Measures of apoptosis [10] as well as the ratio of proliferation to apoptosis have recently been proposed as potential surrogate endpoints. In acquired immunodeficiency syndrome (AIDS) research, CD4 cell counts have been used as surrogates for critical AIDS endpoints [11].

4. *Molecular markers.* A plethora of potential molecular surrogates have been suggested. Examples include specific somatic mutations in cancer-related genes (such as *ras* or *p53*), both DNA *hypo-* and *hyper*methylation of specific genes at various anatomic sites, and gene expression products [12,13]. Chemical–DNA adducts should be considered, not as indicators of exposure (which they might well be; see chapter 1 by Santella), but as markers of a "downstream" integrated metabolic process, that is, one occurring temporally and developmentally closer to the malignant outcome than the exposure itself [14].
5. *Infection.* Infectious processes have been implicated in a number of cancers, and these infections could be viewed as surrogate endpoints. Examples include infections with human papillomavirus (HPV) in cervical carcinogenesis [15] (see chapter 16 by Franco and Ferenczy), *Helicobacter pylori* in gastric cancer [16] (see chapter 8 by Correa), and HTLV1 in adult T-cell leukemia [17].
6. *Bioactive substances in blood and tissue.* Examples here include blood and tissue estrogens or androgens, various antioxidants (again, in both blood and specific tissues), and growth factors. For this category of potential surrogates the marker—blood estrogen levels [18], for example—may not be found directly in the target tissue, but may still properly be considered a potential surrogate endpoint, in this case, for breast cancer.

A key question is how to tell if a particular marker is really a valid surrogate for cancer. Much of this chapter will deal with the logical considerations and empirical investigations pertaining to this question.

Causal Models of Cancer Surrogacy

The logic underlying the evaluation of surrogate validity is well represented by a series of causal pathway models. The simplest causal pathway involving a potential surrogate is depicted in Figure 4.1. E1 represents some "exposure", an environmental or host factor.

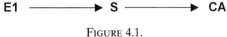

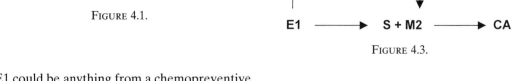

FIGURE 4.3.

(E1 could be anything from a chemopreventive agent to a deleterious risk factor.) According to this idealized model, a change in E1 necessarily alters the surrogate endpoint (S) positivity, which in turn modifies the likelihood of incident cancer. S, by our definition, is a valid surrogate for cancer.

The scenario in Figure 4.1 rarely occurs. Far more realistic are the situations reflected in Figure 4.2. In Figure 4.2, E1 modulates carcinogenesis through two alternative pathways, one through S, the other through another marker (M2). To the extent that E1 operates through the alternative M2 pathway—which means that S is not a necessary component of carcinogenesis—we cannot be assured that S is a valid surrogate in studies involving E1. The reason for this lack of certainty is that E1 might influence M2 in a way that offsets its effect on S, the final effect on cancer simply being unknown. If E1, for example, were to increase M2-positivity, E1 could actually end up *increasing* cancer incidence, while at the same time reducing S-positivity (and thereby giving at least a superficial impression of being anticarcinogenic).

In Figure 4.3, the joint action of two markers (S and M2) is necessary for the development of cancer. E1 may affect either S or M2. Again, we cannot be certain that S is a valid cancer surrogate in studies of exposure E1 because that exposure may affect S and M2 in counterbalancing ways.

The scenarios depicted in Figures 4.2 and 4.3, although qualitatively more complex than that represented in Figure 4.1, are nevertheless

simplified and idealized in their own right. Given the complex, multilevel cascade of events that underlie cell growth and inhibition, one can easily envision still more elaborate combinations of pathways reflected in Figures 4.2 and 4.3.

Although the emphasis here has been on etiologic and intervention studies of incident cancer, the discussion also applies to treatment research in which the focus is not on the occurrence of a malignancy, but rather on the factors contributing to, or preventing, mortality from a given cancer.

Epithelial Hyperproliferation

An extensive literature addresses problems of proliferation biology [19]. (Although I will focus primarily on colorectal epithelial cell proliferation, the arguments presented here apply to hyperproliferation in a variety of tissues.) A number of cell proliferation assays have been developed; these assays have been touted as potential surrogates for cancer in light of the dysregulation of cell growth that characterizes malignancy. Figure 4.4 depicts causal events potentially involved in the relation between hyperproliferation and the neoplastic process. In the upper portion of this diagram, is a single pathway going from normal epithelium to hyperproliferative epithelium to neoplasia/cancer. It is this pathway that implicitly underlies using hyperproliferation as a valid surrogate for cancer.

As the rest of the figure illustrates, though, hyperproliferation may not be necessary by itself for colorectal carcinogenesis. There may be an alternative pathway to neoplasia/cancer that bypasses hyperproliferation. The problem is that the effect of an intervention agent (E1) on this alternative pathway is unknown and may in fact counterbalance its effect through

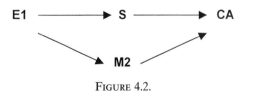

FIGURE 4.2.

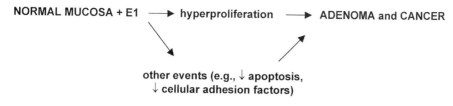

FIGURE 4.4.

the hyperproliferation pathway. Two scenarios here are revealing: (i) The agent (E1) reduces proliferation, but at the same time reduces apoptosis, and therefore has no effect on colorectal cancer; (ii) The agent has no effect on proliferation but does increase apoptosis, thereby reducing colorectal cancer incidence. In both cases, a hyperproliferation assay gives the wrong answer about an intervention's effect on colorectal cancer; by definition, hyperproliferation would not be a valid surrogate for cancer in studies of E1.

It is important to emphasize that the proliferation marker does not necessarily give the wrong answer about the agent's effect on cancer; the proliferation data may, in fact, be giving us the right answer. The problem is the uncertainty that flows from the existence of multiple alternative pathways to cancer. Given this *a priori* theoretical uncertainty for a putative marker like hyperproliferation, how can we evaluate the validity of such a marker?

Evaluating Potential Surrogate Endpoints

The answer is to integrate the marker, in this case, epithelial cell proliferation, into observational epidemiologic studies or clinical trials that have colorectal cancer (or adenomatous polyps–see later discussion) as an endpoint. Such integration can elucidate the causal structure underlying the relationships among interventions (or exposures), potential surrogate endpoints, and cancer. The specific data for revealing this underlying structure come from investigating three questions: (i) Is the intervention (or exposure) associated with the potential surrogate? (ii) Is the potential surrogate endpoint associated with cancer? (iii)

Does the potential surrogate endpoint mediate the relation of the intervention (exposure) to cancer?

Standard epidemiologic measures are pertinent to answering these questions. These measures can be defined with reference to the 2 by 2 table shown in Figure 4.5. (For simplicity of discussion, reference is made here to surrogate endpoints that are either present or absent. The arguments presented here, though, are germane to markers measured as continuous variables.) For a cohort study, the association between the surrogate endpoint (S in Figure 4.5) and cancer would be reflected in the relative risk (RR), defined as $[a/(a + b)]/[c/(c + d)]$. For a case-control study, the RR would be estimated by the odds ratio, defined as ad/bc. A RR (or odds ratio) of 1.0 indicates no association between the potential surrogate endpoint and cancer. The attributable proportion (AP) is an epidemiologic measure that indicates the proportion of cancer that is attributable to surrogate endpoint positivity.

$AP = S(1 - 1/R)$ where $R = RR$ and $S =$ sensitivity, defined as $a/(a + c)$. (*The reader should note that S in this standard formula refers to "sensitivity", not "surrogate".*) An AP of 1.0 means that marker positivity is necessary for the development of cancer; that is, the carcinogenic pathway must go through this positive

		Cancer	
		+	−
S	+	a	b
	−	c	d

FIGURE 4.5.

marker, or to put it another way, there is no alternative pathway bypassing this marker.

Question 1: Intervention (or Exposure) versus Surrogate

For a given potential surrogate marker to be valid with respect to a particular intervention (or exposure), there must be some relation between the intervention (exposure) and the marker. In an experimental setting, we need to see that the intervention changes the marker; in an observational context, we need to observe an association between an exposure and marker positivity.

This question can be addressed in relatively small metabolic intervention studies. Several studies, for example, have examined the effect of dietary change or supplementation on epithelial cell proliferation [20]; others have investigated the effect of fat modification [21] or alcohol consumption [22] on blood or urine estrogen levels. We can also examine this question in the context of a case-control or cohort study. Schiffman et al., for example, showed a strong association between reproductive risk factors, particularly number of sexual partners, and HPV infection [23]. Ecologic studies may also provide indirect information on this question. One could examine, for example, the mean colorectal epithelial cell proliferation index in populations with different average consumptions of dietary fat.

Question 2: Surrogate versus Cancer

For a marker to be a reasonable surrogate for a given cancer, it must have some relation to that cancer. In evaluating a potential surrogate, therefore, we need some way of characterizing the connection between the marker and malignancy.

Ecologic studies may provide useful, if indirect, information on this connection. Studies are considered to be "ecologic", or aggregate, in that individual-level information is not used; rather, an average marker value is obtained for a sample of individuals selected from specific populations (e.g., Seventh Day Adventists versus non-Adventists), which is then related to the overall risk of cancer in those populations. Several studies, for example, have compared mean proliferation indices in groups at varying risk of cancer [24]. In such studies, however, one cannot be certain that those who are marker-positive are the ones with increased incidence of cancer.

This "ecologic" problem is obviated in moving to individual-level observational epidemiologic studies, whether case-control or cohort. Such studies are important tools for examining the relation between a putative surrogate and cancer. Blood estrogen levels have been shown in several studies to be directly associated with breast cancer, a necessary relation before estrogens could be considered a surrogate for breast malignancy [25]. HPV infection, another potential surrogate (for cervical cancer) has been shown to be highly associated with risk of severe cervical neoplasia [26]. Observational studies may also be nested in trials. In trials with adenomatous polyp formation as the primary endpoint, for example, it is possible to examine the relation of colorectal epithelial cell proliferation measures to subsequent adenoma recurrence. In one such study, Baron et al. found no relation between calcium carbonate supplementation and epithelial cell proliferation measured one year later [27], even though calcium did reduce overall adenoma recurrence [28]. This certainly suggests that proliferation measures are problematic surrogates for colorectal neoplasia/cancer in studies with calcium supplements as the main intervention/exposure.

(Note: reference is made here to studies with adenomas or cervical intraepithelial neoplasia (CIN) endpoints. Although these are only neoplastic cancer precursors, for purposes of discussion, they have been considered as proxies for cancer, even though, as discussed below, the validity of these precursor endpoints is not ironclad.)

The epidemiologic parameter AP may be useful in determining the importance of alternative pathways and thereby evaluating the relation between the potential surrogate and cancer. In the simple linear causal model of Figure 4.1, the AP for the surrogate is 1.0. When at least one pathway exists that is alternative to the pathway containing the surrogate, as in

Figure 4.2, then the AP for the surrogate is less than 1.0. If, however, the AP is still relatively high, though less than 1.0, that would suggest that the alternative (M2) pathway plays a small role in the genesis of the cancer. An AP substantially lower than 1.0 for the surrogate implies that one or more alternative pathways is (are) indeed operative.

Question 3: Intervention (Exposure) versus Surrogate versus Cancer

Having investigated Questions (i) and (ii) above, we may have determined (i) the potential surrogate is likely causally linked to cancer, and (ii) the surrogate is indeed linked to a given intervention or exposure. Suppose, however, with reference to Question 1, that the AP is less than 1.0, implying that alternative pathways bypassing the surrogate are operative in carcinogenesis. It would still be valuable to ascertain the *relative* importance of the intervention/exposure → *surrogate* → cancer pathway, as opposed to the alternative intervention/exposure → *other marker(s)* → cancer pathway(s). To do this, we can examine the extent to which the putative surrogate *mediates* the relation between the intervention/exposure and cancer. In other words, we determine the extent to which surrogate-end-point status accounts for any observed intervention effect or exposure association. To carry out such analyses, one must integrate an assay for the surrogate into either clinical trials or observational epidemiologic studies, with information on both the intervention/exposure as well as cancer (or severe neoplasia).

As an example, investigators have used a case-control study to look at the extent to which HPV infection mediated the association between number of sexual partners and dysplasia [29]. As Table 4.1 shows, number of sexual partners and cervical dysplasia risk were strongly and directly associated. When the relation between number of sexual partners and dysplasia was adjusted for HPV infections status (present or absent), the relative risk for number of sexual partners dropped dramatically. This suggests that most of the association

TABLE 4.1. Cervical dysplasia odds ratio for number of sexual partners, unadjusted and adjusted for HPV status (from reference 29).

	Number of sexual partners				
	1	2	3–5	6–9	10+
Unadjusted	1.0	1.7	3.1[1]	4.7[1]	4.4[1]
Adjusted for HPV status	1.0	1.0	1.1	1.5	1.6

[1] p < .05
Source: Schiffman MH and Schatzkin A, 1994, with permission.

between number of partners and cervical dysplasia is due to HPV infection [30].

The same analytic strategy can be used in other study designs of cancer endpoints when assessing intervention or exposure via surrogate mediation. For example, researchers obtaining blood specimens from participants in large cohort studies will be able to investigate whether serum hormone levels mediate the relation between reproductive risk factors and breast cancer. A dietary modification or dietary supplement study of colorectal neoplasia, from which rectal biopsy specimens are obtained for mucosal proliferation assays, can provide information on the extent to which any observed diet/supplement effect is attributable to proliferation changes.

The statistical aspects of mediation analysis are an important area of current research [31,32]. One can investigate whether a potential surrogate marker mediates an intervention/exposure–cancer relation by means of stratified analyses or multiple-regression techniques. As a general rule, the greater the intervention effect or exposure association, the fewer study participants are needed in a mediation analysis. Because the range of exposure among individual participants in an observational study may be wider than the differences between average treatment group exposures in experimental studies (trials), exposure RRs in observational studies tend to be larger than intervention effects observed in trials. It follows that mediation analyses may be more likely to provide interpretable data in the observational epidemiologic setting. Specific genetic mutations or polymorphisms, if they may be shown to yield high relative risks for specific cancers, may prove to be a valuable source of mediation analyses of various potential biochemical or cellular surrogates.

Mediation analyses, in which one adjusts the intervention or exposure RRs for the value of the potential surrogate marker, may yield null results. That is, the adjusted RR may not be materially different from the crude one. Such null findings suggest that the potential surrogate does not mediate the relation between intervention/exposure and cancer. Even with null results, however, there are two possible scenarios under which the surrogate could still be on the causal pathway to cancer. The first, illustrated in Figure 4.2 occurs when there is an alternative pathway from an exposure (E1) to cancer through a second marker. In other words, the surrogate is not a necessary step between E1 and cancer. The degree to which the exposure (E1)–cancer relation is attenuated after adjustment for the surrogate depends on the (probably unknown) relative contributions of the alternative pathways—one through the surrogate, the other through another marker— to the development of cancer.

The second scenario is illustrated in Figure 4.6. Some unknown factor leads to surrogate marker positivity. In addition, the positive surrogate marker requires the exposure E1 as a cofactor for the development of cancer. Thus the surrogate is on the pathway to cancer, but adjustment for surrogate marker status will not necessarily reduce the relative risk of the exposure to 1.0. The surrogate does not mediate the known risk factor but does mediate the unknown risk factor.

It should also be recognized that misclassification of surrogate status will also lead to a situation in which the adjusted estimate is not lower than the crude one (see Chapter 5 by Franco).

The presence of interaction in mediation analyses is also a consideration. In Figure 4.3, an intervention affects both the surrogate and another intermediate marker (M2). It is at least

theoretically possible that the intervention can affect the surrogate and the other marker in offsetting ways. In that instance, the mediation analysis will demonstrate a significant interaction between the intervention and the surrogate marker, that is, the cancer rate among surrogate-positive participants will differ according to whether they are in the intervention (exposed) or control (nonexposed) group. Such an interaction indicates that the surrogate does not fully mediate the intervention effect. The surrogate, however, does indeed lie on a single dominant causal pathway.

Surrogates with High Likelihood of Validity

Unlike putative surrogates, such as epithelial cell proliferation or blood hormone levels, for which validity is problematic (as discussed already), considerable evidence supports the relative validity of a few "downstream" surrogate markers (that is, those close to cancer on the causal pathway).

The overwhelmingly large proportion of cervical cancer requires prior persistent HPV infection. (Some immunologic deficit or nutritional/environmental cofactor may be involved in the development of persistent HPV infection.) HPV persistence results in inactivation, by the E6 and E7 proteins of the HPV genome, of p53 and pRb tumor suppressor genes, leading in turn to increasingly severe intraepithelial neoplasia and, eventually, cancer (see Chapter 16 by Franco). At most, only a very small proportion of cervical cancer can arise as a result of tumor suppressor gene product inactivation occurring by mutation in the absence of HPV infection. Because most cervical cancer does occur through persistent HPV infection, an intervention that eliminates or reduces such infection would have a high likelihood of decreasing cervical cancer incidence.

With regard to cervical cancer, some further consideration of cervical intraepithelial neoplasia (CIN), especially CIN III, is warranted. This histopathologic development is considered a strong surrogate for cancer and has been used as an endpoint in a number of epidemiologic studies. A very high percentage of CIN III will

Unknown risk factor ⟶ S + E1 ⟶ CA

FIGURE 4.6.

progress to cancer in twenty years; only a very small fraction regresses. In fact, CIN III is very close to *being* invasive cancer and is downstream from persistent HPV infection in the causal pathway leading to malignancy.

A second example in this vein is Barrett's esophagus, a metaplastic change from squamous to columnar epithelium in the lower esophagus that is thought to be a necessary precursor to most cases of esophageal adenocarcinoma (see Chapter 7 by Vaugham) [33]. Gastric acid reflux is regarded as the primary precipitant of this metaplastic change; other factors may operate in the transition from Barrett's epithelium through dysplasia to adenocarcinoma. Similar to the persistent HPV infection example, a small proportion of esophageal adenocarcinomas appear to arise from esophageal submucosal glands, independent of the Barrett's epithelium pathway. Nevertheless, an intervention (e.g., photoablation or electrocoagulation) [34] that eradicates the Barrett's epithelium would likely greatly reduce esophageal adenocarcinoma incidence. (The operative word here is "eradication". Some have argued that photoablation causes epithelialization over remaining "nests" of Barrett cells. If that were the case, we would have an instance of misclassification: the apparent disappearance of Barrett cells would lead us to classify the individual as "marker negative" in a subsequent study, when in fact the true state is "marker positive."

The Adenomatous Polyp as Surrogate Endpoint

The marker that has received perhaps the greatest attention as a potential surrogate endpoint in clinical trials—one for which inferences to cancer are considered to be strong—is the adenomatous polyp (adenoma). Colorectal adenomas are attractive candidates for cancer surrogacy in research studies because of their high recurrence rate (at about 10% or more per year, nearly 2 orders of magnitude greater than the incidence of cancer) (see Chapter 9 by Baron). The underlying *biologic* rationale for the use of adenoma endpoints in epidemiologic studies and clinical trials is the strong pathologic, cell biologic, and molecular biologic evidence showing a relation between this marker and colorectal cancer (Question 2). This adenoma–carcinoma sequence is supported by studies demonstrating carcinomatous foci in adenomas and adenomatous foci within carcinomas, by experiments showing the malignant transformation of adenoma cell lines, and by studies identifying common mutations in adenomatous and carcinomatous tissue [3]. An intervention reducing the recurrence of adenomas in the large bowel would therefore likely decrease the incidence of colorectal cancer, thus making adenoma recurrence a reasonably valid surrogate marker.

It is worth noting, however, that even the adenoma is not an ironclad surrogate, and some inferential difficulties remain with adenoma recurrence trials. Recurrent adenomas represent neoplastic changes from normal mucosa through the development of a small adenoma. The results of adenoma recurrence trials may be misleading if the intervention factor operates later in the neoplastic process, that is, affecting the growth of a small into a large adenoma or the transformation of a large adenoma to cancer. A (false) null result for recurrent adenomas may result if the intervention operates only in the later stages of neoplasia. A positive result, though, suggests that cancer would be reduced, because large adenomas and cancers derive from small adenomas.

A second inferential difficulty with adenoma recurrence as a surrogate endpoint flows from the likely biologic heterogeneity of adenomas. Only a relatively small proportion of adenomas go on to cancer. Suppose that one type, the "bad" adenoma that progresses to cancer, is caused by exposures E1 and E2, as in Figure 4.7. The second type, the "innocent"

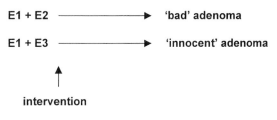

FIGURE 4.7.

adenoma, is caused by the same exposure E1 but in concert with exposure E3. Imagine an intervention that works only on exposure E3. We could reduce the pool of innocent adenomas—thereby yielding a statistically significant reduction in adenoma formation in our trial—but in fact, the incidence of bad adenomas and cancer would be unaffected. This could work the other way as well: we might see at most a small reduction in all adenomas (the bad ones being only a small proportion of all adenomas) even though the intervention truly decreases the formation of bad adenomas and, therefore, reduces the incidence of cancer.

Must a Marker Be a Necessary Step on the Pathway to Cancer to Be a Valid Surrogate?

Markers like persistent HPV infection and adenoma formation are close to being necessary steps on the pathways, respectively, to cervical and colorectal cancer. In other words, alternative pathways bypassing these markers are minor at best. Therefore, it is unlikely that the action of an intervention/exposure through an alternative pathway can offset the action through the surrogate's pathway. Thus, when a marker is a necessary, or close to necessary, step on the causal pathway to cancer, we have *a priori* confidence that the marker is a reasonably valid surrogate (though other inferential difficulties can arise, such as those discussed above for adenoma recurrence).

That is not to say, though, that a marker *must* be a necessary step toward cancer (with an AP of 1.0) for it to be a valid surrogate. Even when alternative pathways bypassing the surrogate do exist, they do not necessarily offset action through the surrogate marker, although the effect of an intervention on such a "non-necessary" surrogate may be substantially less than that on the necessary surrogate. In other words, with cell proliferation as an endpoint, even if there were an alternative pathway through apoptosis, a given intervention agent, such as aspirin or calcium, might not affect apoptosis in any substantial way; the effect on proliferation, therefore, will be translated into some reduction in cancer incidence [35]. The

problem is that we don't know about the possible offsetting pathways in advance; we have to test the marker in large-scale epidemiologic studies or trials.

The virtue of necessary or close-to-necessary markers, like HPV infection or the adenoma, is that we simply don't have to worry much about the offsetting alternative pathways. The causal logic, even without empirical testing in large scale studies, dictates confidence in these markers.

Is a Surrogate Valid for One Intervention Valid for Another?

Figure 4.8 reprises the simple idealized scheme from Figure 4.1, but adds another exposure, E2. (As before, the exposure here can refer to an intervention agent or a risk factor.) In Figure 4.8, both E1 and E2 operate through a single surrogate on the path to cancer. Because, in this scenario, the surrogate is a necessary component of the cancer pathway, the validity of this surrogate is exposure independent. In other words, any other exposure (E2) that affects cancer must operate through the surrogate. The surrogate is valid for studies of E2 as well as those of E1.

In Figure 4.9, with E2 entering into the more complex scenario depicted in Figure 4.2, the existence of a nontrivial alternative pathway (through M2) means that the validity of the surrogate S may be exposure dependent. Even if E1 works primarily through the surrogate and affects M2 minimally, suggesting that the surrogate is reasonably valid for E1–cancer studies, one cannot assume that the E1–M2–cancer pathway plays a similarly minor role in carcinogenesis.

A given agent, for example, might influence colorectal carcinogenesis largely through its

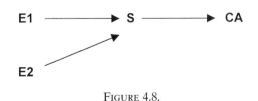

FIGURE 4.8.

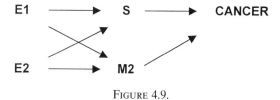

FIGURE 4.9.

influence on cell proliferation (Figure 4.4). Cell proliferation in this scenario is a likely valid surrogate for colorectal cancer. A second agent, though, might have minimal effect on cell proliferation but could increase apoptosis (or activate some other comparable alternative pathway) sufficiently to decrease cancer incidence. Focusing only on cell proliferation would give a falsely pessimistic impression of the efficacy of the second agent. In other words, even if one establishes that proliferation markers are valid surrogates for colorectal cancer in calcium studies, one can't be certain that this marker is a valid surrogate for assessing the effects of vitamin E or aspirin. (This is not to say that the marker *isn't* valid for the effect of these other agents; it's just that the existence of alternative pathways engenders uncertainty that could only be avoided by specific validation studies for these other agents.)

Interpreting Potential Surrogate Marker Data: Epidemiologic and Statistical Considerations

One cannot escape the need to use common sense and judgement in any epidemiologic study or clinical trial involving potential surrogate markers. The traditional epidemiologic causal criteria can be applied to data from these studies involving surrogates. Consider persistent HPV infection as a possible surrogate. Are the results biologically plausible? Yes, there is good reason to think that the strong epidemiologic association between number of sexual partners and cervical neoplasia/cancer is explained by the distribution of HPV infection. Are data from multiple studies consistent? Several studies have now demonstrated the relation between HPV and cervical neopla-

sia/cancer, and at least one has shown that HPV mediates the association between reproductive risk factors and cervical neoplasia. Are the measures of effect (the RR, AP) strong? They are for the connection between HPV and cervical neoplasia/cancer. Is the reduction of RR in the mediation analyses substantial? It was in the reproductive-risk-factors–HPV–cervical-neoplasia mediation analysis. In evaluating the validity of HPV infection as a surrogate, the totality of evidence suggests that this is a reasonably valid surrogate.

All biomarkers are measured with some error. Two important statistical issues need to be considered. First, a potential surrogate is useful (and ultimately valid) only if it can discriminate among study participants, those in the different treatment arms of a trial or the various exposure categories in an epidemiologic study. Discrimination is possible only if the interparticipant variability in the surrogate values is greater than the intraindividual variability. (Intraindividual variability arises from, for example, differences in marker values obtained from different tissue areas, measured at different time points, or read by multiple readers.) This means that the intraclass correlation coefficient (ICC), the proportion of all variability (inter-plus intraparticipant variability) due to interparticipant variability, is reasonably large [36].

$$(ICC = interparticipant\ variability/$$
$$[interparticipant\ variability$$
$$+ intraparticipant\ variability]).$$

Intraparticipant variability may be reduced (and the ICC thereby increased) by taking repeat samples, such as multiple biopsies from different areas or multiple blood draws over time. At a minimum, therefore, data are required on the potential surrogate marker's components of variance to establish the minimum number of marker samples needed for meaningful discrimination among study participants. In the absence of such data, one cannot be certain that null findings for a potential surrogate reflect the true lack of effect (or association) or simply the attenuating influence of random sources of intraindividual variation.

These data have not been routinely collected in marker studies. Few studies have provided data on potential surrogate marker variability, particularly with respect to time-to-time variability. A notable exception are recent investigations attempting to estimate the number of estradiol measurements necessary to reasonably discriminate among individuals [37]. Studies of colorectal epithelial cell proliferation are under way [38]. Quality-control studies designed to obtain data on the variability characteristics of potential surrogate markers are essential.

Second, even if the ICC is acceptable, measurement error will tend to attenuate findings from each of the three studies discussed above. The intervention (exposure)–marker and marker–cancer associations will be attenuated by error in marker measurement. In mediation analyses, the expected attenuation of the intervention effect (exposure association) will itself be attenuated, so the marker-adjusted effect (association) will be inflated.

Additional Issues in Evaluating Potential Surrogate Markers

Comparing one potential surrogate marker assay to another (proliferating cell nuclear antigen to bromodeoxyuridine or tritiated thymidine cell proliferation assays [39]) can provide valuable information on assay characteristics and on the biology of the phenomenon under study. Such a comparison, however, does not constitute surrogate validation. The close association of a newer marker with an older one does not in itself overcome the inferential limitations of the older marker.

A marker not directly on the causal pathway to cancer may still be closely linked to a component of that pathway so that it does constitute a reasonable surrogate marker. One possible example is micronuclei, which have been detected in epithelial cells from oral, esophageal, bronchial, and colorectal tissue [40]. Many micronucleated cells are nonviable and therefore cannot be a direct cellular precursor of a malignant tumor. The overall prevalence of micronucleated cells, though, might strongly reflect genetic damage in other cells

that do eventually undergo malignant transformation and clonal expansion.

An increasingly popular (if not explicit) approach to cancer research is what might be considered a two-stage strategy. In one set of studies, the relation between an intervention agent or exposure and a potential surrogate marker is examined. The marker–cancer relation is investigated in a separate set of studies. For example, investigators have looked (i) at the effect of alcohol consumption on blood estrogen levels in metabolic studies, and (ii) the association between blood estrogen levels and breast cancer in prospective cohort studies. Should strong links be shown for the marker in both sets of studies, this would be at least some evidence that the marker is a valid surrogate for cancer. This two-stage evidence, however, is less than absolute when it comes to surrogate-marker validation. That is because the intervention/exposure may be related to a second marker in a way that offsets the effect through the first marker (a possibility reflected in Figures 4.2 and 4.9). This potential offsetting phenomenon cannot be detected in the two-stage separate studies.

We should also consider this discussion of surrogate markers in a broader context of multiple disease endpoints and intervention or treatment toxicity. A surrogate marker might give the "right" answer about cancer for a given intervention, but nevertheless give little or no information about important adverse events that bear heavily on any overall evaluation of the intervention. Suppose, for example, that we have a valid tissue or blood marker for breast cancer, one that gives us the right answer about a promising hormone modulating intervention. That breast cancer surrogate will tell us nothing about the potential of the intervention to increase the incidence of stroke. One could examine potential surrogates for stroke, but then we are faced with uncertainties about the relation of our surrogate and the actual occurrence of a serious cerebrovascular event. Would we accept, in the absence of clinical trial evidence with explicit stroke endpoints, cholesterol determinations or platelet aggregation studies as definitive proof that our intervention does not raise the risk of cerebrovascular catastrophe? The fairly obvious negative answer to this question illustrates still another dimension of difficulty arising from the exclusive reliance on surrogate-marker studies.

Conclusion

Because studies with surrogate cancer endpoints can be smaller, faster, and substantially less expensive than those with frank cancer outcomes, the use of surrogate endpoints is undeniably attractive. This attractiveness is likely to grow in coming years as the rapidly advancing discoveries in cell and molecular biology generate new therapies requiring testing—and new markers that could plausibly serve as surrogates for cancer.

Surrogate endpoint studies can certainly be suggestive. They continue to play a legitimate role in Phase 2 clinical studies. And they *may* give the right answers about intervention effects on (or exposure associations with) cancer.

The problem is the uncertainty attached to most potential surrogates. Except for those few surrogates that are both necessary for and relatively close developmentally to cancer, the existence of plausible alternative pathways makes inferences to cancer from many surrogates problematic. Merely being on the causal pathway to cancer does not in itself constitute surrogate validity. It is the totality of causal connections that is critical. There is unfortunately a fairly extensive history of quite plausible surrogate markers giving the wrong answer about various chronic disease therapies [41]. There is no reason to believe that cancer surrogacy is immune to such inferential difficulties.

This chapter is in part an invitation, even a plea, for researchers to carry out the investigations necessary to evaluate potential surrogates, particularly surrogate–cancer studies and intervention/exposure–surrogate–cancer mediation analyses. Such studies are needed if we are to generalize from surrogate endpoint findings to cancer. There is, however, an implicit and perhaps unavoidable irony here: the large, long, expensive studies required to fully evaluate potential surrogates are precisely the studies that surrogates were designed to replace. Moreover, the exposure dependence alluded to above complicates matters further: establishing validity for a given surrogate for one intervention/exposure vis-a-vis cancer does not necessarily translate into validity for another intervention/exposure.

One can enhance the inferential strength of surrogacy by using further "downstream" markers. Results of trials with CIN3 as an endpoint are arguably more persuasive than those from intervention studies with HPV infection endpoints. Similarly, one could consider only the advanced adenoma (1 cm, villous elements, or high-grade dysplasia) as the primary endpoint in adenoma recurrence trials. The inferential gain, however, comes with substantial costs: studies with CIN3 endpoints have to be a lot larger than those with HPV infection endpoints; adenoma recurrence trials with sufficient rates of recurrence of advanced adenomas as endpoints will have to be 5 or 6 times larger than trials with any recurrent adenomas as endpoints. A law emerges here: in using surrogate endpoints, inferential certainty is directly associated with study cost. In other words, you get what you pay for.

The problems inherent in using surrogate endpoints need not be regarded as a cause for pessimism in cancer research. If anything, the limitations of surrogacy remind us of the complexity of cancer causation and affirm the continued importance of large clinical trials and observational epidemiologic studies with explicit cancer endpoints.

References

1. Prentice RL. Surrogate endpoints in clinical trials: definition and operational criteria. *Stat Med* 1989; 8:431–40.
2. Women's Health Initiative Study Group. Design of the Women's Health Initiative Clinical Trial and Observational Study. *Control Clin Trials* 1998; 19:61–109.
3. Mitchell MF, Hittelman WN, Hong WK, et al. The natural history of cervical intraepithelial neoplasia: an argument for intermediate endpoint biomarkers. *Cancer Epidemiol Biomarker Prev* 1994; 3:619–26.

4. Schatzkin A, Freedman LS, Dawsey SM, et al. Interpreting precursor studies: what polyp trials tell us about large bowel cancer. *J Natl Cancer Inst* 1994; 86:1053–7.

5. Misset JL, Mathé G, Santelli G, et al. Regression of bronchial epidermoid metaplasia in heavy smokers with etretinate treatment. *Cancer Detect Prev* 1986; 9:167–70.

6. Dawsey SM, Fleischer DE, Wang GQ, et al. Mucosal iodine staining improves endoscopic visualization of squamous dysplasia and squamous cell carcinoma of the esophagus in Linxian, China. *Cancer* 1998; 83:220–31.

7. Saftlas AF, Wolfe JN, Hoover RN, et al. Mammographic parenchymal patterns as indicators of breast cancer risk. *Am J Epidemiol* 1989; 129:518–26.

8. Karlan BY. Screening for ovarian cancer: what are the optimal surrogate endpoints for clinical trials? *J Cell Biochem* 1995; 23 (Suppl):227–32.

9. Baron JA, Wargovich MJ, Tosteson TD, et al. Epidemiological use of rectal proliferation measures. *Cancer Epidemiol Biomarker Prev* 1995; 4:57–61.

10. Bedi A, Pasrich PJ, Akhtar AJ, et al. Inhibition of apoptosis during development of colorectal cancer. *Cancer Res* 1995; 55:1811–16.

11. Tsiatis AA, DeGruttola V, Wulfsohn MS. Modeling the relationship of survival to longitudinal data measured with error. Applications to survival and CD4 counts in patients with AIDS. *J Am Stat Assoc* 1995; 90:27–37.

12. Fearon ER. Genetic alterations underlying colorectal tumorigenesis. *Cancer Surv* 1992; 12: 119–36.

13. Counts JL, Goodman JI. Alterations in DNA methylation may play a variety of roles in carcinogenesis. *Cell* 1995; 83:13–15.

14. Groopman JD, Wogan GN, Roebuck BD, et al. Molecular biomarkers for aflatoxins and their application to human cancer prevention. *Cancer Res* 1994; 54 (Suppl):1907–11.

15. Schiffman MH. Recent progress in defining the epidemiology of human papillomavirus infection and cervical neoplasia. *J Natl Cancer Inst* 1992; 84:394–8.

16. Munoz N. Is *Helicobacter pylori* a cause of gastric cancer? An appraisal of the seroepidemiological evidence. *Cancer Epidemiol Biomarker Prev* 1994; 3:445–51.

17. Blattner WA. Retroviruses. In: Evans AS (ed) *Viral infections in humans*, 3rd ed. New York: Plenum Medical Book Co., 1989, pp. 545–92.

18. Dorgan JF, Longcope C, Stephenson HE, et al. Relations of prediagnostic serum estrogen and androgen levels to breast cancer risk. *Cancer Epidemiol Biomarker Prev* 1996; 5:533–9.

19. Wargovich MJ. Precancer markers and predicition of tumorigenesis. In: Young GP, Rozen P, Levin B (eds) *Prevention and early detection of colorectal cancer*. London: WB Saunders Company, 1996, pp. 89–101.

20. Holt PR, Atillasoy EO, Gilman J, et al. Modulation of abnormal colonic epithelial cell proliferation and differentiation by low-fat dairy foods: a randomized controlled trial. *JAMA* 1998; 280:1074–9.

21. Prentice R, Thompson D, Clifford C, et al. Dietary fat reduction and plasma estradiol concentration in healthy premenopausal women. *J Natl Cancer Inst* 1990; 82:129–34.

22. Reichman ME, Judd JT, Longcope C, et al. Effects of moderate alcohol consumption on plasma and urinary hormone concentrations in premenopausal women. *J Natl Cancer Inst* 1993; 85:722–7.

23. Schiffman MH, Bauer HM, Hoover RN, et al. Epidemiologic evidence showing that human papillomavirus infection causes most cervical intraepithelial neoplasia. *J Natl Cancer Inst* 1993; 85:958–64.

24. Lipkin M, Blattner WA, Gardner EJ, et al. Classification and risk assessment of individuals with familial polyposis, Gardner's syndrome, and familial non-polyposis colon cancer from [³H]thymidine labeling patterns in colonic epithelial cells. *Cancer Res* 1984; 44:4201–7.

25. Toniolo PG, Levitz M, Zeleniuch-Jacquotte A, et al. A prospective study of endogenous estrogens and breast cancer in postmenopausal women. *J Natl Cancer Inst* 1995; 87:190–7.

26. Schiffman MH, Bauer HM, Hoover RN, et al. Epidemiologic evidence showing that human papillomavirus infection causes most cervical intraepithelial neoplasia. *J Natl Cancer Inst* 1993; 85:958–64.

27. Baron JA, Tosteson TD, Wargovich MJ, et al. Calcium supplementation and rectal mucosal proliferation: a randomized controlled trial. *J Natl Cancer Inst* 1995; 87:1303–7.

28. Baron JA, Beach M, Mandel JS, et al. Calcium supplements for the prevention of colorectal adenomas. *N Engl J Med* 1999; 340:101–7.

29. Schiffman MH, Schatzkin A. Test reliability is critically important to molecular epidemiology: an example from studies of human papillomavirus infection and cervical neoplasia. *Cancer Res* 1994; 54 (Suppl):1944–7.

30. Franco EL. The sexually transmitted disease model for cervical cancer: incoherent epidemio-

logic findings and the role of misclassification of human papillomavirus infection. *Epidemiology* 1991; 2:98–106.

31. Freedman LS, Graubard BI, Schatzkin A. Statistical validation of intermediate endpoints for chronic diseases. *Stat Med* 1992; 11:167–78.

32. Buyse M, Molenberghs G. Criteria for the validation of surrogate endpoints in randomized experiments. *Biometrics* 1998; 54:1014–29.

33. Haggitt RC. Barrett's esophagus, dysplasia, and adenocarcinoma. *Hum Pathol* 1994; 25:982–93.

34. Berenson MM, Johnson TD, Markowitz NR, et al. Restoration of squamous mucosa after ablation of Barrett's esophageal epithelium. *Gastroenterology* 1993; 104:1686–91.

35. Schatzkin A, Freedman LS, Schiffman MH, et al. The validation of intermediate endpoints in cancer research. *J Natl Cancer Inst* 1990; 82:1746–52.

36. Fleiss JL. *The design and analysis of clinical experiments*. New York: John Wiley & Sons, 1986, pp. 1–5.

37. Hankinson SE, Manson JE, Spiegelman D, et al. Reproducibility of plasma hormone levels in postmenopausal women over a 2–3-year period. *Cancer Epidemiol Biomarker Prev* 1995; 4:649–54.

38. Lyles CM, Sandler RS, Keku TO, et al. Reproducibility and variability of the rectal mucosal proliferation index using proliferating cell nuclear antigen immunohistochemistry. *Cancer Epidemiol Biomarker Prev* 1994; 3:597–605.

39. Einspahr J, Alberts D, Xie T, et al. Comparison of proliferating cell nuclear antigen *versus* the more standard measures of rectal mucosal proliferation rates in subjects with a history of colorectal cancer and normal age-matched controls. *Cancer Epidemiol Biomarker Prev* 1995; 4:359–66.

40. Garewal HS, Ramsey L, Kaugars G, et al. Clinical experience with the micronucleus assay. *J Cell Biochem* 1993 (Suppl); 17F (Suppl):206–12.

41. Fleming TR, DeMets DL. Surrogate endpoints in clinical trials: are we being misled? *Ann Intern Med* 1996; 125:605–13.

5
Assessing Epidemiological Relations and the Role of Measurement Errors

Eduardo L. Franco and Thomas E. Rohan

Understanding the role of cancer precursors in the natural history of cancer requires careful scrutiny of plausible epidemiologic relations involving remote exposures, intermediate endpoints, correlates of these variables, and, if available for study, the occurrence of cancer per se. To assess the pertinence of etiologic hypotheses in such investigations, one must specify *a priori* models that depict the relations among variables and their directionality in an attempt to reproduce the causal pathway leading to disease. These variables include remote exposure variables—typically measured by questionnaire, such as diet, lifestyle, sexual activity—and genetic susceptibility traits, cancer precursor lesions or their surrogates (for instance, a lesion detected by a cytologic test such as the Pap smear or a biomarker), and the occurrence of clinically evident cancer. Verification of the appropriateness of such models is based on some time-tested statistical analysis tools used in the context of epidemiologic study designs, such as case-control and cohort investigations.

The epidemiologic assessment of etiologic models in cancer causation relies on the verification that estimates of relative risk (RR) for the various exposure–outcome relations being probed change in some expected fashion upon adjustment by other relevant variables in the model. (These RR estimates can be estimated directly in cohort studies as the incidence rate ratio or indirectly, via the odds ratio (OR), in case-control studies.) This provides an empirical demonstration of the putative relation specified in the hypothesized etiological model under consideration.

This chapter illustrates the theoretical basis for some common types of etiologic relations encountered in epidemiologic studies of cancer precursors and the expected outcomes from statistical data analysis that provide empirical evidence in support of the assumed relations (see Chapter 4 by Schatzkin for models involving intermediate endpoints that are relevant in controlled prevention trials). In practice, however, proper interpretation of the outcomes of these analyses must consider the role of misclassification of the remote exposures, genetic susceptibility markers, covariates, and also the cancer precursor itself. A few examples are considered in this chapter to illustrate the impact of misclassification, some of which are based on the literature on the role of human papillomavirus (HPV) infection in cervical carcinogenesis.

Component Relations in Etiologic Models in Cancer Epidemiology

Much has been written concerning disease causation and diagrammatic representation of causes in epidemiology. The interested reader should refer to previous work in this area [1–3]. Figure 5.1 shows some simple theoretical models that are typically entertained in cancer epidemiology studies (independence,

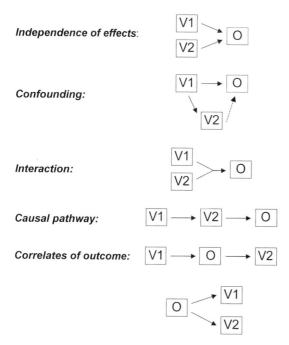

Independence of effects:

Confounding:

Interaction:

Causal pathway:

Correlates of outcome:

FIGURE 5.1. Simple theoretical models specifying some epidemiologic relations of interest in studies involving cancer precursors. V1 and V2 designate any two variables that mediate risk of an outcome (O) in the natural history of disease. V1 and V2 could denote exposure variables or intermediate endpoints. O could denote a cancer outcome or a cancer precursor, depending on the situation. Solid arrows denote causal relations. Dotted arrows denote secondary, non-causal relations.

confounding, and interaction), whereas others (causal pathway, correlates of outcome) are more rarely contemplated, despite their plausibility in natural history studies. V1 and V2 designate any two variables that are believed to mediate risk of an outcome (O) in the natural history of the disease. V1 and V2 could denote candidate exposure variables or intermediate endpoints. O could denote a cancer outcome or even a cancer precursor depending on the situation. The fact that these designations are interchangeable merely implies that the assumed relations do not necessarily represent entire etiologic models but, rather, components of more complex sets of relations that occur in the natural history of different types of cancer. The important aspect here is to have a range of

expected statistical effects of such component relations in empirical research, that is, in case-control and cohort studies (and occasionally also cross-sectional studies) that collect information on the pertinent variables.

Independence of Effects

The first model in Figure 5.1 represents a set of relations that is probably the most commonly entertained scenario in cancer epidemiology: that of independence of causal effects. It simply states that V1 leads to (causes) O, but V2 also causes O independently. V1 and V2 could be two independent intermediate endpoints (for instance two distinct lesions originated from separate etiologic pathways) leading to cancer as nonsufficient, non-necessary precursors of O. Alternatively, V1 and V2 could be two exposures independently affecting the risk of a cancer precursor O, for instance, two separate dietary constituents increasing the risk of adenoma formation in the colon.

Confounding

Assessment of confounding bias and attempts to correct for it are among the most important tasks in the analysis of cancer epidemiology studies. Confounding is best defined as the distortion of the epidemiologic effect for a given exposure of interest by those of one or more extraneous factors (the confounding variables) that are associated with the disease and with the exposure. In consequence, the effect of the exposure of interest may be overestimated or underestimated because of the mixing of effects of the exposure and confounders [2]. In the simple example shown in Figure 5.1, V1 is the true cause or precursor of O, but V1 also leads to V2, which is only statistically related to O (hence the dotted arrow) secondarily via its relation with V1. It is said that the association between V2 and O is confounded by that of V1–O. For instance, V1 could be tobacco smoking, O could represent the onset of oral leukoplakias [an oral cancer precursor (see Chapter 6 by Sankaranarayanan)], and V2 could represent coffee drinking as a lifestyle variable collected by interview via the same questionnaire that elicited information on smoking (V1). In this case, a V1–V2 association exists because smokers tend to consume more coffee than nonsmokers. Alternatively, V2 could designate a biochemical or serological marker of V1, the true precursor event leading to O. For instance, persistent HPV infection, (V1), is the precursor event leading to cervical intraepithelial neoplasia (CIN), (O), (see chapter 16 by Franco), but it also elicits an immune response that can be assessed serologically via detection of anti-HPV capsid antibodies. In the two examples, the associations for coffee drinking and a positive anti-HPV serology in each case are "confounded" by their respective models' genuine causal variables, that is, smoking and cervical HPV infection.

The two examples of factors given above (coffee and HPV serology) are assumed not to play a causal or mediating role in the genesis of their respective outcomes; that is, their presumed associations with risk are entirely confounded by those of their respective confounders, smoking and HPV infection. In practice, however, an exposure could have its own genuine relation with risk and also be confounded. For instance, if coffee drinking had, on its own, a direct oral carcinogenic effect— perhaps as an irritant or because of a hypothetical genotoxic constituent—the estimated association would be the mixing of two effects: one for the direct causal effect of coffee drinking and another secondary to the confounded association with smoking.

Interaction

Cancer epidemiology investigations also devote much energy to assessing interactions among risk factors. As shown in Figure 5.1, V1 and V2 interact to influence the overall risk of O in such a way that their joint effect on risk will be greater (if the interaction is synergistic) or lower (if the interaction is antagonistic) than that estimated by considering their independent effects added together (the scale in which the interaction is investigated is a key issue when investigating interaction). V1 and V2 could be two exposures such as tobacco and

alcohol and O could denote oral dysplasias, also an oral cancer precursor. Alcohol drinking may enhance (promote) the carcinogenic effect of tobacco by a number of mechanisms, such as by increasing the permeability of oral cells to tobacco carcinogens, by inducing cell proliferation, and/or by leading to nutritional deficiencies that increase the oral epithelium's susceptibility to the action of tobacco [4,5]. Interaction is also a mechanism to be entertained in gene–environment studies, in which a genetic susceptibility trait (V2) could affect the relation between a carcinogenic exposure (V1) and a cancer precursor (O). Typical examples include the role of genetic polymorphisms in the major histocompatibility complex [6] or in the p53 tumour suppressor gene [7,8] potentially interacting with HPV infection to affect the overall risk of CIN.

Causal Pathway

The causal pathway model in Figure 5.1 is particularly relevant to studies that collect information on cancer precursors or their surrogates and also on remote as well as "downstream" outcome variables. It states that V1 increases risk of V2, an intermediate endpoint or early event that, with time (and possibly with the influence of additional cofactors), culminates with an increased risk of O. One of the most thoroughly studied examples is that of the genesis of CIN: high risk sexual activity (high number of sexual partners and an early age at first intercourse) leads to a higher risk of HPV infection, which in turn causes CIN (also described in Chapters 4, 16, and 17 by Schatzkin and Franco) [9,10]. Another example could be the model of a genetic polymorphism in V1 that leads to an increased risk of a given precancerous lesion (V2), which in turn places the individual at a higher risk of malignancy (O). For instance, a mutated APC gene confers a higher risk of adenomatous polyposis, a precursor event that increases risk of colorectal carcinoma (see chapter 9 by Baron). Although the model simply uses three variables, one can also envisage a more complex multistep scenario in which several events or variables are in a linear arrangement leading to cancer development. The basic empirical assumptions (to be discussed later) also hold in such more complex causal pathway models.

Correlates of Outcome

The last two types of epidemiologic relations described in Figure 5.1 are frequently neglected in practice. They refer to situations in which the disease outcome leads to (i.e., causes) one or more conditions or states that may be mistaken as intermediate outcomes and not true correlates of disease. The first of the two theoretical examples shows V1 leading directly to O which in turn increases the probability of V2, a single correlate (consequence) of the outcome, whereas the second example shows O directly leading to two correlates of outcome, V1 and V2. Under the category of correlates of outcome one may consider scenarios in which disease development may lead to certain surrogate markers that occur as a consequence of the final outcome being analyzed. In the CIN example described above one might be interested in focusing on the relation between sexual activity (V1) as the exposure and HPV infection as the outcome (O), but data might also have been collected on occurrence of CIN (V2) in the same women. Another plausible situation that may occur in cancer precursor studies is the analysis of multiple histopathological and genetic characteristics of the outcome. Certain genetic instability markers may follow (and thus would be designated as correlates or consequences) rather than precede (which would imply that they are precursors) the development of the neoplastic lesion and should thus be placed "downstream" from O in a causal pathway diagram.

Empirical Demonstration of Different Types of Epidemiologic Relations

The process of analyzing the epidemiologic data collected in observational investigations of the etiology of cancer precursors and cancer requires that the pertinence of the above relations be verified in specific statistical analyses by using suitable regression models or by constructing contingency tables with the Mantel-Haenszel technique. The investigator should have *a priori* expectation that some of the relations depicted in Figure 5.1 may be influencing the joint distribution of observations across all variables on which information was collected in the study. As part of the analytical strategy, such relations can be verified by computing crude (unadjusted) estimates of epidemiologic effect (the RR) for the associations between each of the suspected etiologic variables or key events, that is, V1 or V2, and the outcome (O) of interest in a given situation. A second set of analyses, adjusting each of the associations for the remaining covariate (i.e., V1–O for V2 and V2–O for V1) will aid the investigator in deciding whether or not there is empirical evidence in support of the suspected relation. In some circumstances, computing the crude estimates followed by the adjusted ones and then comparing the two sets for an indication of change is also called mediation analysis (see chapter 4 by Schatzkin).

Table 5.1 shows the expected results from these two sets of analyses under the assumption that the underlying relations follow each of the theoretical etiologic models described in Figure 5.1. These results were obtained by simulation using single-cycle, one- or two-state Markov transition models specifying a range of plausible statistical association scenarios that are likely to occur in practice, all of which assume that the relations under study are not absolute and that V1, V2, and O are binary variables (that is, exposed/nonexposed, positive/negative, or attribute present/absent). A "++" indicates that the relation is identified as present of moderate or high magnitude (as estimated by the RR) and statistically precise (as judged by the width of the 95% confidence interval) depending on the size of the study. A "+" indicates that the relation is appreciably lower in strength than the one indicated by "++" and a minus sign "−" indicates that the association is nonidentifiable, that is, a unity RR. Modeling was done with the EpiMod1M software utility [11].

TABLE 5.1. Possible findings for the statistical associations between V1 and O and between V2 and O under the different models of the natural history of cancer precursors described in Figure 5.1.

Etiologic model	Assumed relations	Association V1–O		Association V2–O	
		Crude	Adjusted for V2	Crude	Adjusted for V1
Independence	V1 → O ← V2	++	++	++	++
Confounding	V2 ← V1 → O	++	++	+	–[1]
Interaction[2]	V1 + V2 → O	+	++/+/–	+	++/+/–
Causal pathway	V1 → V2 → O	+	–	++	++
Correlates of outcome[3]	V1 → O → V2	++	+	++	+
	V1 ← O → V2	++	++/+	++	++/+

[1] A negative sign indicates that the association disappears, i.e., a RR = 1.
[2] Stratification is more informative than adjustment and should thus be the preferred approach.
[3] A change from ++ to + indicates that in some combinations the adjusted estimate is substantially lower than the crude one.

Independence of Effects

In the first situation of Table 5.1 it can be seen that the magnitude of the crude associations V1–O and V2–O are unaffected upon mutual adjustment. Were these results seen in practice, the observer should conclude that it is unlikely that the pathway leading to O from V1 is mediated by V2 or vice versa. For instance, if V1 and V2 were two dietary variables associated with risk of colonic adenomas (O), then in the absence of other information, one would be tempted to conclude that they are possibly affecting the same initiating or promoting step in the development of lesions.

Confounding

The confounded relation (Table 5.1) specifies that V1 is the confounder (the actual cause of O) and V2 is the variable with no causal effect of its own but whose association with O is confounded by that of V1–O. The stronger statistical association for V1–O than for V2–O is the first indication that this could be the case, since V2–O is a spurious, indirect relation. Adjusting V1–O for V2 has no effect on the magnitude of the RR, but the V2–O association disappears after adjustment for V1, which provides empirical evidence for the hypothesis of a confounded relation with a zero effect. In the examples discussed above, the crude association between coffee drinking (V2) and

oral leukoplakias (O) would not persist upon adjustment for smoking (V1), the true risk factor. Similarly, the anti-HPV serological response, described above in the context of a CIN study, will probably be a good statistical marker of the presence of lesions, but adjustment of such an association for persistent cervical HPV infection—should this variable be available and properly measured (see Effect of Measurement Error)—will make it disappear.

The confounding scenario assumed in Table 5.1 is one of a null effect for V2. It is conceivable, however, that V2 could have its own mediating effect on the genesis of O. In that case, the adjusted RR will not necessarily disappear but reveal a net effect that represents the average V2–O association among those exposed to V2 and not exposed to V1.

Interaction

If V1 and V2 interact to produce a modified joint effect on the risk of O, the results will be consistent with the range shown in Table 5.1, which would not be helpful in interpreting the nature of the relation. However, mutual adjustment is not the appropriate strategy for assessing interaction, because the resulting adjusted RRs are simply summary measures of the net effect of these variables and would hide the critical evidence that the strength of the association for either V1–O or V2–O varies according to the categories of the other variable. The appropriate strategy, should interaction be suspected, would be to conduct a stratified analysis that would reveal the association of V1–O in each of the categories of V2 and vice versa. This could also be accomplished in a regression model that included a cross-product term for V1 × V2 in addition to the main effects for V1 and V2. Any of these approaches would reveal effect modification and provide empirical evidence in support of interaction. In the example of tobacco (V1) and alcohol (V2) as risk factors for oral dysplasias (O) the latter analytical approaches (i.e., stratification or fitting a cross-product term) would be equally suitable. On the other hand, in a case-control study collecting information on genetic polymorphisms, it is possible that the investigators might opt to conduct the genetic assays only among cases because of the expense of carrying them out among all subjects. In such gene–environment studies, case-only analyses of the association between an environmental exposure and a genotype treat case subjects without the susceptibility genotype as the control group and the case subjects who were not exposed to the environmental factor serve as the referent group. This type of study design (the case-only design) assumes that the exposure and genetic attribute occur independently in the population, and that the disease is rare. The OR thus obtained is an adequate estimate of the multiplicative interaction effect that would have been measured if the genetic information were available for all subjects [12–14].

Causal Pathway

The simple pathway model in Figure 5.1 specifies that V1 is the remote variable mediating risk of O via V2, the intermediate endpoint. In consequence, a stronger association has to be expected for V2–O than for V1–O, but the latter may be moderate or even large, depending on the strength of the V1–V2 and V2–O relations. More important, however, is the fact that adjustment of V1–O for V2 will necessarily make the association disappear, whereas adjustment of that of V2–O for V1 has no effect (Table 5.1). In the CIN example described above, HPV infection (V2) is in the causal

pathway between sexual behavior (V1) and cervical lesion outcome (O) [9]. Empirical evidence supporting this model was obtained by Schiffman et al. [15], who showed that the OR for sexual activity is considerably attenuated upon adjustment for HPV infection (see chapter 4 by Schatzkin).

It is noteworthy that the fact that the V1–O association was "adjusted away" by V2 may be erroneously interpreted as being caused by confounding, a scenario that is suspected far more frequently by cancer epidemiologists when conducting data analysis. This underscores the importance of considering plausible biological mechanisms that could influence the natural history of the target disease so that an appropriate *a priori* hypothesis of a causal pathway may be formulated beforehand.

Correlates of Outcome

Finally, analysis of the relations in the two situations depicted in Figure 5.1 where correlates of outcome are to be suspected may generate some unexpected results if the underlying causal relations are not considered. In the first of the two examples, the observer may decide that adjustment of the V1–O association for V2 is justifiable perhaps because of a mistaken assumption that V2 would be an intermediate endpoint preceding the outcome (O) in the natural history of the disease (as in the causal pathway described above). The resulting adjusted estimate would show an attenuated association and could lead to the erroneous interpretation that V2 would be in the causal pathway from V1 to O, that is, as a mediator of the effect of V1. A suitable example would be the model of sexual activity as a remote risk factor (V1) leading to HPV infection (considered here as O, the dependent variable in the analysis) and ultimately to CIN (V2). Adjustment of the association between the sexual activity variable and HPV infection for the presence of CIN would lead to spurious results, since CIN is a direct correlate of HPV infection, taken here as the outcome. Likewise, the second example of correlates of outcome would also lead to unpredictable results that could lead to an erroneous interpretation of the underlying biological model. In this more extreme case, the analysis implies that the observer inverted the directionality of the causal relation and undertook an inappropriate adjustment.

In practice, the empirical validation of the types of expected etiological relations described in Figure 5.1 would require accommodating the role of covariates in more complex relations that could involve joint confounding and other potential sources of biases. Nevertheless, the basic premise of how the stated relations would be verified empirically through statistical analysis should follow the range of expectations mentioned previously. Many consumers of information from epidemiologic studies tend to consider adjusted RR estimates in cancer etiology studies as inherently bias-free. As shown above, covariate adjustment has a clear role in mitigating the effects of confounded relations and in revealing mediation in causal pathways but one should refrain from generalizing this strategy indiscriminately without considering the underlying biological models.

Effect of Measurement Error

The etiologic models depicted in Figure 5.1 represent relations in the source populations, that is, structural relations that occur among the variables of interest before a study sample is taken and before exposures, endpoints, and outcome are measured in an investigation. Therefore, such relations are unaffected by random and systematic errors that occur in empirical research. A major caveat in the interpretation of the data analysis results described in the preceding section is the effect of measurement error. The effects of exposure and covariate misclassification are a long-standing interest of statistical methodologists [16–18]. Misclassification bias is among the most serious problems hampering the validity of much of the epidemiologic research on risk factors for cancer and other chronic diseases. Those attempting to assess the effects of dietary or environmental factors on cancer risk are well aware of the difficulties involved. Epidemio-

logic common sense has it that improper ascertainment of an exposure will bias its RR estimate generally towards the null, if the misclassification is random and nondifferential with respect to the outcome (being a case of the disease or not). If the measurement error is not random or nondifferential with respect to the outcome, the direction and degree of the bias are difficult to predict *a priori*.

The following paragraphs describe typical situations that are affected by measurement error of intermediate endpoints or outcomes in epidemiologic studies of cancer precursors. The examples that are described to illustrate specific scenarios of misclassification were produced by simulation of hypothetical cohorts of size 100,000 using single-cycle, one- or two-state Markov models based on a wide range of plausible parameters for transitions. Correction for the presumed misclassification is sometimes feasible if knowledge exists about the performance of techniques used to measure exposure or outcome variables.

Effect on the Prevalence of the Endpoint

Measurement error in the endpoint under study can have a marked biasing effect on the presumed prevalence of the condition [9]. Table 5.2 shows the effect of varying test sensitivity and specificity on the presumed prevalence of cancer precursors or intermediate endpoints in three hypothetical populations with prevalences that vary from 0.1%–10%. As shown, when the endpoint is rare, the presumed prevalence can be a gross overestimation of the true prevalence. The bias always results in an overestimation of the prevalence and is influenced more by a low test specificity than by low sensitivity. Lowering sensitivity has only a moderate biasing effect on the presumed prevalence, an effect that is only evident for conditions that are relatively common.

It is noteworthy that although there is a 10-fold difference in true prevalences between the respective situations shown in Table 5.2, the perceived magnitude of the difference is much lower, particularly if the test produces too many false positive results. For instance, at 10% false

TABLE 5.2. Presumed prevalence (%) of a cancer precursor endpoint resulting from testing for a surrogate marker under different levels of test sensitivity and specificity, in three hypothetical populations, with different prevalence rates of the endpoint.

True prevalence[1]	Specificity	Presumed prevalence (%) at different sensitivity levels		
		99%	90%	70%
0.1%	99%	1.1	1.1	1.1
	90%	10.1	10.1	10.1
	70%	30.1	30.1	30.0
1%	99%	2.0	1.9	1.7
	90%	10.9	10.8	10.6
	70%	30.7	30.6	30.4
10%	99%	10.8	9.9	7.9
	90%	18.9	18.0	16.0
	70%	36.9	36.0	34.0

[1] Assumed free of error.

positives (i.e., 90% specificity) the estimated prevalences will differ by less than twofold, regardless of test sensitivity. This indicates, for example, that a molecular epidemiologic survey may fail to detect important differences in prevalence or incidence of two distinct endpoints that are substantially different in their occurrence in a given population.

When both the sensitivity and specificity of the test used to detect the endpoint are known it is possible to correct the resulting rate to eliminate the bias. The formula [19] is as follows:

$$Pc = (Pu + W - 1)/(S + W - 1)$$

where Pc and Pu are the corrected and uncorrected prevalence rates, respectively, S denotes test sensitivity, and W denotes test specificity.

Effect on the Association between Exposure and Endpoint or Outcome

Figure 5.2 illustrates the biasing effect of measurement error on the estimates of association between an exposure biomarker and its cancer precursor outcome in a cohort study. The two graphs show separately the effects of misclassification of the biomarker (Figure 5.2, top) and of the outcome (Figure 5.2, bottom). Three hypothetical underlying causal relations between these two variables are depicted in

each graph based on the strength of their statistical associations: RRs of 2, 10, and 50. Baseline biomarker prevalence is assumed as 20% and the cumulative risk of the outcome is constrained to be around 2.5%, levels that are consistent with those of natural history studies of HPV infection (taken as the biomarker measured at baseline) and high-grade CIN (taken as outcome, measured by short-term cytological follow-up) in many Western populations [20].

Under conditions of perfect outcome classification, it is possible to observe that increasing misclassification of baseline biomarker status leads to biased estimates of RRs towards unity (Figure 5.2, top). At 10% misclassification, that is, testing for the biomarker with 90% sensitivity and 90% specificity, the original RRs of 2, 10, and 100 are mistakenly estimated as being 1.7, 5.8, and 15.0, respectively. At 30% misclassification, the bias is so severe that the measured RRs are 1.3, 2.3, and 3.3, respectively, values that would be indistinguishable statistically in most epidemiologic studies.

Although the biasing effect of biomarker exposure misclassification may seem appreciable, it is not as damaging to the validity of a study as misclassification of the cancer precursor outcome (Figure 5.2, bottom). Assuming perfect ascertainment of the baseline biomarker, even minor levels of outcome misclas-

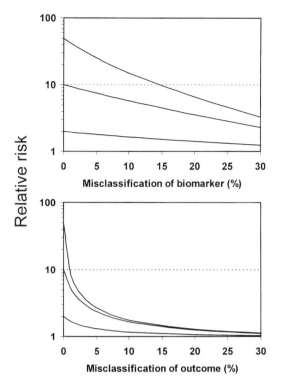

Relative risk

FIGURE 5.2. Biasing effect of misclassification of an exposure biomarker (top graph) or of its resulting cancer precursor outcome (bottom graph) on the RR estimate for the association between the biomarker and the outcome, in a hypothetical cohort study. Baseline prevalence of the biomarker is assumed as 20% and the cumulative risk of the outcome as between 2% and 3%. Three hypothetical relations are assumed based on the strength of the statistical associations (RRs of 2, 10, and 50) for the underlying biomarker-outcome relation.

sification diminish considerably the statistical strength of the underlying associations. With only 5% misclassification, that is, a level equivalent to an impressive cytological performance of 95% sensitivity and 95% specificity to detect high-grade CIN, the RRs of 2, 10, and 50 are mismeasured as 1.3, 2.4, and 2.7, estimates that cannot be distinguished statistically in practice.

It can be generalized that, for the conditions described above, outcome misclassification has a greater impact on study validity than exposure misclassification. Using the HPV–CIN example, had HPV infection been the outcome instead of the biomarker exposure, as is the case in cross-sectional surveys of determinants of HPV infection, the same conclusion would apply, that is, the effect of misclassification of viral status would be more important than if HPV infection had been assumed as the exposure variable.

In practice, study validity is further aggravated by concomitant misclassification of exposure as well as outcome. This is a real concern in cohort studies since they frequently use precancer lesions as endpoints. On the other hand, case-control studies of invasive cancer are far less likely to be affected by outcome misclassification, but are prone to more severe exposure misclassification that can be differential or nondifferential [21].

If the diagnostic performance of the biomarker assay is known (perhaps from a substudy done for validation purposes) separately for cases and noncases in a case-control or cross-sectional study, it is possible to correct for the biasing effect of differential and nondifferential exposure misclassification using a simple formula [19]:

$$OR = \frac{(W_1 n_1 - b)(S_2 n_2 - c)}{(W_2 n_2 - d)(S_1 n_1 - a)}$$

where S = sensitivity, W = specificity, n is the number of subjects, and the subscripts 1 and 2 indicate cases or controls (or noncases), respectively. The frequencies a, b, c, and d represent the cells of the 2 × 2 table in which the frequencies of exposure and outcome are cross-classified as follows: a = biomarker positive cases, b = biomarker negative cases, c = biomarker positive controls, and d = biomarker negative controls.

In the absence of data on the validity of an exposure assessment instrument or for a biomarker assay, one cannot resort to the above formula to correct for the effects of misclassification. If misclassification is known to exist because of test variability—for instance, because of inter-rater disagreement, interlaboratory variation, or similar reasons—one can use latent-class statistical techniques [22–24] that consider the collective information on the multiple results assessing the exposure or biomarker. This permits the computation of RR estimates that are less biased than estimates computed considering the exposure information from a single assessment with error.

A simple illustration of how misclassification bias can be minimized by exploring the interlaboratory assay variability for a genetic susceptibility marker was published recently [25]. An association between codon-72 *p53* polymorphism and risk of HPV-induced cervical cancer (*Arg/Arg* genotype equated to greater risk) has been found [7,8] but this finding has not been replicated by others [26–31]. One possible reason may have been measurement error in the genotyping assay used by most laboratories that have attempted to reproduce the association. This was shown in a case-control study that assessed the impact of interlaboratory variation in *p53* genotyping on the magnitude of the proposed association [25]. This study analyzed codon-72 polymorphism blindly in three different laboratories. The disagreement among laboratories was substantial with Kappa coefficients in the 0.49 to 0.63 range. When disagreement between labs was allowed, the OR for the *Arg/Arg* genotype, compared to other forms, was 1.5 (95%CI: 0.5–3.9). In contrast, the OR increased to 8.0 (95%CI: 2.3–28.5) after exclusion of discordant genotypes, which presumably

restricted the analysis to those subjects in whom measurement error was minimal or nonexistent. This strategy provided empirical evidence for the hypothesis that homozygous codon-72 *p53-Arg* may confer a higher susceptibility to HPV-associated cervical tumorigenesis.

Misclassification of Biomarker as a Covariate

As stated above in the discussion on empirical verification of the causal pathway model, the etiologic role of an intermediate endpoint can be verified by mediation analysis, that is, by using it as a covariate for adjusting the relation between a remote exposure and the cancer precursor outcome. If the intermediate endpoint is truly in the causal pathway between exposure and outcome, the association between the latter two variables should disappear upon adjustment for the endpoint. Table 5.3 shows how this assessment may be hampered by measurement error in the intermediate endpoint. Three hypothetical scenarios are considered that specify different strengths for the relations between exposure and endpoint and between endpoint and outcome (V1–V2, and V2–0, respectively, using the causal pathway scheme in Figure 5.1).

TABLE 5.3. Effect of misclassification of an intermediate endpoint on the adjusted relative risk estimates for the relation[1] between a remote exposure and a cancer precursor outcome that is mediated by the intermediate endpoint.

Underlying RR (exposure-endpoint)	Underlying RR endpoint-outcome)	Resulting Crude RR (exposure-outcome)	Specificity in detecting endpoint	Adjusted RR (exposure-outcome)[2] by sensitivity level		
				99%	90%	70%
10	10	1.74	99%	1.16	1.22	1.36
			90%	1.55	1.58	1.65
			70%	1.68	1.70	1.72
10	50	3.96	99%	1.47	1.68	2.18
			90%	2.98	3.13	3.45
			70%	3.62	3.70	3.84
50	50	17.11	99%	1.82	3.06	5.99
			90%	6.40	7.78	10.83
			70%	11.63	12.81	15.04

[1] Model assumptions: cumulative risk of endpoint among non-exposed = 1%, cumulative risk of outcome among those with endpoint = 1%, prevalence of exposure = 30%.
[2] RR adjusted for the intermediate endpoint measured by a hypothetical assay with stated levels of sensitivity and specificity.

Given the assumptions of strength of association for the latter "connecting relations" and baseline risk, the resulting crude RR between exposure and outcome varies from 1.7 to 17.1. As shown, misclassification of the endpoint as a covariate severely affects the ability to "adjust away" the indirect exposure–outcome association. At moderate levels of misclassification (10% false negatives and false positives), there remains a substantial portion of the original crude effect. In the second scenario shown in Table 5.3 (at 90% sensitivity and specificity), the adjusted RR of 3.1 may be indistinguishable in practice from the crude RR of 4, depending on the size of the study. Upon realizing that the adjusted RR is not materially different from the crude one, the observer may erroneously interpret this as an indication of an independent effect for the remote exposure via a separate mechanism that does not involve the intermediate endpoint. With greater misclassification the efficacy of the adjustment strategy is virtually nonexistent. It can also be seen that test specificity influences the degree of misclassification bias more prominently than sensitivity.

As an illustration using the HPV–CIN model, lifetime number of sexual partners is a predictor of risk for acquiring HPV infection, an intermediate endpoint that influences risk of CIN. In this model the statistical association between sexual activity and CIN should only be present in analyses that do not control for properly ascertained HPV status [9]. This has been empirically demonstrated in studies using polymerase chain reaction techniques to detect HPV infection [15,32,33]. However, earlier molecular epidemiology studies using first generation hybridization assays to detect HPV infection were prone to misclassification and erroneously revealed that number of sexual partners was independently associated with risk of cervical cancer, even after adjustment for HPV infection [34,35].

Misclassification of an Intermediate Endpoint Producing Spurious Interaction

Another deleterious effect of measurement error in the causal pathway model described

above results in the erroneous perception of interaction between the remote exposure and the intermediate endpoint on the risk of the cancer precursor. This situation will occur if an observer is attempting to verify interaction assuming the third model scenario in Figure 5.1, when in reality, the correct underlying model is that of a causal pathway. As part of the empirical verification process, the investigator will probably have calculated adjusted estimates for V1–0 given V2 and for V2–O given V1 and then proceeded to compute stratum-specific RRs for each of these two relations to probe for effect modification, which would have given empirical proof of interaction between V1 and V2 on the risk of O.

The potential findings from such an analysis can be best illustrated by considering the first situation in Table 5.3 at 90% sensitivity and specificity for the testing of V2, the unsuspected intermediate endpoint. In addition to the estimates for V1–O which are shown in Table 5.3 (RR for V1–O: crude = 1.74, V2–adjusted = 1.58) the results for V2–O are as follows: crude RR = 3.19, V1-adjusted RR = 3.08. Taken together, before any supplemental analysis is done, these findings are consistent with independence of effects (with V2 being the stronger determinant of the two) accompanied by mild mutual confounding; but the results are certainly not consistent with the unsuspected, true causal pathway that "drives" those relations. The analysis of a random sample of 500 cases and 500 controls (to simulate a moderately large case-control study) drawn from the source cohort that was used to illustrate these associations reproduces these findings, using ORs to estimate the RRs. The next step is the stratification of the two associations to verify effect modification. The stratum specific ORs for V1–O are 3.24 (95%CI: 1.7–6.2) for V2-positive and 1.10 (95%CI: 0.8–1.5) for V2-negative individuals, with strong evidence of heterogeneity between these two estimates (P = 0.002). The ORs for V2–O after stratification by levels of V1 are 5.15 (95%CI: 3.0–8.8) for V1-positive and 1.74 (95%CI: 1.1–2.8) for V1-negative, with equivalent evidence of heterogeneity between estimates. The conclusion that would be reached by the analyses of this case-control study would point to interaction between V1 and V2 on the risk of O, clearly an erroneous interpretation because the underlying model specified a causal pathway relation scheme. In fact, without the 10% misclassification of the intermediate endpoint V2, the stratum-specific RRs for V1–O are both equal to 1.0, whereas those for V2–O are both equal to 10.0, the actual magnitude of the relation specified in the first scenario of Table 5.3.

Measurement Error Affecting the Assessment of a Necessary Cause

On the basis of epidemiologic theory, it can be expected that the RR between risk factor and disease will tend to infinity (because of a denominator of zero due to the nonexistence of nonexposed cases) if the disease cannot arise from routes other than that initiated by the risk factor, that is, if the latter is a necessary cause for the disease. On the other hand, if a cause is not necessary, the risk of disease among those not exposed to the risk factor will not be negligible, and thus, the magnitude of the RR will be lower, all other conditions being held constant. The difference in the magnitude of RRs between these two situations is a key element in judging whether the results from traditional epidemiologic studies can be used to distinguish a necessary from a non-necessary cause. However, measurement error in ascertaining an exposure or intermediate endpoint will also hamper our ability to assess empirically whether or not such an endpoint is a necessary event in carcinogenesis.

Of the known causes and determinants of cancer, none is considered necessary or sufficient, but recently it has been suggested that HPV infection may be the first determinant of a human cancer that may have characteristics of a necessary cause [10,36,37]. If confirmed, this would have obvious implications for the primary and secondary prevention of cervical cancer. However, misclassification of cumulative exposure to HPV alone makes it impossible to use the magnitude of the RR estimates for the association between HPV and CIN to differentiate between the necessary and non-necessary cause assumptions [11]. Figure

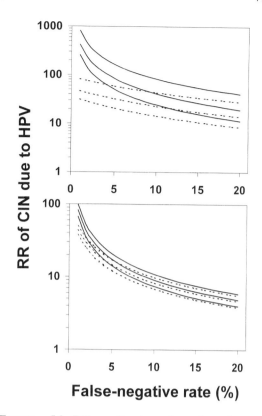

FIGURE 5.3. RR estimates for the human papillomavirus-cervical intraepithelial neoplasia (HPV–CIN) association as a function of the misclassification in HPV exposure, assuming a 50% cumulative risk of CIN among those exposed to HPV and 0.5% or 0% among those unexposed, for non-necessary and necessary cause assumptions, respectively. Continuous lines: cohorts based on the necessary-cause assumption for the HPV–CIN association; broken lines: cohorts based on the assumption that HPV is not a necessary cause of CIN. The three curves in each set represent different specificity levels: 99% (top), 90% (middle), and 80% (bottom). The two graphs differ in the assumed prevalence of HPV exposure: 10% (top), 50% (bottom) (Adapted from Franco EL, Rohan TE, Villa LL, 1999, with permission.)

5.3 illustrates the problem by showing how RRs vary in response to changes in sensitivity (abscissa) and specificity (the three curves in each set), separately, and for two scenarios of HPV exposure prevalence: 10% and 50% [11]. Cumulative risk of CIN among those exposed to HPV is fixed at 50%, resulting in a RR of 100 if HPV exposure ascertainment is free of error and we assume a non-necessary causal relation (that is, the risk of CIN among the unexposed is non-negligible at 0.5%). At an HPV prevalence of 10%, there is substantial overlapping of curves (Figure 5.3, top), with relations becoming of comparable magnitude at sensitivity levels of 90% and lower (i.e., false negative rates of 10% and higher). A nearly complete loss of the ability to distinguish between causality assumptions occurs at the higher HPV prevalence of 50% (Figure 5.3, bottom). Figure 5.3 also shows that the lower the exposure prevalence, the less important the effect of losses in sensitivity in reducing RR estimates. Conversely, specificity takes a more important role at the lower prevalence levels and has an almost negligible effect on the magnitude of the HPV–CIN relation at the relatively high 50% HPV exposure.

Minimizing the Influence of Measurement Error

It is obvious from the preceding demonstrations that epidemiologists and their laboratory collaborators would do well to devote energy and resources towards the improvement of questionnaire instruments to obtain information on exposure to risk factors and towards developing more specific and sensitive assays to detect intermediate endpoints and other biomarkers of cancer risk. In addition, characterizing or quantifying the measurement characteristics of biomarkers and endpoints enables subsequent correction for measurement error. However, even with nearly perfect study instruments, there is another aspect of measurement error that remains critical: that of an incomplete ascertainment of the true exposure and endpoint status due to fluctuations in these variables over time. This is an issue that is particularly important in studies of cancer precursors because of the dynamic changes in early events of the natural history of neoplasia that precede the onset of irreversible lesions [11,38]. Unfortunately, most epidemiologic studies of cancer and precancer are based on only one measurement of exposure to remote determinants, intermediate endpoints, and lesion outcomes. Case-control and cohort investigations thus fail to capture the complete picture of the history of transition events in carcinogenesis.

Statistical modelling by logistic and proportional hazards regression methods enhances the ability to probe associations in epidemiologic datasets by allowing control of confounding, assessment of interaction among variables, and stratification (by design and matching variables, and by time between onset of exposure and outcome). However, behind the added level of insight that multivariate modelling brings to epidemiologic data analysis, the basic 2×2 table correlating exposure and outcome remains the fundamental unit of information used to generate epidemiologic evidence for or against the role of a risk factor. Unfortunately, this central 2×2 table is usually based on a single-specimen assessment of exposure, which combines the sampling and testing errors typical of one testing opportunity with those resulting from temporal fluctuations in detectability of biomarkers during the natural history of cancer.

Therefore, to understand the role of and mechanism for such dynamic changes in the natural history of cancer, one must conduct studies that collect data repeatedly on risk factors, intermediate endpoints, and lesion outcomes on multiple occasions during follow-up. A longitudinal, repeated-measurement cohort study is required to increase the accuracy and to reduce bias in the assessment of cumulative exposure and outcome history. The longitudinal nature of such studies poses new challenges in study conduct, data management [39–41] and analysis [42–44], but greatly enhances our ability to learn about key events leading to cancer development.

Conclusion

As discussed in this chapter, epidemiologic studies coupled with careful, hypothesis-driven data analysis [45,46] can be useful in providing empirical evidence for the role of intermediate endpoints and cancer precursors in the genesis of cancer, and for the role of susceptibility traits and exposures in the development of cancer precursors. The specification of *a priori* models that depict the relations among variables and their directionality requires an eclectic consideration of all aspects of disease biology, histopathology, and genetics within the time-tested epidemiologic framework for assessing causal mechanisms of disease [47]. However, even the most multidisciplinary molecular epidemiology studies must contend with the impact of measurement error in remote exposure, genetic susceptibility markers, intermediate endpoints, and precursor lesions. Although careful consideration of the possible effects of misclassification of key variables helps our understanding of the nature and degree of the ensuing biases on the measures of association, a preventive approach to minimizing misclassification is a preferred solution. This involves not only the development and validation of better survey instruments and laboratory assays, but also the design of epidemiologic studies that can properly measure the dynamic changes occurring as the early events in the natural history of cancer.

References

1. Rothman KJ. Causes. *Am J Epidemiol* 1976; 104:587–92.
2. Rothman KJ, Greenland S. *Modern Epidemiology*, 2nd Edition. Philadelphia: Lipincott-Raven, 1998, pp. 7–28, 115–34.
3. Greenland S, Pearl J, Robins JM. Causal diagrams for epidemiologic research. *Epidemiology* 1999; 10:37–48.
4. Cann CI, Fried MP, Rothman KJ. Epidemiology of squamous cell cancer of the head and neck. *Otolaryngol Clin North Am* 1985; 18:367–88.
5. Schlecht NF, Franco EL, Pintos J, et al. Interaction between tobacco and alcohol consumption and the risk of cancers of the upper aerodigestive tract in Brazil. *Am J Epidemiol* 1999; 150:1129–37.
6. Apple RJ, Erlich HA, Klitz W, et al. HLA DR–DQ associations with cervical carcinoma show papillomavirus-type specificity. *Nat Genet* 1994; 6:157–62.
7. Storey A, Thomas M, Kalita A, et al. Role of a *p53* polymorphism in the development of human Papillomavirus-associated cancer. *Nature* 1998; 393:229–34.
8. Zehbe I, Voglino G, Wilander E, et al. Codon 72 polymorphism of *p53* and its association with cervical cancer. *Lancet* 1999; 354:218–9.
9. Franco EL. The sexually transmitted disease model for cervical cancer: incoherent epidemiologic findings and the role of misclassification of human papillomavirus infection. *Epidemiology* 1991; 2:98–106.
10. Franco EL. Cancer causes revisited: human papillomavirus and cervical neoplasia. *J Natl Cancer Inst* 1995; 87:779–80.
11. Franco EL, Rohan TE, Villa LL. Epidemiologic evidence and human papillomavirus infection as a necessary cause of cervical cancer. *J Natl Cancer Inst* 1999; 91:506–11.
12. Begg CB, Zhang ZF. Statistical analysis of molecular epidemiology studies employing case-series. *Cancer Epidemiol Biomarkers Prev* 1994; 3:173–5.
13. Khoury MJ, Flanders WD. Nontraditional epidemiologic approaches in the analysis of gene-environment interaction: case-control studies with no controls. *Am J Epidemiol* 1996; 144: 207–13.
14. Goldstein AM, Andrieu N. Detection of interaction involving identified genes: available study designs. *J Natl Cancer Inst Monogr* 1999; 26: 49–54.
15. Schiffman MH, Bauer HM, Hoover RN, et al. Epidemiologic evidence showing that human papillomavirus infection causes most cervical intraepithelial neoplasia. *J Natl Cancer Inst* 1993; 85:958–64.
16. Greenland S. The effect of misclassification in the presence of covariates. *Am J Epidemiol* 1980; 112:564–9.
17. Greenland S, Robins JM. Confounding and misclassification. *Am J Epidemiol* 1985; 122:495–506.
18. Armstrong BG. Effect of measurement error on epidemiological studies of environmental and occupational exposures. *Occup Environ Med* 1998; 55:651–6.
19. Franco EL. Measurement errors in epidemiological studies of human papillomavirus and cervical cancer. In: Muñoz N, Bosch FX, Shah KV, et al. (eds) *The epidemiology of human papillomavirus and cervical cancer*. Oxford: Oxford University Press, 1992, pp. 181–97.
20. Franco EL. Statistical issues in studies of human papillomavirus infection and cervical cancer. In: Franco EL, Monsonego J (eds) *New developments in cervical cancer screening and prevention*. London: Blackwell, 1997, pp. 39–50.

21. Wynder EL. Investigator bias and interviewer bias: the problem of reporting systematic error in epidemiology. *J Clin Epidemiol* 1994; 47: 825–7.

22. Liu XH, Liang KY. Adjustment for non-differential misclassification error in the generalized linear model. *Stat Med* 1991; 10:1197–211.

23. Bashir SA, Duffy SW. The correction of risk estimates for measurement error. *Ann Epidemiol* 1997; 7:154–64.

24. Emsley CL, Gao S, Hall KS, et al. Estimating odds ratios adjusting for misclassification in Alzheimer's disease risk factor assessment. *Stat Med* 2000; 19:1523–30.

25. Makni H, Franco EL, Kaiano J, et al. *p53* polymorphism in codon 72 and risk of human papillomavirus-induced cervical cancer: effect of inter-laboratory variation. *Int J Cancer* 2000; 87:528–33.

26. Helland A, Langerod A, Johnsen H, et al. *p53* polymorphism and risk of cervical cancer. *Nature* 1998; 396:530–1.

27. Josefsson AM, Magnusson PK, Ylitalo N, et al. *p53* polymorphism and risk of cervical cancer. *Nature* 1998; 396:531.

28. Hildesheim A, Schiffman M, Brinton LA, et al. *p53* polymorphism and risk of cervical cancer. *Nature* 1998; 396:531–2.

29. Lanham S, Campbell I, Watt P, et al. *p53* polymorphism and risk of cervical cancer. *Lancet* 1998; 352:1631.

30. Klaes R, Ridder R, Schaefer U, et al. No evidence of *p53* allele-specific predisposition in human papillomavirus-associated cervical cancer. *J Mol Med* 1999; 77:299–302.

31. Minaguchi T, Kanamori Y, Matsushima M, et al. No evidence of correlation between polymorphism at codon 72 of *p53* and risk of cervical cancer in Japanese patients with papillomavirus 16/18 infection. *Cancer Res* 1998; 58: 4585–6.

32. Munoz N, Bosch FX, de Sanjose S, et al. Risk factors for cervical intraepithelial neoplasia grade III/carcinoma in situ in Spain and Colombia. *Cancer Epidemiol Biomarkers Prev* 1993; 2:423–31.

33. Kjaer SK, van den Brule AJ, Bock JE, et al. Human papillomavirus—the most significant risk determinant of cervical intraepithelial neoplasia. *Int J Cancer* 1996; 65:601–6.

34. Reeves WC, Brinton LA, Garcia M, et al. Human papillomavirus infection and cervical cancer in Latin America. *N Engl J Med* 1989; 320:1437–41.

35. Donnan SP, Wong FW, Ho SC, et al. Reproductive and sexual risk factors and human papilloma virus infection in cervical cancer among Hong Kong Chinese. *Int J Epidemiol* 1989; 18:32–6.

36. Walboomers JMM, Meijer CJLM. Do HPV-negative cervical carcinomas exist? *J Pathol* 1997; 181:253.

37. Walboomers JM, Jacobs MV, Manos MM, et al. Human papillomavirus is a necessary cause of invasive cervical cancer worldwide. *J Pathol* 1999; 189:12–19.

38. Schiffman MH, Schatzkin A. Test reliability is critically important to molecular epidemiology: an example from studies of human papillomavirus infection and cervical neoplasia. *Cancer Res* 1994; 54 (Suppl):1944–7.

39. Duffy SW, Rohan TE, McLaughlin JR. Design and analysis considerations in a cohort study involving repeated measurement of both exposure and outcome: the association between genital papillomavirus infection and risk of cervical intraepithelial neoplasia. *Stat Med* 1994; 13:379–90.

40. Rothman N, Stewart WF, Schulte PA. Incorporating biomarkers into cancer epidemiology: a matrix of biomarker and study design categories. *Cancer Epidemiol Biomarkers Prev* 1995; 4: 301–11.

41. Franco E, Villa L, Rohan T, et al. Design and methods of the Ludwig-McGill longitudinal study of the natural history of human papillomavirus infection and cervical neoplasia in Brazil. *Panam J Pub Health* 1999; 6:223–33.

42. Zeger SL, Liang KY. Longitudinal data analysis for discrete and continuous outcomes. *Biometrics* 1986; 42:121–30.

43. Zeger SL, Liang KY. An overview of methods for the analysis of longitudinal data. *Stat Med* 1992; 11:1825–39.

44. Ho GY, Burk RD, Klein S, et al. Persistent genital human papillomavirus infection as a risk factor for persistent cervical dysplasia. *J Natl Cancer Inst* 1995; 87:1365–71.

45. Greenland S. Modeling and variable selection in epidemiologic analysis. *Am J Public Health* 1989; 79:340–9.

46. Maldonado G, Greenland S. Simulation study of confounder-selection strategies. *Am J Epidemiol* 1993; 138:923–36.

47. Schulte PA, Rothman N, Schottenfeld D. Design considerations in molecular epidemiology. In: Schulte PA, Perera FP (eds) *Molecular epidemiology: Principles and practices*. San Diego: Academic Press, 1993, pp. 159–98.

Part III
Site-Specific
Precancerous Conditions

6
Upper Aerodigestive Tract

R. Sankaranarayanan and Thara Somanathan

Cancer precursor is a term used to describe lesions or systemic states with a high probability of invasive cancer occurrence compared to that in the absence of these conditions. Cancer precursors may consist of morphologically- or genetically-altered localized tissue in which cancer is more likely to occur than in its apparently normal counterpart, or of precancerous conditions, which refer to a generalized state associated with an increased risk of cancer. Identifying those patients with precursors offers a potential strategy to prevent cancer or to detect it early.

The upper aerodigestive tract (UADT) consists of those anatomical regions of the body with shared alimentary and respiratory functions. These include the oral cavity, pharynx, and larynx. Precursors of the UADT are mostly clinically defined entities (Table 6.1). Leukoplakia, erythroplakia and oral submucous fibrosis (OSF) are clinically identifiable oral cancer precursors, which on histology may reveal areas of dysplasia. Laryngeal keratosis and erythrokeratosis are precancerous mucosal changes in the larynx, particularly in the vocal cords, with great similarity to oral leukoplakia. Plummer-Vinson syndrome is a precancerous condition for hypopharyngeal cancer, particularly post cricoid malignancy, and upper esophageal cancer. Plummer-Vinson syndrome is now observed rarely thanks to general improvements in nutrition.

The need for clear definition of the precursors in order to achieve consistency in diagnosis and comparison has long been recognized.

There have been efforts to achieve consensus in the definition of oral precursors such as leukoplakia and erythroplakia. Considerable progress has been made in understanding the biology and natural history of cervical cancer precursors. However, this is not the case with UADT precursors. There is a certain paucity of knowledge of the underlying biology and the progression of these lesions. Most of the current understanding of UADT precursors is based on selected case-series from hospitals in different geographical locations, with few population-based studies on oral precancers.

Precursors in the Oral Cavity

Clinical Definition

The term *leukoplakia* was first used in 1877 by Schwimmer to denote white lesions of the oral cavity. It is now used as a clinical term, without any histological connotation, to characterize a wide range of white, and red and white oral lesions that cannot be rubbed off or diagnosed as another specific disease entity. Leukoplakia has been defined as "a white patch or plaque that cannot be characterized, clinically or histopathologically, as any other disease", by the WHO Collaborating Center for Oral Precancerous lesions [1].

An international consultation in 1983 modified the above definition as: "Leukoplakia is a whitish patch or plaque that cannot be characterized clinically or pathologically as any other

TABLE 6.1. Precursors of the upper aerodigestive tract (UADT) cancers.

Cancer site	Precursors
Oral cavity	Homogeneous leukoplakia
	Nonhomogeneous leukoplakia
	Erythroplakia
	Oral submucous fibrosis (OSF)
	Palatal keratosis and red lesions
	?Toombak-associated lesions
	Sideropenic anemia
	Syphillitic glossitis
	?Lichen planus
Oro and hypopharynx	Erythroplakia
	Submucous fibrosis
	Plummer-Vinson syndrome
Larynx	Laryngeal keratosis
	Erythroplakia
	Erythrokeratosis
	?Recurrent papilloma

disease and it is not associated with any physical or chemical causative agent except the use of tobacco" [2]. This implies that the term leukoplakia should be avoided when there is a known etiological factor other than tobacco use. Thus lesions associated with friction, dental restorations, cheek biting, and so on, should not be designated as leukoplakia. It was also proposed that an etiological and clinical description for leukoplakia [2] be established. Etiologically, lesions resulting from tobacco use were designated as "tobacco-associated leukoplakia" and those with unknown etiology as "idiopathic leukoplakia". Clinically, leukoplakia was categorized as being homogeneous or non-homogeneous, with three subtypes of the latter (erythroleukoplakia, nodular lesions, and verrucous lesions). White lesions with a smooth, corrugated, or wrinkled surface were termed homogeneous leukoplakia, and those with white, or red and white lesions having irregular flat, nodular, or exophytic surfaces were termed as nonhomogeneous.

A new set of guidelines and a clinical staging procedure for oral leukoplakia were proposed in 1994 [3]. The new definition of oral leukoplakia reads as "a predominantly white lesion of the oral mucosa that cannot be characterized as any other definable lesion; some oral leukoplakia will transform into cancer". Two clinical subtypes were recognized:

1. Homogeneous leukoplakia: A predominantly white lesion with a uniformly flat, thin appearance, that may exhibit shallow cracks. It has a smooth, wrinkled, or corrugated surface with a consistent texture throughout.

2. Nonhomogeneous leukoplakia: A predominantly white, or white and red lesion (erythroleukoplakia) that may be irregularly flat, nodular, or exophytic. The nodular lesions have slightly raised, rounded, red and/or white excrescences, and the exophytic lesions have irregular blunt or sharp projections.

It was also proposed that oral leukoplakia could be diagnosed provisionally or definitively, depending on the circumstances under which subjects are examined. The provisional diagnosis is always a clinical diagnosis, while definitive diagnosis is based on histopathological examination and exclusion of other definable lesions. If carcinoma-*in-situ* or invasive carcinoma, or other definable lesions such as lichen planus, papilloma, or pseudomembranous candidiasis are found in a biopsy of oral leukoplakia, then a provisional diagnosis of oral leukoplakia should be replaced by the definitive diagnosis obtained histopathologically.

In spite of these attempts to formulate uniform terms and definitions, other terms such as preleukoplakia (white lesions of less than 5 mm), ulcerative leukoplakia, speckled and erosive leukoplakia (the latter three are nonhomogeneous lesions) have been frequently used by workers in different countries. Many reports in the literature do not specify whether a diagnosis of leukoplakia has been reached on the basis of a clinical examination only, or after a histopathology report on a biopsy. It is likely that most reports contained both, with a predominance of clinically diagnosed lesions.

We prefer to classify oral leukoplakia mainly as homogeneous or nonhomogeneous, since these are clinically more definite categories, without any further attempt to subclassify nonhomogeneous lesions. This may result in descriptive categories with considerable misclassification between the subcategories. However, we do encourage the identification of nonhomogeneous lesions with nodular or exophytic (verrucous) surface characteristics, as these are more likely to harbour malignancy or high-grade dysplasia histologically.

Erythroplakia is used to denote lesions of the oral mucosa that present as bright red patches or plaques, that cannot be characterized clinically or pathologically as any other condition. Histological examination is mandatory to exclude malignancy and to arrive at a definite diagnosis.

Oral submucous fibrosis (OSF) is a generalized pathological state of the oral mucosa. It takes the form of an insidious, chronic disease in which the oral mucosa becomes stiff due to fibroelastic transformation of the juxtaepithelial layer. This leads to progressive inability to open the mouth, difficulty in protruding the tongue, as well as difficulty in eating, swallowing, and phonation. The clinical criteria for diagnosis of this condition vary between clinicians. While some diagnose OSF based on earlier signs and symptoms such as pain, history of vesicles and ulcers, and blanching of oral mucosa, others palpate for fibrous bands to establish a clinical diagnosis.

Descriptive Epidemiology

The information available on the incidence and prevalence of leukoplakia over different time periods is limited, and the information that exists is based on a few prevalence surveys and intervention studies in selected populations in a few geographic regions. The prevalence of leukoplakia in populations with a high risk of oral cancer varies between 0.2–12.9% in various reports [4–8]. The age-adjusted (world standard population of 1960) annual incidence rate of oral leukoplakia among 20,358 villagers in Kerala, India, was reported to be 3.3/1,000 in males and 1.9/1,000 in females in the late 1960s and early 1970s [9]. In an ongoing oral cancer screening study in Kerala, India, preliminary results indicate the incidence to be approximately 5.5/1,000 in males and 3.6/1,000 in females [10]. The variations in incidence and prevalence seem to be due to the differing characteristics of the populations studied, including risk factor prevalence, and the varying methodologies used. In spite of efforts for uniformity

TABLE 6.2. Age specific prevalence (per 1,000 persons) of oral leukoplakia in two community studies.

Age group	Ernakulam district, Kerala, 1969	Trivandrum district, Kerala, 2000
15–24	3.9	
25–34	19.5	
35–44	45.7	38.8
45–54	71.0	71.4
55–64	78.2	83.3
65–74	54.8	57.0
75+	46.1	42.3

Sources: Sankaranarayanan R, Mathew B, Jacob BJ, et al., 2000, and Mehta FS, Pindborg JJ, Gupta PC, et al., 1969.

of clinical definition of lesions, the lesions included under leukoplakia differ and vary considerably from study to study. The age-specific prevalence of lesions in two populations in the state of Kerala, India, surveyed in the 1960s and late 1990s, are given in Table 6.2 [10,11]. The prevalence rates increased with advancing age, with peak age frequency in persons in their fifties, but the peak incidence rate for oral cancer is observed in people in their sixties in most populations. A higher frequency is observed in males, due to a higher prevalence of risk factors as compared to females. The age-specific prevalence of homogeneous and nonhomogeneous leukoplakia, as a proportion of the peak age frequency, is shown in Figure 6.1. It is not possible to address trends in incidence and prevalence of oral precursors, in view of the very limited data available in relation to time and place and also due to the inconsistency in diagnostic criteria used in various studies.

Erythroplakia is a much less frequently occurring lesion than leukoplakia, and its prevalence and incidence are not well known. Quite often, a reddish-white lesion (the so called erythroleukoplakia) is confused with erythroplakia. OSF occurs predominantly among people of Indian subcontinent origin and occasionally among other Asians. Sporadic cases have been reported among non-Asians. The prevalence of OSF in India varies from 0.2–1.2% [4,6,12,13]. In a 10-year follow-up study of oral precancer in the 1970s in India,

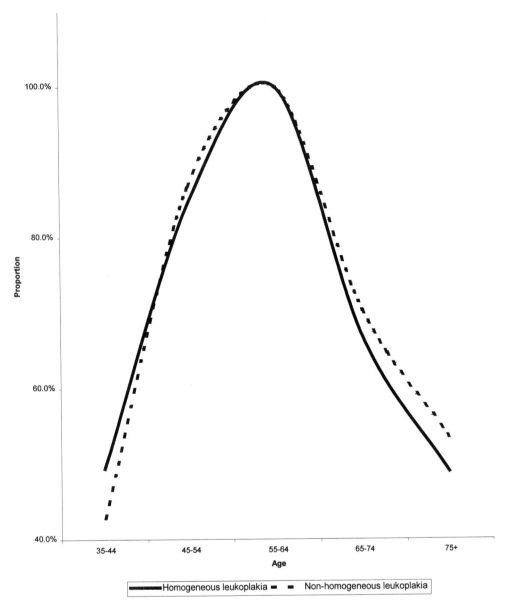

FIGURE 6.1. Prevalence of homogeneous and nonhomogeneous leukoplakia as a proportion of peak prevalence, both sexes, Trivandrum District, Kerala, India.

the incidence rate of OSF varied from 8–21.3/100,000 in men and 29–45.7/100,000 in women [4]. The variations in prevalence in different surveys are due to variations in risk factor prevalence and differences in disease definition. While some investigators adhered to earlier signs and symptoms (such as pain, history of vesicles and ulcers, and blanching of the mucosa) for diagnosis of OSF, others used palpation of fibrous bands in the oral mucosa as their diagnostic basis. The female preponderance in incidence may be related to a higher prevalence of nutritional deficiencies among women in the subcontinent.

The most common intraoral site of leukoplakias is the buccal mucosa and commissural aspects, which account for more than three-fourths of all intraoral lesions, followed by labial mucosa, gingiva, tongue, and floor of mouth [10–14]. OSF is initiated more or less as a localized lesion, mostly in the buccal or labial mucosa, progressing later to involve the oral mucosa symmetrically and entirely.

Etiology

Oral Leukoplakia

All forms of tobacco use have been well established as major risk factors for oral leukoplakia [4,5,11,12,15–24]. The association between oral leukoplakia and tobacco habits has been addressed in several epidemiological studies, and the findings satisfy the criteria of causality. The association is strong, consistent, reproducible, biologically plausible, and demonstrates a significant dose–response relationship. Finally, when tobacco habits are discontinued, a significant increase in the regression of leukoplakia has been observed [16,17].

In a recent case-control study, involving 927 subjects with oral leukoplakia (a mix of provisionally and definitely diagnosed lesions) and 47,773 controls (identified in a screening intervention trial in Kerala, India), the odds ratio (OR) of leukoplakia for ever having chewed tobacco in the betel quid was 7.0 (95%CI: 5.9–8.3) when controlled for age, sex, education, body mass index (BMI), smoking and drinking [22]. When stratified by sex, the adjusted OR for ever chewing tobacco was 37.7 (95%CI: 24.2, 58.7) for women and 3.4 (95%CI: 2.8, 4.1) for men. The adjusted OR for current chewers (OR = 9.4, 95%CI: 8.0–11.2) was higher than for past chewers (OR = 3.9, 95%CI: 2.8–5.6) and occasional chewers (OR = 2.4, 95%CI: 1.7–3.3). A dose–response relationship was seen for both the frequency and duration of chewing with the risk of oral leukoplakia. The adjusted OR for chewers who swallowed the chewing tobacco fluid (OR = 13.3, 95%CI: 9.0, 16.9) was higher than the adjusted OR for chewers who did not swallow the chewing tobacco fluid (OR = 7.5, 95%CI: 6.4–8.8). Chewers who kept the chewing tobacco quid in their mouths overnight also had a higher

adjusted OR (OR = 13.8, 95%CI: 9.3, 20.3) than chewers who did not (OR = 7.6, 95%CI: 6.5, 8.9). Subjects who had ever smoked bidis (local hand rolled cigarettes) had an OR of 3.0 (95%CI: 2.5–3.7) after controlling for age, sex, education, body mass index, chewing and drinking. The adjusted OR for persons who had ever smoked was 3.3 (95%CI: 2.5, 4.3) for men and 2.0 (95%CI: 1.5, 2.9) for women. Current smokers had the highest adjusted OR (OR = 3.4, 95%CI: 2.8–4.2), followed by occasional smokers (OR = 2.0, 95%CI: 1.4–2.8), and then past smokers (OR = 1.7, 95%CI: 1.0–2.7). Dose–response relationships were seen for the frequency, duration, and pack–years of smoking with the risk of oral leukoplakia.

In a case-control study, involving 127 incident cases of oral precursors with histologically proven oral epithelial dysplasia and matched controls in Connecticut, USA, the adjusted OR for subjects who had ever smoked cigarettes was 2.0 (95%CI: 1.1–3.9) after adjusting for drinking, mouth-wash use, denture status, and education; the OR for exsmokers was 1.0 (95%CI: 0.5–2.2), and the OR for current smokers was 4.1 (95%CI: 1.8–9.1) [20]. The risk also increased with increased pack–years of smoking and the average number of cigarettes smoked per day. Tobacco smoking has been found to be an important risk factor for oral epithelial dysplasia in Europe [23,24].

In a recent case-control study involving 100 Taiwanese patients with oral leukoplakia, betel nut (arecanut) chewing without tobacco emerged as a strong risk factor (OR = 17.4; 95%CI: 1.9–156.3) [25].

Contrary to studies addressing the role of tobacco in oral precursors, the role of alcohol as a risk factor has received only minimal attention in the past, with inconsistent findings [18,19,26,27]. The results from other recently concluded case-control studies indicate that alcohol is an independent risk factor for oral leukoplakia [22–24]. In a case-control study in the context of an oral cancer screening trial in Southern India, subjects who had ever drunk alcohol had an adjusted OR of 1.4 (95%CI: 1.2–1.7) [22]. A dose–response relationship between alcohol drinking and the risk of oral leukoplakia was also shown. The type of alcohol was also a factor. The adjusted OR was 1.3 (95%CI: 1.0, 1.7) for subjects who drank arrack (locally made spirit) only, 2.0 (95%CI: 1.3, 3.3) for subjects who drank arrack and foreign liquor (drinks such as whisky, rum, brandy etc), and 1.4 (95%CI: 1.1, 1.8) for subjects who drank toddy (fermented wine from palm sap), arrack and foreign liquor. When alcohol drinking was examined as a risk factor among subjects without tobacco habits, the adjusted OR for subjects who had ever drunk alcohol was 1.8 (95%CI: 1.3, 2.5) among nonchewers and 2.1 (95%CI: 1.3, 3.4) among nonsmokers. A dose–response relationship was seen for both the frequency and duration of drinking.

An inverse dose–response association was shown between BMI and the risk of oral leukoplakia in the above study (Table 6.3) [22]. Though BMI is reportedly inversely associated with the risk of oral cancer [28], the association with oral leukoplakia is reported for the first time in this study [22]. The highest quartile of BMI appeared to have a potentially protective effect on oral leukoplakia compared to the lowest quartile. When stratified by sex, the crude analysis showed an inverse dose–response relationship. An inverse dose–response relationship was suggested among subjects without tobacco habits and among subjects without drinking habits. It is likely that lower BMI may be confounded by the more direct influence of lower socioeconomic status and malnutrition on risk of disease.

The role of diet in the etiology of oral precursors has not been studied extensively. A recent population-based case-control study from India reported a protective effect of fiber for oral leukoplakia, with a 10% reduction in risk per gram of fiber consumed per day [29]. Ascorbic acid appeared to be protective against leukoplakia, halving the risk in the two highest quartiles of intake versus the lowest quartile: OR 0.46 and 0.44 respectively. A protective effect of tomato consumption was also observed in leukoplakia. In another recent population-based case-control study from Kerala, India, after controlling for tobacco use, intake of fruits, vegetables, and β carotene showed a reduction in risk [30]. A protective effect of iron and ascorbic acid intake was also observed.

Oral Submucous Fibrosis

Arecanut chewing seems to be an independent risk factor for OSF [31,32]. Arecanut is chewed alone or as an ingredient in the betel quid or pan. In a case-control study in Karachi, Pakistan, involving 157 cases of OSF and an equal number of controls, an increased risk was observed for arecanut chewing [31]. This habit, when practiced alone, appeared to have the highest risk (RR = 154.0). In another case-control study in India, arecanut chewing, either alone (OR = 29.9) or as an ingredient of betel quid without tobacco (OR = 78.0), emerged as a major risk factor for OSF. The OR for chewing betel quid mixtures containing tobacco was 106.4 [32].

Recent data from India indicate an increased risk of OSF in association with the use of pan masala, a dry powdered chewing mixture of arecanut, catechu, lime, spices and flavoring

TABLE 6.3. Body mass index and the risk of leukoplakia.

	Total cases	Total controls	Adjusted OR[1]	(95% Cl)
Continuous (kg/m^2)			0.974	(0.956, 0.993)
Quartile 1[2]	320	11,869	1.0	
Quartile 2	285	11,835	1.1	(0.9, 1.2)
Quartile 3	191	11,791	0.9	(0.7, 1.1)
Quartile 4	126	11,852	0.8	(0.6, 1.0)
P for trend			0.0075	

[1] OR adjusted for age, sex, education, smoking, drinking and tobacco chewing.
[2] quartile 1: BMI < 18.26 kg/m^2, quartile 2: 18.25 < BMI < 20.93, quartile 3: 20.94 < BMI < 23.87, quartile 4: BMI > 23.88.
Source: Hashibe M, Sankaranarayanan R, Thomas G, et al., 2000.

agents [33–37]. The chewing of pan masala is becoming increasingly popular in the Indian subcontinent.

While chewing betel nut is considered a risk factor for OSF, the effect of BMI, cigarette smoking and alcohol drinking have not been well established. In a case-control study, involving 177 OSF cases and 47,773 controls, in the context of an oral cancer screening trial, low BMI ($\leq$20 kg/m^2) was a risk factor for OSF with an OR of 1.8 (95%CI: 1.2–2.9) when adjusted for age, sex, education, tobacco chewing, smoking and drinking (38). An inverse dose–response relationship was shown between BMI as a continuous variable and the risk of OSF, even when the risk was adjusted for fruit and vegetable intake (P for trend = 0.0319). The OR for ever chewing tobacco was 68.4 (95%CI: 21.2–220.5) with a dose–response relationship between years of chewing tobacco and risk of OSF. No significant effects were observed for ever drinking (OR = 1.5, 95%CI: 0.7–3.3) or ever smoking (OR = 1.07, 95%CI: 0.5–2.1).

A population-based case-control study from India reported that fiber has a protective effect for OSF, resulting in a 10% reduction in risk per gram consumed per day [29]. Wheat consumption was also observed to have protective effect. Another population-based case-control study from Kerala, India, showed a reduction in risk [30], for intake of fruits, vegetables, and β-carotene after controlling for tobacco use. A protective effect of iron and ascorbic acid intake was also observed.

There is clinical and experimental evidence to support an autoimmune etiology in OSF. High frequency of antinuclear antibodies, with autoantibodies to gastric parietal cells, thyroid microsomes, reticulin and smooth muscle, and human leukocyte antigen (HLA) haplotypic pairs A10/DR3, B8/DR3, and A10/B8, are associated with this disease [13].

Pathology

The histopathological aspects of provisionally diagnosed oral leukoplakia may vary, from atrophy of the epithelium to hyperplasia, with or without varying types and degrees of hyperkeratosis. In tobacco-associated leukoplakia, the so-called chevron type of keratinisation may be observed. Some lesions reveal exophytic architecture, that is, papillomatous or verrucous hyperplasia without evidence of dysplasia.

The lesions may contain varying grades of epithelial dysplasia (Figures 6.2 and 6.3). The various changes that occur in epithelial dyspla-

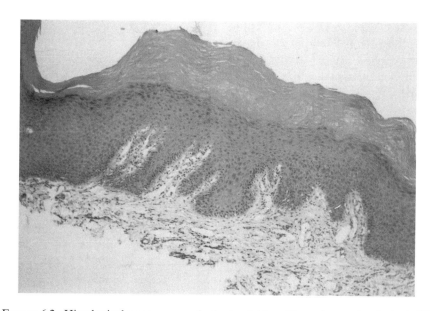

FIGURE 6.2. Histological appearance of a leukoplakia with moderate dysplasia (×63).

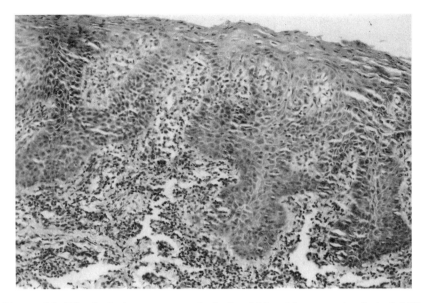

FIGURE 6.3. Histological appearance of a leukoplakia with severe dysplasia (×160).

sia (Table 6.4) are well documented [1,39–42]. Almost all dysplasias that occur in oral leukoplakia are of the keratinising type [42]. Based on the histopathological features, epithelial dysplasia is subdivided into three categories: mild, moderate and severe. However, the absence of a formal scheme for grading the severity of epithelial dysplasia leads to inconsistencies in grading [43–45]. Notwithstanding this difficulty, the presence or absence of epithelial dysplasia and its severity should be mentioned in a histopathological report on oral leukoplakia. A higher frequency of dysplasia is observed with nonhomogeneous lesions and lesions located in the tongue and floor of mouth. A variant of oral epithelial dysplasia, koilocytic dysplasia, with koilocytes and other features predictive of human papillomavirus (HPV) infection has been described [46]. The clinical significance and potential for malignant transformation of koilocytic dysplasia remain to be investigated.

Some provisionally diagnosed leukoplakic lesions may reveal carcinoma *in situ* or early invasive squamous cell or verrucous carcinoma on histological examination. The distribution of histological findings in provisionally diagnosed leukoplakia in the first prevalence round of screening in an oral cancer intervention trial in

South India is given in Table 6.2 [10]. The high proportion of dysplasia (36.7% in homogeneous and 59.7% in nonhomogeneous lesions) is due to the selection of cases for biopsy; 7.5% of the provisionally nonhomogeneous lesions had early malignancy.

The genetic changes observed in oral leukoplakias include loss of tumour suppressor genes

TABLE 6.4. Histopathological features of epithelial dysplasia in oral leukoplakia.

Loss of polarity of cells
Presence of more than one layer of cells having a
  basaloid appearance
Increased nuclear-cytoplasmic ratio
Drop-shaped rete process
Irregular epithelial stratification
Increased number of mitotic figures with a few abnormal
  mitosis
Presence of mitotic figures in the superficial half of the
  epithelium
Cellular pleomorphism
Reduction in cellular cohesion
Nuclear hyperchromatism
Enlarged nucleoli
Keratinization of single cells or cell groups in prickle cell
  layer
Increase in the number of subepithelial lymphocytes,
  plasma cells, Langerhans' cells and interepithelial cells
Presence of *Candida* organisms
Microvascularisation

on chromosomes 3p, 9p and 17p; aberrations of *erbB-1* and *erbB-2* oncogenes, and genotypic polymorphisms, such as polymorphisms in glutathione S-transferase M1 (GSTM1) and cytochrome P450 (CYP450A1) [47–53].

More than two-thirds of biopsy specimens from erythroplakia show areas of dysplasia, carcinoma *in situ* or invasive cancer [54–56]. A biopsy is mandatory in the case of oral erythroplakia, as it is safer to consider the lesion an early clinical manifestation of carcinoma rather than a precursor lesion. The histological appearance of a leukoplakic lesion with early malignancy is shown in Figure 6.4.

In the case of OSF, the oral epithelium is atrophic and may show atypia and dysplasia [3,13,40,41,57]. Epithelial hyperplasia may be observed in very early disease before atrophy becomes evident. It is not clear though, whether the epithelial atrophy is the aftermath of heavy fibrosis in the underlying connective tissue as a result of stretching and thinning, or as a result of malnutrition. The underlying connective tissue shows hyalinization and homogenization of collagen bundles. It is generally agreed that the pathological alteration begins in the lamina propria, and the epithelium responds to it only secondarily [58,59]. A vascular response due to inflammation, apart

from the connective tissue repair process, is found in early cases. Blood vessels are obliterated or narrowed, muscle fibers undergo progressive atrophy, and chronic inflammatory cell infiltration may be seen. The narrowing of the vessels begins in the upper mucosa and gradually spreads to deeper vessels. The inflammatory cells seen are mainly lymphocytes and plasma cells. Circulating immune complexes and serum antibodies in OSF probably aggravate the pathological changes in OSF. The histological appearance of OSF is shown in Figure 6.5.

Natural History

It is not clear whether homogeneous and non-homogeneous leukoplakias, as well as erythroplakia, represent independent disease entities or a continuum of progressive clinical phases of the underlying disease process. In a follow-up study in India, nonhomogeneous nodular leukoplakias that progressed to malignancy were often preceded by other lesions, such as ulcerated and homogeneous leukoplakia [60]. The nodular appearance of the leukoplakic lesions reportedly preceded the development of invasive cancer in this study. A quarter of the nodular leukoplakia in this study regressed to

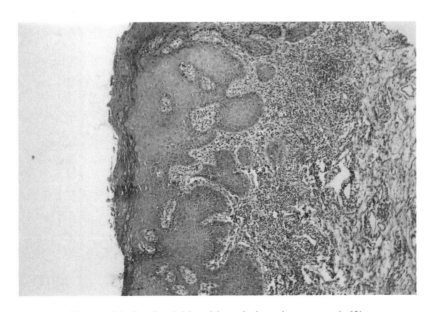

FIGURE 6.4. Leukoplakia with early invasive cancer (×63).

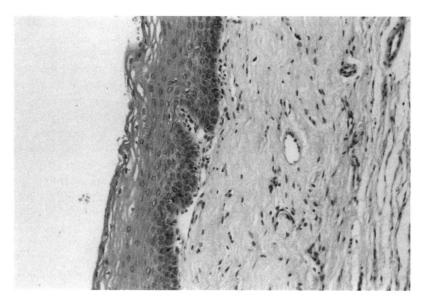

FIGURE 6.5. Histological appearance of oral submucous fibrosis (×63).

normal or homogeneous leukoplakia in an average follow-up period of 2.8 years. We hypothesize that homogeneous leukoplakia, nonhomogeneous leukoplakia, and erythroplakia represent successive and progressive clinical phases of oral carcinogenesis. Erythroplakia and nodular lesions probably indicate the earliest clinical sign of oral cancer.

It is well known that oral leukoplakias undergo regression, but there is only limited information on the rate of regression. It is often difficult to interpret the results reported, as many studies have been hospital-based. The cumulative regression rates of leukoplakia range from 20–30% over follow-up periods of 1 to 30 years (Table 6.5) [4,61–63,66]. An increase in the rate of regression of leukoplakia after cessation or reduction of tobacco habits has been reported in a few primary prevention studies in India [16,17]. Preliminary findings from an ongoing oral cancer screening trial in Kerala, India, indicate a cumulative regression rate of 63.1% of the leukoplakic lesions during a follow-up period ranging from 1 to 3 years. This surprisingly high rate seems to be due to both the effect of stopping or reducing the frequency of tobacco/alcohol habits, and the outcome of natural regression of lesions. There is also the possibility of diagnostic misclassification. This ongoing study is likely to provide further insight into the natural history of oral precursors.

TABLE 6.5. Histological findings in subjects with provisionally diagnosed oral leukoplakia in community-based study.

Histology findings	Homogeneous leukoplakia ($N = 71$)	Nonhomogeneous leukoplakia ($N = 226$)
Benign lesions	4	7
Hyperplasia/hyperkeratosis	37	33
Submucous fibrosis	0	2
Mild dysplasia	17	60
Moderate dysplasia	12	88
Severe dysplasia	0	19
Invasive cancer	1	17

Source: Sankaranarayanan R, Mathew B, Jacob BJ, et al., 2000 [10], with permission.

The rate of reported malignant transformation in different studies varies from 0.1–17.5% over follow-up periods ranging from 1 to 30 years [4,25,60–70]. The transformation rates found in hospital-based studies vary from 4.4%–17.5% whereas they range from 0.13%–2.2% in community-based studies (Table 6.6). It is difficult to assess to what an extent these differences are due to variations in natural history as opposed to selection of cases. It is also likely that invasive cancers confirmed histologically within a short period (<6–12 months) after clinical diagnosis of precursors had been classified as 'malignant transformation' in many of these studies, particularly in hospital-based studies. This might account for some of the high risk of such transformation in such studies. The relatively low proportion of biopsy procedures in population-based studies might have resulted in under-reporting of risk of malignant transformation. The risk of malig-

nant transformation is reportedly higher in females, and with nonhomogeneous lesions, lesions in intraoral locations such as the tongue and the floor of the mouth, multiple lesions, lesions not associated with tobacco habits, as well as in the presence of *Candida albicans*, or epithelial dysplasia [4,12,39,61–72].

The proportion of oral cancers which arise from precursor lesions is not accurately known. It has been suggested that, in India, most oral cancers arise from precursor lesions [17,60], but the proportion of oral cancers arising de novo is reportedly greater in Western countries [72,73]. The frequency of carcinoma *in-situ* and invasive cancer in preexisting leukoplakia varies from 4–18% [10,74]. Oral leukoplakias reportedly coexist in 20–80% of patients diagnosed with invasive oral cancer [4,60,72–75]. In a follow-up study in Kerala, 79% of oral cancers arose from preexisting leukoplakia [60].

TABLE 6.6. The frequency of malignant transformation in oral leukoplakia.

Country (source ref.)	Study base	Number of cases	Follow-up period	Cumulative regression, %	Cumulative malignant transformation, %
Sweden (64)	Hospital	782	1–20 years	—	4.0
USA (65)	Hospital	105	1–11 years	—	6.7
Denmark (61)	Hospital	248	1–10 years	20.1	4.4
India (62)	Factory workers	4,762	2 years	31.6	0.13
Hungary (63)	Hospital	670	1–30 years	31	6
India (4)	Community	410	1–10 years	4.6/1,000 p.a	2.2, 4.4/1,000 p.a
USA (66)	Hospital	257	Mean 7.2 years	28.6	17.5
Norway (67)	Hospital	157	6–16 years	—	8.9
Netherlands (68)	Hospital	46	1–8 years	—	6.5
India (60)	Cohort of tobacco users	489 homogeneous	Mean 4.8 years	—	0.13 p.a
India (60)	Cohort of tobacco users	13 nodular	Mean 2.8 years	—	16.5 p.a
India (60)	Cohort of tobacco users	105 ulcerated	Mean 4.4 years	—	0.22 p.a
USA (69)	Hospital	54 proliferative verrucous	Mean 7.7 years	—	70.3
Netherlands (70)	Hospital	166	Median 2.5 years	—	2.9 annual
India	Screening trial	161 dysplasia	1–3 years	—	1.9%
India	Screening trial	1,743 leukoplakia	1–3 years	—	0.3%

No spontaneous regression is believed to occur in the case of OSF. The reported malignant transformation rates vary from 2 to 7.6% over a follow-up period ranging from 4 to 17 years [4,13,58,76].

There are no specific molecular markers that predict malignant transformation in oral cancer precursors.

Diagnosis and Treatment

Oral leukoplakia and erythroplakia do not produce symptoms and are often painless. On the other hand, OSF is symptomatic. The prodromal symptoms in OSF include a burning sensation in the mouth while consuming spicy food, recurrent appearance of blisters in the mouth, ulceration and inflammation of the oral mucosa, excessive salivation, altered taste, and, finally, dryness of mouth. There are periods of exacerbation manifested by the appearance of small vesicles in the mouth at intervals of a few months to a few years. As the disease progresses, the oral mucosa becomes blanched and opaque, with fibrous bands. Pain and the dense fibrosis lead to varying degrees of trismus, deglutition, and phonation problems.

An oral visual examination carefully performed under adequate light by physicians and/or trained healthcare auxilliary personnel can lead to the detection of oral precursors [10,77–83]. The procedure for an oral examination with acceptable sensitivity and specificity to detect disease has been well established [*http://www.tambcd.edu/oralexam/nidroc05.htm*].

Oral self-examination has also been shown to be useful in the detection of oral precursors [84]. Out of the approximately 22,000 subjects taught mouth self-examination (MSE), 8,028 (36%) practiced it, and 247 of them reported to the clinics. Seven of these had oral cancer, and 85 had oral precancerous lesions. Six of the 7 subjects with oral cancer had stage I disease, and five of these accepted treatment and were alive disease-free 5 years later.

Unlike management of cervical intraepithelial lesions, management of oral precursors is often challenging, and results are far from satisfactory [85]. There are no widely accepted guidelines for the specific management of these lesions, although control of tobacco and alcohol habits should be an integral part of their management [86,87]. Surgical excision is the most widely used treatment for localized oral leukoplakia and erythroplakia [85,88,89]. Other treatment procedures include laser vaporization, photodynamic therapy, cryotherapy, chemoprevention with carotenoids and retinoids, and topical application of retinoids or bleomycin [90–98]. The role of chemoprevention in long-term control and oral cancer prevention has not yet been established [96–98]. There are several instances in which active treatment of oral leukoplakia can hardly be instituted because the lesions may be quite extensive. There is no evidence that active management of oral leukoplakia with specific procedures such as surgery or laser therapy, over and above efforts toward tobacco/alcohol control, contributes to long-term control of lesions and prevents further progression into cancer. However, the authors advocate routine excision of localized nonhomogeneous lesions with nodular or exophytic surface and of erythroplakia, along with the control of causative factors.

It is mandatory to do biopsies of all cases of nonhomogeneous lesions, erythroplakia, multiple large lesions, and lesions in sites such as the tongue and floor of the mouth, to exclude carcinoma *in situ*, invasive cancer, and dysplasia. It is advisable to excise lesions demonstrating dysplasia [39].

Management strategies in OSF include control of arecanut chewing and tobacco/alcohol use, and nutritional support with diets high in protein, calories, vitamin B complex, and minerals [13]. Use of supplementary multivitamins has reportedly improved symptoms due to OSF and interincisor distance [99,100]. The value of other therapies such as surgery, local and systemic administration of corticosteroids, hyaluronidase, and placental extract is not established.

Other Oral Precursors

Palatal keratosis and red areas are established oral cancer precursor in subjects practicing reverse smoking [4,101]. A large scale follow-up study in India revealed that reverse smoking and other tobacco habits were associated with palatal precancerous lesions and palatal cancer [4,102]. Epithelial dysplasia was found in 23% of 101 biopsies of palatal lesions in reverse smokers [103]. All new palatal cancers developed in individuals with a prior diagnosis of precancerous lesions in the palate [16]. In a follow-up study of 12,038 individuals in the Srikakulam district in India, 10 of the 11 new oral cancers had developed among individuals with palatal changes, and 1 in an individual with oral leukoplakia [17]. A significant reduction in the incidence of palatal red lesions has been demonstrated as a result of health education intervention [17]. Since the palatal precursors have been shown to be the point of origin of palatal cancers, a decrease in the risk of palatal red areas may be considered as a surrogate for the decrease in the risk of palatal cancer.

Lichen planus is a mucocutaneous disease of unknown cause that has its principal clinical manifestations in the skin and mucosa of the oral cavity. The natural history of the cutaneous form is one of spontaneous resolution over time, but oral lichen planus pursues a much more chronic course with a low rate of regression. Malignant change in oral lichen planus does occur and seems to be prompted by carcinogenic cofactors [103,104]. However, there is no increased risk of developing carcinoma in cutaneous lichen planus. In a 10-year follow-up study of 702 patients with oral lichen planus in the Ernakulam district of India, carcinoma developed in 3 (0.4%) patients [103]. The annual incidence rate of oral cancer among lichen planus cases in this cohort was estimated to be 83/100,000, against an expected incidence rate of 25/100,000, thus yielding a relative risk (RR) of 3.3. This RR did not reach statistical significance, assuming poisson distribution for the occurrence of 3 oral cancer cases. Although this study could not confirm the precancerous nature of this disease with a high degree of certainty, the disease does not appear to be innocuous either. In another follow-up study in New Zealand involving 832 patients with lichen planus, 7 (0.8%) developed intraoral squamous

cell carcinoma, including 3 cases of carcinoma *in situ* [104]. It is possible that epithelial atrophy, the predominant histological feature, probably renders the mucosa more vulnerable to the carcinogenic action of tobacco.

The use of toombak (a mixture of tobacco and sodium bicarbonate) in Sudan is reportedly associated with oral cancer [105]. Though toombak-associated oral mucosal lesions (while or yellowish-white lesions with wrinkling and thickening) demonstrate a low frequency of epithelial dysplasia, the premalignant nature of these lesions remains to be established [106].

Other precancerous conditions, such as sideropenic anemia with dysphagia, and syphilitic glossitis, are now very rare. Plummer-Vinson syndrome is associated with iron-deficiency, nutritional deficits, and autoimmunity [107]. It is believed that the decline of this disease parallels the improvement of dietary status and the treatment of sideropenic anemia with iron supplements [107,108]. Widespread use of antibiotic therapy for infections, particularly penicillin, seems to be responsible for the decline of syphilitic glossitis.

Precursors of cancers of the Oro and Hypopharynx

The precursors of cancers of the oro and hypopharynx include erythroplakia and Plummer-Vinson (Paterson-Kelly) syndrome. The pathologic process in OSF may extend into the pharynx as well, particularly to the tonsillar pillars and soft palate oropharyngeal mucosa. Plummer-Vinson (Paterson-Kelly) syndrome refers to the association of iron-deficiency anemia with dysphagia secondary to a post-cricoid or upper esophageal web and glossitis. The other associated findings may include cheilosis, koilonychia, brittle finger nails and splenomegaly. Approximately 10% of patients with this syndrome develop neoplasms in the oesophagus or hypopharynx, particularly post-cricoid carcinoma [109]. Dysphagia improves with correction of iron deficiency and dilation of the web. Thanks to the general improvement in nutrition, this syndrome is rarely observed nowadays.

Precursors of Laryngeal Cancer

Laryngeal keratosis is a precursor of laryngeal cancer that bears great similarity to oral leukoplakia [110]. This is clinically a white keratotic plaque in the larynx. Other precursors include erythroplakia and erythrokeratosis or speckled keratosis, which is a mucosal plaque in the larynx having areas of red and white lesions intermixed. Malignant transformation of laryngeal papilloma has been reported, particularly in recurrent cases [111–113]. More than four-fifths of laryngeal cancer precursors are found in men, the peak age frequency occurring in men in their fifties. Laryngeal keratosis is almost always found on the vocal cords and is usually bilateral. Laryngeal cancer precursors are causally associated with tobacco smoking and alcohol drinking [110]. Laryngeal keratosis is found adjacent to 18–43% of laryngeal cancers diagnosed [110]. Histologically, two types are identified: keratosis without atypia (KWOA), and keratosis with atypia (KWA). Dysplasia is observed in the vast majority of lesions [108,112,113]. The malignant transformation rate varies between 1 and 40% in hospital-based studies; the transformation rate in KWA varies from 5.6%–40%, but it is less than 16% in KWOA [110,113–116]. Surgical excision is the preferred method of treatment of laryngeal precursors.

Prevention of UADT Cancer Precursors

It is well established that the vast majority of UADT precursors are caused by tobacco use and alcohol drinking. Thus, primary prevention by control of these risk factors is the most potentially useful strategy to prevent UADT cancer precursors and reduce the risk of UADT cancers. Primary prevention studies in India have established the reduction in incidence of oral leukoplakia and OSF after health education interventions [16,17,71,87,117]. In the 10-year follow-up study of 36,000 individuals in India, 23 of 24 oral cancers detected were associated with oral precancerous lesions [17]. Thus the evidence is quite strong that a decrease in the incidence of oral precursors represents a potential decrease in the risk of oral cancer [16]. It is estimated, based on a recent study in Taiwan, that elimination of the habit of betel nut chewing may reduce the incidence of leukoplakia by 62% and reduce the rate of malignant transformation by 26% in the underlying population [25].

Nutritional factors are also important, and a diet rich in vegetables and fruits also contributes to prevention. The role of supplementation with chemopreventive agents such as retinoids and carotenoids is not clear. The increased risk of death from lung cancer, from cardiovascular causes, and from any cause associated with supplementation of carotenoids in smokers (in intervention trials) [118,119] is of concern, as smoking is a major risk factor for UADT cancers and precursors.

Screening for oral precursors by visual examination of the oral cavity has proved to be effective in the early detection of these lesions [10,77–81]. Since stopping or reducing tobacco use has been shown to result in regression of oral precursors [16,17,87,117], detection of these lesions and control of risk factors should contribute to a reduction in the overall risk of oral cancers in this high-risk group. While screening the high risk group of tobacco/alcohol users in routine health care interactions is recommended, a policy on routine general population screening should await evidence on cost-effectiveness.

Educational, fiscal, legislative, and advocacy measures, when applied in concert and in a sustained fashion rather than in isolation, seem to be the means by which long term changes in the prevalence of risk factors may be effected. Initiatives related to primary prevention are mainly dealt with as ad hoc measures in many countries. Sustained primary prevention efforts, based on health education and improved awareness, through health services, social welfare activities, educational establishments, voluntary and cultural organizations, and advocacy groups, is the most cost-effective means of preventing UADT precursors, cancers, and other related chronic diseases.

References

1. World Health Organization Collaborating Centre for Oral Precancerous Lesions. Definition of leukoplakia and related lesions: an aid to studies on oral precancer. *Oral Surg Oral Med Oral Pathol* 1978; 46:518–39.

2. Axell T, Holmstrup P, Kramer IRH, et al. International seminar on oral leukoplakia and associated lesions related to tobacco habits. *Community Dent Oral Epidemiol* 1984; 12: 145–54.

3. Axell, T, Pindborg JJ, Smith CJ, et al. Oral white lesions with particular reference to precancerous and tobacco-related lesions: Conclusions of an international symposium held in Uppsala, Sweden, May 18–21, 1994. *J Oral Pathol Med* 1996; 25:49–54.

4. Gupta PC, Mehta FS, Daftary DK, et al. Incidence of oral cancer and natural history of oral precancerous lesions in a 10-year follow-up study of Indian villagers. *Community Dent Oral Epidemiol* 1980; 8:287–333.

5. Tobacco habits other than smoking; betel-quid and areca-nut chewing; and some related nitrosamines. *IARC monographs on the evaluation of the carcinogenic risk of chemicals to humans*, Vol. 37. Lyon: International Agency for Research on Cancer, 1985.

6. Mehta FS, Pindborg JJ, Hamner JE, et al. *Report on investigations of oral cancer and precancerous conditions in Indian rural populations, 1966–1969.* Copenhagen: Munksgaard, 1971, pp. 48, 68, 89, 107, 120.

7. Kleinman DV, Swango PA, Niesson LC. Epidemiologic studies of oral mucosal conditions-methodological issues. *Community Dent Oral Epidemiol* 1991; 19:129–40.

8. Zain RB, Ikeda N, Razak IA, et al. A national epidemiological survey of oral mucosal lesions in Malaysia. *Community Dent Oral Epidemiol* 1997; 25:377–83.

9. Mehta FS, Pindborg JJ, Bhonsle RB, et al. Incidence of oral leukoplakias among 20,358 Indian villagers in a 7-year period. *Br J Cancer* 1976; 33:549–54.

10. Sankaranarayanan R, Mathew B, Jacob BJ, et al. Early findings from a community-based cluster-randomized controlled oral cancer screening trial in Kerala, India. *Cancer* 2000; 88:664–73.

11. Mehta FS, Pindborg JJ, Gupta PC, et al. Epidemiologic and histologic study of oral cancer and leukoplakia among 50,915 villagers in India. *Cancer* 1969; 24:832–49.

12. Mehta FS, Gupta PC, Daftary DK, et al. An epidemiologic study of oral cancer and precancerous conditions among 101,761 villagers in Maharashtra, India. *Int J Cancer* 1972; 10:134–41.

13. Rajendran R. Oral submucous fibrosis: etiology, pathogenesis, and future research. *Bull WHO* 1994; 72:985–96.

14. Silverman S Jr, Bilimoria KF, Bhargava K, et al. Cytologic, histologic and clinical correlations of precancerous and cancerous oral lesions in 57,518 industrial workers of Gujarat, India. *Acta Cytol* 1977; 21:196–8.

15. Gupta PC. A study of dose-response relationship between tobacco habits and oral leukoplakia. *Br J Cancer* 1984; 50:527–31.

16. Mehta FS, Aghi MB, Gupta PC, et al. An intervention study of oral cancer and precancer in rural Indian populations. A preliminary report. *Bull WHO* 1982; 60:441–6.

17. Gupta PC, Pindborg JJ, Bhonsle RB, et al. Intervention study for primary prevention of oral cancer among 36,000 Indian tobacco users. *Lancet* 1986; 1:1235–9.

18. Macigo FG, Mwaniki DL, Guthua SW. The association between oral leukoplakia and use of tobacco, alcohol and khat based on relative risk assessment in Kenya. *Eur J Oral Sci* 1995; 103:268–73.

19. Macigo FG, Mwaniki DL, Guthua SW. Influence of dose and cessation of kiraiku, cigarettes and alcohol use on the risk of developing oral leukoplakia. *Eur J Oral Sci* 1996; 104: 498–502.

20. Morse DE, Katz RV, Pendrys DG, et al. Smoking and drinking in relation to oral epithelial dysplasia. *Cancer Epidemiol Biomarkers Prevention* 1996; 5:769–77.

21. Walsh PM, Epstein JB. The oral effects of smokeless tobacco. *J Can Dent Assoc* 2000; 66:22–5.

22. Hashibe M, Sankaranarayanan R, Thomas G, et al. Alcohol drinking, body mass index and the risk of oral leukoplakia in an Indian population. *Int J Cancer* 2000; 88:129–34.

23. Kulasegaram R, Downer MC, Julien JA, et al. Case-control study of oral dysplasia and risk habits among patients of a dental hospital. *Eur J Cancer Oral Oncol* 1995; 31B:227–31.

24. Jaber MA, Porter SR, Gilthorpe MS, et al. Risk factors for oral epithelial dysplasia—the role of smoking and alcohol. *Oral Oncol* 1999; 35:151–6.

25. Shiu MN, Chen THH, Chang SH, et al. Risk factors for leukoplakia and malignant transformation to oral carcinoma: a leukoplakia cohort in Taiwan. *Br J Cancer* 2000; 82:1871–4.

26. Gupta PC. Epidemiologic study of the association between alcohol habits and oral leukoplakia. *Community Dent Oral Epidemiol* 1984; 12:47–50.

27. Evstifeeva TV, Zaridze DG. Nass use, cigarette smoking, alcohol consumption and risk of oral and oesophageal precancer. *Eur J Cancer Oral Oncol* 1992; 28B:29–35.

28. Kabat CG, Chang CJ, Wynder EL. The role of tobacco, alcohol use, and body mass index in oral and pharyngeal cancer. *Int J Epidemiol* 1994; 23:1137–44.

29. Gupta PC, Hebert JR, Bhonsle RB, et al. Dietary factors in oral leukoplakia and submucous fibrosis in a population-based case control study in Gujarat, India. *Oral Dis* 1998; 4:200–6.

30. Gupta PC, Hebert JR, Bhonsle RB, et al. Influence of dietary factors on oral precancerous lesions in a population-based case-control study in Kerala, India. *Cancer* 1999; 85:1885–93.

31. Maher R, Lee AJ, Warnakulasuriya, et al. Role of arecanut in the causation of oral submucous fibrosis: a case-control study in Pakistan. *J Oral Pathol Med* 1994; 23:65–9.

32. Sinor PN, Gupta PC, Murti PR, et al. A case-control study of oral submucous fibrosis with special reference to the etiologic role of arecanut. *J Oral Pathol Med* 1990; 19:94–8.

33. Gupta PC, Sinor PN, Bhonsle RB, et al. Oral submucous fibrosis in India: a new epidemic? *Natl Med J India* 1998; 11:113–16.

34. Misra SP, Misra V, Dwivedi M, et al. Oesophageal subepithelial fibrosis: an extension of oral submucous fibrosis. *Postgrad Med J* 1998; 74:733–6.

35. Shah N, Sharma PP. Role of chewing and smoking habits in the etiology of oral submucous fibrosis (OSF): a case-control study. *J Oral Pathol Med* 1998; 27:475–9.

36. Hazare VK, Goel RR, Gupta PC. Oral submucous fibrosis, areca nut and pan masala use: a case-control study. *Natl Med J India* 1998; 11:299.

37. Chaudhry K. Is pan masala-containing tobacco carcinogenic? *Natl Med J India* 1999; 12:21–7.

38. Hashibe M, Sankaranarayanan R, Thomas G, et al. Body Mass Index, Tobacco Chewing and the Risk of Oral Submucous Fibrosis. *Proc Am Assoc Cancer Res* 2000; 41:593.

39. Van der Wall I, Schepman KP, van der Meij EH, et al. Oral leukoplakia: a clinicopathological review. *Eur J Cancer Oral Oncol* 1997; 33: 291–301.

40. Cawson RA, Binnie WH, Speight P, et al. *Lucas pathology of tumours of the oral tissues.* 5th ed. London: Harcourt Brace, 1998, pp. 221–2.

41. World Health Organization. *International Classification of Tumours. Histological Typing of Cancer and Precancer of the Oral Mucosa.* Berlin: Springer-Verlag, 1997.

42. Crissman JD, Visscher DW, Sakr W. Premalignant lesions of the upper aerodigestive tract: pathologic classification. *J Cell Biochem* 1993; 17 (Suppl):49–56.

43. Pindborg JJ, Reibel J, Holmstrup P. Subjectivity in evaluating oral epithelial dysplasia, carcinoma in situ and initial carcinoma. *J Oral Pathol* 1985; 14:698–708.

44. Karabalut A, Reibel J, Therikildsen MH, et al. Observer variability in the histologic assessment of oral premalignant lesions. *J Oral Pathol Med* 1995; 24:198–200.

45. Abbey LM, Kaugars GE, Gunsolley JC, et al. Intraexaminer and interexaminer reliability in the diagnosis of oral epithelial dysplasia. *Oral Surg Oral Med Oral Path* 1995; 80:188–91.

46. Fornatora M, Jones AC, Kerpel S, et al. Human papillomavirus-associated oral epithelial dysplasia (koilocytic dysplasia): an entity of unknown biologic potential. *Oral Surg Oral Med Oral Pathol* 1996; 82:47–56.

47. Prime SS, Eveson JW, Guest PG, et al. Early genetic and functional events in the pathogenesis of oral cancer. *Radiat Oncol Investig* 1997; 5:93–6.

48. Chang KW, Lin SC, Kwan PC, et al. Association of aberrant p53 and p21 (WAF1) immunoreactivity with the outcome of oral verrucous leukoplakia in Taiwan. *Oral Pathol Med* 2000; 29:56–62.

49. Saranath D, Tandle AT, Teni TR, et al. p53 inactivation in chewing tobacco-induced oral cancers and leukoplakias from India. *Oral Oncol* 1999; 35:242–50.

50. Mao EJ, Schwartz SM, Daling JR, et al. Human papilloma viruses and p53 mutations in normal premalignant and malignant oral epithelia. *Int J Cancer* 1996; 69:152–8.

51. Schwartz JL. Biomarkers and molecular epidemiology and chemoprevention of oral carcinogenesis. *Crit Rev Oral Biol Med* 2000; 11:92–122.

52. Nair UJ, Nair J, Mathew B, et al. Glutathione S-transferase M1 and T1 null genotypes as risk factors for oral leukoplakia in ethnic Indian betel quid/tobacco chewers. *Carcinogenesis* 1999; 20:743–8.

53. Werkmeister R, Brandt B, Joos U. Aberrations of *erbB-1* and *erbB-2* oncogenes in non-dysplastic leukoplakias of the oral cavity. *Br J Oral Maxillofac Surg* 199; 37:477–80.

54. Shafer WG, Waldron CA. Erythroplakia of the oral cavity. *Cancer* 1975; 36:1021–8.

55. Shear M. Erythroplakia of the mouth. *Int Dent J* 1972; 22:460–73.

56. Katz HC, Shear M, Altini M. A critical evaluation of epithelial dysplasia in oral mucosal lesions using Smith-Pindborg method of standardization. *J Oral Pathol* 1985; 14:476–82.

57. Pindborg JJ, Sirsat SM. Oral submucous fibrosis. *Oral Surg Oral Med Oral Pathol* 1966; 22: 764–79.

58. Pindborg JJ, Murti PR, Bhonsle RB, et al. Oral submucous fibrosis as a precancerous condition. *Scand J Dent Res* 1984; 92:224–9.

59. Rajendran R, Vijayakumar T, Vasudevan DM. An alternative pathogenetic pathway for oral submucous fibrosis (OSMF). *Med Hypotheses* 1989; 30:35–7.

60. Gupta PC, Bhonsle RB, Murti PR. An epidemiologic assessment of cancer risk in oral precancerous lesions in India with special reference to nodular leukoplakia. *Cancer* 1989; 63:2247–52.

61. Pindborg JJ, Jolst O, Renstrup G, et al. Studies in oral leukoplakia: a preliminary report on the period prevalence of malignant transformation in leukoplakia based on a follow-up study of 248 patients. *J Am Dent Assoc* 1968; 76:767–71.

62. Silverman S Jr, Bhargava K, Smith LW, et al. Malignant transformation and natural history of oral leukoplakia in 57,518 industrial workers of Gujarat, India. *Cancer* 1976; 38:1790–5.

63. Banoczy J. Follow-up studies in oral leukoplakia. *J Maxillofac Surg* 1977; 5:69–75.

64. Einhorn J, Wersall J. Incidence of oral carcinoma in patients with leukoplakia of the mucosa. *Cancer* 1967; 20:2189–93.

65. Silverman S Jr. Observations on the clinical characteristics and natural history of oral leukoplakia. *J Am Dent Assoc* 1968; 76:772–7.

66. Silverman S Jr, Gorsky M, Lozada F. Oral leukoplakia and malignant transformation. A follow-up study of 257 patients. *Cancer* 1984; 53:563–8.

67. Lind PO. Malignant transformation in oral leukoplakia. *Scand J Dent Res* 1987; 95:449–55.

68. Hogewind WF, van der Kwast WA, van der Waal I. Oral leukoplakia with emphasis on malignant transformation. A follow-up of 46 patients. *J Craniomaxillofac Surg* 1989; 17: 128–33.

69. Silverman S Jr, Gorsky M. Proliferative verrucous leukoplakia: a follow-up study of 54 cases. *Oral Surg Oral Med Oral Pathol* 1997; 84:154–7.

70. Schepman KP, van der Meij EH, et al. Malignant transformation of oral leukoplakia: a follow-up study of a hospital-based population of 166 patients with oral leukoplakia from the Netherlands. *Eur J Cancer Oral Oncol* 1998; 34:270–5.

71. Saito T, Sugiura C, Hirai A, et al. High malignant transformation rate of wide spread multiple oral leukoplakias. *Oral Dis* 1999; 5:15–19.

72. Sankaranarayanan R. Oral cancer in India: an epidemiologic and clinical review. *Oral Surg Oral Med Oral Path* 1990; 69:325–30.

73. Johnson NW, Ranasinghe AW, Warnakulasuriya KA. Potentially malignant lesions and conditions of the mouth and oropharynx: natural history—cellular and molecular markers of risk. *Eur J Cancer Prev* 1993; 2:31–51.

74. Waldron CA, Shafer WG. Leukoplakia revisited. A clinicopathologic study of 3,256 leukoplakias. *Cancer* 1975; 36:1386–92.

75. Hogewind WF, van der Waal I, van der Kwast WA, et al. The association of white lesions with oral squamous cell carcinoma. A retrospective study of 212 patients. *Int J Oral Maxillofac Surg* 1989; 18:163–4.

76. Murti PR, Bhonsle RB, Pindborg JJ, et al. Malignant transformation rate in oral submucous fibrosis over a 17-year period. *Community Dent Oral Epidemiol* 1985; 13:340–1.

77. Warnakulasuriya KAAS, Ekanayake ANI, Sivayoham S, et al. Utilization of primary care workers for early detection of oral cancer and precancer cases in Sri Lanka. *Bull WHO* 1984; 62:243–50.

78. Mehta FS, Gupta PC, Bhonsle RB, et al. Detection of oral cancer using basic health workers in an area of high oral cancer incidence in India. *Cancer Detect Prev* 1986; 9:219–25.

79. Warnakulasuriya KAAS, Nanayakara BG. Reproducibility of an oral cancer and precancer detection program using primary health care model in Sri Lanka. *Cancer Detect Prev* 1991; 15:331–4.

80. Mathew B, Sankaranarayanan R, Sunilkumar KB, et al. Reproducibility and validity of oral visual inspection by trained health workers in the detection of oral precancer and cancer. *Br J Cancer* 1997; 76:390–4.

81. Fernandez-Garrote L, Sankaranarayanan R, Lence-Anta JJ, et al. An evaluation of the oral cancer control programme in Cuba. *Epidemiology* 1995; 6:428–31.

82. Mashberg A, Barsa P. Screening for oral and oropharyngeal squamous cell carcinomas. *CA Cancer J Clin* 1984; 34:262–8.

83. Sankaranarayanan R. Healthcare auxiliaries in the detection and prevention of oral cancer. *Oral Oncol* 1997; 33B:149–54.

84. Mathew B, Sankaranarayanan R, Wesley R, et al. Evaluation of mouth self-examination in the control of oral cancer. *Br J Cancer* 1995; 71:397–9.

85. Tradati N, Grigolat R, Calabrese L, et al. Oral leukoplakias: to treat or not? *Eur J Cancer Oral Oncol* 1997; 33B:317–21.

86. Scully C, Cawson RA. Potentially malignant oral lesions. *J Epidemiol Biostat* 1996; 1:3–12.

87. Gupta PC, Murti PR, Bhonsle RB, et al. Effect of cessation of tobacco use on the incidence of oral mucosa lesions in a 10-yr follow-up study of 12,212 users. *Oral Dis* 1995; 1:54–8.

88. Pandey M, Thomas G, Somanathan T, et al. Evaluation of surgical excision of non-homogeneous oral leukoplakia in a screening intervention trial, Kerala, India. *Oral Oncol* 2001; 37:103–9.

89. Vedtofte P, Holmstrup P, Hjorting-Hansen E, et al. Surgical treatment of premalignant lesions of the oral mucosa. *Int J Oral Maxillofac Surg* 1987; 16:656–64.

90. Schoelch ML, Sekandari N, Regezi JA, et al. Laser management of oral leukoplakias: a follow-up study of 70 patients. *Laryngoscope* 1999; 109:949–53.

91. Kubler A, Haase T, Rheinwald M, et al. Treatment of oral leukoplakia by topical application of 5-aminolevulinic acid. *Int J Oral Maxillofac Surg* 1998; 27:466–9.

92. Epstein JB, Gorsky M. Topical application of vitamin A to oral leukoplakia: A clinical case series. *Cancer* 1999; 86:921–7.

93. Epstein JB, Gorsky M, Wong FL, et al. Topical bleomycin for the treatment of dysplastic oral leukoplakia. *Cancer* 1998; 83:629–34.

94. Sankaranarayanan R, Mathew B. Retinoids as cancer-preventive agents. In: Stewart BW, McGregor D, Kleihues P, (eds) *Principles of chemoprevention,* IARC Scientific Publications No. 139, Lyon: International Agency for Research on Cancer, 1996, pp. 47–59.

95. Sankaranarayanan R, Mathew B, Nair PP, et al. Chemoprevention of the cancers of the oral cavity and head and neck. In: Hakama M, Beral V, Buiatti E, et al. (eds) *Chemoprevention in cancer control,* IARC Scientific Publications No. 136. Lyon: International Agency for Research on Cancer, 1996, pp. 13–22.

96. *IARC handbooks of cancer prevention. Vol. 2. Carotenoids.* Lyon: International Agency for Research on Cancer, 1998.

97. *IARC handbooks of cancer prevention. Vol. 3. Vitamin A.* Lyon: International Agency for Research on Cancer, 1998.

98. *IARC handbooks of cancer prevention. Vol. 4. Retinoids.* Lyon: International Agency for Research on Cancer, 1999.

99. Maher R, Aga P, Johnson NW, et al. Evaluation of multiple micronutrient supplementation in the management of oral submucous fibrosis in Karachi, Pakistan. *Nutr Cancer* 1997; 27: 41–7.

100. Maher R, Sankaranarayanan R, Johnson NW, et al. Evaluation of inter-incisor distance as an objective criterion of the severity of oral submucous fibrosis in Karachi, Pakistan. *Oral Oncol Eur J Cancer* 1996; 32B:362–4.

101. Pindborg JJ, Mehta FS, Gupta PC, et al. Reverse smoking in Andhra Pradesh, India: A study of palatal lesions among 10,169 villagers. *Br J Cancer* 1971; 25:10–20.

102. Mehta FS, Jalnawalla PN, Daftary DK, et al. Reverse smoking in Andhra Pradesh, India: variability of clinical and histologic appearances of palatal changes. *Int J Oral Surg* 1977; 6:75–83.

103. Murti PR, Daftary DK, Bhonsle RB, et al. Malignant potential of oral lichen planus: observations in 722 patients from India. *J Oral Pathol* 1986; 15:71–7.

104. Rajentheran R, McIlean NR, Kelly CG, et al. Malignant transformation of oral lichen planus. *Eur J Surg Oncol* 1999; 25:520–3.

105. Idris AM, Ahmed HM, Malik MO. Toombak dipping and cancer of the oral cavity in the Sudan: a case-control study. *Int J Cancer* 1995; 63:477–80.

106. Idris AM, Warnakulasuriya KAAS, Ibrahim YE, et al. Toombak-associated oral mucosal lesions in Sudanese show a low prevalence of epithelial dysplasia. *J Oral Pathol Med* 1996; 25:239–44.

107. Chen TS, Chen PS. Rise and fall of the Plummer-Vinson syndrome. *J Gastroenterol Hepatol* 1994; 9:654–8.
108. Larsson LG, Sandstrom A, Westling P. Relationship of Plummer-Vinson disease to cancer of the upper alimentary tract in Sweden. *Cancer Res* 1975; 35:3308–16.
109. Shamma MH, Benedict EB. Esophageal webs. *N Engl J Med* 1958; 259:378–82.
110. Bouquot JE, Gnepp DR. Laryngeal precancer: a review of the literature, commentary, and comparison with oral leukoplakia. *Head Neck* 1991; 13:488–97.
111. Klozar J, Taudy M, Bekta J, et al. Laryngeal papilloma-precancerous condition? *Acta Otolaryngol* 1997; 527 (Suppl):100–2.
112. Sugar J, Vereczkey I, Toth J, et al. New aspects in the pathology of the preneoplastic lesions of the larynx. *Acta Otolaryngol* 1997; 527 (Suppl):52–6.
113. Pich J, Par I, Navratilova I, et al. Long term follow-up study of laryngeal precancer. *Auris Nasus Larynx* 1998; 25:407–12.
114. Cuchi A, Bombi JA, Avellaneda R, et al. Precancerous lesions of the larynx: clinical and pathologic correlations and prognostic aspects. *Head Neck* 1994; 16:545–9.
115. Velasco JRR, Nieto CS, de Bustos CP, et al. Premalignant lesions of the larynx; pathological prognostic factors. *J Otolaryngol* 1987; 16:367–70.
116. Hojslet PE, Nielsen VM, Palvio D. Premalignant lesions of the larynx. A follow-up study. *Acta Otolaryngol* 1989; 107:150–5.
117. Murti PR, Gupta PC, Bhonsle RB, et al. Effect on the incidence of oral submucous fibrosis of intervention in the areca nut chewing habit. *J Oral Pathol Med* 1990; 19:99–100.
118. The Alpha-Tocopherol, Beta Carotene Cancer Prevention Study Group. The effect of vitamin E and beta carotene on the incidence of lung cancer and other cancers in male smokers. *N Engl J Med* 1994; 330:1029–35.
119. Omenn GS, Goodman GE, Thornquist MD, et al. Effects of a combination of beta carotene and vitamin A on lung and cardiovascular disease. *N Engl J Med* 1996; 334:1150–5.

7
Esophagus

Thomas L. Vaughan

Cancer of the esophagus is a major health problem throughout the world. It is estimated that 316,000 people were diagnosed with the disease in 1990, making it the eighth most common cancer worldwide [1]. Unfortunately, treatment is largely ineffective, and it remains one of the least survivable cancers; for example, in the United States, median survival is nine months, with only 7.3% surviving five years [2].

Esophageal cancer is a fascinating disease for the epidemiologist to study, as it exhibits some of the most striking secular and geographic variations in incidence of any cancer [3]. Two major histologies are observed, squamous cell carcinoma and adenocarcinoma, each with its own characteristic pattern of incidence and constellation of risk factors.

Most esophageal cancers occurring in the world are squamous cell carcinomas, and the majority of these occur in developing countries. Areas with extremely high mortality have long been noted in areas of North Central China, Central Asia and Southern Africa [4]. Some of the areas with the highest mortality rates are remarkably well circumscribed, with large variations over relatively short distances. In the United States, incidence rates for squamous cell carcinoma are relatively low, with little recent change over time; however, blacks experience six-fold higher incidence rates than whites [5]. In general, in high-risk populations, rates are similar in males and females, whereas in low-risk populations, the majority of cases occur in males.

The incidence pattern of adenocarcinoma contrasts markedly with that for squamous cell carcinoma. This cancer tends to be much more common in developed nations, where it has increased dramatically over the past two decades and now accounts for the majority of new esophageal cases in many countries. In the United States, an increase of over 350% was observed among white males between 1974 and 1994 [5]. Although the disease is substantially more common among white males, increasing rates have also been noted recently among white females and black males in the United States [5]. Some of the highest incidence rates in the world are observed in Scotland and other parts of the United Kingdom, with increasing incidence also reported in numerous other areas of Western, but not Eastern, Europe [6].

Further differentiating these histologic types of cancer are the specific precursor lesions that can be observed in the esophageal epithelium during neoplastic progression towards invasive cancer. Therefore, precursors of squamous cell carcinoma and adenocarcinoma are discussed separately throughout this chapter.

Precursor Lesions in Esophageal Cancer

The term "precursor lesion" is used to refer to an abnormality at the tissue, cellular, or molecular level, that can be detected in the esophageal epithelium before the development of invasive carcinoma, and that confers or is associated with increased risk of invasive carcinoma [7]. It does not imply inevitability in progression to cancer and does not exclude the possibility of regression.

Background

Several characteristics of the esophagus and of esophageal neoplasia make it an ideal organ system not only for studying the natural history of esophageal cancer and its precursor lesions, but for understanding more generally the neoplastic process in humans. First, it is easily visualized with minimally invasive endoscopic procedures, and multiple biopsies can be taken safely [8]. Second, as yet no medical or surgical treatment has been proven to safely reduce the likelihood of progression to either type of esophageal cancer in persons with identifiable precursor lesions. Consequently, there is currently little that the clinician can do beyond careful surveillance until the disease has progressed to cancer or to a near-cancerous condition that would justify the hazards of surgery or other aggressive treatments that attempt a cure. This is in contrast to carcinomas occurring in the colon or cervix, for which surgical treatment of precursor lesions clearly decreases risk of the development of invasive cancer. Finally, attention to landmarks during endoscopy allows biopsies to be taken in approimately the same area throughout surveillance. Thus, precursor lesions can be localized to a specific region and followed over time to identify the evolution of the original abnormality as well as the serial development of new abnormalities [9].

Types of Precursor Lesions

The microscope and specialized staining procedures have been the traditional tools used to identify and classify visible abnormalities of individual cells and of tissue composition and organization that develop during neoplastic progression. Recent advances in biotechnology afford additional perspectives on the neoplastic process, perspectives that potentially reflect more closely the genetic and epigenetic events that eventually lead to loss of control of cell division, widespread genetic instability, and the ability of cells to invade and metastasize.

Histologic Abnormalities

One early histologic abnormality, commonly found in populations at risk of both types of esophageal carcinoma, is esophagitis, which is characterized by basal cell hyperplasia and infiltration of inflammatory cells [10]. It can be classified as mild, moderate, or severe depending on the extent of abnormalities [11].

The esophagitis observed early in the pathogenesis of adenocarcinoma usually develops in response to chronic gastroesophageal reflux and is frequently complicated by additional pathology such as ulcers, erosions and strictures [4,12]. Grading systems have been developed to facilitate reliable assessment of its severity, emphasizing the presence and extent of mucosal breaks [12,13].

In a minority of persons with chronic gastroesophageal reflux, Barrett's esophagus develops, in which the normal squamous epithelium is replaced by a specialized intestinal metaplasia consisting of a villous columnar epithelium containing goblet cells [14,15]. Although other types of columnar epithelium can be found in the esophagus, including fundic and cardiac types, it is generally thought that only specialized intestinal metaplasia is associated with increased risk of adenocarcinoma [14,15]. There is some evidence, however, that the presence of cardiac mucosa, containing only mucous and columnar cells, may be an earlier marker of chronic reflux, preceding specialized intestinal metaplasia [15–17].

The most severe histologic abnormality is unquestionably dysplasia, characterized by distorted crypt architecture, and enlarged and hyperchromatic nuclei that vary in size and shape [14]. Based on the degree of these abnormalities, dysplasias can be classified into low and high grades, although intra- and interobserver variation can be a problem, especially in instances where the abnormalities are mild or indefinite in nature [14,18].

Cell Cycle Abnormalities

Abnormalities of the cell cycle also may be useful predictors of cancer risk. DNA content flow cytometry and multiparameter flow cytometry using the monoclonal antibody Ki67, which identifies proliferating cells, allows the determination of the total fraction of cells that are proliferating, the fraction of cells in each specific phase of the cell cycle (G0, G1, S and G2), and the presence of aneuploid cell populations [9,19].

Genetic Abnormalities

The identification of highly polymorphic markers at closely spaced intervals throughout the genome now allows rapid genome-wide assays for allelic loss (loss of heterozygosity, LOH). Such assays are useful in determining the role of specific tumor suppressor genes in neoplastic progression, since LOH is one important way in which function of a tumor suppressor gene can be eliminated. Allelic loss studies are also useful for identifying regions of the genome which may harbor undiscovered tumor suppressor genes. Tumor suppressor genes can also be silenced by mutation and by methylation of promoter regions. These abnormalities now can be detected using extremely small tissue samples and relatively high-throughput techniques [20].

Descriptive Epidemiology

Squamous Cell Carcinoma

Histologic Precursors

Several authors have suggested a progression of histologic abnormalities leading to esophageal squamous cell carcinoma similar to that described in Figure 7.1 [11,21].

The possibility that esophagitis may be a useful precursor lesion is suggested by the high frequency with which it is found in populations at high risk of esophageal squamous cell carcinoma, and the apparent correlation between prevalence of esophagitis and mortality rates of squamous cell carcinoma in specific populations. For example, in areas of high mortality in northern Iran (Turkoman) and Linxian, China (Henan Province), esophagitis was found in at least one biopsy in 83.1% and 65.0% of men (respectively) and in at least one biopsy in 76.2% and 63.5% of women (respectively). Whereas lower prevalence was seen in intermediate- and lower-risk populations, including France, Argentina, and other areas in China [4,11,21]. In contrast, esophagitis in persons without symptoms of gastroesophageal reflux is uncommon in the United States.

However, not all studies show a correlation between esophagitis prevalence and cancer incidence. Qiu and Yang analyzed biopsies from 300 randomly selected individuals from a high-incidence population (Huixian, with annual mortality rates from esophageal squamous cell carcinoma of 120.9 per 100,000 men and 68.0 per 100,000 women) and 300 randomly selected individuals from a low-incidence population (Fanxian, with annual mortality rates of 26.5 per 100,000 men and 7.49 per 100,000 women) [22]. They reported no significant differences between groups in the prevalence of histopathological findings characterizing esophagitis. The overall presence of endoscopically diagnosed esophagitis in males (74.1% in Huixian versus 83.5% in Fanxian) and females (53.9% in Huixian versus 47.3% in Fanxian) was also similar in the two samples, although the severity of the esophagitis was somewhat higher among men from Huixian. A more recent study involving 754 residents of Linxian reported a prevalence of esophagitis lower than in most previous studies of high-incidence populations

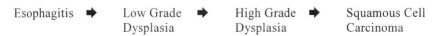

FIGURE 7.1. Sequence of histologic abnormalities in the development of esophageal squamous cell carcinoma. (Adapted from Munoz and Day, 1996 [4]).

[23]. Normal histology was found in 71.1% of biopsies, representing 43.5% of subjects.

There is good evidence that esophagitis occurs at an early age, suggesting the importance of factors acting early in life. A study among persons aged 15–26 years in Huixian, China included two groups of persons: 166 young persons from households with a case of esophageal cancer over the previous six years (case households), and 372 randomly selected from households without a esophageal cancer (control households) [24]. In those from case households, histologic evidence for esophagitis was noted in 58.6% of males and 35.8% of females, compared to 37.6% of males and 35.9% of females from control households. The study by Qiu and Yang included persons as young as 21; they found little difference in overall esophagitis prevalence by age, although severe esophagitis was more common among the older participants [22].

Interpretation of studies reporting esophagitis prevalence is limited, however, by several factors that make comparisons difficult. First is the issue of representativeness of the persons sampled in each study relative to the general population. In the study in Iran, persons were initially invited to participate if they had gastrointestinal symptoms, or if they had a close relative with esophageal cancer [11]. Overall, 33% of persons who participated had a family history of esophageal cancer, and 48% had gastrointestinal symptoms. Similarly, in Argentina, subjects were recruited among persons attending gastroenterology clinics for various gastrointestinal symptoms [25]. The early studies in Linxian, Huixian, Fanxian, and Jiaoxian, China involved more representative samples of the population [21,22,26], whereas the later studies in Linxian [27] involved persons who had been screened positive (by balloon cytology) (see section on Detection for a description of this technique) for dysplasia approximately four years earlier.

Another issue is comparability of histologic evaluation. This issue was reviewed by Dawsey and Lewin [28], who concluded that the differences reported in the prevalence of esophagitis may largely be due to differences in definition, and that apparently small changes in criteria could result in relatively large reported differences in prevalence. Also, most of the earlier studies reported the prevalence of esophagitis independent of other abnormalities that might be present (e.g., dysplasia or cancer); whereas in the later studies, only the worst histologic diagnosis for an individual was reported [28]. In the later study in Linxian [27], only 4.6% of persons were given a diagnosis of esophagitis. However, as the study population included only persons with previous cytologic evidence of dysplasia, those with a subsequent biopsy-based diagnosis of dysplasia or cancer were not reported as having esophagitis. Thus the prevalence reported would likely be substantially higher if the same method of calculating prevalence were used as in most earlier studies. Evidence for this is the finding that in a subset of biopsies that could be examined in a second review, 17% of dysplasias and 78% of cancers showed evidence of esophagitis.

More directly addressing the usefulness of esophagitis as a precursor lesion are prospective studies that examine subsequent risk of developing more advanced lesions or cancer. One such study followed up 682 persons from Linxian who underwent endoscopy with biopsies in 1987 and did not have cancer at that time [29]. Of these, 33 had esophagitis without evidence of dysplasia. None of these developed symptomatic esophageal cancer over a period of approximately 3.5 years. However, the conclusions that can be drawn from this study are limited by the small number of subjects with "pure" esophagitis, the short follow-up time, and the requirement for symptomatic cancer as an outcome, as opposed to outcomes determined endoscopically. In a separate study of persons from high-incidence areas of China, 124 persons with chronic esophagitis (without more advanced lesions), five (4.0%) developed esophageal cancer [22]. Finally, in a study of 12,693 residents of Linxian who had been screened by balloon cytology in 1974, Dawsey et al. [27] reported 37 incident cancers occurring over 15 years of follow up among 318 persons with a baseline diagnosis of esophagitis, representing a 50% (relative risk (RR) = 1.5, 95% CI: 1.1–2.1) increase in risk compared to those with normal cytology at baseline.

In summary, esophagitis appears to be of only modest value as a precursor lesion for squamous cell carcinoma. While it is clearly quite common in high-incidence populations in China and Iran, it is also seen quite frequently in areas of China with relatively low incidence. More definitive conclusions are difficult given the methodologic problems mentioned above. The follow-up studies that have examined the predictive potential of esophagitis have been few, and suggest that it has only limited predictive ability for cancer.

In contrast, there is strong evidence that dysplasia is associated with a very high risk of subsequent esophageal squamous cell carcinoma. First, relatively large differences in prevalence between high- and low-incidence areas for esophageal cancer have been consistently reported across studies, although the absolute values of the prevalence estimates have varied widely. In studies of randomly selected participants from Huixian (high-incidence) and Fanxian (low-incidence), among men the prevalence was 36.5% and 6.0% respectively, with similar levels among women [22]. Dawsey et al. [27] reported that 22.7% of 754 subjects from Linxian had dysplasia, although it should be noted that all of them already had evidence of dysplasia from balloon cytology screening several years before their endoscopy.

The most convincing evidence regarding dysplasia originates from longitudinal studies. In one investigation from Henan province, 21 (33.9%) of 62 persons with dysplasia at baseline endoscopy developed cancer, as detected by periodic endoscopy with biopsy of visible lesions, after a period of 30 to 78 months [22]. In a follow-up study of persons in Linxian, 31 (22.0%) of 141 with dysplasia at baseline endoscopy developed symptomatic cancer over 3.5 years of follow-up, compared to 10 (1.9%) of 525 without dysplasia [29]. In comparison to persons without any histologic abnormalities at baseline endoscopy, and after adjustment for age, sex and other possible confounding variables, they reported RRs of 2.2 (95% CI: 0.7–7.5) for mild dysplasia, 15.8 (95% CI: 5.9–42.2) for moderate dysplasia, and 72.6 (95% CI: 29.8–177) for severe dysplasia. In follow up of persons

screened by balloon cytology in 1974, RRs of 1.5 (95% CI: 1.1–2.1) and 1.9 (95% CI: 1.5–2.4) were reported for "dysplasia 1" and "dysplasia 2" respectively [27].

While standardization of the definition of the various grades of dysplasia remains a problem, and the predictive value of a dysplasia varies considerably depending on the source of tissue (e.g., balloon cytology *versus* biopsy), there remains little doubt of the importance of dysplasia, particularly high-grade dysplasia, as a precursor to esophageal squamous cell carcinoma.

Cell Cycle Abnormalities

Only a few studies have investigated the prevalence of cell cycle abnormalities in the development of squamous cell carcinoma. The importance of aneuploidy is suggested by the finding of this abnormality in cancerous tissue from 21 of 23 patients, of which 7 had multiple aneuploid populations [30]. The most poorly differentiated cancers had the highest fraction of aneuploid cells. in a study of esophagectomy specimens from 80 persons with squamous cell carcinoma from Thailand, the prevalence of aneuploidy increased according to the severity of histologic abnormalities: 0% in normal or mild dysplasia, 11% in moderate dysplasia, 29% in severe dysplasia and 84% in cancer [31]. The S-phase fraction was also found to increase with increasing severity of dysplasia.

Munoz et al. [32] examined patterns of cellular proliferation within the epithelium, and reported that increased proliferation was found to reach the upper layers more frequently in biopsies from high-incidence areas than from low-incidence ones. Measurement of proliferation in Linxian biopsies using tritiated-thymidine labeling indicated somewhat higher levels in esophagitis and dysplasia than in normal esophagus [33].

Genetic Abnormalities

The tumor suppressor gene, *p53*, plays a critical role in the cell's DNA damage response pathway as well as in other processes important in maintaining genetic stability [34]. Mutations in *p53* are one of the most common genetic abnormalities detected in human solid tumors; it is estimated that approximately 50% of human solid tumors harbor at least one of over 10,000 mutations of this gene that have now been identified [35–37]. *P53* abnormalities are important in the development of esophageal cancers as well. The prevalence of *p53* mutation in squamous cell carcinomas is thought to be at least 45% [38], with frequencies as high as 84% reported [39]. Loss of function of *p53* usually occurs through mutation of one allele and loss of the other. Consistent with this is the observation that allelic loss of the *p53* locus at 17p13 also occurs quite frequently, estimated at 43% to 65% of squamous cell carcinomas [38]. Similar patterns of *p53* abnormalities are observed in high incidence areas of China as well [40–43].

There is good evidence that *p53* abnormalities occur relatively early in the neoplastic process leading to squamous cell carcinoma. Both *17p* LOH and *p53* mutations have been demonstrated in dysplastic as well as normal appearing tissue adjacent to squamous cell carcinomas [38,42,44, 45]. In some cases, multiple clones containing different *p53* mutations have been detected in nearby epithelium [38,45,46].

Another abnormality found frequently in esophageal squamous cell carcinomas is *9p* LOH [38]. *9p* LOH was detected in 57% of 93 Japanese cases [47], and in a high incidence area of China, in 88% of tumors [48]. There is some evidence that this loss targets the *p16* gene, which is involved in cell cycle regulation [46]. The *p16* gene can also be inactivated by mutation and promoter hypermethylation; each has been found in esophageal squamous cell carcinomas, although at relatively low frequencies (10–20%) [38,49,50].

An inherited susceptibility to esophageal squamous cell carcinoma has long been recognized as part of the rare tylosis syndrome (focal nonepidermolytic pamoplantar keratoderma) [4,51]. Recently, the putative susceptibility gene (*TOC*) has been mapped through linkage analysis to 17q23 [51]. Interestingly, recent studies have observed frequent allelic loss near this locus in sporadic esophageal squamous cell carcinomas. Iewaya et al. [52] examined 52 cases in a Japanese population; 37 (71%) had

17q LOH, of which 33 involved the TOC locus. Similarly, von Brevern et al. reported that 69% of 35 sporadic cases had LOH at one or more loci near *TOC* on *17q* [53]. These results suggest an important role for the *TOC* gene in cases of esophageal squamous cell carcinomas arising in the general population as well as in high-risk families.

Although several additional chromosomes have been noted to be frequent sites of allelic loss in esophageal squamous cell carcinoma, in most cases, specific tumor suppressor genes that may be targeted have not been identified [38,46,54].

In summary, strong evidence exists for *p53* mutation and *17p* LOH as important predictors of subsequent risk of progression to esophageal squamous cell carcinoma. Nevertheless, prospective studies are needed to more clearly define the role of *p53* abnormalities, including the RR associated with the abnormalities, the sequence of events leading to *17p* LOH and *p53* mutation, and their interactions with other precursor lesions, such as dysplasia and the loss of other alleles. Of the other genetic abnormalities that have been noted in tumors or in adjacent tissue, the most promising are those that appear to target the *p16* and *TOC* genes.

Adenocarcinoma

Histologic Precursors

The sequence of histologic abnormalities believed to precede esophageal adenocarcinoma is described in Figure 7.2 [55].

The prevalence of reflux esophagitis in higher-incidence areas such as the United States and western Europe is difficult to estimate since population-based screening has not been carried out. It can be estimated through indirect means, however. Among adult men and women (mean age 63) who participated in a multi-center population-based case-control study in the United States [56], 6.0% reported severe heartburn or regurgitation on a daily basis, which is similar to other estimates [12]. The reported prevalence of esophagitis among persons with symptoms of chronic reflux has ranged from 16% to more than 50% [57–60].

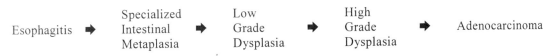

FIGURE 7.2. Sequence of histologic abnormalities in the development of esophageal adenocarcinoma.

Combining these estimates suggests a prevalence of reflux esophagitis in the general population of the United States and western Europe of between 1% and 3%, which is similar to that calculated from a Swedish study of endoscopy reports in a defined population [12,61].

Among persons with chronic reflux, an estimated 10% to 15% will develop Barrett's esophagus [62,63]. It is thought that most adenocarcinomas arise in metaplastic epithelium, although it is often difficult to identify such precursors adjacent to larger tumors [64,65]. Persons with Barrett's esophagus have long been recognized to be at high risk of adenocarcinoma, approximately 1% per year, representing a 30 to 40-fold increase over the incidence rate in the general population [66–69]. Similar or higher incidence rates of progression to other precursor lesions, including high-grade dysplasia and aneuploidy, have also been observed [67,69,70]. There is currently considerable controversy regarding the risk of developing adenocarcinoma among persons with short (less than 3 cm) segments of visible Barrett's esophagus. Available evidence suggests that a short segment does confer excess risk, although probably somewhat less than a longer segment [69]. The significance of specialized intestinal epithelium detected at the gastroesophageal junction in the absence of visible columnar epithelium is presently unknown.

The development of dysplasia implies a much higher level of risk than metaplasia alone [71]. In the largest study published thus far, the 5-year cumulative incidence of adenocarcinoma among persons with high-grade dysplasia was

estimated to be 59% (95%CI: 44–74), compared to 12.0% (95%CI: 4.0–34.0) among persons with low-grade dysplasia [70]. Among persons with Barrett's esophagus but without high-grade dysplasia, the 5-year cumulative incidence was 4.0% (95%CI: 1.6–9.0).

Cell Cycle Abnormalities

From the perspective of flow cytometry, development of esophageal adenocarcinoma occurs through a series of abnormalities described in Figure 7.3 [9,55,72,73].

Reflux esophagitis and subsequent development of metaplasia are typically associated with an increased fraction of proliferating cells, which is sometimes associated with an increased S-phase fraction [72,74,75]. Examination of the pattern of proliferation suggests that increasing severity of histologic abnormalities is associated with increased proliferation in the surface epithelium and upper crypt [74,75]. However, the utility of these early precursor lesions and their pattern of occurrence in predicting risk of subsequent adenocarcinoma has not yet been demonstrated. In contrast, there is stronger evidence that an elevated G2/4N fraction is associated with an increased risk of developing aneuploidy [73], as well as adenocarcinoma, for which a RR of 7.5 (95%CI: 4.0–14.0) has been measured [70]. Interpretation of increased G2/4N fractions is complicated by the fact that it is difficult to separate aneuploid populations with near 4N DNA content from true G2 populations [69].

There is abundant evidence implicating aneuploidy as a key precursor lesion. It is present

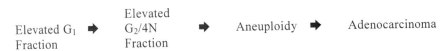

FIGURE 7.3. Sequence of flow cytometric abnormalities in the development of esophageal adenocarcinoma.

in approximately 90% of adenocarcinomas, as well as in the majority of biopsies of high-grade dysplasia [9,77,78]. It is found much less frequently in metaplasia without dysplasia or with only indefinite or low-grade dysplasia [77]. When biopsies are taken at different levels along the segment with Barrett's metaplasia, multiple clones with different aneuploid populations can be found in metaplastic and dysplastic tissue, and occasionally, identical ploidy abnormalities can be found over extensive areas [77,79]. These findings suggest that aneuploidy may be associated with an overall increase in genetic instability over a wide area (e.g., field cancerization), and that aneuploid populations may have a proliferative advantage [77]. Longitudinal follow-up of persons with aneuploid populations on one or more biopsies demonstrates a significantly higher risk of developing adenocarcinoma [69,70,80,81]. Five-year cumulative cancer incidence has been estimated at 43% (95%CI: 28–62) [70].

Genetic Abnormalities

From the genetics perspective (Figure 7.4), esophageal adenocarcinoma arises through a series of somatic genetic abnormalities, some of which lead to gene silencing or inactivation of key genes involved in the cell cycle and DNA repair [9].

Somatic abnormalities of the *p53* gene are especially common in esophageal adenocarcinoma, occurring in an estimated 90% of tumors [82–84]. As with squamous cell carcinoma, the gene is usually inactivated by mutation of one allele and loss of the other. Evidence of *p53* mutation and/or loss can be detected in approximately half of patients with high-grade dysplasia, and less frequently in low-grade/indefinite dysplasia or in uncomplicated metaplasia [85–90]. *p53* mutation and *17p* LOH can be found in diploid as well as in aneuploid cell populations suggesting that these abnormalities

may serve as relatively early markers of esophageal adenocarcinoma risk [86,91–93].

It is likely that development of *p53* abnormalities confers substantial risk of further progression to cancer. Although no large prospective studies have been published that allow estimation of cancer incidence in this group, a small study based on protein accumulation (a marker of missense *p53* mutation) reported that 5 (56%) of 9 persons with low-grade dysplasia and *p53*-positive immunohistochemistry developed high-grade dysplasia or cancer, compared with none among those with *p53*-negative biopsies [94]. Consistent with this are preliminary results from long-term follow-up of a large cohort of persons with Barrett's esophagus (described in [70]), which indicate that *17p* LOH is associated with a significant increase in risk of developing adenocarcinoma, as well as aneuploidy (B. Reid, personal communication).

Loss of function of the *p16* gene is also a very frequent occurrence in esophageal adenocarcinoma and its precursor lesions [9,95–99]. *p16* can be inactivated not only by allelic loss of the 9p21 locus, and by mutation, but by a progressive process of CpG island methylation [95,96]. *9p* LOH was found in 24 (75%) of 32 persons with aneuploidy, and was detected in endoscopies taken before the diagnosis of aneuploidy in 13 (87%) of 15 persons with available tissue [82]. Similarly, among 59 patients with high-grade dysplasia (some of whom also had aneuploidy), *9p* LOH was reported in 59% [99]. Interestingly *9p* LOH appears to occur earlier than *17p* LOH; among diploid biopsy samples with normal G2/4N fractions, *9p* LOH was found in 42%, compared to 20% with *17p* LOH [99]. Promoter methylation has been reported in 38% of aneuploid populations from persons with adenocarcinoma or precanerous lesions [98], whereas *p16* mutation tends to be found less frequently [96].

| 9p LOH | ➡ | 17p LOH | ➡ | Other LOH | ➡ | Adenocarcinoma |
| p16 inactivation | | p53 inactivation | | (5q, 13q, 18q) | | |

FIGURE 7.4. Sequence of genetic abnormalities in the development of esophageal adenocarcinoma.

Frequent losses of other chromosome arms, including *4q*, *5q*, *13q* and *18q*, have been reported in esophageal adenocarcinoma, but the gene targets of these losses have not yet been identified [9,82,100].

While it is apparent that no direct (one-to-one) correspondence exists among the histologic, cell cycle and genetic abnormalities described in Figures 7.2 through 7.4, and that no single precursor lesion is a necessary step in the development of adenocarcinoma, it is also evident that these abnormalities tend to develop together over time. This suggests that a combination of them may hold the best hope of defining high-risk subsets for clinical care research [70,86].

Etiology

Squamous Cell Carcinoma

Cancer

In the United States and other developed countries, the two major contributors to the incidence of esophageal squamous cell carcinoma are tobacco use and alcohol intake. Each has been shown to increase risk independently and in a dose-dependent manner; together they are estimated to account for 90% of cases of esophageal squamous cell carcinoma [4,101–103]. Among current smokers, the RR is approximately 5; cessation results in a relatively rapid decrease in RR to levels half that of current smokers after approximately 10 years [4,104]. Among heavy drinkers, RRs of 7 to 10 have been estimated [4,103,104]. The other major determinant of risk of squamous cell carcinoma in western countries is diet. In particular, a diet high in fruit and vegetables has been quite consistently associated with significant reduction in risk [105–107].

In contrast to western countries, the role of tobacco and alcohol in Asia is less important, and varies by region. In moderate-incidence areas, cigarette and alcohol use are still significant risk factors, but their RRs are weaker than in western countries. In Shanghai, for example,

these two factors together are estimated to account for 50% of esophageal squamous cell carcinomas [108]. However, in the high-incidence areas of China, alcohol consumption does not appear to play a significant role, and cigarette smoking is only modestly associated with cancer risk [4,109–112]. Thus the underlying reasons for the extremely high incidence in specific areas of China and Central Asia remain somewhat of a mystery. It is generally thought that overall poor nutritional status drives much of the incidence. Studies investigating nutritional deficiencies, including low intake of fruits and vegetables, have generally demonstrated an increased risk [4]. However, attempts to identify particular nutrients have not yielded clear results. Specific dietary practices, such as consumption of pickled or moldy foods containing nitrosamines or their precursors, also have been associated with increased risk in some [109,113] but not all studies [110–112]. In other pockets of high risk in South America, Iran, and elsewhere, increased risk has been documented among consumers of very hot tea and other beverages [4]. Inherited susceptibility may also play a role in certain high-risk areas [4,109–114].

A growing body of evidence indicates that aspirin and other nonsteroidal anti-inflammatory drugs (NSAIDs) may be protective against colon cancer and its precursors, probably through their inhibition of the COX-2 enzymes. More recent evidence also suggests a similar role against both types of esophageal cancer [115]. Another possible protective factor is green-tea consumption, which may act via a number of pathways [116,117].

Precursor Lesions

While a number of prevention trials have investigated precursor lesions as outcomes (see later discussion), there are few observational studies of risk factors for precursors of esophageal squamous cell carcinoma. In one of the largest studies, risk factors for esophagitis were examined in a cross-sectional study among persons aged 15 to 26 years in the high-incidence area of Huixian, China [24]. Approximately one-third of subjects were chosen from households in which a case of esophageal cancer had occurred in a first-degree relative. Esophagitis was graded visually as very mild, mild or moderate; none had severe esophagitis. In a multivariate analysis comparing subjects with mild or moderate esophagitis to those with very mild or no esophagitis, increased risk was associated with a family history of esophageal cancer (OR = 1.8; 95%CI: 1.0–3.4) and intake of very hot beverages (OR = 4.7; 95%CI: 1.8–12.3), while a decreased risk was observed for frequent intake of fresh fruits (OR = 0.3; 95%CI: 0.2–0.6) and wheat flour products (OR = 0.4; 95%CI: 0.2–0.8).

A cross-sectional study in Brazil also investigated the association between histologically confirmed esophagitis and consumption of hot beverages, in particular *maté* tea [118]. In a comparison of 30 daily consumers and 30 nonconsumers, the daily consumers had approximately a 2-fold increase in risk.

The few studies relevant to the etiology of genetic abnormalities that are precursors to esophageal squamous cell carcinoma have examined risk factors for *p53* mutations. These were based on cross-sectional analyses among persons already diagnosed with esophageal squamous cell carcinoma, under the assumption that most of the mutations occurred before the cancer [38,42,44,45]. There is some evidence to suggest that *p53* mutation occurs more frequently among persons with a history of exposure to tobacco products and alcohol. In univariate analyses of 91 cases of carcinoma available worldwide with smoking and alcohol information, *p53* mutations were found in 80% of those who smoked more than 20 cigarettes per day at the time of diagnosis, 50% of light smokers, and 20% of nonsmokers [119,120]. A somewhat higher prevalence of mutations was also found among alcohol drinkers [119]. However, the results regarding cigarettes were not supported in a study of 29 persons with esophageal squamous cell carcinoma from the high-incidence area of Guangzhou, China [40]. In this case series, *p53* mutations were found in 20 (69%), with the fraction somewhat higher in nonsmokers (7 of 9) than in smokers (13 of 20).

Thus, at present, there is no convincing evidence that tobacco or alcohol use is associated with increased risk of *p53* mutation in the esophagus.

Adenocarcinoma

Cancer

Although the rapid rise in incidence of esophageal adenocarcinoma has been recognized only since the mid-1980s, a good deal of progress has already been made in understanding its etiology. A key risk factor is gastroesophageal reflux; persons with long-term and severe symptomatic reflux experience an approximately 5-fold to 8-fold higher risk of esophageal adenocarcinoma, with a clear dose-response relationship [56,65]. Besides reflux, the strongest and most consistent risk factor is increased body mass; those in the highest quartile have an approximately 3-fold increase in risk [65,121,122]. The RRs associated with symptomatic reflux and increased body mass are little changed after adjustment for the other risk factor [65,121].

Cigarette smoking only modestly increases risk of adenocarcinoma [104,122]. Interestingly, it appears that the effect of smoking cessation does not manifest itself for 20 to 30 years, in contrast to the effect of smoking cessation on squamous cell carcinoma [104,122]. This suggests that smoking may act relatively early in the pathogenesis of adenocarcinoma, possibly by causing mutation or loss of the *p53* or *p16* genes, and that other factors, such as chronic reflux, may be important in later stages. Also in contrast to squamous cell carcinoma, there appears to be only a modest association with alcohol intake [104,122]. Several studies suggest that a diet high in fat and low in fruits and vegetables increases risk of adenocarcinoma [123,124].

Precursor Lesions

Potential causes of the gastroesophageal reflux that underlies esophagitis and Barrett's esophagus are many. Chief among them are hiatal hernia and reduced lower esophageal sphincter pressure [125]. Contributors to reduced sphincter pressure include a number of drugs that are in common use, including calcium channel blockers, certain asthma medications, and tricyclic antidepressants [126]. Overweight, a condition that is increasing markedly in prevalence in many western countries, also plays a significant role in reflux and reflux esophagitis [127–129]. This is thought to occur through increased intraabdominal pressure. Another contributor to reflux is diet. In particular, fat intake can exacerbate reflux by reducing the effectiveness of the lower esophageal sphincter, as well as delaying gastric emptying (thereby prolonging the time during which reflux can occur) [130]. Tobacco and alcohol can also increase reflux through reduced lower esophageal sphincter pressure [131].

As described previously, reflux and reflux esophagitis are common conditions in western countries. However, only a minority with chronic reflux develop the specialized intestinal metaplasia characteristic of Barrett's esophagus. The factors that determine which persons with reflux and esophagitis are likely to develop Barrett's esophagus remain largely unknown. One factor that does appear important is male gender. In particular, among all of the precursor lesions, it appears to be in the development of Barrett's esophagus that the male and Caucasian predominance characteristic of esophageal adenocarcinoma first manifests [58,132]. However, it is not known whether the male predominance at this step is explained by differing susceptibility, gender-specific exposures or a combination of the two.

Duration and severity of reflux, and cigarette use also appear to be predictors of Barrett's esophagus among persons with gastroesophageal reflux [132–134]. Consistent with these results are cross-sectional analyses from our studies of persons with Barrett's esophagus, which indicate a two-fold risk of developing Barrett's esophagus among the highest quartile of body mass index (BMI) compared to the lowest, and a 40% increase among cigarette smokers. Both animal and human data support the concept that the presence of bile in the refluxate is also associated with an increased

risk of developing Barrett's esophagus [135–137]. Some studies, but not all, have suggested that infection with *H. pylori* might be associated with reduced risk of Barrett's esophagus and esophageal adenocarcinoma, possibly through reduced acid production as a consequence of gastritis and gastric atrophy [58,125,132,138].

Among persons with Barrett's esophagus, several potential risk factors for the development of high-grade dysplasia have been identified, including size of hiatal hernia and length of the Barrett's metaplasia segment [139]. Increased Barrett's segment length has also been associated with increased risk of aneuploidy [69]. Persons with longer segment lengths may be at increased risk of more advanced lesions such as aneuploidy, high-grade dysplasia, and cancer because they have more proliferating cells, which are more vulnerable to genetic damage.

Moe et al. examined the relationship between diet and nutritional status and two proliferative abnormalities in a cross-sectional analysis of biopsies taken from persons with Barrett's esophagus [140]. Weight gain since age 25 was found to be positively correlated with the G2/4N fraction ($r = 0.39$), but there was no association between current BMI and G2/4N fraction. This suggests that persons who gain significant weight during adulthood may be at higher risk than those who were overweight since early adulthood. This might occur by causing functional changes in the effectiveness of the lower esophageal sphincter or by promoting the development of a hiatal hernia [140]. It may also reflect a lack of physical activity, with subsequent decline in GI motility and delayed gastric emptying.

In cross-sectional analyses of serum selenium concentration in 261 persons with Barrett's esophagus, we found a strong negative association (trend p-value = 0.004) between selenium levels and risk of concurrent high-grade dysplasia. A similar strong trend was found with aneuploidy, whereas the associations with other precursor lesions, including *9p* LOH, *17p* LOH, and increased G2/4N fraction were weaker. These results, while preliminary, suggest that selenium may offer its greatest protection at more advanced stages of neoplastic progression.

In preliminary analyses, we also examined NSAID use at baseline among persons with reflux and Barrett's esophagus. NSAID use appeared to be protective (OR = 0.4; 95%CI: 0.2–0.8) for development of Barrett's esophagus among persons with reflux, and also for development of *17p* LOH and aneuploidy, but not for *9p* LOH. These results were supported by short-term longitudinal analyses using aneuploidy as an endpoint.

Detection

Squamous Cell Carcinoma

An effective screening program for the detection of early esophageal squamous cell carcinoma and its precursors, using currently available technologies, requires the identification of a high-risk subpopulation in order to justify the considerable costs, inconvenience, and risk. Thus most screening efforts have focused on high incidence areas of China. Esophageal balloon cytology, which was developed in China, is one technique that has been used frequently in studies of etiology and prevention [141]. In this simple procedure, a mesh-covered balloon is swallowed, inflated, and withdrawn, with collected cells smeared onto slides before fixing and staining [141]. Thus it can be accomplished safely, quickly, and inexpensively, and with only minimal technical training.

There is some evidence that balloon cytology is effective as well. In a study of participants in a prevention trial in Linxian, China, in which this technique yielded 12,649 persons with usable slides containing squamous cells, 29% were diagnosed with dysplasia (graded 1, 2 and "near cancer"), and 2% were diagnosed with cancer [142]. Follow-up over 7.5 years revealed an increasing RR of subsequent cancer according to grade of dysplasia (ranging from 2.2–6.0) [143]. A later study in this area also found that cytologic results could identify high risk individuals [27]. However, comparison of cytologic results from balloon cytology with results from endoscopy with biopsies indicates a relatively low sensitivity for the balloon method, ranging from 14% to 47% for detecting squamous cell carcinoma or dysplasia [141,144].

In other parts of the world with lower incidence of esophageal cancer, screening of the general population using currently available techniques is not justifiable. Conceivably, screening could be effective among high-risk individuals identified on the basis of environmental exposures. In fact several studies have explored this issue. Jacob et al. [145] carried out balloon-mesh cytology on 255 asymptomatic persons with a significant history of alcohol and tobacco use, and found 37 (14.5%) with dysplasia. Short-term (maximum 36 months) follow-up with endoscopy at 6 month intervals revealed one who developed esophageal squamous cell carcinoma. Ban et al. [146] carried out endoscopy with iodine staining and targeted biopsy on 255 alcoholics in Japan. They found 10 (3.9%) with superficial squamous cell carcinoma.

Balloon cytology and endoscopy with biopsy of visible lesions are both capable of detecting early cancers as well as precursor lesions that have been demonstrated to predict subsequent cancer risk. While endoscopy with biopsy, especially when guided by mucosal iodine staining [147,148], is clearly more sensitive than balloon cytology, it is also a much more expensive and time-consuming procedure, and thus more difficult to carry out in the very areas with the highest incidence of esophageal cancer. Unfortunately, there has been little research effort, either in high-incidence areas of China or in high-risk persons elsewhere, directed towards evaluating the effect of screening programs on mortality rates, or towards evaluating the feasibility and effectiveness of periodic surveillance of persons with precursor lesions such as dysplasia. Aside from identifying worthwhile preventive interventions in these populations, screening and surveillance represent the best hope of reducing their considerable burden of esophageal squamous cell carcinoma.

Adenocarcinoma

The detection of precursors of esophageal adenocarcinoma is facilitated by the fact that a substantial proportion of high-risk persons can be identified on the basis of symptoms of gastroesophageal reflux. As described above, persons with long-standing and frequent reflux experience substantially increased risk of adenocarcinoma, roughly comparable in magnitude to the associations between heavy cigarette and alcohol use and squamous cell carcinoma [56,65]. Furthermore, the precursor lesions typically develop several years before an invasive carcinoma and thus provide a substantial time window during which they can be identified by endoscopic screening. Those persons found to have Barrett's metaplasia or other precursors can then enter a periodic surveillance program to detect the development of more advanced lesions such as *p53* mutation, high-grade dysplasia or aneuploidy [9,71,149]. The incidence of cancer associated with each precursor lesion is beginning to be estimated more precisely; when combined with information on environmental and host factors that are important during each stage of neoplastic progression, this eventually will allow a schedule of surveillance that is specific to an individual.

Unfortunately, the potential for surveillance of persons with Barrett's esophagus to detect more advanced precursor lesions and early, curable adenocarcinoma remains largely unrealized in the general population. This is evidenced by three observations: the vast majority of persons with Barrett's esophagus remain undiagnosed, virtually all new cases (over 96%) of esophageal adenocarcinoma occur in persons who had never been previously diagnosed with Barrett's esophagus, and there has been little shift in the general population towards earlier stage of diagnosis of adenocarcinoma [2,56,150].

It is notable that a sizable fraction of persons presenting with esophageal adenocarcinoma do not report a significant history of reflux symptoms [56,65]. In a large United States population-based study, 40.4% of newly diagnosed cases reported severe heartburn or acid regurgitation less than twice per year, compared to 33.8% who reported such symptoms more than twice per week [56]. Similarly, in a Swedish study of esophageal adenocarcinoma,

40% of cases reported heartburn or regurgitation less than once per week [65]. Thus, as long as investigation of reflux symptoms remains the sole avenue for identifying individuals with precursor lesions of esophageal adenocarcinoma, a large proportion will be missed.

In order to identify those with "silent" Barrett's esophagus, less invasive techniques that do not initially depend on endoscopy will need to be developed. For example, measurement of circulating p53 protein or anti-p53 antibodies has been suggested as a screening method for esophageal and other cancers [151–153]. The development of a Barrett's esophagus risk factor profile, which might include such factors as gender, ethnicity, BMI, weight change, cigarette use, and family history, in addition to reflux symptoms, might also help identify persons at risk of esophageal adenocarcinoma who would benefit from screening.

Prevention

Squamous Cell Carcinoma

Cancer

Investigations into methods of preventing squamous cell carcinoma have focused largely on high-risk populations in China. In a 6-year trial among 3,318 persons in Linxian with evidence of dysplasia from balloon cytology screening, the RR among those taking daily supplementation with 14 vitamins and 12 minerals was 0.84 (95%CI: 0.54–1.29) for esophageal cancer mortality, and 0.94 (95%CI: 0.73–1.20) for esophageal cancer incidence, compared to those taking a placebo [154]. Interim endoscopies with biopsies on a sample of participants did not show a significant reduction in the prevalence of esophageal cancer at 30 months (4.1% versus 5.3% in active versus placebo respectively) or at 72 months (4.1% versus 2.7%) [155].

In a concurrent trial in Linxian, 29,584 adults were randomized to one of 7 treatment arms containing various combinations of vitamins and minerals, or a placebo arm [156]. There was little difference in esophageal cancer mortality or incidence among the groups over a 63 month period. In this general population trial, 391 persons underwent endoscopy at the end of the study. There was a suggestion of a decreased risk (RR = 0.58; 95%CI: 0.19–1.76) among those in the arm with β-carotene, vitamin E and selenium, but not the other arms.

Precursor Lesions

The two Linxian trials also evaluated the effect of the interventions on several precursor lesions. In the dysplasia trial, interim endoscopies did not show evidence of an important protective effect on the prevalence of severe dysplasia, esophagitis, or any abnormal esophageal diagnosis, although there was a modest and nonsignificant reduction in the prevalence of any dysplasia [155]. Interim balloon cytologic examinations were also carried out at 30 and 72 months on subjects in the dysplasia trial without known cancer. While there was no evidence of a beneficial effect on cancer risk, those in the treatment arm were slightly more likely (RR = 1.2; 95%CI: 1.1–1.4) to have no evidence for dysplasia on follow up [157]. Biopsies taken at 30 months from 512 subjects in the dysplasia trial were also analyzed for proliferative activity. There was no difference by intervention status in total labeling index, although those in the active arm had a modestly lower fraction of proliferating cells in the lower layers of the epithelium [158]. In the general population trial, those on the arm with β-carotene, vitamin E and selenium had slightly higher prevalence (80.4% versus 75.2%) of a normal esophageal biopsy (i.e., no evidence of acanthosis, esophagitis or dysplasia) than those not on that arm [159]; however, there was no clear or statistically significant decrease in any particular esophageal precancerous lesion.

Several other smaller and short-term studies have investigated possible means of preventing precursor lesions or causing their regression. In a randomized trial of 610 persons selected from among the general population in Henan province who received either a once weekly supplement containing retinol, riboflavine, and zinc, or placebo, there was no difference after 1 year in the prevalence of esophagitis, atrophy or dysplasia by treatment group [32]. In another trial from the same area, 200 persons were randomized to receive either a calcium supplement or placebo, and followed with endoscopy at 11 months [160]. Again, there was no evidence of reduced prevalence of cellular proliferation abnormalities, hyperplasia or dysplasia.

Finally, in a trial in a moderately high-incidence area of Uzbekistan, 461 men with a histologic diagnosis of chronic esophagitis were randomized to one of three treatment arms containing various combinations of riboflavin, vitamin A, vitamin E and β-carotene, or a placebo group [161]. After 20 months, 292 underwent a repeat endoscopy with biopsy. Overall, no statistically significant differences were observed by treatment arm in the prevalence of esophagitis or the likelihood of progressing to a more severe form of esophagitis, although those taking a combination of retinol, β-carotene, and vitamin E were somewhat less likely to progress (OR = 0.66; 95%CI: 0.37–1.16).

Thus far, attempts to prevent progression to more advanced precursor lesions or esophageal squamous cell carcinoma in high-risk individuals have tested specific vitamins or minerals, without notable success. It now seems more likely that effective interventions will focus on improving overall diet, especially increasing daily intake of fruit and vegetables, rather than particular micronutrients. The recent decline in esophageal cancer incidence in Shanghai, by over 50% within a relatively short 18-year period, while not proven to be diet-related, suggests the unrealized potential for such an effect [162]. The recent reports suggesting protective effects of NSAIDs also suggest a prevention strategy in high-risk persons, although little is known about their effect on esophageal squamous cell carcinoma precursors. In other parts of the world, where the overwhelming role of cigarettes and alcohol in esophageal squamous cell carcinoma has been demonstrated so clearly, the possibility for substantial reduction in incidence by reducing exposure is equally clear. However there has been little research into the effects of smoking and alcohol cessation on the prevalence of dysplasia or esophagitis.

Adenocarcinoma

Prevention research on esophageal adenocarcinoma and its precursors is at an early stage, and little has been published on the subject. The interventions most likely to have a substantial impact include measures aimed at reducing reflux, such as weight loss, reduction of dietary fat, and avoidance of certain medications; measures directed towards reducing likelihood of DNA damage, such as smoking cessation, and increasing intake of foods containing selenium and other antioxidants; and increased intake of NSAIDs, especially the newer COX-2 inhibitors. Several such prevention trials among persons with Barrett's esophagus are already underway.

Conclusion

The high incidence rate of and poor survival from esophageal cancer provide a compelling rationale for identifying precursor lesions that distinguish individuals at high risk of developing invasive carcinoma. Such biomarkers are potentially useful in two major ways. First, they can be employed as intermediate outcomes for observational studies and prevention trials. Using an intermediate endpoint, as opposed to a cancer endpoint, can substantially reduce the number of participants and length of follow-up needed to test hypotheses. It can also allow the determination of the stage(s) at which specific risk factors act, which can shed light on mechanisms of action and help identify specific interventions that are most effective for a particular precancerous disease state. Second, they can identify persons who would be most likely to benefit from cancer prevention activities. These might include modification of exposure to risk or preventive factors, medical or surgical interventions aimed at eliminating precancerous lesions before they progress to cancer, and surveillance programs designed to identify cancer-

ous or near-cancerous lesions at an early, treatable stage.

References

1. Parkin DM, Pisani P, Ferlay J. Estimates of the worldwide incidence of 25 major cancers in 1990. *Int J Cancer* 1999; 80:827–41.
2. Farrow DC, Vaughan TL. Determinants of survival following the diagnosis of esophageal adenocarcinoma (United States). *Cancer Causes Control* 1996; 7:322–7.
3. Pisani P, Parkin DM, Bray F, et al. Estimates of the worldwide mortality from 25 cancers in 1990. *Int J Cancer* 1999; 83:18–29.
4. Munoz N, Day NE. Esophageal cancer. In: Schottenfeld D, Fraumeni JF Jr (eds) *Cancer epidemiology and prevention*, 2nd ed. New York: Oxford University Press, 1996, pp. 681–706.
5. Devesa SS, Blot WJ, Fraumeni JF Jr. Changing patterns in the incidence of esophageal and gastric carcinoma in the United States. *Cancer* 1998; 83:2049–53.
6. Parkin DM, Whelan SL, Ferlay J, et al. *Cancer Incidence in Five Continents Vol VII. IARC Scientific Publication No. 143*. Lyon: International Agency for Research on Cancer, 1997, p. 821.
7. Correa P. Morphology and natural history of cancer precursers. In: Schottenfeld D, Fraumeni JF Jr (eds) *Cancer epidemiology and prevention*, 2nd ed. New York: Oxford University Press, 1996, p. 45.
8. Levine DS, Blount PL, Rudolph RE, et al. Safety of a systematic endoscopic biopsy protocol in patients with Barrett's esophagus. *Am J Gastroenterol* 2000; 98:1152–7.
9. Barrett MT, Sanchez CA, Prevo LJ, et al. Evolution of neoplastic cell lineages in Barrett oesophaus. *Nature Genet.* 1992; 22:106–9.
10. Dawsey SM, Lewin KJ. Histologic precursors of squamous esophageal cancer. *Pathol Ann* 1995; 30(Pt 1):209–26.
11. Crespi M, Munoz N, Grassi A, et al. Oesophageal lesions in northern Iran: a premalignant condition? *Lancet* 1979; 2:217–21.
12. Sonnenberg A, El-Serag HB. Clinical epidemiology and natural history of gastroesophageal reflux disease. *Yale J Biol Med* 1999; 72: 81–92.
13. Lundell LR, Dent J, Bennett JR, et al. Endoscopic assessment of oesophagitis: clinical and functional correlates and further validation of the Los Angeles classification. *Gut* 1999; 45:172–80.

14. Haggitt RC. Barrett's esophagus, dysplasia, and adenocarcinoma. *Hum Pathol* 1994; 25:982–93.
15. DeMeester SR, DeMeester TR. Columnar mucosa and intestinal metaplasia of the esophagus: fifty years of controversy. *Ann Surg* 2000; 231:303–21.
16. Oberg S, Peters JH, DeMeester TR, et al. Inflammation and specialized intestinal metaplasia of cardiac mucosa is a manifestation of gastroesophageal reflux disease. *Ann Surg* 1997; 226:522–30.
17. Chandrasoma P. Pathophysiology of Barrett's esophagus. *Semin Thorac Cardiovasc Surg* 1997; 9:270–8.
18. Reid BJ, Haggitt RC, Rubin CE, et al. Observer variation in the diagnosis of dysplasia in Barrett's esophagus. *Hum Pathol* 1988; 19: 166–78.
19. Rabinovitch PS. DNA content histogram and cell-cycle analysis. *Methods Cell Biol* 1994; 41: 263–96.
20. Paulson TG, Galipeau PC, Reid BJ. Loss of heterozygosity analysis using whole genome amplification, cell sorting, and fluorescence-based PCR. *Genome Res* 1999; 9:482–91.
21. Munoz N, Crespi M, Grassi A, et al. Precursor lesions of oesophageal cancer in high-risk populations in Iran and China. *Lancet* 1982; 1:876–9.
22. Qiu SL, Yang GR. Precursor lesions of esophageal cancer in high-risk populations in Henan Province, China. *Cancer* 1988; 62:551–7.
23. Dawsey SM, Lewin KJ, Liu FS, et al. Esophageal morphology from Linxian, China. Squamous histologic findings in 754 patients. *Cancer* 1994; 73:2027–37.
24. Chang-Claude JC, Wahrendorf J, Liang QS, et al. An epidemiological study of precursor lesions of esophageal cancer among young persons in a high-risk population in Huixian, China. *Cancer Res* 1990; 50:2268–74.
25. Castelletto R, Munoz N, Landoni N, et al. Precancerous lesions of the oesophagus in Argentina: prevalence and association with tobacco and alcohol. *Int J Cancer* 1992; 51:34–7.
26. Crespi M, Munoz N, Grassi A, et al. Precursor lesions of oesophageal cancer in a low-risk population in China: comparison with high-risk populations. *Int J Cancer* 1984; 34:599–602.
27. Dawsey SM, Yu Y, Taylor PR, et al. Esophageal cytology and subsequent risk of esophageal cancer. A prospective follow-up study from Linxian, China. *Acta Cytol* 1994; 38:183–92.
28. Dawsey SM, Lewin KJ. Histologic precursors of squamous esophageal cancer. *Pathol Ann* 1995; 30(Pt 1):209–26.
29. Dawsey SM, Lewin KJ, Wang GQ, et al. Squamous esophageal histology and subsequent risk of squamous cell carcinoma of the esophagus. A prospective follow-up study from Linxian, China. *Cancer* 1994; 74:1686–92.
30. Robaszkiewicz M, Reid BJ, Volant A, et al. Flow-cytometric DNA content analysis of esophageal squamous cell carcinomas. *Gastroenterology* 1991; 101:1588–93.
31. Chanvitan A, Puttawibul P, Casson AG. Flow cytometry in squamous cell esophageal cancer and precancerous lesions. *Dis Esoph* 1997; 10: 206–10.
32. Munoz N, Wahrendorf J, Bang LJ, et al. No effect of riboflavine, retinol, and zinc on prevalence of precancerous lesions of oesophagus. Randomised double-blind intervention study in high-risk population of China. *Lancet* 1985; 2:111–4.
33. Liu FS, Dawsey SM, Wang GQ, et al. Correlation of epithelial proliferation and squamous esophageal histology in 1185 biopsies from Linxian, China. *Int J Cancer* 1993; 55:577–9.
34. Harris CC. p53 tumor suppressor gene: at the crossroads of molecular carcinogenesis, molecular epidemiology, and cancer risk assessment. *Environ Health Perspect* 1996; 104 (Suppl)3:435–9.
35. Hollstein M, Hergenhahn M, Yang Q, et al. New approaches to understanding *p53* gene tumor mutation spectra. *Mutat Res* 1999; 431:199–209.
36. Harris CC. Structure and function of the *p53* tumor suppressor gene: clues for rational cancer therapeutic strategies. *J Natl Cancer Inst* 1996; 88:1442–55.
37. Hussain SP, Harris CC. Molecular epidemiology and carcinogenesis: endogenous and exogenous carcinogens. *Mutat Res* 2000; 462:311–22.
38. Montesano R, Hollstein M, Hainaut P. Genetic alterations in esophageal cancer and their relevance to etiology and pathogenesis: a review. *Int J Cancer* 1996; 69:225–35.
39. Audrezet MP, Robaszkiewicz M, Mercier B, et al. *TP53* gene mutation profile in esophageal squamous cell carcinomas. *Cancer Res* 1993; 53:5745–9.
40. Bennett WP, von Brevern MC, Zhu SM, et al. *p53* mutations in esophageal tumors from a high incidence area of China in relation to patient diet and smoking history. *Cancer Epidemiol Biomarkers Prev* 1997; 6:963–6.

41. Liang YY, Esteve A, Martel-Planche G, et al. *p53* mutations in esophageal tumors from high-incidence areas of China. *Int J Cancer* 1995; 61:611–4.

42. Gao H, Wang LD, Zhou Q, et al. *p53* tumor suppressor gene mutation in early esophageal precancerous lesions and carcinoma among high-risk populations in Henan, China. *Cancer Res* 1994; 54:4342–6.

43. Wang GQ, Dawsey SM, Li JY, et al. Effects of vitamin/mineral supplementation on the prevalence of histological dysplasia and early cancer of the esophagus and stomach: results from the General Population Trial in Linxian, China. *Cancer Epidemiol Biomarkers Prev* 1994; 3: 161–6.

44. Bennett WP. *p53* alterations in progenitor lesions of the bronchus, esophagus, oral cavity, and colon. *Cancer Detect Prev* 1995; 19:503–11.

45. Bennett WP, Hollstein MC, Metcalf RA, et al. *p53* mutation and protein accumulation during multistage human esophageal carcinogenesis. *Cancer Res* 1992; 52:6092–7.

46. Montesano R, Hainaut P. Molecular precursor lesions in oesophageal cancer. *Cancer Surv* 1998; 32:53–68.

47. Aoki T, Mori T, Du X, et al. Allelotype study of esophageal carcinoma. *Genes, Chromosom Cancer* 1994; 10:177–82.

48. Hu N, Roth MJ, Emmert-Buck MR, et al. Allelic loss in esophageal squamous cell carcinoma patients with and without family history of supper gastrointestinal tract cancer. *Clin Cancer Res* 1999; 5:3476–82.

49. Maesawa C, Tamura G, Nishizuka S, et al. Inactivation of the *CDKN2* gene by homozygous deletion and de novo methylation is associated with advanced stage esophageal squamous cell carcinoma. *Cancer Res* 1996; 56:3875–8.

50. Esteve A, Martel-Planche G, Sylla BS, et al. Low frequency of *p16/CDKN2* gene mutations in esophageal carcinomas. *Int J Cancer* 1996; 66:301–4.

51. Kelsell DP, Risk JM, Leigh IM, et al. Close mapping of the focal non-epidermolytic palmoplantar keratoderma (*PPK*) locus associated with oesophageal cancer (*TOC*). *Hum Mol Genet* 1996; 5:857–60.

52. Iwaya T, Maesawa C, Ogasawara S, et al. Tylosis esophageal cancer locus on chromosome 17q25.1 is commonly deleted in sporadic human esophageal cancer. *Gastroenterology* 1998; 114:1206–10.

53. von Brevern M, Hollstein MC, Risk JM, et al. Loss of heterozygosity in sporadic oesophageal tumors in the tylosis oesophageal cancer (TOC) gene region of chromosome 17q. *Oncogene* 1998; 17:2101–5.

54. Hu N, Roth MJ, Polymeropolous M, et al. Identification of novel regions of allelic loss from a genomewide scan of esophageal squamous-cell carcinoma in a high-risk Chinese population. *Genes, Chromosom Cancer* 2000; 27:217–28.

55. Mueller J, Werner M, Siewert JR. Malignant progression in Barrett's esophagus: pathology and molecular biology. *Recent Results Cancer Res* 2000; 155:29–41.

56. Farrow DC, Vaughan TL, Sweeney C, et al. Gastroesophageal reflux disease, use of H_2 receptor antagonist, and risk of esophageal and gastric cancer. *Cancer Causes Control* 2000; 11:231–8.

57. Haggitt RC. Histopathology of reflux-induced esophageal and supraesophageal injuries. *Am J Med* 2000; 108 (Suppl)4a:109–11.

58. Voutilainen M, Sipponen P, Mecklin JP, et al. Gastroesophageal reflux disease: prevalence, clinical, endoscopic and histopathological findings in 1,128 consecutive patients referred for endoscopy due to dyspeptic and reflux symptoms. *Digestion* 2000; 61:6–13.

59. Stein HJ, Barlow AP, DeMeester TR, et al. Complications of gastroesophageal reflux disease. Role of the lower esophageal sphincter, esophageal acid and acid/alkaline exposure, and duodenogastric reflux. *Ann Surg* 1992; 216: 35–43.

60. Achem SR. Endoscopy-negative gastroesophageal reflux disease. The hypersensitive esophagus. *Gastroenterol Clin North Am* 1999; 28:893–904, vii.

61. Loof L, Gotell P, Elfberg B. The incidence of reflux oesophagitis. A study of endoscopy reports from a defined catchment area in Sweden. *Scand J Gastroenterol* 1993; 28:113–18.

62. Morales TG. Sampliner RE. Barrett's esophagus: update on screening, surveillance, and treatment. *Arch Intern Med* 1999; 159:1411–16.

63. Phillips RW, Wong RK. Barrett's esophagus. Natural history, incidence, etiology, and complications. *Gastroenterol Clin North Am* 1991; 20:791–816.

64. Cameron AJ, Lomboy CT, Pera M, et al. Adenocarcinoma of the esophagogastric junction and Barrett's esophagus. *Gastroenterology* 1995; 109:1541–6.

65. Lagergren J, Bergstrom R, Lindgren A, et al. Symptomatic gastroesophageal reflux as a risk

factor for esophageal adenocarcinoma. *N Engl J Med* 1999; 340:825–31.

66. O'Connor HJ. Review article: *Helicobacter pylori* and gastro-oesophageal reflux disease-clinical implications and management. *Aliment Pharmacol Therap* 1999; 13:117–27.

67. Weston AP, Badr AS. Hassanein RS. Prospective multivariate analysis of clinical, endoscopic, and histological factors predictive of the development of Barrett's multifocal high-grade dysplasia or adenocarcinoma. *Am J Gastroenterol* 1999; 94:3413–19.

68. Cameron AJ, Ott BJ, Payne WS. The incidence of adenocarcinoma in columnar-lined (Barrett's) esophagus. *N Engl J Med* 1985; 313:857–9.

69. Rudolph RE, Vaughan T, Storer BE, et al. Effect of segment length on risk for neoplastic progression in patients with Barrett esophagus. *Ann Intern Med* 2000; 132:612–20.

70. Reid BJ, Levine DS, Longton G, et al. Predictors of progression to cancer in Barrett's esophagus: baseline histology and flow cytometry identify low and high risk patient subsets. *Am J Gastroenterol* 2000; 95:1669–76.

71. Sampliner RE. Practice guidelines on the diagnosis, surveillance, and therapy of Barrett's esophagus. The Practice Parameters Committee of the American College of Gastroenterology. *Am J Gastroenterol* 1998; 93: 1028–32.

72. Reid BJ, Barrett MT, Galipeau PC, et al. Barrett's esophagus: ordering the events that lead to cancer. *Eur J Cancer Prev* 1996; 5 (Suppl 2):57–66.

73. Galipeau PC, Cowan DS, Sanchez CA, et al. 17p (p53) allelic losses, 4N (G2/tetraploid) populations, and progression to aneuploidy in Barrett's esophagus. *Proc Natl Acad Sci USA* 1996; 93:7081–4.

74. Gulizia JM, Wang H, Antonioli D, et al. Proliferative characteristics of intestinalized mucosa in the distal esophagus and gastroesophageal junction (short-segment Barrett's esophagus): a case control study. *Hum Pathol* 1999; 30:412–8.

75. Reid BJ, Sanchez CA, Blount PL, et al. Barrett's esophagus: cell cycle abnormalities in advancing stages of neoplastic progression. *Gastroenterology* 1993; 105:119–29.

76. Hong MK, Laskin WB, Herman BE, et al. Expansion of the Ki-67 proliferative compartment correlates with degree of dysplasia in Barrett's esophagus. *Cancer* 1995; 75:423–9.

77. Reid BJ. Barrett's esophagus and esophageal adenocarcinoma. *Gastroenterol Clin North Am* 1991; 20:817–34.

78. Krishnadath KK, Tilanus HW, van Blankenstein M, et al. Accumulation of genetic abnormalities during neoplastic progression in Barrett's esophagus. *Cancer Res* 1995; 55: 1971–6.

79. Rabinovitch PS, Reid BJ, Haggitt RC, et al. Progression to cancer in Barrett's esophagus is associated with genomic instability. *Lab Invest* 1989; 60:65–71.

80. Reid BJ, Blount PL, Rubin CE, et al. Flow-cytometric and histological progression to malignancy in Barrett's esophagus: prospective endoscopic surveillance of a cohort. *Gastroenterology* 1992; 102(4 Pt 1):1212–19.

81. Teodori L, Gohde W, Persiani M, et al. DNA/protein flow cytometry as a predictive marker of malignancy in dysplasia-free Barrett's esoplagus: thirteen-year follow-up study on a cohort of patients. *Cytometry* 1998; 34:257–63.

82. Barrett MT, Galipeau PC, Sanchez CA, et al. Determination of the frequency of loss of heterozygosity in esophageal adenocarcinoma by cell sorting, whole genome amplification and microsatellite polymorphisms. *Oncogene* 1996; 12:1873–8.

83. Gleeson CM, Sloan JM, McManus DT, et al. Comparison of *p53* and DNA content abnormalities in adenocarcinoma of the oesophagus and gastric cardia. *Br J Cancer* 1998; 77:277–86.

84. Hamelin R, Flejou JF, Muzeau F, et al. *TP53* gene mutations and p53 protein immunoreactivity in malignant and premalignant Barrett's esophagus. *Gastroenterology* 1994; 107:1012–8.

85. Prevo LJ, Sanchez CA, Galipeau PC, et al. *P53*-mutant clones and field effects in Barrett's esophagus. *Cancer Res* 1999; 59:4784–7.

86. Younes M, Lechago J, Chakraborty S, et al. Relationship between dysplasia, p53 protein accumulation, DNA ploidy, and Glut1 overexpression in Barrett metaplasia. *Scand J Gastroenterol* 2000; 35:131–7.

87. Campomenosi P, Conio M, Bogliolo M, et al. p53 is frequently mutated in Barrett's metaplasia of the intestinal type. *Cancer Epidemiol Biomarkers Prev* 1996; 5:559–65.

88. Gimenez A, Minguela A, Parrilla P, et al. Flow cytometric DNA analysis and p53 protein expression show a good correlation with histologic findings in patients with Barrett's esophagus. *Cancer* 1998; 83:641–51.

89. Ramel S, Reid BJ, Sanchez CA, et al. Evaluation of p53 protein expression in Barrett's esophagus by two-parameter flow cytometry. *Gastroenterology* 1992; 102(4 Pt 1):1220–8.

90. Casson AG, Manolopoulos B, Troster M, et al. Clinical implications of *p53* gene mutation in the progression of Barrett's epithelium to invasive esophageal cancer. *Am J Surg* 1994; 167:52–7.

91. Galipeau PC, Prevo LJ, Sanchez CA, et al. Clonal expansion and loss of heterozygosity at chromosomes 9p and 17p in premalignant esophageal (Barrett's) tissue. *J Natl Cancer Inst* 1999; 91:2087–95.

92. Neshat K, Sanchez CA, Galipeau PC, et al. p53 mutations in Barrett's adenocarcinoma and high-grade dysplasia. *Gastroenterology* 1994; 106:1589–95.

93. Blount PL, Galipeau PC, Sanchez CA, et al. 17p allelic losses in diploid cells of patients with Barrett's esophagus who develop aneuploidy. *Cancer Res* 1994; 54:2292–5.

94. Younes M, Ertan A, Lechago LV, et al. p53 Protein accumulation is a specific marker of malignant potential in Barrett's metaplasia. *Diges Dis Sci* 1997; 42:697–701.

95. Wong DJ, Foster SA, Galloway DA, et al. Progressive region-specific de novo methylation of the p16 CpG island in primary human mammary epithelial cell strains during escape from M-0 growth arrest. *Mol Cell Biol* 1999; 19:5642–51.

96. Barrett MT, Sanchez CA, Galipeau PC, et al. Allelic loss of *9p21* and mutation of the *CDKN2/p16* gene develop as early lesions during neoplastic progression in Barrett's esophagus. *Oncogene* 1996; 13:1867–73.

97. Tarmin L, Yin J, Zhou X, et al. Frequent loss of heterozygosity on chromosome 9 in adenocinoma and squamous cell carcinoma of the esophagus. *Cancer Res* 1994; 1;54:6094–6.

98. Wong DJ, Barrett MT, Stoger R, et al. p16INK4a promoter is hypermethylated at a high frequency in esophageal adenocarcinomas. *Cancer Res* 1997; 57:2619–22.

99. Galipeau PC, Prevo LJ, Sanchez CA, et al. Clonal expansion and loss of heterozygosity at chromosomes 9p and 17p in premalignant esophageal (Barrett's) tissue. *J Natl Cancer Inst* 1999; 91:2087–95.

100. Hammoud ZT, Kaleem Z, Cooper JD, et al. Allelotype analysis of esophageal adenocarcinomas: evidence for the involvement of sequences on the long arm of chromosome 4. *Cancer Res* 1996; 56:4499–502.

101. La Vecchia C, Negri E. The role of alcohol in oesophageal cancer in non-smokers, and of tobacco in non-drinkers. *Int J Cancer* 1989; 43:784–5.

102. Cheng KK, Duffy SW, Day NE, et al. Oesophageal cancer in never-smokers and never-drinkers. *Int J Cancer* 1995; 60:820–2.

103. Blot WJ, McLaughlin JK. The changing epidemiology of esophageal cancer. *Semin Oncol* 1999; 26 (5 Suppl 15):2–8.

104. Gammon MD, Schoenberg JB, Ahsan H, et al. Tobacco, alcohol, and socioeconomic status and adenocarcinomas of the esophagus and gastric cardia. *J Natl Cancer Inst* 1997; 89:1277–84.

105. Cheng KK, Day NE. Nutrition and esophageal cancer. *Cancer Causes Control* 1996; 7:33–40.

106. Steinmetz KA, Potter JD. Vegetables, fruit, and cancer. I. epidemiology. *Cancer Causes Control* 1991; 2:325–57.

107. Brown LM, Swanson CA, Gridley G, et al. Dietary factors and the risk of squamous cell esophageal cancer among black and white men in the United States. *Cancer Causes Control* 1998; 9:467–74.

108. Gao YT, McLaughlin JK, Blot WJ, et al. Risk factors for esophageal cancer in Shanghai, China. I. Role of cigarette smoking and alcohol drinking. *Int J Cancer* 1994; 58:192–6.

109. Wang YP, Han XY, Su W, et al. Esophageal cancer in Shanxi Province, People's Republic of China: a case-control study in high and moderate risk areas. *Cancer Causes Control* 1992; 3:107–13.

110. Li JY, Ershow AG, Chen ZJ, et al. A case-control study of cancer of the esophagus and gastric cardia in Linxian. *Int J Cancer* 1989; 43:755–61.

111. Guo W, Blot WJ, Li JY, et al. A nested case-control study of oesophageal and stomach cancers in the Linxian nutrition intervention trial. *Int J Epidemiol* 1994; 23:444–50.

112. Yu Y, Taylor PR, Li JY, et al. Retrospective cohort study of risk-factors for esophageal cancer in Linxian, People's Republic of China. *Cancer Causes Control* 1993; 4:195–202.

113. Cheng KK, Day NE, Duffy SW, et al. Pickled vegetables in the aetiology of oesophageal cancer in Hong Kong Chinese. *Lancet* 1992; 339:1314–8.

114. Hu N, Dawsey SM, Wu M, et al. Familial aggregation of oesophageal cancer in Yangcheng County, Shanxi Province, China. *Int J Epidemiol* 1992; 21:877–82.

115. Farrow DC, Vaughan TL, Hansten PD, et al. Use of aspirin and other nonsteroidal anti-

inflammatory drugs and risk of esophageal and gastric cancer. *Cancer Epidemiol Biomarkers Prev* 1998; 7:97–102.

116. Kuroda Y, Hara Y. Antimutagenic and anticarcinogenic activity of tea polyphenols. *Mutat Res* 1999; 436:69–97.

117. Gao YT, McLaughlin JK, Gridley G, et al. Risk factors for esophageal cancer in Shanghai, China. II. role of diet and nutrients. *Int J Cancer* 1994; 58:197–202.

118. Munoz N, Victora CG, Crespi M, et al. Correa P. Hot *maté* drinking and precancerous lesions of the oesophagus: an endoscopic survey in southern Brazil. *Int J Cancer* 1987; 39:708–9.

119. Montesano R, Hollstein M, Hainaut P. Genetic alterations in esophageal cancer and their relevance to etiology and pathogenesis: a review. *Int J Cancer* 1996; 69:225–35.

120. Hollstein M, Shomer B, Greenblatt M, et al. Somatic point mutations in the p53 gene of human tumors and cell lines: updated compilation. *Nucleic Acids Res* 1996; 24:141–6.

121. Chow WH, Blot WJ, Vaughan TL, et al. Body mass index and risk of adenocarcinomas of the esophagus and gastric cardia. *J Natl Cancer Inst* 1998; 90:150–5.

122. Vaughan TL, Davis S, Kristal A, et al. Obesity, alcohol and tobacco as risk factors for cancers of the esophagus and gastric cardia: Adenocarcinoma versus squamous cell carcinoma. *Cancer Epidemiol Biomarkers Prev* 1995; 4:85–92.

123. Brown LM, Swanson CA, Gridley G, et al. Adenocarcinoma of the esophagus: role of obesity and diet. *J Natl Cancer Inst* 1995; 87:104–9.

124. Kabat GC, Ng SK, Wynder EL. Tobacco, alcohol intake, and diet in relation to adenocarcinoma of the esophagus and gastric cardia. *Cancer Causes Control* 1993; 4:123–32.

125. Richter J. Do we know the cause of reflux disease? *Eur J Gastroenterol Hepatol* 1999; Suppl 1:3–9.

126. Vaughan TL, Farrow DC, Hansten PD, et al. Risk of esophageal and gastric adenocarcinomas in relation to use of calcium channel blockers, asthma drugs, and other medications that promote gastroesophageal reflux. *Cancer Epidemiol Biomarkers Prev* 1998; 7:749–56.

127. Day JP, Richter JE. Medical and surgical conditions predisposing to gastroesophageal reflux disease. *Gastroenterol Clin North Am* 1990; 19:587–607.

128. Wilson KT, Fu S, Ramanujam KS, et al. Increased expression of inducible nitric oxide synthase and cyclooxygenase-2 in Barrett's esophagus and associated adenocarcinomas. *Cancer Res* 1998; 58:2929–34.

129. Ruhl CE, Everhart JE. Overweight, but not high dietary fat intake, increases risk of gastroesophageal reflux disease hospitalization: the NHANES I Epidemiologic Followup Study. First National Health and Nutrition Examination Survey. *Ann Epidemiol* 1999; 9:424–35.

130. Becker DJ, Sinclair J, Castell DO, et al. A comparison of high and low fat meals on postprandial esophageal acid exposure. *Am J Gastroenterol* 1989; 84:782–6.

131. Orlando RC. Reflux esophagitis. In: Yamada T, et al. (eds). *Textbook of Gastroenterology* Vol. 1. 1123–47, 1991. Philadelphia: Lippincott.

132. Hirota WK, Loughney TM, Lazas DJ, et al. Specialized intestinal metaplasia, dysplasia, and cancer of the esophagus and esophagogastric junction: prevalence and clinical data. *Gastroenterology* 1999; 116:277–85.

133. Eisen GM, Sandler RS, Murray S, et al. The relationship between gastroesophageal reflux disease and its complications with Barrett's esophagus. *Am J Gastroenterol* 1997; 92:27–31.

134. Coenraad M, Masclee AA, Straathof JW, et al. Is Barrett's esophagus characterized by more pronounced acid reflux than severe esophagitis? *Am J Gastroenterol* 1998; 93:1068–72.

135. Vaezi MF, Richter JE. Bile reflux in columnar-lined esophagus. *Gastroenterol Clin North Am* 1997; 26:565–82.

136. Stein HJ, Kauer WK, Feussner H, et al. Bile reflux in benign and malignant Barrett's esophagus: effect of medical acid suppression and nissen fundoplication. *J Gastrointest Surg* 1998; 2:333–41.

137. Nehra D, Howell P, Williams CP, Pye JK, Beynon J. Toxic bile acids in gastro-oesophageal reflux disease: influence of gastric acidity. *Gut* 1999; 44:598–602.

138. Chow WH, Blaser MJ, Blot WJ, et al. An inverse relation between cagA+ strains of *Helicobacter pylori* infection and risk of esophageal and gastric cardia adenocarcinoma. *Cancer Res* 1998; 58:588–90.

139. Weston AP, Badr AS, Hassanein RS. Prospective multivariate analysis of clinical, endoscopic, and histological factors predictive of the development of Barrett's multifocal high-grade dysplasia or adenocarcinoma. *Am J Gastroenterol* 1999; 94:3413–9.

140. Moe GL, Kristal AR, Levine DS, et al. Waist-to-hip ratio, weight gain, and dietary and serum selenium are associated with DNA content flow

cytometry in Barrett's esophagus. *Nutr Cancer Int J* 2000; 36:7–13.

141. Dawsey SM, Shen Q, Nieberg RK, et al. Studies of esophageal balloon cytology in Linxian, China. *Cancer Epidemiol Biomarkers Prev* 1997; 6:121–30.

142. Shen O, Liu SF, Dawsey SM, et al. Cytologic screening for esophageal cancer: results from 12,877 subjects from a high-risk population in China. *Int J Cancer* 1993; 54:185–8.

143. Liu SF, Shen Q, Dawsey SM, et al. Esophageal balloon cytology and subsequent risk of esophageal and gastric-cardia cancer in a high-risk Chinese population. *Int J Cancer* 1994; 57:775–80.

144. Roth MJ, Liu SF, Dawsey SM, et al. Cytologic detection of esophageal squamous cell carcinoma and precursor lesions using balloon and sponge samplers in asymptomatic adults in Linxian, China. *Cancer* 1997; 80:2047–59.

145. Jacob P, Kahrilas PJ, Desai T, et al. Natural history and significance of esophageal squamous cell dysplasia. *Cancer* 1990; 65:2731–9.

146. Ban S, Toyonaga A, Harada H, et al. Iodine staining for early endoscopic detection of esophageal cancer in alcoholics. *Endoscopy* 1998; 10:253–7.

147. Dawsey SM, Fleischer DE, Wang GQ, et al. Mucosal iodine staining improves endoscopic visualization of squamous dysplasia and squamous cell carcinoma of the esophagus in Linxian, China. *Cancer* 1998; 83:220–31.

148. Freitag CP, Barros SG, Kruel CD, et al. Esophageal dysplasias are detected by endoscopy with Lugol in patients at risk for squamous cell carcinoma in southern Brazil. *Dis Esoph* 1999; 12:191–5.

149. Reid BJ, Blount PL, Feng Z, et al. Optimizing endoscopic biopsy detection of early cancers in Barrett's high-grade dysplasia. *Am J Gastroenterol* 2000; 95:3089–96.

150. Cameron AJ, Zinsmeister AR, Ballard DJ, et al. Prevalence of columnar-lined (Barrett's) esophagus. Comparison of population-based clinical and autopsy findings. *Gastroenterology* 1990; 99:918–22.

151. Soussi T. p53 Antibodies in the sera of patients with various types of cancer: a review. *Cancer Res* 2000; 60:1777–88.

152. Chiang PW, Beer DG, Wei WL, et al. Detection of *erbB-2* amplifications in tumors and sera from esophageal carcinoma patients. *Clin Cancer Res* 1999; 5:1381–6.

153. Cawley HM, Meltzer SJ, De Benedetti, et al. Anti-p53 antibodies in patients with Barrett's esophagus or esophageal carcinoma can predate cancer diagnosis. *Gastroenterology* 1998; 115:19–27.

154. Li LY, Taylor PR, Li B, et al. Nutrition intervention trials in Linxian, China: multiple vitamin/mineral supplementation, cancer incidence, and disease-specific mortality among adults with esophageal dysplasia. *J Natl Cancer Inst* 1993; 85:1492–8.

155. Dawsey SM, Wang GQ, Taylor PR, et al. Effects of vitamin/mineral supplementation on the prevalence of histological dysplasia and early cancer of the esophagus and stomach: results from the Dysplasia Trial in Linxian, China. *Cancer Epidemiol Biomarkers Prev* 1994; 3:167–72.

156. Blot WJ, Li JY, Taylor PR, et al. Nutrition intervention trials in Linxian, China: supplementation with specific vitamin/mineral combinations, cancer incidence, and disease-specific mortality in the general population. *J Natl Cancer Inst* 1993; 5:1483–92.

157. Mark SD, Liu SF, Li JY, et al. The effect of vitamin and mineral supplementation on esophageal cytology: results from the Linxian Dysplasia Trial. *Int J Cancer* 1994; 57:162–6.

158. Rao M, Liu FS, Dawsey SM, et al. Effects of vitamin/mineral supplementation on the proliferation of esophageal squamous epithelium in Linxian, China. *Cancer Epidemiol Biomarkers Prev* 1994; 3:277–9.

159. Wang GQ, Dawsey SM, Li JY, et al. Effects of vitamin/mineral supplementation on the prevalence of histological dysplasia and early cancer of the esophagus and stomach: results from the General Population Trial in Linxian, China. *Cancer Epidemiol Biomarkers Prev* 1994; 3:161–6.

160. Wang LD, Qiu SL, Yang GR, et al. A randomized double-blind intervention study on the effect of calcium supplementation on esophageal precancerous lesions in a high-risk population in China. *Cancer Epidemiol Biomarkers Prev* 1993; 2:71–8.

161. Zaridze D, Evstifeeva T, Boyle P. Chemoprevention of oral leukoplakia and chronic esophagitis in an area of high incidence of oral and esophageal cancer. *Ann Epidemiol* 1993; 3:225–34.

162. Zheng W, Jin F, Devesa SS, et al. Declining incidence is greater for esophageal than gastric cancer in Shanghai, People's Republic of China. *Br J Cancer* 1993; 68:978–82.

8
Stomach

Pelayo Correa

It has long been recognized that in most cases, gastric carcinoma develops against a background of drastically modified gastric mucosa. The original mucosa is replaced by glandular structures bearing an intestinal phenotype, namely intestinal metaplasia. Such a lesion was observed by Kupfer in 1883 [1] and later characterized in detail by pathologists in several countries [2–5]. It has also been determined that intestinal metaplasia is one of several steps in a prolonged precancerous process. The cascade of events identifiable by histopathological means consists of the following sequential steps: chronic gastritis, gland loss (atrophy), intestinal metaplasia, dysplasia and finally invasive carcinoma [6].

In 1983, Warren and Marshall published observations linking the bacterium *Helicobacter pylori* to the process of chronic gastritis [7]. This connection had been postulated as the first identifiable step in the gastric precancerous process. Since that discovery, extensive research has been conducted which has established the bacterium as a major player in the process.

Types of Gastric Carcinoma

Gastric carcinoma is not a homogenous entity. At least 5 types have been recognized by epidemiologic and histopathological means [8]. Each type differs from others in terms of its precursors. The predominant type in most countries has been described as "intestinal type" mostly because it is preceded by "intestinalization" (metaplasia) of the gastric mucosa. This chapter deals with the precursors of this type of gastric carcinoma. For the sake of completeness, the other major types will be briefly mentioned.

1. The "diffuse" type differs from the intestinal type in failing to replicate glandular structures resembling intestinal glands that are the hallmark of the intestinal type. The adhesion molecules which bind epithelial neoplastic cells to each other, allowing them to form tubular glandular structures, are either lacking or functionally defective in the neoplastic cells of the diffuse type. No clearly defined and universally accepted precursors have been reported for diffuse carcinomas. It has been postulated that the lack of adhesion molecules facilitates the spread of neoplastic cells from the site of initiation, bypassing intermediate steps which characterize other types [9].

2. The "stump" carcinoma arises in surgical gastroenteric anastomoses which favor duodenal reflux, especially the Billroth II anastomosis. The precursor lesion is characterized by polypoid formations with prominent papillary structures and dysplastic cysts which eventually become malignant and invade the muscularis propria. Such lesion has been named "gastritis cystica polyposa" [10].

3. Carcinomas associated with the pernicious anemia syndrome characteristically arise in the oxyntic mucosa which has previously become diffusely atrophic and metaplastic.

Markers of such lesions are well known, especially very high blood concentrations of gastrin and the presence of anti-parietal cell antibody [11].

4. Adenocarcinomas of the gastric cardia have been increasing in incidence in recent decades, especially in white males of affluent populations. They appear to share epidemiological features with adenocarcinomas of the lower esophagus and may not be separable from such adenocarcinomas when discovered in an advanced stage. Reflux esophagitis and Barrett's esophagus have been linked to such tumors.

Histopathology

The precancerous process for the intestinal type of gastric carcinoma consists of the following steps identifiable in histopathological terms: chronic gastritis, atrophy, intestinal metaplasia and dysplasia.

1. Chronic gastritis. The most frequent cause of chronic inflammation of the gastric mucosa is infection with *Helicobacter pylori*. Although all infected subjects have chronic gastritis identifiable in histopathological terms, there is great diversity in terms of topographic localization, intensity, mucosal damage, and leukocytic infiltrate [12]. Most infections are subclinical and presumably only display a mild infiltration by lymphocytes and plasma cells. Other patients develop nonatrophic diffuse antral gastritis (DAG) which can be accompanied by duodenal ulcer. This does not increase their risk of gastric cancer above that of the general population [13]. The type of gastritis found predominantly in populations at high risk of gastric cancer involves mainly the antrum and is associated with multifocal gland loss (multifocal atrophic gastritis, MAG). This type of gastritis may lead to intestinal metaplasia and dysplasia.

2. Intestinal metaplasia. Two types of intestinal metaplasia have been recognized. The most frequent, called complete or type I metaplasia, resembles the small intestine in that it is composed of groups of absorptive enterocytes with a brush border alternating with mucin-filled goblet cells [14]. Less frequently, all metaplastic cells resemble colon epithelium, but they have more irregularly shaped crypts lined by goblet cells of different sizes and shapes and lack a brush border [15]. This type has been called "incomplete" (because it lacks digestive enzymes) or "Type III" intestinal metaplasia. Complete metaplasia produces only sialomucins. Incomplete (Type III) metaplasia produces sialo- and sulfo-mucins [16]. Incomplete metaplasia is frequently associated with frank dysplasia and early carcinoma, and is considered by some investigators to represent some form of dysplasia.

3. Dysplasia. More advanced stages in the precancerous process are characterized by partial or complete loss of differentiation, partially manifested by decrease or loss of mucin secretion. Additionally the nuclei become enlarged, hyperchromatic, irregular in shape, and displaced towards the lumen of the gland (pseudostratification). The lesion is considered noninvasive neoplasia because its cells have neoplastic characteristics but remain within the basal membrane of the gland. When the neoplastic cells become able to penetrate the basal membrane, invasive neoplasia develops.

After many attempts to reach an international classification of dysplasia, a recent proposal from a group of gastrointestinal pathologists from Europe, Asia and the Americas provides a consensus that reconciles most of the previous semantic misunderstandings [17]. The agreement was reached in a final meeting in Padova, Italy in 1998. The Padova International Classification especially addressed differences in nomenclature between Western and Japanese pathology schools. The Western hallmark of malignancy is the stromal invasion. Japanese pathologists pay more attention to cytological aytpia. Table 8.1 displays the categories of the Padova International Classification, which will be addressed below.

The categorization "indefinite for dysplasia" is reserved for cases in which the pathologist is unable to determine whether the lesion being considered represents a neoplastic or non-

TABLE 8.1. Padova international classification of gastric dysplasia and related lesions.

1 *Negative for dysplasia*
  1.0 Normal
  1.1 Reactive foveolar hyperplasia
  1.2 Intestinal metaplasia
    1.2.1 Intestinal metaplasia, complete type
    1.2.2 Intestinal metaplasia, incomplete type

2 *Indefinite for dysplasia*
  2.1 Foveolar hyperproliferation
  2.2 Hyperproliferative intestinal metaplasia

3 *Dysplasia or noninvasive neoplasia* (flat or elevated [synonym adenoma])
  3.1 Low-grade
  3.2 High-grade
    3.2.1 Including suspicious for carcinoma without invasion (intraglandular)
    3.2.2 Including carcinoma without invasion (intraglandular)

4 *Suspicious for invasive carcinoma*

5 *Invasive carcinoma*

neoplastic cell. This situation may arise because the biopsy material provided is inadequate or because architectural distortion and nuclear atypia are present to the point of creating doubts about the dysplastic nature of the proliferating cells. In such cases, these doubts may be resolved with new, more-adequate biopsies or after removing possible sources of cellular hyperproliferation or atypia, such as *Helicobacter pylori* infection or nonsteroid anti-inflammatory drugs (NSAIDs) exposure [18,19]. In such cases, atypical, tortuous glandular structures are lined by mucus-depleted epithelial cells with large, hyperchromatic nuclei having thickened nuclear membranes and prominent nucleoli. Mitosis may be very prominent.

A similar situation arises in patients with intestinal metaplasia, usually when the metaplasia has incomplete components such as deep portions of the metaplastic glands are closely packed and lined by large irregular cells with large, hyperchromatic nuclei with frequent mitosis. Some glands show elongated and pseudostratified nuclei. Such lesions have been called "hyperplastic" or "hyperproliferative" or "deep" metaplasia. The excessive prolifer-

ative activity of such glands contrasts with the normal nuclei, which are basal, small, and normochromatic.

The term *dysplasia* has been used in publications referring to gastric precancerous lesions in Japan [20] and in Western countries. It is not part of the official Japanese classification system (Japanese Classification of Gastric Carcinoma; Japanese Research Society for Gastric Cancer, 1995). It was adopted by a World Health Organization (WHO) expert committee and has since become more accepted in some publications [21,22]. In this chapter it refers to phenotypically neoplastic epithelium confined to glandular structures inside the basement membrane. When such proliferation forms a discrete macroscopic mass that protrudes into the lumen, it is called "adenoma." In both situations, it should be divided into two subcategories: low-grade and high-grade. This dichotomy has been followed for the classification of dysplasia associated with ulcerative colitis, in which case management guidelines have been adopted for each category [23]. In general, high-grade dysplasia is equivalent to the carcinoma in situ category of squamous epithelia and has therapeutic implications of resection.

Although low-grade gastric dysplasia is not an absolute indicator for resection, the management guidelines are less clear. In low-grade dysplasia, multiple, small, round glandular structures are identified that resemble adenomatous polyps of the colon. The dysplastic glands are lined by crowded, elongated cells with large, hyperchromatic nuclei, which have been compared with cigar packs. The nuclei are pseudostratified. The secretion of mucins is minimal to none. The dysplastic cells extend to the surface epithelium, a feature absent in non-neoplastic proliferations. In high-grade dysplasia, the tubular structures are irregular in shape, with thick membranes and prominent amphophilic nucleoli. No neoplastic epithelium having any degree of stromal invasion is included in this category. For Western pathologists, invasion is the hallmark of carcinoma. For Japanese pathologists, definitive neoplastic epithelia, even in the absence of proven invasion, are grounds for a diagnosis of carcinoma. In Japan, this diagnosis may lead to endoscopic resection, which provides additional material for diagnosis. In the West, a diagnosis of carcinoma is almost always an indication for gastrectomy.

The biological forces which promote (or inhibit) the progression to more advanced stages have not been identified. There is evidence suggesting that regression from a more advanced to a less advanced stage may take place. The evidence is based on gastric biopsies taken at different time intervals.

Epidemiology

It has been shown that in most subjects, the precancerous process takes several decades. Migrant studies reported by Haenszel have shown that the risk of gastric cancer in populations is largely determined by experiences in the first years of life [24]. This "Haenszel" phenomenon was described in the 1960s; at that time it was not explainable with the available epidemiologic knowledge. An explanation is presently available, based on the epidemiology of *Helicobacter pylori* infection. Such infections are known to be acquired mostly in childhood and to persist for life in populations at high cancer risk [25]. In populations at lower risk, a "delay in the initiation" of the precancerous process has been proposed [26].

The multifocal atrophic gastritis (MAG) complex is geographically distributed similarly to gastric carcinoma. It is most frequent in East Asia (China, Japan, Korea), in Russia, in eastern and southern Europe, and in the Andean populations of Latin America.

The prevalence of MAG (atrophy and metaplasia) and its correlation with gastric cancer risk has been documented in several populations. In a comparison of autopsy specimens collected in Japan from 1958 to 1962 with autopsy specimens collected in Minnesota between 1937 and 1947, a prevalence of atrophy/metaplasia was reported in subjects 20 years of age or older of 73.60% in Japan and 21.37% in Minnesota [27]. A decrease in the prevalence of MAG has been documented in Japan in autopsy series from 1957 to 1962 compared with series from 1978 to 1980. The prevalence of metaplasia was 69.95% in the first period and 39.21% in the second. The drop in prevalence was of greater magnitude in persons under 40 years of age [28], thus following a birth cohort pattern.

In Colombia, a positive correlation has been reported between gastric cancer rates (age-adjusted to the world population) and the prevalence of atrophy and intestinal metaplasia in gastric mucosa of adults using gastroscopic biopsy series shown in Table 8.2 [29].

In China, a gastroscopic survey of adults in Shandong province shows that the prevalence of intestinal metaplasia and dysplasia is significantly greater in the high-gastric-cancer region of Linqu (30% and 15.1%) compared with the low-risk region of Cangshan (7.9% and 5.6%) ($p < 0.01$) [30].

Analytical epidemiology studies in the pre-*Helicobacter pylori* era, carried out in Japan, Hawaii, Colombia and New Orleans, identified risk factors for atrophic gastritis and intestinal

TABLE 8.2. Stomach cancer incidence and prevalence of metaplasia in gastric biopsies.

Population	Estimated cancer incidence per 100,000	Prevalence (%) of MAG[1]
High risk		
Nariño mountains	150	56.3
Low risk		
Nariño coast	40	33.3
Cali natives	23	26.3
Cartagena	6	13.4

[1] Multifocal atrophic gastritis.

metaplasia mostly related to diet. Excessive salt intake has been found to increase the risk of metaplasia. Stemmerman reported a relative risk of 6.9 (p = 0.01) for patients with extensive metaplasia in a case-control study of gastric ulcer and gastric carcinomas in Japanese from Hawaii [31]. Consistent negative associations have been reported for fresh fruits and vegetables. A case-control study of atrophic gastritis in Louisiana reported an odds ratio of 0.40, 95% CI: 0.30–0.99 associated with above-median consumption of fruits and fresh vegetables; in the same study an odds ratio of 0.40, 95% CI: 0.22–0.74 was found for vitamin C. Similar factors had been identified in studies of gastric cancer and of gastric ulcer. A positive association with smoking was reported in Louisiana (odds ratio ranging from 1.3 to 2.38 for several pack/year categories) [32]. The search for carcinogens in the diet has considered pyrolytic products in treated fish and meat, and nitrosamines in different foods. Intragastric nitrosation of amines, amides, and ureas can take place in patients with atrophic gastritis. However, definitive proof of carcinogenesis by these compounds is lacking.

Since the rediscovery of *Helicobacter pylori* and its characterization as a human pathogen [7] and especially after the recognition of this infection as a carcinogen [33], the role of this bacterium as a cancer precursor has been studied. Analytical epidemiology studies have reported positive associations with atrophy and metaplasia [32]. There is general agreement that the bacterium is the most common cause of chronic gastritis. In some populations, however, high prevalence of the infection is not accompanied by high cancer rates. This phenomenon, first described in Africa and called the "African enigma" [34], is also observed in Hindu populations and in low elevations in tropical countries. It would appear that the infection is not a sufficient cause for gastric cancer. Only when the infection leads to gland loss (MAG), does it increase cancer risk. The forces which modulate the infection may be crucial in determining a cancer outcome, and such forces may be of diverse natures. Host susceptibility may be related to the mucin geno-

type of the individual [35]. Differences in bacterial virulence may be involved, especially those associated with the Cag A and the Vac A genotypes [36]. Dietary factors are probably also involved as suggested by recent studies carried out in Shandong, China. The population in high-cancer-risk regions (Linqu) has high prevalence rates of MAG and metaplasia; low-risk regions (Cangshan) have low prevalence rates of atrophy and metaplasia, low prevalence of *Helicobacter pylori* infection, and abundant consumption of garlic [30]. Garlic extracts inhibit the growth of *Helicobacter pylori* cultures.

Helicobacter pylori infection may play a role in different stages of the precancerous process. The bacteria may damage the mucus barrier which protects the gastric mucosa, exposing it to carcinogens and irritants in the lumen. *Helicobacter pylori* infection also increases the rate of proliferation of the gastric epithelium, and lowers the concentration of ascorbic acid in the gastric juice [37]. Special attention is being given presently to the role of the inflammation brought about by the bacteria as a potential carcinogen. Inflammatory cells, especially polynuclear leukocytes and macrophages, may synthesize the enzyme inducible nitric-oxide synthase. This may result in excessive production of nitric oxides and related species which are mutagenic. They are delivered in the immediate vicinity of actively replicating epithelial cells, making the cells vulnerable to mutagenic (and carcinogenic) influences related to oxidative radicals [38,39].

Detection

Knowledge about the histopathology and epidemiology of gastric cancer precursors has been gained mostly by using techniques based on flexible fiber-optic endoscopes. They have been of great help, especially to clinicians taking care of individual patients. In Japan, where the incidence of gastric cancer is very high, extensive screening programs for the detection of early cancer have been launched.

These programs are based on double-contrast X-ray of the stomach with special mobile equipment, which is rotated to factories and other places where workers can be screened. Abnormal X-ray patterns (seen in approximately 18% of screenees) are used as indications for gastroscopy and biopsy of suspicious lesions [40,41]. This strategy has been effective in Japan, where specialized endoscopy centers are available in a large number of hospitals. In these centers, lesions suspected to be early cancer development are resected endoscopically and studied histopathologically to determine if more radical surgical procedures (gastrectomy) are required. This multistage set-up has been very successful and may account for the drastic reduction in mortality (but not incidence) rates in the country. Such screening and early detection programs have not been established in other countries where the incidence is lower and the monetary resources more limited. An attempt to establish a similar program has been made in the state of Tachina in Venezuela. A small number of early cancers has been detected and cured with surgical interventions. There is no clear evidence that it has impacted the population in terms of incidence and mortality rates [42].

Timidly, the use of other techniques for early detection of cancer and precancerous lesions has been attempted. One technique of potential value is the study of serum pepsinogens. Pepsinogen I (or A in the European literature) is secreted especially by the chief cells of the gastric corpus. Their loss in atrophic gastritis results in a gradual decrease of serum levels of pepsinogen I. Pepsinogen II is secreted by antral glands and by fovelar epithelial cells. Its levels may be increased in *Helicobacter* infection. The ratio of pepsinogen I/II has also been used as a marker of gastric atrophy. Low levels of pepsinogen I or of the I/II ratio are good indicators of extensive atrophy and intestinal metaplasia. Following up detection of low levels of pepsinogen I (or low I/II ratio) by endoscopy may lead to detection of early gastric cancers and gastric dysplasia [43]. This approach, identifying individuals at high risk, is promising in countries where endoscopy and monetary resources are limited, as well as in populations in which the incidence rates are not so high.

Prevention

Epidemiologic studies have identified the main etiologic factors in gastric cancer. Increasing the risk are mostly irritants, especially excessive dietary intake of salt (NaCl) and infection with *Helicobacter pylori*. There has been a universal tendency to decrease salt intake in most populations, mostly directed to lowering rates of hypertensive cardiovascular disease. Low risk of gastric cancer has also been linked to adequate intake of fresh vegetables and fruits.

The emphasized strategies to reduce the incidence of gastric cancer have been to control *Helicobacter pylori* infection and to increase intake of dietary antioxidants. There are approximately 10 trials being conducted at the present time in Europe, the United States, China, Japan and Latin America [44]. Some trials have cancer as an endpoint, and so require large populations followed for decades. Other trials take advantage of the fact that the different stages of the precancerous lesions have been well characterized. These trials attempt to document the effects of intervention on the dynamics of the precancerous process. Determination of progression, regression, or no change in the precancerous stages is documented by the status of the gastric mucosa before and after the intervention. This is done by comparing multiple biopsies at the two points of the study.

The only trial that has been completed and partially reported at the present time was conducted in the high-risk population of Nariño, in the Andes mountains of Colombia. Six-hundred-thirty subjects with multifocal atrophic gastritis were randomized following a 2^3 factorial design to receive triple therapy directed to *Helicobacter pylori* infection and/or dietary supplementation with antioxidant micronutrients for 6 years. The antioxidants used were ascorbic acid and/or β-carotene. Rates of progression, regression, or no change were determined by comparing histopathologic findings at baseline and at 72 months of

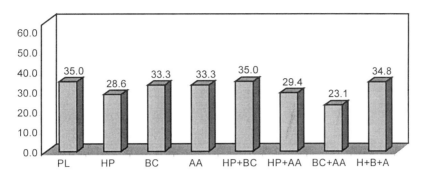

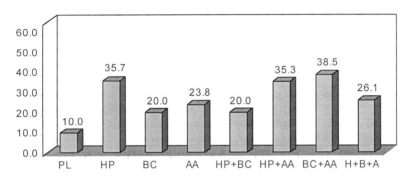

FIGURE 8.1. Progression and regression rates by treatment in subjects with non-metaplastic multifocal atrophic gastritis (MAG). PL, placebo; HP, anti-Helicobacter triple therapy; BC, β-carotene; AA, ascorbic acid. (*Source*: Correa P, Fontham ETH, Bravo JC, et al., 2000 [45], with permission.)

intervention. Figure 8.1 shows rates of progression and regression for subjects with MAG but no metaplasia. No difference was detected in progression rates but a significant higher rate of regression was seen in all groups receiving anti-*Helicobacter* treatment and/or antioxidant dietary supplementation. Figure 8.2 shows the effects of these treatments for patients with intestinal metaplasia. Significantly lower rates of progression and higher rates of regression are seen in subjects receiving the active intervention ingredients compared to placebo [45].

This study shows beneficial effects of anti-*Helicobacter* treatment and antioxidant micronutrient dietary supplementation in slowing the gastric precancerous process. The results may be useful in designing prevention strategies. At the present time, there is a debate about the cost-effectiveness of treating the infection in the general population. It has been estimated that more than half of the world population is infected with *Helicobacter pylori*. However, in the great majority of infected subjects, no identifiable disease can be linked to the infection. It would appear that there is a need to identify the subjects in whom the infection may lead to disease, especially to neoplasia.

The benefit of adequate intake of fresh vegetables and fruits has been documented for gastric cancer as well as other chronic diseases.

Progression Rates, Metaplasia Score

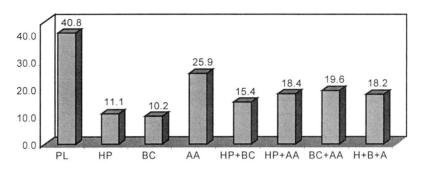

Regression Rates, Metaplasia Score

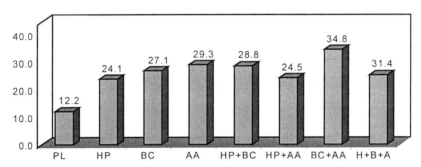

FIGURE 8.2. Progression and regression rates by treatment in subjects with MAG and intestinal metaplasia. (*Source*: Correa P, Fontham ETH, Bravo JC, et al., 2000 [45], with permission.)

Which specific antioxidants are causally associated with which disease is still incompletely understood. Whether those antioxidants should be supplied as pills or as fresh vegetables and fruits is also debatable. This author's preference is the latter.

References

1. Kupfer C. Festschrift. *Arz Verein Munch* 1883: 7.
2. Schmidt A. Untersuchungen uber des mensliche Magenepithel unter normalen und pathologischen Werhaltnissen. *Virchows Arch Pathol Anat* 1896; 143:477–508.
3. Masson P. *Tumeurs Humaines*, 1923. Kobernick O (translator). Detroit: Wayne University Press, 1970, pp. 643–6.
4. Lauren P. The two histological main types of gastric carcinoma: diffuse and so-called intestinal-type carcinoma: an attempt at a his-
   toclinical classification. *Acta Pathol Microbiol Scand* 1965; 64:31–49.
5. Michalany J. Metaplasia intestinal da mucosa gastrica. *Rev Assoc Med Brasil* 1959; 5:25–36.
6. Correa P, Haenszel W, Cuello C, et al. A model for gastric cancer epidemiology. *Lancet* 1975; 2:58–60.
7. Warren JR. Unidentified curved bacilli on gastric epithelium in active chronic gastritis (Letter to the Editor). *Lancet* 1983; i:1273 and Marshall BJ. Unidentified curved bacilli on gastric epithelium in active chronic gastritis (letter). *Lancet* 1983; i:1273–5.
8. Correa P, Chen VW. Gastric Cancer. *Cancer Surv* 1994; 19/20:55–76.
9. Tahara E. Molecular mechanisms of gastric carcinogenesis. *J Cancer Res Clin Oncol* 1983; 119:265–72.
10. Appelman H. Localized and extensive expansions of the gastric mucosa: mucosal polyps and giant folds. In: Appelman H (ed) *Pathology*

of the esophagus, stomach and duodenum. New York: Churchill Livingston, 1984, pp. 79–119.

11. Correa P. The epidemiology and pathogenesis of chronic gastritis: three etiologic entities. *Front Gastroenterol Res* 1980; 6:98–108.

12. Correa P. *Helicobacter pylori* and gastric carcinogenesis. *Am J Surg Pathol* 1995; 19 (suppl):37–43.

13. Hansson LE, Nyren O, Hsing A, et al. The risk of stomach cancer in patients with gastric or duodenal ulcer disease. *N Engl J Med* 1996; 335:242–8.

14. Filipe I, Muñoz N, Matko I, et al. Intestinal metaplasia types and the risk of gastric cancer. A cohort study in Slovenia. *Int J Cancer* 1994; 57:324–9.

15. Heilmann KL, Hopker WW. Loss of differentiation intestinal metaplasia in cancerous stomachs. A comprehensive morphologic study. *Pathol Res Pract* 1979; 164:249–58.

16. Sipponen P, Seppala K, Varis K, et al. Intestinal metaplasia with colonic type sulfomucins: its association with gastric carcinoma. *Acta Pathol Microbiol Scand* 1981; 88:217–24.

17. Rugge M, Correa P, Dixon MF, et al. Gastric dysplasia: the Padova International Classification. *Am J Surg Pathol* 2000; 24:167–76.

18. Brenes F, Ruiz B, Correa P, et al. Helicobacter pylori causes hyperproliferation of the gastric epithelium. Pre and post-eradication indices of proliferating cell nuclear antigen (PCNA). *Am J Gastroenterol* 1993; 88:1870–5.

19. el-Zimaity HM, Genta RM, Graham DY. Histological features do not define NSAID-induced gastritis. *Hum Pathol* 1996; 27:1348–54.

20. Nagayo T. Dysplasia of the gastric mucosa and its relation to the precancerous process. *Gann* 1981; 72:813–23.

21. Morson BC, Sobin LH, Grundmann E, et al. Precancerous conditions and epithelial dysplasia in the stomach. *J Clin Pathol* 1980; 33:711–21.

22. Rugge M, Farinati F, Baffa R, et al. Gastric epithelial dysplasia in the natural history of gastric cancer: a multicenter prospective follow-up study. Interdisciplinary Group on Gastric Epithelial Dysplasia. *Gastroenterology* 1994; 107:1288–96.

23. Riddell RH, Goldman H, Ransoholl DF, et al. Dysplasia in inflammatory bowel disease: standardized classification with provisional clinical applications. *Hum Pathol* 1983; 14:931–68.

24. Haenszel W, Kurihara M. Studies of Japanese migrants. Mortality from cancer and other diseases among Japanese in the United States. *J Natl Cancer Inst* 1968; 40:43–68.

25. Goodman K, Correa P. Transmission of *Helicobacter pylori* among siblings. *Lancet* 2000; 385:358–62.

26. Blaser M, Chyou DH, Nomura A. Age at establishment of *Helicobacter pylori* infection and gastric carcinoma, gastric ulcer, and duodenal ulcer risk. *Cancer Res* 1995; 55:562–5.

27. Imai T, Kub T, Watanabe H. Chronic gastritis in Japanese with reference to high incidence of gastric carcinoma. *J Natl Cancer Inst* 1971; 47: 179–95.

28. Imai T, Murayama H. Time trends in the prevalence of intestinal metaplasia in Japan. *Cancer* 1983; 52:353–61.

29. Correa P, Cuello C, Dugue E, et al. Gastric cancer in Colombia. III. natural history of precursor lesions. *J Natl Cancer Inst* 1976; 57: 1027–35.

30. You WC, Zhang L, Gail M, et al. Precancerous lesions in two counties of China with contrasting gastric cancer risk. *Int J Epidemiol* 1998; 27: 945–8.

31. Stemmerman GN, Haenszel W, Locke F. Epidemiologic pathology of gastric ulcer and gastric carcinoma among Japanese in Hawaii. *J Natl Cancer Inst* 1977; 58:13–20.

32. Fontham ETH, Ruiz B, Perez A, et al. Determinants of *Helicobacter pylori* infection and chronic gastritis. *Am J Gastroenterol* 1995; 90: 1094–101.

33. Schistosomes, liver flukes and *Helicobacter pylori*. International Agency for Research on Cancer monographs on the evaluation of carcinogenic risks to humans. Vol 61. Lyon: International Agency for Research on cancer, France, 1994, pp. 177–240.

34. Holcombe C. *Helicobacter pylori*: The African enigma. *Gut* 1999; 33:429–31.

35. Reis CA, David L, Correa P, et al. Intestinal metaplasia of human stomach displays distinct patterns of mucin (MuC1, MuC2, Mu5AC, MuC6) expression. *Cancer Res* 1999; 59:1003–7.

36. Van Doorn L, Figueiredo C, Megraud F, et al. Geographic distribution of vac A allelic types of *Helicobacter pylori*. *Gastroenterology* 1999; 116:823–30.

37. Rood JC, Ruiz B, Fontham E, et al. *Helicobacter pylori* associated gastritis and the ascorbic acid concentrations in gastric juice. *Nutr Cancer* 1994; 22:65–72.

38. Mannick EE, Bravo LE, Zarama G, et al. Inducible nitric oxide synthase, nitrotyrosine,

and apoptosis in *Helicobacter pylori* gastritis: effect of antibiotics and antioxidants. *Cancer Res* 1996; 56:3238–43.

39. Correa P, Miller MJS. Carcinogenesis, apoptosis and cell proliferation. *Br Med Bull* 1998; 54: 151–62.

40. Parkin DM, Pisani P. Gastric Cancer. In: *Cancer screening theory and practice*. Kramer BS, Gohagen JK and Prorok PC (eds) New York: Marcel Dekker Inc., 1999; pp. 516–27.

41. Miller A. Screening for gastrointestinal cancer. *Oncology* 1995; 7:373–6.

42. Pisani P, Oliver WE, Parkin DM, et al. Case-control study of gastric cancer screening. *Br J Cancer* 1994; 69:1102–5.

43. Varis K, Sipponen P, Laxen F, et al. Implications of serum pepsinogen I in early endoscopic diagnosis of gastric cancer and dysplasia. *Scand J Gastroenterol* 2000; 35:950–60.

44. Forman D. Lessons from ongoing intervention studies. In: *Helicobacter pylori. Basic mechanisms to clinical cure*. Hunt RH and Tytgat NJ (eds) Dordrecht: Kluwer Academic Publishers, 1998, pp. 354–61.

45. Correa P, Fontham ETH, Bravo JC, et al. Chemoprevention of gastric dysplasia: randomized trial of antioxidant supplements and anti-*Helicobacter pylori* therapy. *J Natl Cancer Inst* 2000; 92:1881–8.

9
Colon and Rectum

John A. Baron

Carcinogenesis pathways in the large bowel have been studied extensively, and much is known about the lesions which may develop into invasive carcinoma. It is generally thought that most colorectal cancers emerge from a progression that includes adenomatous tissue at some point in an evolution from normal mucosa to invasive cancer. However, such an "adenoma-carcinoma sequence" clearly does not explain everything: the nature of the adenomatous step can vary, and there is a possibility that colorectal cancer can develop directly from normal tissue. Moreover, nonadenomatous preinvasive tumors have been identified in the bowel (Table 9.1).

The first section of this chapter considers adenomatous polyps—the "classical" preinvasive lesion of the large bowel. Subsequent sections discuss other colorectal tumors that have been implicated in neoplastic progression.

Adenomatous Polyps

Colorectal adenomas are well-demarcated tumors of the large bowel mucosa, comprised of crypts containing cells showing features of epithelial dysplasia [1] (Figure 9.1). This histological definition implies nothing about the gross appearance of the lesion, although commonly it is polypoid, protruding into the lumen of the bowel, sometimes on a stalk. Such polyps are easily visible under endoscopy and (unless very large) can be removed endoscopically. Histologically, adenomas are usually well

demarcated from normal tissue and may display architectural disturbances such as glandular branching or infolding, reduction of stroma, or projection of frond-like villous folds from the luminal surface (Figure 9.2). The latter characteristic is used to define villous or tubulovillous histology, depending on the extent of the villous change [1].

The Adenoma-Carcinoma Sequence

It is thought that the overwhelming majority of colorectal cancers arise from adenomatous tissue. However, evidence for such an adenoma–carcinoma sequence is largely indirect. The association of adenomatous polyps with metachronous and synchronous cancers has been noted above. It is also relevant that a substantial proportion of colorectal cancers have contiguous adenomatous tissue, suggesting that the former grow out of the latter [2,3]. The distribution of adenomas within the bowel differs from that of colorectal cancer [2], but large adenomas (with a greater risk of harboring malignancy) have a site distribution similar to that of cancer [4,5]. Polyps (albeit with unknown histology) have been observed to grow in locations in which cancer was later found [6].

Perhaps the strongest evidence for the preinvasive nature of adenomatous polyps is the spectrum of somatic genetic changes seen in them. These changes fit clearly into a progression, sitting between normal mucosa and invasive carcinoma [7,8]. There is a similarly high

TABLE 9.1. Known and purported preinvasive lesions of the large bowel.

	Familial syndrome	Pathological features	Comments
Adenomas			
Adenomatous Polyp	Familial adenomatous	Decreased cytoplasmic mucin	Villous histology displays
Flat Adenoma	polyposis	Enlarged, stratified,	frondlike mucosal folds
	Flat Adenoma	hyperchromatic nuclei	
	syndrome		
Hamartomas			
Peutz-Jeghers	Peutz-Jeghers	Cytologically normal mucosal cells	It is not clear if the Peutz-
	syndrome	Crowded crypts with scant stroma	Jeghers polyps themselves
		which contains prominent	explain the increased
		muscle fascicles	colorectal cancer risk in
			affected patients
Juvenile polyp	Familial juvenile	Cytologically normal mucosal cells	Solitary juvenile polyps are
	polyposis	Extensive lamina propria,	probably not pre-invasive
		without smooth muscle	In juvenile polyposis, the
		Widely separated crypts, often	responsible mutation is in the
		large and dilated, lined with	stromal cells
		mucin-filled cells	
Other Polyp types			
Hyperplastic polyp		Mature, non-dysplastic epithelium,	Small hyperplastic polyps in the
		with mucosal infolding	rectum unlikely to be pre-
		("serratation")	invasive
			Larger, right-sided hyperplastic
			polyps may be pre-malignant
Serrated adenoma		Serrated crypt architecture with	Serrated adenomas appear to
		dysplastic epithelial cells	be related to hyperplastic
			polyps
Mixed polyp		Distinct areas of hyperplastic	
		and adenomatous tissue	

prevalence of mutation in the adenomatous polyposis coli (APC) gene in colorectal cancer and in adenomas (even small adenomas) [7,9,10]; mutations in this gene seem to be important in turning individual cells onto a dysplastic path. The prevalence of K-ras and p53 mutations increases as one considers progressively small adenomas (<1 cm), large adenomas (≥1 cm), and invasive carcinoma (40–50% of sporadic colorectal cancers) [7,10]. Various genetic changes have been seen at the transition from normal mucosa to small adenoma (APC), and from adenoma to severe dysplasia or carcinoma (p53, TGF-β in tumors with microsatellite instability) [10–12]. However, outside of genetic syndromes, substantial degrees of microsatellite instability are uncommon in adenomatous polyps [13,14].

Adenomas and carcinomas also share metabolic disturbances, including abnormalities in DNA ploidy, mucins, metabolic enzymes, and cytoskeletal proteins [15]. In each case, these changes follow what appears to be a progression of changes from normal mucosa through adenoma to carcinoma.

Assuming that colorectal cancers grow out of large adenomas, and that large polyps were first small polyps, then small adenomas can qualify as precancerous lesions. Nonetheless, except in the setting of genetic syndromes, only a small proportion of adenomas progress to carcinoma even if left in place for decades [2,16,17]. Also, some polyps (of unknown histology) regress or disappear [17–22]. It isn't known if large advanced adenomas grow from small advanced adenomas, or whether the advanced features are acquired with growth (or both). It is also not clear that all large bowel adenocarcinomas have progressed through a stage of adenoma that could be distinctly recognized as such (and potentially removed before malignant conversion) [23]. However, removing adenomatous polyps within the reach of a sigmoidoscope reduces the subsequent risk of cancer in the

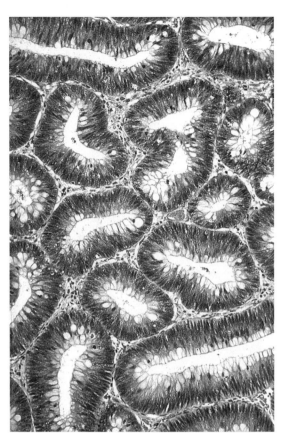

FIGURE 9.1. High-power view of tubular adenoma, with moderately dysplastic glands. Nuclei are crowded and enlarged and are seen at variable distances from the basement membrane. Mucin secretion by goblet cells is reduced in some crypts.

same region of the bowel [24–27], and hemoccult testing (presumably with detection and removal of adenomas) has been associated with a reduced risk of colorectal cancer [28]. These data provide evidence that at least a substantial proportion of cancers grew from the small adenomas detected and removed by the endoscopists.

In carriers of germline mutations in DNA mismatch repair genes [that is, in hereditary nonpolyposis colorectal cancer (HNPCC)], there is evidence that the adenoma–carcinoma sequence may be accelerated. Adenomas in mutation carriers have a higher prevalence of microsatellite instability than those in other patients, and these adenomas are more likely to occur at young ages, to be villous, and to have higher grades of dysplasia [29–31]. Molecular analysis of neoplasms in HNPCC provides powerful confirmation of the adenoma–carcinoma sequence: carcinomas and adjacent adenomatous tissue have been shown to share particular changes in DNA microsatellites [30].

Flat Adenomas

The adenoma–carcinoma sequence is a histopathological description of large bowel carcinogenesis, reflecting the progression of dysplasia to carcinoma. The term *polyp*, a gross description, has no particular histopathological meaning. The adenoma–carcinoma sequence does not necessarily imply a polyp–carcinoma sequence as well [32].

Flat adenomas are discrete areas of adenomatous tissue that are not substantially raised above the mucosal surface, with growth above the muscularis no more than two times the thickness of the normal mucosa [33,34]. Flat adenomas typically have tubular histology, with dysplastic glands superficial to nondysplastic glands, at least at the lesion periphery [34]. These adenomas have a higher prevalence of severe dysplasia than adenomatous polyps of similar size [34,35], and seem to have a more proximal distribution than polypoid adenomas [36–38]. Flat adenomas have been described to follow an hereditary pattern in the flat adenoma syndrome—a possible variant of familial adenomatous polyposis [39].

Flat adenomas have been noted most often in Asia, but have also been seen in North America and Europe [33,35,36,38]. The reasons for the differences in reported prevalences are not clear. Flat adenomas may be difficult to detect endoscopically [38], but it seems unlikely that Western endoscopists have overlooked substantial numbers of premalignant bowel tumors [33].

It is not known if flat adenomas represent a histopathological process distinct from that for polypoid or typical sessile adenomas. Flat adenomas may evolve into polypoid adenomas [40]; however, the detection of flat adenomas at

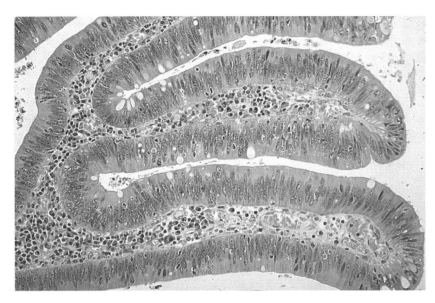

FIGURE 9.2. High-power view of a villous adenoma. Villi are covered by moderately dysplastic epithelium.

the margin of flat carcinomas suggest that at least some flat adenomas may progress to carcinoma without formation of a raised lesion [33]. Several groups of investigators have found that flat adenomas contain *ras* mutations less often than adenomatous polyps observed in the same patient series [37,41].

Flat adenomas do not necessarily suggest an alternative to the adenoma–carcinoma sequence, but the presence of small, flat invasive cancers without surrounding adenomatous tissue has raised the possibility of cancer arising from normal tissue without an intervening adenomatous stage. Flat cancers seem to lack contiguous adenoma more frequently than polypoid cancers [23,42,43], suggesting either growth de novo or very rapid substitution of the parent adenoma with invasive carcinoma. Like flat adenomas, flat cancers have been reported more frequently in Japan than in Western countries. It is possible that there are distinct disease processes in the Orient and in the West, or there may be differences in pathological interpretation [33,44]. Indeed, some Japanese investigators have labeled as "cancer" lesions confined to the mucosa [42,43,45], pathology which would be called severe dysplasia in the West.

Descriptive Epidemiology

The descriptive epidemiology of adenomatous polyps is generally similar to that of colorectal cancer. The prevalence of adenomatous polyps increases with age, and has been found to be 50% or higher after age 65 or so in high-risk populations such as the United States [46]. A male predominance may be seen at older ages [2]. The geographic variation in the prevalence of adenomas seems to be similar to that of colorectal cancer itself [2].

Colonoscopic and autopsy studies have suggested somewhat different anatomic subsite distributions for colorectal adenomas. In autopsy series, the proportion of adenomas proximal to the splenic flexure has been relatively high—sometimes greater than 60%. This is in contrast with the more distal pattern for colorectal cancer in the same geographic areas [46]. Colonoscopic studies, however, have tended to show a subsite distribution with greater proportions of tumors distal to the splenic flexure [46,47]. Both autopsy and colonoscopic studies have found the anatomic distribution of large (≥ 1 cm) or more dysplastic adenomas to more closely mirror that for cancers, with greater proportions in the descending colon, sigmoid colon, and rectum [2,4,46].

Adenomatous polyps anywhere in the large bowel indicate an increased risk of synchronous (that is, simultaneous) neoplasia elsewhere in the bowel. Individuals with adenomas in the distal bowel (for example, within the reach of a sigmoidoscope) have an increased risk of more proximal neoplasia [48,49]. Advanced adenomas—those with larger size (typically >1 cm), villous histology, or advanced dysplasia—are stronger markers of synchronous neoplasia than adenomas without such features [49–52]. Histology and number of polyps are independent predictors of risk; size probably is not [49,53]. In a high proportion of large adenomas (particularly large villous adenomas) there are foci of carcinoma [47,54,55].

An increased risk of later (metachronous) adenomas or cancer is also seen in patients with large bowel adenomas [6,53,56,57]. This excess risk is concentrated in patients with large or multiple adenomas, or with polyps that display villous histology or higher degrees of dysplasia [53,56,58–61]. Advanced histology appears to explain the association of size with risk of metachronous tumors [53,56]. The risks of later cancer in patients with adenomas has probably been understated, since risk comparisons have been made to the general population, rather than to individuals screened as intensively for colorectal cancer as the subjects with adenomas.

These data show that the association between adenomatous polyps and synchronous or metachronous neoplasia depends on the characteristics of the presenting polyp [53,62]. Advanced adenomas are associated with an increased risk of both synchronous and metachronous advanced (that is, high–risk) lesions. However, adenomas without advanced features do not seem to be strongly associated with more advanced adenomas or with cancer. Thus, it is possible that advanced and simple adenomas reflect somewhat different biological pathways.

Risk Factors for Adenomatous Polyps

In general, risk factors for adenomatous polyps closely resemble those for colorectal cancer itself [63,64]. Risk factors also seem to be similar for small adenomas and larger ones, as well as for adenomas in the proximal and distal bowel. These issues have not been well investigated, however, and some exceptions to these patterns are noted below.

Diet

In observational studies, intake of vegetables and fruits has often been inversely associated with adenoma risk. However, details have not been consistent. Some studies have found vegetable consumption to be more strongly associated with colorectal adenoma risk than intake of fruits [65–67], while others reported that fruits show a stronger association [68,69]. Findings regarding cruciferous vegetables have been conflicting, although some studies have suggested that high intake may be protective [65,66,69–71]. The association of dietary fiber intake with adenoma risk is also not clear; some studies have shown no association [72], others weak or inconsistent effects [69,70], and a few studies pronounced inverse associations with risk [65,73]. In most studies, cereals or cereal fiber have not been strongly inversely associated with risk of adenomas [65,68,69,72,74], although this has been reported [66,70,75]. Intake of refined sugar and sweets may be a risk factor [65,74].

There are some indications that dietary fat intake is directly associated with the risk of adenomas [68,73,76,77], but several studies have reported contrary findings [65,70,74,78]. Some investigations have reported that intake of saturated fat is a risk factor [75,76], but that has also been disputed [65,70]. Results regarding polyunsaturated fat have been inconsistent [65,68,70,76]. Intake of red meat or beef has had a direct association with risk of adenomas in some studies [68,75,76,79], although this has not been a universal finding [65,70,77]. Well-done meat in particular may be a risk factor [79,80].

In some epidemiological studies there have been findings suggesting that micronutrients may be related to adenoma risk. Folate intake has been reported to have a protective effect, particularly in association with high alcohol consumption [81–83]. In observational studies, calcium intake has been variably, but suggestively, related to risk of both cancer and adenomas [84,85]. Intake of carotenoids [70,81,86,87] and vitamin E [70,81,88] has not been associated with adenomas in most observational studies, although on both accounts, there have been a few dissenting reports [65,74,78,88].

Investigations of the association of estimated iron intake with risk of adenomas have not been conclusive, but in general, studies have suggested no association or a reduction in risk [65,70,74,88–90]. On the other hand, serum ferritin, a measure of iron stores, may be directly associated with risk [89–91]. Observational data regarding the association between plasma selenium and risk of adenoma are mixed [92–95].

In several studies, coffee drinking has been inversely related to colorectal adenoma occurrence [67,96–100], and also inversely related, perhaps less strongly, to rectal adenomas [67]. This has not been a universal finding [101,102], however. Tea, on the other hand, seems not to be related to adenoma risk [98–101].

Metabolic Factors and Drugs

There are clear indications that various metabolic factors are related to adenoma risk. Exercise seems inversely related to colon adenomas, but in some studies the relationship with adenomas of the rectum has been weaker than that for colonic adenomas, or even absent [63,64,67,103–107]. Although data are not entirely consistent, obesity appears to be a risk factor for colorectal adenoma [2,104,106,108–110]. Some studies have found this effect to be stronger for adenomas in more proximal portions of the large bowel [106], although others have not [104,109]. A high waist-to-hip ratio may also be a risk factor for colon adenomas, at least in men [104–106]. Cholecystectomy may also be a risk factor for colorectal adenomas, but questions of confounding by diet and obesity remain [2].

Although some investigations have reported an association between high total cholesterol levels and adenoma risk, in aggregate, the data are conflicting [111–113]. There are similar inconsistencies in findings regarding lipoprotein fractions [89,113]. Part of the reason for the varying results may be the difficulty of separating out independent associations in the face of confounding with lifestyle factors such as obesity, exercise, and alcohol intake.

In women, menopausal hormone therapy has been inversely related to risk of both colorectal cancer and large bowel adenomas [114–116]. Data regarding associations between parity or age of menopause and adenoma risk are inconsistent [114,117,118]. Use of nonsteroidal antiinflammatory drugs (NSAIDs) is very clearly inversely associated with risk of adenomas [119]. Aside from aspirin, there are little data pertaining to any one particular NSAID, but the effect seems to be one that is shared by cyclooxygenase inhibitors generally. The fact that use of acetaminophen is not similarly inversely related to risk provides reassurance that the findings are not due to bias.

Cigarette Smoking and Alcohol Intake

Cigarette smoking, particularly current smoking, has been found to be a risk factor for colorectal adenomas in most studies that have examined this issue [120–122], although there are a few dissenting reports [83,123]. Findings regarding alcohol intake have been less consistent. While some studies have shown increased adenoma risks with high alcohol intake [81,83,97,124–127], many other studies have reported only weak or frankly negative findings [65,98,102,121–123,128–133].

Genetic Factors

Relatives, particularly first-degree relatives, of patients with colorectal cancer have an increased risk of colorectal adenomas, presumably because of inherited factors [67,134–136]. Nonetheless, in several studies there have been no differences between adenoma cases and controls in reported family history of colorectal cancer [75,114,137,138].

There are only limited data available regarding the association of various metabolic polymorphisms and the risk of colorectal adenomas. Overall, N-acetyltransferase-1 or N-acetyltransferase-2 variants appear unrelated to adenoma risk [139]. Cigarette smoking seems not to modify this association substantially, but there may be a more pronounced association among individuals who eat greater amounts of red meat [139,140]. The situation regarding glutathione S-transferase M null genotype and adenoma risk is similar: there appears to be no overall association, and cigarette smoking does not appear to modify the relationship [141,142].

Methylenetetrahydrofolate reductase is an important enzyme in folate metabolism; a common polymorphism (C677T) results in enzyme thermolability [143] with reduced activity. Individuals who carry the TT genotype do not have a substantially altered risk of colorectal adenomas overall [143–145]. However, there appears to be an interaction with dietary folate intake, such that among those with higher folate intake, the TT genotype confers a lower risk, while among those with lower folate intake, that genotype is associated with a higher risk [143,144]. The mechanisms underlying such an interaction are not understood.

Prevention of Adenomatous Polyps: Clinical Trial Findings

Because adenoma patients are convenient subjects for chemoprevention trials, and since adenomas themselves are suitable endpoints for these trials [146], there have been a large number of adenoma prevention trials, almost all conducted among patients with a history of these tumors. These trials have all selected patients with a recent history of colorectal adenomas and who have no known polyps left in the bowel; subsequent adenomas are the endpoints, and typically the intervention has been applied for about 3 to 4 years. Other studies have focused on patients with familial adenomatous polyposis (FAP), many of whom had had colectomy with ileorectal anastomosis. In these investigations, typically the polyps at baseline are not removed; rather, the change in the numbers from baseline is recorded. Thus, these investigations study combined effects on existing and incident tumors.

Dietary Change or Fiber Supplements

Several adenoma prevention trials have used dietary interventions. One study of cereal fiber supplements, conducted among patients with FAP, found suggestions of benefit [147]; two others, conducted among patients with sporadic adenomas, were more or less negative [148,149]. Trials that used low-fat/high-fiber dietary instruction [150,151] or low-fat dietary advice [148] have not suggested a benefit [148, 151].

Micronutrients

Antioxidants have been used in several trials that studied patients with sporadic adenomatous polyps. β-carotene is ineffective when given for up to four years [148, 152], and vitamin E also appears to have no effect [152,153]. For vitamin C, two studies conducted among patients with FAP were essentially negative [147,154] as were two other studies of patients with sporadic adenomas [152,153]. A preliminary trial of folate supplementation suggested that there may be benefits, but the study was too small to yield statistically secure results [155].

A recent clinical trial confirmed a modest beneficial effect of calcium supplementation on adenoma occurrence. Over a 4-year treatment period, the risk of an individual having a recurrent adenoma was decreased by about 15%, and the number of adenomas reduced by around 25% [156]. A smaller European trial reported a similar relative risk reduction, although with the limited sample size, the findings were not statistically significant [157].

Nonsteroidal Antiinflammatory Drugs

With few exceptions, epidemiological studies have pointed to a chemoprotective effect of nonsteroidal antiinflammatory drugs (NSAIDs). Trials in FAP patients have uniformly found that sulindac can lead to polyp regression and prevention of new polyps [158–160]. A Cox-2 inhibitor, Celecoxib, has shown some efficacy in reducing polyp burden in FAP, although the drug is apparently less effective than sulindac [161]. In patients with sporadic adenomas, there have been some hints of efficacy in inducing regression of existing polyps, but the effect appears to be less striking than in patients with FAP [162–164]. A randomized trial of low-dose aspirin found only suggestions of a modest effect on adenomas after a mean treatment period of 5 years [165].

Prospects for (Chemo)prevention of Colorectal Adenomas

Clinical trial data, together with strong observational findings, suggest that NSAIDs may be effective agents for the prevention of colorectal neoplasia. In contrast, clinical trial data do not provide support for the idea that increased intake of fruits, vegetables, cereal fiber or antioxidants are effective chemopreventive agents in the large bowel. However, the interpretation of negative adenoma trials is not straightforward. The endpoints in these trials were small adenomas—typically less than 0.5 mm. Thus these investigations studied relatively early phases of carcinogenesis, possibly missing effects on later stages. Also, as in any clinical trial, it is possible that more intense or prolonged intervention might be required for an effect.

Screening for Colorectal Adenomas

Colorectal adenomas can easily be detected by endoscopy, and, as noted previously, there is evidence that removal of adenomatous polyps decreases the risk of subsequent invasive carcinoma. Nonetheless, colorectal screening is usually considered in terms of early detection of invasive carcinoma, with detection of adenomas a potential added benefit. Currently, it is not clear to what extent the detection of adenomas per se will reduce colorectal mortality.

The sensitivity of stool testing for occult blood is poor for adenomatous polyps: adenomas less than about 1–2 cm do not bleed enough to be detected with any reliability in this manner whatever the specific test used [166–170]. Examination of stool [171–173] and even blood [174] for mutations and other molecular changes characteristic of colorectal neoplasia holds promise for screening, but these modalities remain under development.

Hyperplastic Polyps and Serrated Adenomas

Hyperplastic polyps (HPs) are mucosal nodules, typically less than about 5 mm in diameter, that consist of focal areas of crypt elongation with intact overall mucosal architecture [175] (Figure 9.3). In unselected series, HPs are usually found in the distal bowel, especially in the rectum [176–181]. In terms of ultrastructure and cell kinetics, HPs appear to be hypermature, with a slowing of migration of cells up the crypt [175,182], and lower proliferative indices than in adenomas [183–187]. A relationship to chronic inflammation or relative ischemia has been proposed [188,189]. In general, HPs are not thought to have significant malignant potential [190], although some investigators have found them to be markers of risk of adenomas [177,179,181,191,192]. The prevalence of HPs appears to increase with age [179], although after age 50, prevalence seems not to rise [177,180].

The little research that has been published regarding risk factors for hyperplastic polyps suggests many similarities with those for adenomatous polyps. Individuals who drink alcohol or smoke cigarettes appear to have an increased risk of hyperplastic polyps [193,194]. Total dietary fiber has been inversely associated with risk [193,194], possibly because of the associated folate intake [193]. Dietary fat appears unrelated to risk [193,194], while folate and calcium may be protective micronutrients [193,194]. Obesity may be risk factor, and exercise may be protective [194].

Polyps with distinct areas of hyperplastic and adenomatous tissue are called mixed polyps (Figure 9.4). In some cases, the contiguous hyperplastic and adenomatous tissues in these polyps have shared particular microsatellite changes (with additional genetic changes in the latter) [195]. This pattern suggests that the hyperplastic tissue developed adenomatous

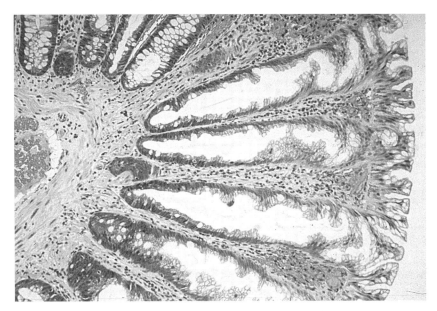

FIGURE 9.3. Medium-power view of a hyperplastic polyp. There are well-formed glands lined by well-differentiated cells and containing a high proportion of goblet cells. The serrated appearance is generated by infolding of the crowded epithelial cells, particularly evident at the luminal (top) ends of the crypts.

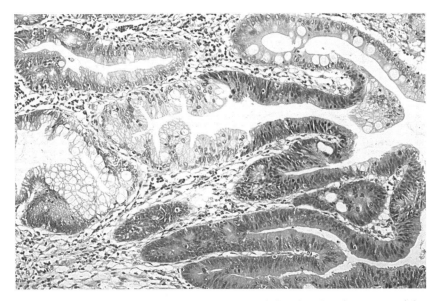

FIGURE 9.4. Medium-power view of mixed hyperplastic/tubular adenoma, showing distinct areas of hyperplastic and adenomatous tissue. In the central and lower part of the image, the hyperplastic epithelium displays numerous goblet cells and a serrated border. In the upper right, the adenomatous epithelium contains dysplastic cells with virtually no goblet cells; nuclei are pleomorphic and are at varying distances form the basement membrane.

changes, rather than vice versa. The possibility that hyperplastic polyps may evolve into neoplastic tumors is supported by repeated reports of what have been described as hyperplastic polyps with foci of dysplasia or even invasive malignancy. Some of these lesions have been identified in patients with hyperplastic polyposis—a syndrome of multiple large hyperplastic polyps in the large bowel (often in the proximal colon) and an apparent increased risk of colorectal cancer [196–203]. The dysplasia that develops in hyperplastic polyposis may evolve along a "mutator" pathway, with low or high levels of microsatellite instability [200,204]. The hyperplastic polyps themselves may have neoplastic molecular features, including K-ras mutations (<10%) [204], low levels of microsatellite instability [205], or other clonal changes [204].

Hyperplastic polyps in other settings may also have neoplastic molecular features. K-ras mutations have been seen in substantial proportions of apparently sporadic HPs [206–209], and much less commonly, mutation or overexpression of p53 [187,206,210,211]. More rarely, low levels of microsatellite instability may be seen [195,210]. Not surprisingly, in HNPCC patients, hyperplastic polyps may also have microsatellite instability [205,212].

The differences in cancer associations and molecular characteristics, between the common (that is, distal and small) hyperplastic polyps, and the larger, often more proximal tumors, in hyperplastic polyposis suggests that hyperplastic histology may be a heterogeneous category, or that other features of these tumors may have been overlooked. Indeed it has been proposed that the polyps in hyperplastic polyposis are actually a neoplastic tumor, the serrated adenoma. These tumors are characterized by the presence of hyperplastic architecture and adenomatous (dysplastic) features combined in the same histological areas (Figure 9.5). The "serrated" description derives from their appearance on low-power microscopy: these polyps share the serrated ("saw-toothed") architecture of HPs. Their endoscopic appearance resembles that of hyperplastic polyps as well [213].

Serrated adenomas (SAs) have malignant potential; carcinomatous change has been seen in these tumors [185,214,215]. The prevalence of K-ras mutations in SAs has generally been found to be low [204,215,216]. p53 overexpres-

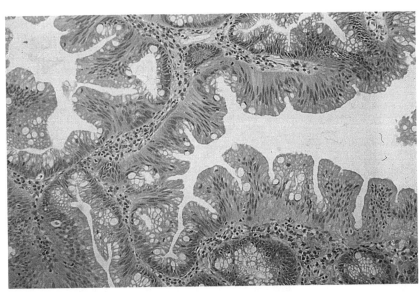

FIGURE 9.5. Medium-power view of a serrated adenoma. There is architectural complexity (branching and villosity), reduced goblet cell numbers (in comparison to a hyperplastic polyp), and nuclear characteristics as in a dysplastic polyp. Infolding ("serration") of the epithelium is evident.

sion in a substantial proportion of SAs has been reported in some series [206,211,217,218], but this has not been a consistent finding [185,187]. In one study, the same p53 mutation was seen in adenocarcinomas and in the adjacent SAs [206]. Low levels of microsatellite instability (MSI-L) have also been identified in SAs [195,219]. In terms of markers of proliferation and apoptosis, SAs resemble HPs much more than adenomas [187].

The basic epidemiology of serrated adenomas has not been well investigated, although they appear to occur predominately in the sigmoid colon and rectum [185,213,220]. In several studies, SAs have accounted for a few percent of neoplastic polyps [185,213,220], although in one smaller study from Sweden, SAs comprised 46% of all adenomas [213].

In retrospect, at least some of the polyps called "hyperplastic" in hyperplastic polyposis are likely to have been serrated adenomas [200,211]. However, the genesis of these large polyps is not clear. It is possible that small serrated adenomas grow into the large lesions that have been associated with cancer. Alternatively, but perhaps less likely [214], hyper-

plastic polyps themselves may have the potential to evolve in a neoplastic evolution, perhaps involving serrated adenomas [200].

Aberrant Crypt Foci

Aberrant crypt foci (ACF) are groups of morphologically altered crypts that are delineated from the adjacent glands, larger than normal, and often with dilated lumina [221] (Figure 9.6). The lesions are histologically heterogenous, variably including hyperplastic and dysplastic crypts. Determination of the hyperplastic/dysplastic nature of ACF may require serial sectioning, and mixed foci are common [222–224]. The multiplicity of ACF (that is, the number of crypts that they contain) can vary from one to as many as several hundred.

ACF, first described in rats treated with carcinogens, display neoplastic characteristics [223,225,226]. In experimental animals, ACF are not commonly seen in the absence of treatment with bowel carcinogens, but after such treatment, the number, size, and dysplastic

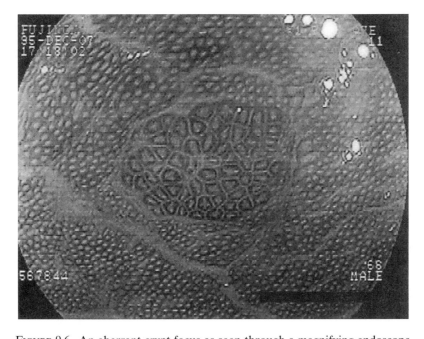

FIGURE 9.6. An aberrant crypt focus as seen through a magnifying endoscope.

characteristics of ACF increase over time. Agents that promote or inhibit colorectal carcinogenesis seem to have the corresponding effects on the number and multiplicity of the ACF [226,227]. A natural history study found that after administration of carcinogen, areas in which there were ACF were later shown to contain adenomas or carcinoma; nonetheless, some ACF clearly regressed [228]. In one large-scale investigation of various chemopreventive agents, the response of ACF to the interventions correlated reasonably well with earlier efficacy studies of the same agents [229,230].

ACF can also be seen in vivo in the human colorectal mucosa with magnifying endoscopy and methylene blue staining of the mucosa [231], particularly in patients with familial adenomatous polyposis or sporadic colorectal cancer [221,222,232,233]. The numbers of ACF are progressively higher in the more distal regions of the bowel [232,234–236], although dysplastic ACF may be preferentially found more proximally [222,237]. The endoscopic appearance of the lumina of hyperplastic and dysplastic ACF tend to be distinct [221,231,232].

In humans, ACF have been found to display characteristics of colorectal carcinogenesis. ACF with carcinoma-in-situ have been observed [224,238], and the numbers of ACF in a patient may correlate with the numbers of adenomas [231]. ACF may show monoclonality, hyperproliferation, overexpression of carcinoembryonic antigen, MSI phenotype, and acquisition of somatic mutations of APC or k-ras [186,221,234,239–242]. Indeed, k-ras mutations are very common (in various studies ranging up to 100% [221]), although APC and p53 mutations are relatively uncommon [207,221,236,243–246]. APC mutation may correlate with dysplastic histology in ACF [245].

The place of ACF in neoplastic progression has not been completely clarified. Dysplastic ACF may be precursors of adenomas, and it is possible that hyperplastic ACF may evolve into dysplastic ACF [247]. It has also been suggested that ACF are precursors of both adenomas and hyperplastic polyps [221].

Hamartomatous Polyps

A hamartoma is a tumor containing an overgrowth of mature cells and with disordered architecture and organization [248]. Hamartomatous polyps occur in the large bowel in several inherited syndromes that confer an increased risk of colorectal cancer, including Peutz-Jeghers Syndrome, Juvenile Polyposis Syndrome, and Hereditary Mixed Polyposis Syndrome [248].

The Peutz-Jeghers Syndrome is an autosomal dominant syndrome caused by a mutation in the serine/threonine kinase 11 (LKB-1/STK-11) gene on chromosome 19p. Clinically, the syndrome is characterized by abnormal mucocutaneous pigmentation and the presence of hamartomatous polyps throughout the gastrointestinal (GI) tract. In the large bowel, the polyps appear to be approximately uniformly distributed in the colon and rectum [248]. Histologically, they contain crowded crypts and a sparse stroma characterized by the prominence of smooth muscle [1] (Figure 9.7).

An increased risk of colorectal cancer in Peutz-Jeghers syndrome is accompanied by apparent increases in the risks of cancers of the duodenum, the small intestine, and probably breast and other gynecological cancers as well [249–251]. Neoplastic transformation has been observed in duodenal Peutz-Jeghers polyps as well as in those from the large bowel [252–255]. The hamartomas exhibit allelic loss at the LKB-1/STK-11 locus, suggesting that the gene functions as a tumor suppressor; the neoplastic progression occurs in the epithelium itself, apparently in a hamartoma–adenoma–carcinoma sequence [1,256,257]. However, adenomatous polyps have been found in the large bowel of patients with Peutz-Jeghers syndrome, and it is possible that some of the increased risk of large bowel cancer derives from these tumors [254,258].

Juvenile polyps are another type of hamartomatous polyp of the GI tract; these are characterized by a predominant stroma, cystic crypts, and lamina propria lacking smooth muscle [1] (Figure 9.8). These polyps may

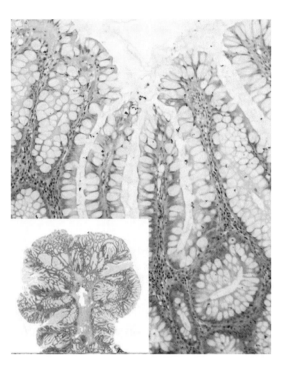

FIGURE 9.7. A: Low-power view of a polyp removed from the colon a patient with Peutz-Jegher's Syndrome. The stroma is sparse and the central core contains abundant smooth muscle. B: A high-power view of crypts from the part of the polyp shown in 9.7A. Note the normal-appearing mucosa, with many goblet cells and lack of nuclear enlargement. The nuclei are seen at a fairly uniform distance from the basement membrane.

the polyps, apparently as part of a progressive sequence from hamartoma to carcinoma [1,262,263]. In contrast to Peutz-Jeghers syndrome, the clonal genetic changes seem to occur in the stroma of the polyps, rather than in the epithelium (in which the malignancy actually develops) [248,256,264]. The genetic changes in tumors from patients with Juvenile Polyposis seem to resemble those in sporadic colorectal carcinogenesis: mutations in APC, K-ras and p53 have been seen in juvenile polyps [265].

Conclusions

Several types of colorectal lesions appear to be premalignant. The most widely recognized is the adenomatous polyp. The adenoma–carcinoma sequence is well established, and the risk factor epidemiology of colorectal adenomas resembles that of colorectal cancer. Not surprisingly, removal of adenomatous polyps appears to reduce the risk of colorectal cancer. Flat adenomas are a variant of the adenomatous polyp that do not necessarily imply any novel carcinogenic pathways. Serrated adenomas are a recently described lesion that are not well characterized epidemiologically. These polyps may participate in a variant of the adenoma–carcinoma progression. Alternatively—or in addition—these tumors may be part of an evolution that involves hyperplastic polyps.

A hamartoma–carcinoma sequence, quite distinct from the adenoma–carcinoma progression, appears to occur among individuals with Juvenile Polyposis. The underlying genetic pathology involves stromal rather than epithelial mutations. Peutz-Jeghers hamartomas seem also to be preinvasive; here the molecular progression occurs in the epithelium itself.

At this juncture, there remains uncertainty about the molecular changes in these neoplastic progressions, and how these different pathways may combine or inter-relate. Clarifying these issues will be an important step in understanding neoplasia—particularly preinvasive lesions—in the large bowel.

occur in isolation, particularly in children, and in this context have not been associated with increased risks of colorectal cancer [259,260]. In Juvenile Polyposis there are multiple juvenile polyps throughout the GI lumen, most commonly in the colorectum; this syndrome may be inherited in an autosomal dominant manner [248,260]. At least some cases of inherited Juvenile Polyposis are due to mutations in the *SMAD4* and perhaps *PTEN* genes [256] although other genes seem also to be involved in the phenotype [261].

An increased risk of carcinoma of the colorectum has been observed in Juvenile Polyposis [260]. As in Peutz-Jeghers syndrome, increasing degrees of dysplasia may be seen in

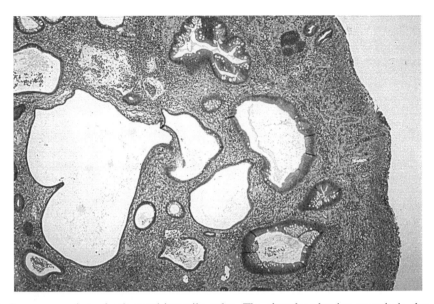

FIGURE 9.8. Low power view of colorectal juvenile polyp. The abundant lamina propria is abundant, there are cystic glands lined by non-neoplastic epithelium, and superficial ulceration is present.

References

1. Compton C. Incipient neoplasia of the large intestine. In: Henson DE, Albores-Saavedra J (eds) The pathology of incipient neoplasia. New York: Oxford University Press, 2000, pp. 174–206.
2. Peipins LA, Sandler RS. Epidemiology of colorectal adenomas. *Epidemiol Rev* 1994; 16:273–97.
3. Eide TJ. Remnants of adenomas in colorectal carcinomas. *Cancer* 1983; 51:1866–72.
4. Konishi F, Morson BC. Pathology of colorectal adenomas: a colonoscopic survey. *J Clin Pathol* 1982; 35:830–41.
5. Matek W, Hermanek P, Demling L. Is the adenoma–carcinoma sequence contradicted by the differing location of colorectal adenomas and carcinomas? *Endoscopy* 1986; 18:17–9.
6. Stryker SJ, Wolff BG, Culp CE, et al. Natural history of untreated colonic polyps. *Gastroenterology* 1987; 93:1009–13.
7. Kinzler KW, Vogelstein B. Lessons from hereditary colorectal cancer. *Cell* 1996; 87:159–70.
8. Potter JD. Colorectal cancer: molecules and populations. *J Natl Cancer Inst* 1999; 91:916–32.
9. Powell SM, Zilz N, Beazer-Barclay Y, et al. APC mutations occur early during colorectal tumorigenesis. *Nature* 1992; 359:235–7.
10. Boland CR, Sato J, Appelman HD, et al. Microallelotyping defines the sequence and tempo of allelic losses at tumour suppressor gene loci during colorectal cancer progression. *Nat Med* 1995; 1:902–9.
11. Ahuja N, Li Q, Mohan AL, et al. Aging and DNA methylation in colorectal mucosa and cancer. *Cancer Res* 1998; 58:5489–94.
12. Grady WM, Rajput A, Myeroff L, et al. Mutation of the type II transforming growth factor-beta receptor is coincident with the transformation of human colon adenomas to malignant carcinomas. *Cancer Res* 1998; 58: 3101–4.
13. Samowitz WS, Slattery ML. Microsatellite instability in colorectal adenomas. *Gastroenterology* 1997; 112:1515–19.
14. Young J, Leggett B, Gustafson C, et al. Genomic instability occurs in colorectal carcinomas but not in adenomas. *Hum Mutat* 1993; 2: 351–4.
15. Tierney RP, Ballantyne GH, Modlin IM. The adenoma to carcinoma sequence. *Surg Gynecol Obstet* 1990; 171:81–94.
16. Eide TJ. Risk of colorectal cancer in adenoma-bearing individuals within a defined population. *Int J Cancer* 1986; 38:173–6.
17. Knoernschild H. Growth rate and malignant potential of colonic polyps: early results. *Surg Forum* 1963; 14:137.

18. Welin S, Youker J, Spratt J. The rates and patterns of growth of 375 tumors of the large intestine and rectum observed serially by double contrast enema study (Malmo technique). *Am J Roentgenol Radium Ther Nucl Med* 1963; 90:673–87.
19. Nicholls RJ, Springall RG, Gallagher P. Regression of rectal adenomas after colectomy and ileorectal anastomosis for familial adenomatous polyposis. *Br Med J Clin Res Ed* 1988; 296:1707–8.
20. Hofstad B, Vatn M, Larsen S, et al. Growth of colorectal polyps: recovery and evaluation of unresected polyps of less than 10 mm, 1 year after detection. *Scand J Gastroenterol* 1994; 29:640–5.
21. Cole JW, Holden WD, Cleveland MD. Postcolectomy regression of adenomatous polyps of the rectum. *AMA Arch Surg* 1959; 41:385–92.
22. Hoff G, Foerster A, Vatn MH, et al. Epidemiology of polyps in the rectum and colon. Recovery and evaluation of unresected polyps 2 years after detection. *Scand J Gastroenterol* 1986; 21:853–62.
23. Bedenne L, Faivre J, Boutron MC, et al. Adenoma–carcinoma sequence or "de novo" carcinogenesis? A study of adenomatous remnants in a population-based series of large bowel cancers. *Cancer* 1992; 69:883–8.
24. Murakami R, Tsukuma H, Kanamori S, et al. Natural history of colorectal polyps and the effect of polypectomy on occurrence of subsequent cancer. *Int J Cancer* 1990; 46:159–64.
25. Selby JV, Friedman GD, Quesenberry CP Jr, et al. A case-control study of screening sigmoidoscopy and mortality from colorectal cancer. *N Engl J Med* 1992; 326:653–7.
26. Muller AD, Sonnenberg A. Prevention of colorectal cancer by flexible endoscopy and polypectomy. A case-control study of 32,702 veterans. *Ann Int Med* 1995; 123:904–10.
27. Newcomb PA, Norfleet RG, Storer BE, et al. Screening sigmoidoscopy and colorectal cancer mortality. *J Natl Cancer Inst* 1992; 84:1572–5.
28. Mandel JS, Church TR, Bond JH, et al. The effect of fecal occult-blood screening on the incidence of colorectal cancer. *N Engl J Med* 1603; 343:1603–7.
29. Ahlquist DA. Aggressive polyps in hereditary nonpolyposis colorectal cancer: targets for screening. *Gastroenterology* 1995; 108:1590–2.
30. Jacoby RF, Marshall DJ, Kailas S, et al. Genetic instability associated with adenoma to carcinoma progression in hereditary nonpolyposis colon cancer. *Gastroenterology* 1995; 109:73–82.
31. Jarvinen HJ, Aarnio M, Mustonen H, et al. Controlled 15-year trial on screening for colorectal cancer in families with hereditary nonpolyposis colorectal cancer. *Gastroenterology* 2000; 118: 829–34.
32. Morson BC. The polyp story. *Postgrad Med J* 1984; 60:820–4.
33. Owen DA. Flat adenoma, flat carcinoma, and de novo carcinoma of the colon. *Cancer* 1996; 77:3–6.
34. Muto T, Kamiya J, Sawada T, et al. Small "flat adenoma" of the large bowel with special reference to its clinicopathologic features. *Dis Colon Rectum* 1985; 28:847–51.
35. Wolber RA, Owen DA. Flat adenomas of the colon. *Hum Pathol* 1991; 22:70–4.
36. Lanspa SJ, Rouse J, Smyrk T, et al. Epidemiologic characteristics of the flat adenoma of Muto. A prospective study. *Dis Colon Rectum* 1992; 35:543–6.
37. Fujimori T, Satonaka K, Yamamura-Idei Y, et al. Non-involvement of ras mutations in flat colorectal adenomas and carcinomas. *Int J Cancer* 1994; 57:51–5.
38. Jaramillo E, Watanabe M, Slezak P, et al. Flat neoplastic lesions of the colon and rectum detected by high-resolution video endoscopy and chromoscopy. *Gastrointest Endosc* 1995; 42:114–22.
39. Lynch HT, Smyrk TC, Watson P, et al. Hereditary flat adenoma syndrome: a variant of familial adenomatous polyposis? *Dis Colon Rectum* 1992; 35:411–21.
40. Kubota O, Kino I. Minute adenomas of the depressed type in familial adenomatous polyposis of the colon. A pathway to ordinary polypoid adenomas. *Cancer* 1993; 72:1159–64.
41. Yamagata S, Muto T, Uchida Y, et al. Lower incidence of K-ras codon 12 mutation in flat colorectal adenomas than in polypoid adenomas. *Jap J Cancer Res* 1994; 85:147–51.
42. Shimoda T, Ikegami M, Fujisaki J, et al. Early colorectal carcinoma with special reference to its development de novo. *Cancer* 1989; 64:1138–46.
43. Kuramoto S, Oohara T. How do colorectal cancers develop? *Cancer* 1995; 75 (6 Suppl): 1534–8.
44. Driman DK, Riddell RH. Flat adenomas and flat carcinomas: do you see what I see? [editorial]. *Gastrointest Endosc* 1994; 40:106–9.

45. Minamoto T, Sawaguchi K, Ohta T, et al. Superficial-type adenomas and adenocarcinomas of the colon and rectum: a comparative morphological study. *Gastroenterology* 1994; 106:1436–43.

46. Neugut AI, Jacobson JS, DeVivo I. Epidemiology of colorectal adenomatous polyps. *Cancer Epidemiol Biomarkers Prev* 1993; 2: 159–76.

47. Shinya H, Wolff WI. Morphology, anatomic distribution and cancer potential of colonic polyps. *Ann Surg* 1979; 190:679–83.

48. Lieberman DA, Smith FW. Screening for colon malignancy with colonoscopy. *Am J Gastroenterol* 1991; 86:946–51.

49. Levin TR, Palitz A, Grossman S, et al. Predicting advanced proximal colonic neoplasia with screening sigmoidoscopy. *JAMA* 1999; 281: 1611–7.

50. Schoen RE, Corle D, Cranston L, et al. Is colonoscopy needed for the nonadvanced adenoma found on sigmoidoscopy? The Polyp Prevention Trial. *Gastroenterology* 1998; 115: 533–41.

51. Wallace MB, Kemp JA, Trnka YM, et al. Is colonoscopy indicated for small adenomas found by screening flexible sigmoidoscopy? *Ann Int Med* 1998; 129:273–8.

52. Zarchy TM, Ershoff D. Do characteristics of adenomas on flexible sigmoidoscopy predict advanced lesions on baseline colonoscopy? *Gastroenterology* 1994; 106:1501–4.

53. Atkin WS, Morson BC, Cuzick J. Long-term risk of colorectal cancer after excision of rectosigmoid adenomas. *N Engl J Med* 1992; 326:658–62.

54. Gatteschi B, Costantini M, Bruzzi P, et al. Univariate and multivariate analyses of the relationship between adenocarcinoma and solitary and multiple adenomas in colorectal adenoma patients. *Int J Cancer* 1991; 49:509–12.

55. Muto T, Bussey HJ, Morson BC. The evolution of cancer of the colon and rectum. *Cancer* 1975; 36:2251–70.

56. Simons BD, Morrison AS, Lev R, et al. Relationship of polyps to cancer of the large intestine. *J Natl Cancer Inst* 1992; 84:962–6.

57. Lotfi AM, Spencer RJ, Ilstrup DM, et al. Colorectal polyps and the risk of subsequent carcinoma. *Mayo Clinic Proc* 1986; 61:337–43.

58. Yang G, Zheng W, Sun QR, et al. Pathologic features of initial adenomas as predictors for metachronous adenomas of the rectum. *J Natl Cancer Inst* 1998; 90:1661–5.

59. Winawer SJ, Zauber AG, O'Brien MJ, et al. Randomized comparison of surveillance intervals after colonoscopic removal of newly diagnosed adenomatous polyps. The National Polyp Study Workgroup. *N Engl J Med* 1993; 328: 901–6.

60. Grossman S, Milos ML, Tekawa IS, et al. Colonoscopic screening of persons with suspected risk factors for colon cancer: II. Past history of colorectal neoplasms. *Gastroenterology* 1989; 96(2 Pt 1):299–306.

61. van Stolk RU, Beck GJ, Baron JA, et al. Adenoma characteristics at first colonoscopy as predictors of adenoma recurrence and characteristics at follow-up. The Polyp Prevention Study Group. *Gastroenterology* 1998; 115:13–8.

62. Aubert H, Treille C, Faure H, et al. [Interest for colonic cancer prevention of the follow-up of patients after endoscopic resection of colorectal polyps: 123 cases (author's transl)]. *Gastroenterol Clin Biol* 1982; 6:183–7.

63. Potter JD. Nutrition and colorectal cancer. Cancer Causes & Control 1996; 7:127–46.

64. World Cancer Research Fund, American Institute for Cancer Research. *Food, nutrition and the prevention of cancer: a global perspective.* Washington, DC: American Institute for Cancer Research, 1997, passim.

65. Benito E, Cabeza E, Moreno V, et al. Diet and colorectal adenomas: a case-control study in Majorca. *Int J Cancer* 1993; 55:213–9.

66. Witte JS, Longnecker MP, Bird CL, et al. Relation of vegetable, fruit, and grain consumption to colorectal adenomatous polyps. *Am J Epidemiol* 1996; 144:1015–25.

67. Kato I, Tominaga S, Matsuura A, et al. A comparative case-control study of colorectal cancer and adenoma. *Jap J Cancer Res* 1990; 81:1101–8.

68. Sandler RS, Lyles CM, Peipins LA, et al. Diet and risk of colorectal adenomas: macronutrients, cholesterol, and fiber. *J Natl Cancer Inst* 1993; 85:884–91.

69. Platz EA, Giovannucci E, Rimm EB, et al. Dietary fiber and distal colorectal adenoma in men. *Cancer Epidemiol Biomarkers Prev* 1997; 6:661–70.

70. Little J, Logan RF, Hawtin PG, et al. Colorectal adenomas and diet: a case-control study of subjects participating in the Nottingham faecal occult blood screening programme. *Br J Cancer* 1993; 67:177–84.

71. Hoff G, Moen IE, Trygg K, et al. Colorectal adenomas and food. A prospective study of

change in volume and total mass of adenomas in man. *Scand J Gastroenterol* 1988; 23:1253–8.

72. Fuchs CS, Giovannucci EL, Colditz GA, et al. Dietary fiber and the risk of colorectal cancer and adenoma in women. *N Engl J Med* 1999; 340:169–76.

73. Martinez ME, McPherson RS, Annegers JF, et al. Association of diet and colorectal adenomatous polyps: dietary fiber, calcium, and total fat. *Epidemiology* 1996; 7:264–8.

74. Macquart-Moulin G, Riboli E, Cornee J, et al. Colorectal polyps and diet: a case-control study in Marseilles. *Int J Cancer* 1987; 40:179–88.

75. Haile RW, Witte JS, Longnecker MP, et al. A sigmoidoscopy-based case-control study of polyps: macronutrients, fiber and meat consumption. *Int J Cancer* 1997; 73:497–502.

76. Giovannucci E, Stampfer MJ, Colditz G, et al. Relationship of diet to risk of colorectal adenoma in men. *J Natl Cancer Inst* 1992; 84:91–8.

77. Neugut AI, Garbowski GC, Lee WC, et al. Dietary risk factors for the incidence and recurrence of colorectal adenomatous polyps. A case-control study. *Ann Int Med* 1993; 118:91–5.

78. Olsen J, Kronborg O, Lynggaard J, et al. Dietary risk factors for cancer and adenomas of the large intestine. A case-control study within a screening trial in Denmark. *Eur J Cancer* 1994; 30A:53–60.

79. Sinha R, Chow WH, Kulldorff M, et al. Well-done, grilled red meat increases the risk of colorectal adenomas. *Cancer Res* 1999; 59:4320–4.

80. Probst-Hensch NM, Sinha R, Longnecker MP, et al. Meat preparation and colorectal adenomas in a large sigmoidoscopy-based case-control study in California (United States). *Cancer Causes Control* 1997; 8:175–83.

81. Giovannucci E, Stampfer MJ, Colditz GA, et al. Folate, methionine, and alcohol intake and risk of colorectal adenoma. *J Natl Cancer Inst* 1993; 85:875–84.

82. Bird CL, Swendseid ME, Witte JS, et al. Red cell and plasma folate, folate consumption, and the risk of colorectal adenomatous polyps. *Cancer Epidemiol Biomarkers Prev* 1995; 4: 709–14.

83. Baron JA, Sandler RS, Haile RW, et al. Folate intake, alcohol consumption, cigarette smoking, and risk of colorectal adenomas. *J Natl Cancer Inst* 1998; 90:57–62.

84. Bergsma-Kadijk JA, van't Veer P, Kampman E, et al. Calcium does not protect against colorectal neoplasia. *Epidemiology* 1996; 7:590–7.

85. Martinez ME, Willett WC. Calcium, vitamin D, and colorectal cancer: a review of the epidemiologic evidence. *Cancer Epidemiol Biomarkers Prev* 1998; 7:163–8.

86. Enger SM, Longnecker MP, Chen MJ, et al. Dietary intake of specific carotenoids and vitamins A, C, and E, and prevalence of colorectal adenomas. *Cancer Epidemiol Biomarkers Prev* 1996; 5:147–53.

87. Shikany JM, Witte JS, Henning SM, et al. Plasma carotenoids and the prevalence of adenomatous polyps of the distal colon and rectum. *Am J Epidemiol* 1997; 145:552–7.

88. Tseng M, Murray SC, Kupper LL, et al. Micronutrients and the risk of colorectal adenomas [published erratum in *Am J Epidemiol* 1997; 146:788]. *Am J Epidemiol* 1996; 144:1005–14.

89. Bird CL, Ingles SA, Frankl HD, et al. Serum lipids and adenomas of the left colon and rectum. *Cancer Epidemiol Biomarkers Prev* 1996; 5:607–12.

90. Tseng M, Sandler RS, Greenberg ER, et al. Dietary iron and recurrence of colorectal adenomas [published erratum appears in *Cancer Epidemiol Biomarkers Prev* 1988; 7:556]. *Cancer Epidemiol Biomarkers Prev* 1997; 6:1029–32.

91. Nelson RL, Davis FG, Sutter E, et al. Body iron stores and risk of colonic neoplasia. *J Natl Cancer Inst* 1994; 86:455–60.

92. Clark LC, Hixson LJ, Combs GF Jr, et al. Plasma selenium concentration predicts the prevalence of colorectal adenomatous polyps. *Cancer Epidemiol Biomarkers Prev* 1993; 2:41–6.

93. Dworkin BM, Rosenthal WS, Mittelman A, et al. Selenium status and the polyp-cancer sequence: a colonoscopically controlled study. *Am J Gastroenterol* 1988; 83:748–51.

94. Nelson RL, Davis FG, Sutter E, et al. Serum selenium and colonic neoplastic risk. *Dis Colon Rectum* 1995; 38:1306–10.

95. Russo MW, Murray SC, Wurzelmann JI, et al. Plasma selenium levels and the risk of colorectal adenomas. *Nutr Cancer* 1997; 28:125–9.

96. Giovannucci E. Meta-analysis of coffee consumption and risk of colorectal cancer. *Am J Epidemiol* 1998; 147:1043–52.

97. Cope GF, Wyatt JI, Pinder IF, et al. Alcohol consumption in patients with colorectal adenomatous polyps. *Gut* 1991; 32:70–2.

98. Olsen J, Kronborg O. Coffee, tobacco and alcohol as risk factors for cancer and adenoma

of the large intestine. *Int J Epidemiol* 1993; 22:398–402.

99. Kono S, Shinchi K, Ikeda N, et al. Physical activity, dietary habits and adenomatous polyps of the sigmoid colon: a study of self-defense officials in Japan. *J Clin Epidemiol* 1991; 44: 1255–61.

100. Kono S, Imanishi K, Shinchi K, et al. Relationship of diet to small and large adenomas of the sigmoid colon. *Jap J Cancer Res* 1993; 84:13–9.

101. Baron JA, Greenberg ER, Haile R, et al. Coffee and tea and the risk of recurrent colorectal adenomas. *Cancer Epidemiol Biomarkers Prev* 1997; 6:7–10.

102. Lee WC, Neugut AI, Garbowski GC, et al. Cigarettes, alcohol, coffee, and caffeine as risk factors for colorectal adenomatous polyps. *Ann Epidemiol* 1993; 3:239–44.

103. Sandler RS, Pritchard ML, Bangdiwala SI. Physical activity and the risk of colorectal adenomas. *Epidemiology* 1995; 6:602–6.

104. Kono S, Handa K, Hayabuchi H, et al. Obesity, weight gain and risk of colon adenomas in Japanese men. *Jap J Cancer Res* 1999; 90:805–11.

105. Giovannucci E, Ascherio A, Rimm EB, et al. Physical activity, obesity, and risk for colon cancer and adenoma in men. *Ann Intern Med* 1995; 122:327–34.

106. Giovannucci E, Colditz GA, Stampfer MJ, et al. Physical activity, obesity, and risk of colorectal adenoma in women (United States). *Cancer Causes Control* 1996; 7:253–63.

107. Enger SM, Longnecker MP, Lee ER, et al. Recent and past physical activity and prevalence of colorectal adenomas. *Br J Cancer* 1997; 75:740–5.

108. Davidow AL, Neugut AI, Jacobson JS, et al. Recurrent adenomatous polyps and body mass index. *Cancer Epidemiol Biomarkers Prev* 1996; 5:313–5.

109. Neugut AI, Lee WC, Garbowski GC, et al. Obesity and colorectal adenomatous polyps. *J Natl Cancer Inst* 1991; 83:359–61.

110. Bird CL, Frankl HD, Lee ER, et al. Obesity, weight gain, large weight changes, and adenomatous polyps of the left colon and rectum. *Am J Epidemiol* 1998; 147:670–80.

111. Mannes GA, Maier A, Thieme C, et al. Relation between the frequency of colorectal adenoma and the serum cholesterol level. *N Engl J Med* 1986; 315:1634–8.

112. Kono S, Ikeda N, Yanai F, et al. Serum lipids and colorectal adenoma among male self-defence officials in northern Kyushu, Japan. *Int J Epidemiol* 1990; 19:274–8.

113. Bayerdorffer E, Mannes GA, Richter WO, et al. Decreased high-density lipoprotein cholesterol and increased low-density cholesterol levels in patients with colorectal adenomas. *Ann Intern Med* 1993; 118:481–7.

114. Peipins LA, Newman B, Sandler RS. Reproductive history, use of exogenous hormones, and risk of colorectal adenomas. *Cancer Epidemiol Biomarkers Prev* 1997; 6:671–5.

115. Chen MJ, Longnecker MP, Morgenstern H, et al. Recent use of hormone replacement therapy and the prevalence of colorectal adenomas. *Cancer Epidemiol Biomarkers Prev* 1998; 7:227–30.

116. Grodstein F, Newcomb PA, Stampfer MJ. Postmenopausal hormone therapy and the risk of colorectal cancer: a review and meta-analysis. *Am J Med* 1999; 106:574–82.

117. Platz EA, Martinez ME, Grodstein F, et al. Parity and other reproductive factors and risk of adenomatous polyps of the distal colorectum (United States). *Cancer Causes Control* 1997; 8:894–903.

118. Potter JD, Bostick RM, Grandits GA, et al. Hormone replacement therapy is associated with lower risk of adenomatous polyps of the large bowel: the Minnesota Cancer Prevention Research Unit Case-Control Study. *Cancer Epidemiol Biomarkers Prev* 1996; 5:779–84.

119. Garcia Rodriguez LA, Huerta-Alvarez C. Reduced incidence of colorectal adenoma among long-term users of nonsteroidal antiinflammatory drugs: a pooled analysis of published studies and a new population-based study. *Epidemiology* 2000; 11:376–81.

120. Giovannucci E, Martinez ME. Tobacco, colorectal cancer, and adenomas: a review of the evidence. *J Natl Cancer Inst* 1996; 88:1717–30.

121. Longnecker MP, Chen MJ, Probst-Hensch NM, et al. Alcohol and smoking in relation to the prevalence of adenomatous colorectal polyps detected at sigmoidoscopy. *Epidemiology* 1996; 7:275–80.

122. Nagata C, Shimizu H, Kametani M, et al. Cigarette smoking, alcohol use, and colorectal adenoma in Japanese men and women. *Dis Colon Rectum* 1999; 42:337–42.

123. Breuer-Katschinski B, Nemes K, Marr A, et al. Alcohol and cigarette smoking and the risk of colorectal adenomas. *Digest Dis Sci* 2000; 45:487–93.

124. Kikendall JW, Bowen PE, Burgess MB, et al. Cigarettes and alcohol as independent risk factors for colonic adenomas. *Gastroenterology* 1989; 97:660–4.

125. Kono S, Ikeda N, Yanai F, et al. Alcoholic beverages and adenomatous polyps of the sigmoid colon: a study of male self-defence officials in Japan. *Int J Epidemiol* 1990; 19:848–52.

126. Martinez ME, McPherson RS, Annegers JF, et al. Cigarette smoking and alcohol consumption as risk factors for colorectal adenomatous polyps. *J Natl Cancer Inst* 1995; 87:274–9.

127. Boutron-Ruault MC, Senesse P, Faivre J, et al. Folate and alcohol intakes: related or independent roles in the adenoma-carcinoma sequence? *Nutr Cancer* 1996; 26:337–46.

128. Honjo S, Kono S, Shinchi K, et al. The relation of smoking, alcohol use and obesity to risk of sigmoid colon and rectal adenomas. *Jap J Cancer Res* 1995; 86:1019–26.

129. Todoroki I, Kono S, Shinchi K, et al. Relationship of cigarette smoking, alcohol use, and dietary habits with sigmoid colon adenomas. *Ann Epidemiol* 1995; 5:478–83.

130. Sandler RS, Lyles CM, McAuliffe C, et al. Cigarette smoking, alcohol, and the risk of colorectal adenomas. *Gastroenterology* 1993; 104:1445–51.

131. Riboli E, Cornee J, Macquart-Moulin G, et al. Cancer and polyps of the colorectum and lifetime consumption of beer and other alcoholic beverages. *Am J Epidemiol* 1991; 134:157–66.

132. Jacobson JS, Neugut AI, Murray T, et al. Cigarette smoking and other behavioral risk factors for recurrence of colorectal adenomatous polyps (New York City, NY, USA). *Cancer Causes Control* 1994; 5:215–20.

133. Lubin F, Rozen P, Arieli B, et al. Nutritional and lifestyle habits and water-fiber interaction in colorectal adenoma etiology. *Cancer Epidemiol Biomarkers Prev* 1997; 6:79–85.

134. Burt RW, Bishop DT, Cannon LA, et al. Dominant inheritance of adenomatous colonic polyps and colorectal cancer. *N Engl J Med* 1985; 312:1540–4.

135. Cannon-Albright LA, Skolnick MH, Bishop DT, et al. Common inheritance of susceptibility to colonic adenomatous polyps and associated colorectal cancers. *N Engl J Med* 1988; 319:533–7.

136. Nakama H, Zhang B, Fukazawa K, et al. Family history of colorectal adenomatous polyps as a risk factor for colorectal cancer. *Eur J Cancer* 2000; 36:2111–4.

137. Demers RY, Neale AV, Demers P, et al. Serum cholesterol and colorectal polyps. *J Clin Epidemiol* 1988; 41:9–13.

138. Kune GA, Kune S, Read A, et al. Colorectal polyps, diet, alcohol, and family history of colorectal cancer: a case-control study. *Nutr Cancer* 1991; 16:25–30.

139. Brockton N, Little J, Sharp L, et al. N-acetyltransferase polymorphisms and colorectal cancer: a HuGE review. *Am J Epidemiol* 2000; 151:846–61.

140. Roberts-Thomson IC, Ryan P, Khoo KK, et al. Diet, acetylator phenotype, and risk of colorectal neoplasia. *Lancet* 1996; 347:1372–4.

141. Cotton SC, Sharp L, Little J, et al. Glutathione S-transferase polymorphisms and colorectal cancer: a HuGE review. *Am J Epidemiol* 2000; 151:7–32.

142. Inoue H, Kiyohara C, Marugame T, et al. Cigarette smoking, CYP1A1 MspI and GSTM1 genotypes, and colorectal adenomas. *Cancer Res* 2000; 60:3749–52.

143. Levine AJ, Siegmund KD, Ervin CM, et al. The methylenetetrahydrofolate reductase 677C → T polymorphism and distal colorectal adenoma risk. *Cancer Epidemiol Biomarkers Prev* 2000; 9:657–63.

144. Ulrich CM, Kampman E, Bigler J, et al. Colorectal adenomas and the C677T MTHFR polymorphism: evidence for gene-environment interaction? *Cancer Epidemiol Biomarkers Prev* 1999; 8:659–68.

145. Marugame T, Tsuji E, Inoue H, et al. Methylenetetrahydrofolate reductase polymorphism and risk of colorectal adenomas. *Cancer Lett* 2000; 151:181–6.

146. Baron JA. Large bowel adenomas: markers of risk and endpoints. *J Cellular Biochem—Suppl* 1996; 25:142–8.

147. DeCosse JJ, Miller HH, Lesser ML. Effect of wheat fiber and vitamins C and E on rectal polyps in patients with familial adenomatous polyposis. *J Natl Cancer Inst* 1989; 81:1290–7.

148. MacLennan R, Macrae F, Bain C, et al. Randomized trial of intake of fat, fiber, and beta carotene to prevent colorectal adenomas. The Australian Polyp Prevention Project. *J Natl Cancer Inst* 1995; 87:1760–6.

149. Alberts DS, Elena M, Roe DJ, et al. Lack of effect of a high-fiber cereal supplement on the recurrence of colorectal adenomas. *N Engl J Med* 2000; 342:1156–62.

150. McKeown-Eyssen GE, Bright-See E, Bruce WR, et al. A randomized trial of a low fat high

fibre diet in the recurrence of colorectal polyps. Toronto Polyp Prevention Group [published erratum in *J Clin Epidemiol* 1995; 48:i]. *J Clin Epidemiol* 1994; 47:525–36.

151. Schatzkin A, Lanza E, Corle D, et al. Lack of effect of a low-fat, high-fiber diet on the recurrence of colorectal adenomas. *N Engl J Med* 2000; 342:1149–55.

152. Greenberg ER, Baron JA, Tosteson TD, et al. A clinical trial of antioxidant vitamins to prevent colorectal adenoma. Polyp Prevention Study Group. *New Engl J Med* 1994; 331:141–7.

153. McKeown-Eyssen G, Holloway C, Jazmaji V, et al. A randomized trial of vitamins C and E in the prevention of recurrence of colorectal polyps. *Cancer Res* 1988; 48:4701–5.

154. Bussey HJ, DeCosse JJ, Deschner EE, et al. A randomized trial of ascorbic acid in *polyposis coli*. *Cancer* 1982; 50:1434–9.

155. Paspatis G, Xourgias B, Mylonakou E, et al. A prospective clinical trial to determine the influence of folate supplementation on the formation of recurrent colonic adenomas (abstr.). *Gastroenterology* 1994; 106:A425.

156. Baron JA, Beach M, Mandel JS, et al. Calcium supplements for the prevention of colorectal adenomas. Calcium Polyp Prevention Study Group. *N Engl J Med* 1999; 340:101–7.

157. Bonithon-Kopp C, Kronborg O, Giacosa A, et al. Calcium and fibre supplementation in prevention of colorectal adenoma recurrence: a randomised intervention trial. *Lancet* 2000; 356:1300–6.

158. Labayle D, Fischer D, Vielh P, et al. Sulindac causes regression of rectal polyps in familial adenomatous polyposis. *Gastroenterology* 1991; 101:635–9.

159. Giardiello FM, Hamilton SR, Krush AJ, et al. Treatment of colonic and rectal adenomas with sulindac in familial adenomatous polyposis. *N Engl J Med* 1993; 328:1313–16.

160. Nugent KP, Farmer KC, Spigelman AD, et al. Randomized controlled trial of the effect of sulindac on duodenal and rectal polyposis and cell proliferation in patients with familial adenomatous polyposis. *Brit J Surg* 1993; 80: 1618–19.

161. Steinbach G, Lynch PM, Phillips RK, et al. The effect of celecoxib, a cyclooxygenase-2 inhibitor, in familial adenomatous polyposis. *N Engl J Med* 2000; 342:1946–52.

162. Hixson LJ, Earnest DL, Fennerty MB, et al. NSAID effect on sporadic colon polyps. *Am J Gastroenterol* 1993; 88:1652–6.

163. Ladenheim J, Garcia G, Titzer D, et al. Effect of sulindac on sporadic colonic polyps. *Gastroenterology* 1995; 108:1083–7.

164. DiSario J, Alberts DS, Tietze CC, et al. Sulindac Induces Regression and Prevents Progression of Sporadic Colorectal Adenomas. *Gastroenterology* 1997; 112:A555.

165. Gann PH, Manson JE, Glynn RJ, et al. Low-dose aspirin and incidence of colorectal tumors in a randomized trial. *J Natl Cancer Inst* 1993; 85:1220–4.

166. Demers RY, Stawick LE, Demers P. Relative sensitivity of the fecal occult blood test and flexible sigmoidoscopy in detecting polyps. *Prev Med* 1985; 14:55–62.

167. Ransohoff DF, Lang CA. Small adenomas detected during fecal occult blood test screening for colorectal cancer. The impact of serendipity. *JAMA* 1990; 264:76–8.

168. St John DJ, Young GP, Alexeyeff MA, et al. Evaluation of new occult blood tests for detection of colorectal neoplasia. *Gastroenterology* 1993; 104:1661–8.

169. Ahlquist DA, Wieand HS, Moertel CG, et al. Accuracy of fecal occult blood screening for colorectal neoplasia. A prospective study using Hemoccult and HemoQuant tests. *JAMA* 1993; 269:1262–7.

170. Hope RL, Chu G, Hope AH, et al. Comparison of three faecal occult blood tests in the detection of colorectal neoplasia. *Gut* 1996; 39: 722–5.

171. Villa E, Dugani A, Rebecchi AM, et al. Identification of subjects at risk for colorectal carcinoma through a test based on K-ras determination in the stool. *Gastroenterology* 1996; 110:1346–53.

172. Dutta SK, Nair PP. Noninvasive detection of colorectal cancer by molecular tools: coming of age. *Gastroenterology* 1998; 114:1333–5.

173. Ahlquist DA, Skoletsky JE, Boynton KA, et al. Colorectal cancer screening by detection of altered human DNA in stool: feasibility of a multitarget assay panel. *Gastroenterology* 2000; 119:1219–27.

174. Kopreski MS, Benko FA, Borys DJ, et al. Somatic mutation screening: identification of individuals harboring K-ras mutations with the use of plasma DNA. *J Natl Cancer Inst* 2000; 92:918–23.

175. Williams G. Metaplastic polyposis. In: Spigelman A, Thomson J, (eds) Familial adenomatous polyposis and other polyposis syndromes. London: Arnold, 1994, pp. 174–87.

176. Spjut H, Estrada RG. The significance of epithelial polyps of the large bowel. *Pathol Ann* 1977; 12(Pt 1):147–70.

177. Williams AR, Balasooriya BA, Day DW. Polyps and cancer of the large bowel: a necropsy study in Liverpool. *Gut* 1982; 23:835–42.

178. Correa P, Strong JP, Reif A, et al. The epidemiology of colorectal polyps: prevalence in New Orleans and international comparisons. *Cancer* 1977; 39:2258–64.

179. Clark JC, Collan Y, Eide TJ, et al. Prevalence of polyps in an autopsy series from areas with varying incidence of large-bowel cancer. *Int J Cancer* 1985; 36:179–86.

180. DiSario JA, Foutch PG, Mai HD, et al. Prevalence and malignant potential of colorectal polyps in asymptomatic, average-risk men. *Am J Gastroenterol* 1991; 86:941–5.

181. Jass JR, Young PJ, Robinson EM. Predictors of presence, multiplicity, size and dysplasia of colorectal adenomas. A necropsy study in New Zealand. *Gut* 1992; 33:1508–14.

182. Hayashi T, Yatani R, Apostol J, et al. Pathogenesis of hyperplastic polyps of the colon: a hypothesis based on ultrastructure and in vitro cell kinetics. *Gastroenterol* 1974; 66:347–56.

183. Kikuchi Y, Dinjens WN, Bosman FT. Proliferation and apoptosis in proliferative lesions of the colon and rectum. *Virchows Archiv* 1997; 431: 111–7.

184. Barletta A, Marzullo F, Pellecchia A, et al. DNA flow cytometry, p53 levels and proliferative cell nuclear antigen in human colon dysplastic, precancerous and cancerous tissues. *Anticancer Res* 1998; 18:1677–82.

185. Iwabuchi M, Sasano H, Hiwatashi N, et al. Serrated adenoma: a clinicopathological, DNA ploidy, and immunohistochemical study. *Anticancer Res* 2000; 20:1141–7.

186. Shpitz B, Bomstein Y, Mekori Y, et al. Proliferating cell nuclear antigen as a marker of cell kinetics in aberrant crypt foci, hyperplastic polyps, adenomas, and adenocarcinomas of the human colon. *Am J Surg* 1997; 174:425–30.

187. Kang M, Mitomi H, Sada M, et al. *Ki-67, p53*, and *Bcl-2* expression of serrated adenomas of the colon. *Am J Surg Pathol* 1997; 21:417–23.

188. Araki K, Ogata T, Kobayashi M, et al. A morphological study on the histogenesis of human colorectal hyperplastic polyps. *Gastroenterology* 1995; 109:1468–74.

189. Frazin G, Zamboni G, Scarpa A, et al. Hyperplastic (metaplastic) polyps of the colon. A his-tologic and histochemical study. *Am J Surg Pathol* 1984; 8:687–98.

190. Bensen S, Cole B, Mott L, et al. Colorectal hyperplastic polyps and risk of recurrence of adenomas and hyperplastic polyps. *Lancet* 1999; 354:1873–4.

191. Imperiale TF, Wagner DR, Lin CY, et al. Risk of advanced proximal neoplasms in asymptomatic adults according to the distal colorectal findings. *N Engl J Med* 2000; 343:169–74.

192. Croizet O, Moreau J, Arany Y, et al. Follow-up of patients with hyperplastic polyps of the large bowel. *Gastrointest Endoscopy* 1997; 46:119–23.

193. Kearney J, Giovannucci E, Rimm EB, et al. Diet, alcohol, and smoking and the occurrence of hyperplastic polyps of the colon and rectum (United States). *Cancer Causes Control* 1995; 6:45–56.

194. Martinez ME, McPherson RS, Levin B, et al. A case-control study of dietary intake and other lifestyle risk factors for hyperplastic polyps. *Gastroenterology* 1997; 113:423–9.

195. Iino H, Jass JR, Simms LA, et al. DNA microsatellite instability in hyperplastic polyps, serrated adenomas, and mixed polyps: a mild mutator pathway for colorectal cancer? *J Clin Pathol* 1999; 52:5–9.

196. Cooper HS, Patchefsky AS, Marks G. Adenomatous and carcinomatous changes within hyperplastic colonic epithelium. *Dis Colon Rectum* 1979; 22:152–6.

197. Franzin G, Novelli P. Adenocarcinoma occurring in a hyperplastic (metaplastic) polyp of the colon. *Endoscopy* 1982; 14:28–30.

198. McCann BG. A case of metaplastic polyposis of the colon associated with focal adenomatous change and metachronous adenocarcinomas. *Histopathology* 1988; 13:700–2.

199. Teoh HH, Delahunt B, Isbister WH. Dysplastic and malignant areas in hyperplastic polyps of the large intestine. *Pathology* 1989; 21:138–42.

200. Jass J, Iino H, Ruszkiewicz A, et al. Neoplastic progression occurs through mutator pathways in hyperplastic polyposis of the colorectum. *Gut* 2000; 47:43–9.

201. Orii S, Nakamura S, Sugai T, et al. Hyperplastic (metaplastic) polyposis of the colorectum associated with adenomas and an adenocarcinoma. *J Clin Gastroenterol* 1997; 25:369–72.

202. Azimuddin K, Stasik JJ, Khubchandani IT, et al. Hyperplastic Polyps: "More than Meets the Eye"? *Dis Colon Rectum* 2000; 43:1309–13.

203. Jorgensen H, Mogensen AM, Svendsen LB. Hyperplastic polyposis of the large bowel.

Three cases and a review of the literature. *Scand J Gastroenterol* 1996; 31:825–30.

204. Rashid A, Houlihan P, Booker S, et al. Phenotypic and molecular characteristics of hyperplastic polyposis. *Gastroenterology* 2000; 119: 323–32.

205. Iino H, Simms L, Young J, et al. DNA microsatellite instability and mismatch repair protein loss in adenomas presenting in hereditary non-polyposis colorectal cancer. *Gut* 2000; 47:37–42.

206. Hiyama T, Yokozaki H, Shimamoto F, et al. Frequent p53 gene mutations in serrated adenomas of the colorectum. *J Pathol* 1998; 186: 131–9.

207. Jen J, Powell SM, Papadopoulos N, et al. Molecular determinants of dysplasia in colorectal lesions. *Cancer Res* 1994; 54:5523–6.

208. Otori K, Oda Y, Sugiyama K, et al. High frequency of K-ras mutations in human colorectal hyperplastic polyps. *Gut* 1997; 40:660–3.

209. Nucci MR, Robinson CR, Longo P, et al. Phenotypic and genotypic characteristics of aberrant crypt foci in human colorectal mucosa. *Hum Pathol* 1997; 28:1396–407.

210. Lothe RA, Andersen SN, Hofstad B, et al. Deletion of 1p loci and microsatellite instability in colorectal polyps. *Genes, Chromosomes Cancer* 1995; 14:182–8.

211. Torlakovic E, Snover DC. Serrated adenomatous polyposis in humans. *Gastroenterology* 1996; 110:748–55.

212. Konishi M, Kikuchi-Yanoshita R, Tanaka K, et al. Molecular nature of colon tumors in hereditary nonpolyposis colon cancer, familial polyposis, and sporadic colon cancer. *Gastroenterology* 1996; 111:307–17.

213. Jaramillo E, Watanabe M, Rubio C, et al. Small colorectal serrated adenomas: endoscopic findings. *Endoscopy* 1997; 29:1–3.

214. Longacre TA, Fenoglio-Preiser CM, Mixed hyperplastic adenomatous polyps/serrated adenomas. A distinct form of colorectal neoplasia. *Am J Surg Pathol* 1990; 14:524–37.

215. Ajioka Y, Watanabe H, Jass JR, et al. Infrequent *K-ras* codon 12 mutation in serrated adenomas of human colorectum. *Gut* 1998; 42: 680–4.

216. Uchida H, Ando H, Maruyama K, et al. Genetic alterations of mixed hyperplastic adenomatous polyps in the colon and rectum. *Jap J Cancer Res* 1998; 89:299–306.

217. Yao T, Kouzuki T, Kajiwara M, et al. "Serrated" adenoma of the colorectum, with reference to its gastric differentiation and its malignant potential. *J Pathol* 1999; 187:511–17.

218. Rubio CA, Rodensjo M. *p53* overexpression in flat serrated adenomas and flat tubular adenomas of the colorectal mucosa. *J Cancer Res Clin Oncol* 1995; 121:571–6.

219. Jass JR, Biden KG, Cummings MC, et al. Characterisation of a subtype of colorectal cancer combining features of the suppressor and mild mutator pathways. *J Clin Pathol* 1999; 52: 455–60.

220. Matsumoto T, Mizuno M, Shimizu M, et al. Clinicopathological features of serrated adenoma of the colorectum: comparison with traditional adenoma. *J Clin Pathol* 1999; 52: 513–16.

221. Fenoglio-Preiser C, Noffsinger A. Aberrant crypt foci: a review. *Toxicol Pathol* 1999; 27:632–42.

222. Nascimbeni R, Villanacci V, Mariani PP, et al. Aberrant crypt foci in the human colon: frequency and histologic patterns in patients with colorectal cancer or diverticular disease. *Am J Surg Pathol* 1999; 23:1256–63.

223. Pretlow TP. Aberrant crypt foci and *K-ras* mutations: earliest recognized players or innocent bystanders in colon carcinogenesis? *Gastroenterology* 1995; 108:600–3.

224. Siu IM, Pretlow TG, Amini SB, et al. Identification of dysplasia in human colonic aberrant crypt foci. *Am J Pathol* 1997; 150:1805–13.

225. McLellan EA, Medline A, Bird RP. Sequential analyses of the growth and morphological characteristics of aberrant crypt foci: putative preneoplastic lesions. *Cancer Res* 1991; 51:5270–4.

226. Bird RP. Role of aberrant crypt foci in understanding the pathogenesis of colon cancer. *Cancer Lett* 1995; 93:55–71.

227. Pretlow TP, O'Riordan MA, Pretlow TG, et al. Aberrant crypts in human colonic mucosa: putative preneoplastic lesions. *J Cell Biochem* 1992; (16G Suppl):55–62.

228. Shpitz B, Hay K, Medline A, et al. Natural history of aberrant crypt foci. A surgical approach. *Dis Colon Rectum* 1996; 39:763–7.

229. Wargovich MJ, Chen CD, Jimenez A, et al. Aberrant crypts as a biomarker for colon cancer: evaluation of potential chemopreventive agents in the rat. *Cancer Epidemiol Biomarkers Prev* 1996; 5:355–60.

230. Olivo S, Wargovich MJ. Inhibition of aberrant crypt foci by chemopreventive agents. *In Vivo* 1998; 12:159–66.

231. Takayama T, Katsuki S, Takahashi Y, et al. Aberrant crypt foci of the colon as precursors of adenoma and cancer. *N Engl J Med* 1998; 339:1277–84.

232. Roncucci L, Medline A, Bruce WR. Classification of aberrant crypt foci and microadenomas in human colon. *Cancer Epidemiol Biomarkers Prev* 1991; 1:57–60.

233. Roncucci L, Scalmati A, Ponz de Leon M. Pattern of cell kinetics in colorectal mucosa of patients with different types of adenomatous polyps of the large bowel. *Cancer* 1991; 68: 873–8.

234. Shpitz B, Bomstein Y, Mekori Y, et al. Aberrant crypt foci in human colons: distribution and histomorphologic characteristics. *Hum Pathol* 1998; 29:469–75.

235. Bouzourene H, Chaubert P, Seelentag W, et al. Aberrant crypt foci in patients with neoplastic and nonneoplastic colonic disease. *Hum Pathol* 1993; 30:66–71.

236. Yamashita N, Minamoto T, Ochiai A, et al. Frequent and characteristic K-ras activation and absence of p53 protein accumulation in aberrant crypt foci of the colon. *Gastroenterology* 1995; 108:434–40.

237. Roncucci L, Modica S, Pedroni M, et al. Aberrant crypt foci in patients with colorectal cancer. *Brit J Cancer* 1998; 77:2343–8.

238. Konstantakos AK, Siu IM, Pretlow TG, et al. Human aberrant crypt foci with carcinoma in situ from a patient with sporadic colon cancer. *Gastroenterology* 1996; 111:772–7.

239. Augenlicht LH, Richards C, Corner G, et al. Evidence for genomic instability in human colonic aberrant crypt foci. *Oncogene* 1996; 12:1767–72.

240. Polyak K, Hamilton SR, Vogelstein B, et al. Early alteration of cell-cycle-regulated gene expression in colorectal neoplasia. *Am J Pathol* 1996; 149:381–7.

241. Heinen CD, Shivapurkar N, Tang Z, et al. Microsatellite instability in aberrant crypt foci from human colons. *Cancer Res* 1996; 56:5339–41.

242. Siu IM, Robinson DR, Schwartz S, et al. The identification of monoclonality in human aberrant crypt foci. *Cancer Res* 1999; 59:63–6.

243. Pretlow TP, Brasitus TA, Fulton NC, et al. K-ras mutations in putative preneoplastic lesions in human colon. *J Natl Cancer Inst* 1993; 85:2004–7.

244. Smith AJ, Stern HS, Penner M, et al. Somatic *APC* and *K-ras* codon 12 mutations in aberrant crypt foci from human colons. *Cancer Res* 1994; 54:5527–30.

245. Otori K, Konishi M, Sugiyama K, et al. Infrequent somatic mutation of the adenomatous polyposis coli gene in aberrant crypt foci of human colon tissue. *Cancer* 1998; 83:896–900.

246. Losi L, Roncucci L, di Gregorio C, et al. K-ras and p53 mutations in human colorectal aberrant crypt foci. *J Pathol* 1996; 178:259–63.

247. Otori K, Sugiyama K, Hasebe T, et al. Emergence of adenomatous aberrant crypt foci (ACF) from hyperplastic ACF with concomitant increase in cell proliferation. *Cancer Res* 1995; 55:4743–6.

248. Guillem JG, Smith AJ, Calle JP, et al. Gastrointestinal polyposis syndromes. *Curr Probl Surg* 1999; 36:217–323.

249. Giardiello FM, Welsh SB, Hamilton SR, et al. Increased risk of cancer in the Peutz-Jeghers syndrome. *N Engl J Med* 1987; 316:1511–14.

250. Boardman LA, Thibodeau SN, Schaid DJ, et al. Increased risk for cancer in patients with the Peutz-Jeghers syndrome. *Ann Int Med* 1998; 128:896–9.

251. Giardiello FM, Brensinger JD, Tersmette AC, et al. Very high risk of cancer in familial Peutz-Jeghers syndrome. *Gastroenterology* 2000; 119: 1447–53.

252. Flageole H, Raptis S, Trudel JL, et al. Progression toward malignancy of hamartomas in a patient with Peutz-Jeghers syndrome: case report and literature review. *Can J Surg* 1994; 37:231–6.

253. Miller LJ, Bartholomew LG, Dozois RR, et al. Adenocarcinoma of the rectum arising in a hamartomatous polyp in a patient with Peutz-Jeghers syndrome. *Digest Dis Sci* 1983; 28: 1047–51.

254. Hizawa K, Iida M, Matsumoto T, et al. Neoplastic transformation arising in Peutz-Jeghers polyposis. *Dis Colon Rectum* 1993; 36:953–7.

255. Niimi K, Tomoda H, Furusawa M, et al. Peutz-Jeghers syndrome associated with adenocarcinoma of the cecum and focal carcinomas in hamartomatous polyps of the colon: a case report. *Jap J Surg* 1991; 21:220–3.

256. Bosman FT. The hamartoma-adenoma-carcinoma sequence. *J Pathol* 1999; 188:1–2.

257. Wang ZJ, Ellis I, Zauber P, et al. Allelic imbalance at the LKB1 (STK11) locus in tumours from patients with Peutz-Jeghers' syndrome provides evidence for a hamartoma-(adenoma)-carcinoma sequence. *J Pathol* 1999; 188:9–13.

258. Perzin KH, Bridge MF. Adenomatous and carcinomatous changes in hamartomatous polyps of the small intestine (Peutz-Jeghers syndrome): report of a case and review of the literature. *Cancer* 1982; 49:971–83.

259. Nugent KP, Talbot IC, Hodgson SV, et al. Solitary juvenile polyps: not a marker for subsequent malignancy. *Gastroenterology* 1993; 105: 698–700.

260. Desai DC, Neale KF, Talbot IC, et al. Juvenile polyposis. *Br J Surg* 1995; 82:14–17.

261. Howe JR, Roth S, Ringold JC, et al. Mutations in the SMAD4/DPC4 gene in juvenile polyposis. *Science* 1998; 280:1086–8.

262. Jarvinen H, Franssila KO. Familial juvenile polyposis coli; increased risk of colorectal cancer. *Gut* 1984; 25:792–800.

263. O'Riordain DS, O'Dwyer PJ, Cullen AF, et al. Familial juvenile polyposis coli and colorectal cancer. *Cancer* 1991; 68:889–92.

264. Jacoby RF, Schlack S, Cole CE, et al. A juvenile polyposis tumor suppressor locus at 10q22 is deleted from nonepithelial cells in the lamina propria. *Gastroenterology* 1997; 112:1398–403.

265. Wu TT, Rezai B, Rashid A, et al. Genetic alterations and epithelial dysplasia in juvenile polyposis syndrome and sporadic juvenile polyps. *Am J Pathol* 1997; 150:939–47.

10
Anus

Joel M. Palefsky

Unlike incidence rates of cervical cancer, which have declined, incidence rates of anal cancer have been increasing among both men and women in the last few decades. In the general population anal cancer is more common among women than men, but men who have sex with men (MSM) are among the groups at highest risk, especially MSM who are infected with the human immunodeficiency virus (HIV). Like cervical cancer, anal cancer is associated with human papillomavirus (HPV) infection, and risk factors for the two cancers are similar. Studies from the era prior to the introduction of highly active antiretroviral therapy (HAART) have shown that the prevalence of anal HPV infection was very high among HIV-positive MSM and lower among HIV-negative MSM. Prospective cohort studies also showed that the incidence of high-grade squamous intraepithelial lesions (HSIL), the putative invasive-cancer-precursor lesion, was high among both HIV-positive and HIV-negative MSM. Recent data have portrayed a similar picture for HIV-positive women and for HIV-negative women at high risk of HIV infection, that is, women with a history of intravenous drug use and commercial sex work. In findings consistent with these data, studies have also demonstrated increased risk of anal cancer among HIV-positive women compared to the general population of women.

For HIV-positive men and women, the advent of HAART therapy, with its potential for control of HIV replication and for immune reconstitution, raised the possibility that the risk of anal HSIL and cancer would fall to levels found among HIV-negative MSM and women. However, early data suggest that most anal HSIL lesions do not regress after an individual initiates HAART. Since progression of anal HSIL to invasive anal cancer may require several years, the improvement in survival associated with HAART may paradoxically lead to an increased risk of anal cancer. Like cervical cancer, anal cancer is probably preventable. Although it has not been proven that anal cancer is preceded by anal HSIL, if the analogy with cervical cancer and cervical cytology screening is valid, then detection and treatment of anal HSIL should lead to reduction in the incidence of anal cancer.

Cervical Cancer as a Model for Anal Cancer

The approach to the study of the natural history of anal cancer and its precursors is modeled after the approach to cervical cancer, as is the use of screening and treatment to prevent anal cancer. These are based on strong biological similarities between cervical and anal cancer. Both cervical and anal cancer frequently arise in the transformation zone where the columnar epithelium transitions to squamous epithelium [1]. In the cervix, this is where the endocervical columnar epithelium meets the exocervical squamous epithelium. In the anal canal, the transformation zone is located at the junction between the columnar epithelium of the rectum and the squamous epithelium of the anus. The location of the anal transformation zone varies from individual to individual, but it is usually two to four centimeters from the anal verge.

Both cervical and anal cancer are frequently associated with overlying squamous intraepithelial lesions (SIL), also known as "dysplasia" or "intraepithelial neoplasia". In the cervix, SIL, particularly high-grade SIL (HSIL) has been shown to be the lesion from which cervical cancer arises [2]. There are no published studies, to date, of the natural history of anal HSIL demonstrating directly that anal HSIL progresses to invasive anal cancer, but anal cancer has been shown to be preceded by anal HSIL in several cases (R. Cranston, J. Palefsky, manuscript in preparation). Anal cancer also is often found with overlying anal HSIL. Together, these data support the idea that anal HSIL represents the true precursor lesion to anal cancer, a role similar to that of cervical HSIL as the precursor lesion to cervical cancer.

SIL spans a spectrum of disease in both the cervix and anus. Low-grade SIL (LSIL) is characterized by relatively little basal cell proliferation and atypia, and, in the case of condyloma, by koilocytes (cells with an irregular, enlarged nucleus with a clear "halo"). In contrast, HSIL is characterized by increasingly severe cellular atypia, by abnormal mitotic activity in the more superficial cell layers, and by replacement of the normal epithelium with immature basaloid cells [3]. In the Bethesda system, LSIL includes both condyloma and mild dysplasia. HSIL includes "moderate and severe dysplasia" "intraepithelial neoplasia grades 2 and 3" and "carcinoma-in-situ".

While cervical HSIL is known to be a precursor to invasive cervical cancer, the transition time may vary widely, ranging from a few months to years to as long as several decades. The transition time from anal HSIL to invasive cancer is not known, but is likely to be at least as long in the anal canal as in the cervix in immunocompetent individuals. Transition times in immunocompromised individuals may be shorter, as suggested by the observation that the relative risk of anal cancer is particularly high among HIV-positive women under the age

of 39 years (relative risk [RR] = 134) compared to the general population (Table 10.1). Unlike HSIL, LSIL is not believed to be a direct precursor to invasive cancer, but rather the clinical manifestation of active HPV replication and virion formation. However, as described later in this chapter, LSIL does have the potential to progress to HSIL, and therefore the patient with LSIL must either be treated or followed carefully. Thus, though LSIL is not believed to progress to cancer directly, and many of these lesions regress spontaneously, they may also be considered to be precancerous if they progress to HSIL. In addition to LSIL and HSIL, there is an intermediate category of disease known as atypical squamous cells of undetermined significance (ASCUS). Primarily a cytologic diagnosis rather than a histopathologic diagnosis, this classification is used to describe lesions that have some of the features of LSIL or HSIL but do not fully meet the diagnostic criteria for these lesions. In the cervix, some, but not all, samples classified as ASCUS truly reflect the presence of an HPV-associated lesion, and ASCUS is therefore relatively nonspecific for the presence of a true cervical lesion. However, in the anal canal, the predictive value for anal SIL (ASIL) of a report of ASCUS on anal cytology is higher [4] (Table 10.2).

Finally, cervical and anal cancer share a strong association with HPV [5,6], although the prevalence of HPV infection in anal cancers from men is lower than that in anal cancers from women [6]. Over 100 different types of HPV have been identified on the basis of unique DNA sequences, and a subset of 10 to

TABLE 10.1. Standardized incidence ratios of anal cancer among HIV-positive men and women in United States AIDS–cancer registry match study[1,2].

Age (years)	HIV + women	HIV + men
<30	134	163
30–39	12.2	40
≥40	2.6	32
All ages	6.8	37

[1] Compared to expected incidence in men and women in the general population.
[2] *Source*: Frisch et al., International AIDS Malignancy Conference; 2000 May; Bethesda, MD [19], with permission.

TABLE 10.2. Sensitivity, specificity, positive predictive value, and negative predictive value of anal cytology in HIV-positive and HIV-negative men, with ASCUS classified in the abnormal or normal cytology category.

	HIV-negative		HIV-positive	
	ASCUS abnormal	ASCUS normal	ASCUS abnormal	ASCUS normal
Sensitivity	50%	27%	81%	56%
Specificity[1]	92%	98%	63%	81%
PPV	43%	50%	70%	78%
NPV	92%	90%	79%	70%

[1] Includes specimens with normal histology in the "no lesion" category for defining specificity.
ASCUS, atypical squamous cells of undetermined significance; PPV, positive predictive value; NPV, negative predictive value.

15 types are associated with almost all anogenital cancers [7]. HPV types 6 and 11 have been classified as "low-risk" and are associated with lesions such as condyloma acuminatum, which rarely if ever progress to invasive cancer. "High-risk" HPV types 16 and 18 are associated with invasive anogenital cancers and HSIL. HPV DNA has been identified in more than 99% of cervical squamous cell carcinomas [7]. In the largest study of anal cancer published to date, 84% of these cancers were found to contain an oncogenic HPV type, mostly HPV 16 [6]. HPV type 16 is also the type most frequently detected in cervical cancer and, together with type 18, accounts for 64% of cervical cancer cases [7,8]. Types 31, 33, 35, 45, 51, 52, and 56 are also detected in anogenital cancers but less commonly than HPV 16 or 18. Consistent with the ability of HSIL to progress to cancer in both the cervix and the anus, almost all of the HPV types found in HSIL lesions at these sites are oncogenic HPV types [6,9].

Incidence of Anal Cancer in HIV-Negative and HIV-Positive Men and Women

The introduction of cervical cytology screening has resulted in a substantial reduction in the annual age-standardized incidence rate of cervical cancer in the United States, causing it to decline from approximately 40/100,000 to approximately 8/100,000 [10]. The incidence rate of anal cancer is higher among women (approximately 9/1,000,000) than among men in the general population [11]. However, it has become clear that the incidence of anal cancer varies widely by risk group. Among men with a history of receptive anal intercourse, the annual incidence rate of anal cancer was estimated to be as high at 35/100,000 [12], rendering the incidence of anal cancer in this group similar to that of cervical cancer among women prior to the introduction of routine cervical cytology screening.

Risk factors for anal cancer have been shown to include history of receptive anal intercourse, history of anal warts (presumably reflecting exposure to HPV), and conditions associated with chronic irritation [12–14]. Several studies have shown that having cervical or vulvar cancer is a risk factor for anal cancer [15,16], consistent with both a common etiologic link and the possibility of common exposure to HPV at multiple anogenital sites. To this list must be added immunosuppression, currently most often associated with HIV infection. The data used to generate the above estimates predated the onset of the HIV epidemic and thus reflect the incidence of anal cancer among HIV-negative MSM. The impact of the HIV epidemic on the incidence of anal cancer remains unclear. However, recent data suggest that the incidence rate of anal cancer among HIV-positive MSM may be about twice that of HIV-negative MSM [17]. These data are consistent with those in a more recent report presented at the Fourth International AIDS Malignancy Conference in Bethesda, Maryland, on May 16–18, 2000, showing an increased relative risk for anal cancer among HIV-positive men from an AIDS–cancer registry match (Table 10.1).

The association between these cancers and HIV infection in women is not yet clear. While some studies have shown an increased risk of cervical cancer in HIV-positive women [18], most have not shown a significant increase in risk [17]. Among HIV-positive women, the absolute incidence of anal cancer is not known. However, at the Fourth International AIDS Malignancy Conference, data on the incidence of anal cancer in HIV-positive women were presented by Dr. Morton Frisch for the first time [19]. These data in HIV-positive women were obtained from the U.S. AIDS–Cancer registry match, which showed that the relative risk for anal cancer was 134 for HIV-positive women under the age of 30, 12 for HIV-positive women of ages 30 to 39, and 6.8 for HIV-positive women of all ages (Table 10.1). In summary, current data suggest that, though the incidence of anal cancer is low in the general population, it is at least as high in high-risk groups as the rates of cervical cancer that have been used to justify cervical cancer screening.

Anal HPV Infection and ASIL in HIV-Negative and HIV-Positive MSM

Compared to cervical SIL, ASIL has only recently been recognized as a clinical entity, and its natural history is not as well understood. However, several recent studies performed in San Francisco and Seattle have begun to provide an emerging picture of the prevalence and natural history of anal HPV infection, LSIL, and HSIL. Most of these data were collected before the introduction of highly active antiretroviral therapy (HAART). With respect to anal HPV infection, the results of these studies are striking: nearly all HIV-positive MSM had anal HPV infection, as do the majority of HIV-negative MSM [20,21]. In one study in San Francisco, 93% of the HIV-positive men and 61% of the HIV-negative men had anal HPV infection detectable by polymerase chain reaction (PCR) in a single sampling for cross-sectional analysis. HPV 16, the type most commonly found in cervical [8] and anal cancer [6], was the most common anal HPV type in both groups of men. Infection with multiple types of HPV was more frequent in HIV-positive men (73%) than in HIV-negative men (23%) and was more common among those with lower CD4+ levels [21]. The average number of HPV types detected per person was also striking: approximately 3.5 types for HIV-positive MSM and 2.0 for HIV-negative MSM.

Consistent with the anal HPV data, the prevalence of ASIL was also higher among HIV-positive MSM than among HIV-negative MSM, particularly among those with lower CD4+ levels [22]. Either LSIL or HSIL was present in 36% of HIV-positive MSM and 7% of HIV-negative MSM. Among the HIV-positive MSM, the risk of ASIL was inversely associated with CD4+ levels.

In prospective cohort studies, the incidence and progression of ASIL were shown to be high and to be associated with HIV status and lower CD4+ level. In a Seattle study of MSM with no anal lesions at baseline, HSIL developed within 21 months in 24 (15%) HIV-positive and 8 (5%) HIV-negative men [23]. In a more recent study, performed in San Francisco among men having no anal lesions, ASCUS, or LSIL at baseline, HSIL developed in 49% of the HIV-positive MSM and 17% of the HIV-negative MSM over a 4-year period [24]. In results consistent with the role of LSIL and ASCUS as HSIL precursors, men who had LSIL or ASCUS at baseline were more likely to develop HSIL compared to those with no evidence of any anal lesion at baseline. Risk factors for progression to HSIL were similar among HIV-positive and HIV-negative MSM and included infection with multiple HPV types, persistent anal infection, and high-level infection with oncogenic HPV types. After two years of follow-up, 62% of HIV-positive and 36% of HIV-negative men with LSIL at baseline progressed to HSIL, clearly demonstrating the potential for LSIL to progress to a lesion with higher potential for malignant transformation [25].

Although detection of an oncogenic HPV type is clearly associated with increased risk of anogenital cancer, recent studies of cervical lesions suggest that subtle differences in the genome sequence within variants of a given HPV type such as 16 may substantially affect the level of that risk. Thus, "European" or "prototype" variants of HPV 16 were associated with lower risks of cervical HSIL and cervical cancer than were "non-European" or "nonprototype" variants [26]. Recently this was shown to be the case for ASIL as well: compared to MSM with "prototype" HPV 16 variants, MSM with anal "nonprototype" HPV 16 variants were more than three times likelier to develop anal carcinoma-in-situ [27]. The biological basis for the more aggressive behavior of the nonprototype HPV 16 variants is not yet understood.

Anal HPV Infection and ASIL in HIV-Negative and HIV-Positive Women

Compared to the data regarding HIV-positive and HIV-negative MSM, relatively little is known about anal HPV infection and ASIL in HIV-positive or HIV-negative women. In the first such published study, anal HPV infection was more frequent than cervical infection in both HIV-positive women and women at high risk of acquiring HIV infection [28]. High-risk HIV-negative women were defined as those with a history of intravenous drug use or commercial sex work. These findings were confirmed in a later study of HIV-positive women in Denmark [29]. In the largest study of anal HPV infection in women performed to date, 76% of HIV-positive and 42% of high-risk HIV-negative women were determined to have anal HPV DNA using PCR [30]. In findings consistent with the earlier studies, among women with concurrent anal and cervical HPV data, anal HPV infection was more common than cervical HPV infection in both HIV-positive (79% versus 53%) and high-risk HIV-negative women (43% versus 24%). In multivariate analysis of data for HIV-positive women, lower CD4+ levels, cervical HPV infections, younger ages, and being Caucasian were significant and independent risk factors for anal HPV infection. Analysis of the HPV types in the anal canal and the cervix, in women infected at both sites, showed little difference in the overall spectrum of types at these sites. Notably, however, in only 50% of the women were the same HPV types found in the anus and cervix. Neither higher HIV viral load nor a history of anal intercourse were risk factors for anal HPV infection [30]. Nevertheless, receptive anal intercourse is likely to be an important route by which HPV infection is established in the anal canal, as suggested by a study of adolescent women (J Palefsky, unpublished data). Insertion of inert objects or fingers exposed to other HPV-infected tissues of the individual or their sexual partner may also result in anal HPV infection. Interestingly, anal HPV infection is nearly as prevalent in HIV-positive and high-risk HIV-negative women as it is in MSM, despite the likelihood that the women have many fewer anal sex partners and much lower frequency of anal intercourse than the men.

Less is known about the natural history of ASIL in women than in MSM. Anal HPV infection was an independent risk factor for anal cytologic abnormalities in adolescent women [31]. In earlier studies of adult women, anal cytologic abnormalities were more common among HIV-positive women than among high-risk HIV-negative women [26,27]. In a larger, more-recent study of 61 high-risk HIV-negative women and 235 HIV-positive women, abnormal anal cytology was found in 26% of HIV-positive women and 8% of high-risk HIV-negative women [32]. Risk factors for abnormal anal cytology included anal HPV infection, lower CD4+ level, cervical HPV infection, and history of anal intercourse. Prospective data on the natural history of ASIL in women are still very limited, but early indications from our own studies are that HIV-positive women develop HSIL at rates similar to those of HIV-positive MSM (JM Palefsky, unpublished data).

In summary, data collected on anal HPV infection and ASIL in HIV-positive and high-risk HIV-negative women demonstrate a surprisingly high prevalence of anal HPV infection and ASIL, as well as a high incidence of anal HSIL. Combined with new evidence that the risk of anal cancer is elevated in HIV-positive women, these data point to a need for anal screening in this population similar to that proposed for MSM. Further data on women are clearly needed, as are studies in other populations such as HIV-positive heterosexual men, HIV-negative heterosexual men, HIV-negative women with high-grade cervical or vulvar disease and cancer, and low-risk women. Further studies are also needed to delineate the relationship between cervical and anal HPV infection.

Effect of HAART on the Natural History of ASIL

HAART has been shown to substantially reduce the incidence of diseases associated with viral opportunistic infections in HIV-positive men and women, such as human herpes-virus-8 (HHV-8)–associated Kaposi's sarcoma and cytomegalovirus-induced retinitis. This is presumably due to HAART-associated reconstitution of immune response to these viruses. The impact of HAART on the natural history of HPV-associated anogenital lesions is not yet known [33]. It is possible that successful suppression of HIV replication by HAART may be accompanied by restitution of immune response to HPV and regression of HSIL to normal. If so, then it would be expected that the risk of anal cancer among HIV-positive MSM and women would decline to levels seen in HIV-negative MSM and women. Conversely, if HAART has little impact on regression of HSIL or progression of LSIL to HSIL, there may be increased opportunity for HSIL to progress to invasive cancer, since progression from HSIL to cancer may take many years, and individuals with HSIL may live longer as a result of their treatment. In the absence of screening and treatment for ASIL, a paradoxical increase in the risk of invasive anal cancer among HIV-positive MSM and women might therefore be observed.

It is not yet clear which of these two scenarios is correct, since follow-up is still limited among men with HSIL who have initiated HAART. The experience thus far with cervical disease suggests that HAART will have a limited impact. In one small study, there was evidence that some women with cervical SIL improved after beginning HAART [34]. Ahdieh et al. [35] reported at the Barcelona International Papillomavirus Conference that women on HAART were statistically more likely to show regression of cervical cytology, but as in the Heard study [34], the majority of women on HAART did not regress. In another study presented at the AIDS Conference in Durban, a group from Italy showed no regression of cervical disease among women on HAART [36]. In results consistent with these data, we have seen little regression of anal HSIL among MSM who have had undetectable HIV viral load due to HAART and increased CD4+ levels, and we continue to see high rates of progression from LSIL to HSIL among these men (JM Palefsky, unpublished data). Interestingly, however, the few men with HSIL that did regress to LSIL were those who had the highest CD4+ counts at the time of initiation of HAART.

In summary, further knowledge of the impact of HAART on the natural history of ASIL is needed, but preliminary data suggest that the impact will be limited. The reason for the lack of impact on HPV-associated lesions compared to lesions associated with other viruses such as HHV-8 or CMV is not clear. However, the observation that the most marked effects of HAART on the natural history of ASIL are found among those with higher CD4+ counts suggests that HAART-associated immune reconstitution may be playing an important role in HPV-infected individuals with ASIL who initiate HAART. In this context it is interesting to note that guidelines for initiation of HAART do not routinely call for initiation of therapy in HIV-positive individuals when their immune system might be most intact, that is, when their CD4+ level is above 500 cells/mm^3 and stable. Rather, the current recommendation is to defer HAART initiation until individuals have a plasma HIV RNA level higher than 30,000 copies/mL or a rate of CD4+ cell count decline in excess of 85 cells/mm^3 per year [37]. If widely adopted, these guidelines might exacerbate problems associated with anogenital HPV infection for the reasons described above.

Screening and Treatment Algorithms for Anal HSIL

The data presented above indicate a high prevalence of ASIL, a high incidence of HSIL, and a relatively high incidence of anal cancer among HIV-positive MSM, HIV-negative MSM, and HIV-positive women. Given the many similarities between cervical and anal cancer, it is possible that an anal cytology screening program with treatment of anal HSIL may reduce the incidence of anal cancer. Unlike cervical screening, which is targeted to all women, we propose that an anal cytology screening program for men should be targeted to those at particularly high risk, such as MSM. Other risk groups that could be considered for screening include all HIV-positive women, regardless of whether or not they have engaged in anal intercourse, and all women with high-grade cervical or vulvar lesions and cancer. However, insufficient data exist at this time to support screening in the latter groups.

It is likely that the elements of an anal screening program would closely resemble those of a screening program for cancer of the cervix (Figure 10.1). Every patient should first undergo a complete history and physical examination that includes visual inspection of the perianal region for lesions. Questions to ask in the history include history of bleeding, discharge, and pain. Pain is an uncommon symptom of HSIL and should be considered suspicious for the presence of invasive cancer. On physical examination, enlarged lymph nodes, which may indicate metastasis of anal cancer, should be sought in the inguinal region. The perianal region and anal canal should be digitally examined to palpate anal masses, but this should follow the anal cytology since insertion of a gloved finger requires lubrication, and cytology is best performed before the anal canal is lubricated. Anal cytology and high resolution anoscopy (HRA) would be performed as described previously [4,38]. The sensitivity, specificity, negative predictive value, and positive predictive value have been described for anal cytology as a screening tool (Table 10.2), and these are similar to those of cervical cytology [4]. In our proposed anal screening algorithm, all patients with abnormal anal cytology, including those with ASCUS, should be referred for HRA. This is because of the high proportion of *bona fide* ASIL detected on biopsy of individuals with ASCUS on cytology [4].

HRA is performed by inserting a lubricated plastic disposable anoscope into the anal canal, after which a gauze soaked in 3% acetic acid is inserted through the anoscope as far as it will go. The scope is then removed to allow the gauze to stay in contact with the anal mucosa for one minute or more. Then the gauze is removed and the anoscope is reinserted. The

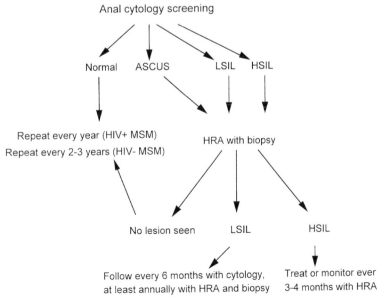

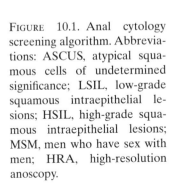

FIGURE 10.1. Anal cytology screening algorithm. Abbreviations: ASCUS, atypical squamous cells of undetermined significance; LSIL, low-grade squamous intraepithelial lesions; HSIL, high-grade squamous intraepithelial lesions; MSM, men who have sex with men; HRA, high-resolution anoscopy.

anal canal and perianal region are then visualized with magnification such as that provided by a standard colposcope. The aim of the procedure is to identify cancer or HSIL, and areas that appear suspicious for HSIL should be biopsied. Criteria used to distinguish low-grade lesions from high-grade lesions that have been validated in the cervix also appear to be useful in the anal canal [38]. Areas that appear to be low-grade, including condylomas, should also be considered for biopsy because they often contain foci of HSIL within them, especially in HIV-positive individuals. Consideration should also be given to referring patients with especially large condylomas to anal surgeons for aggressive biopsying, since such large condylomas sometimes harbor invasive cancers at their base. These large lesions should be biopsied in an ambulatory surgery setting for better anesthesia and control of bleeding than can be achieved in a typical office setting.

In most situations, performing an anal biopsy is a relatively simple procedure (we typically use small biopsy forceps), but training is required. Biopsies of most anal canal lesions do not require anesthetic. Perianal biopsies, which do require local lidocaine injection, can be performed with scissors and forceps or punch biopsy sets. Complications such as serious bleeding or infection are very uncommon if good technique is employed.

There is currently no accepted standard of care for treatment of ASIL, and the medical literature is very limited on this subject. As with cervical lesions, patients with HSIL should be routinely recommended for treatment, particularly those with the most advanced forms, such as severe dysplasia. We do not routinely recommend treatment of LSIL because there is a high likelihood of pain associated with the treatment, a high recurrence rate, and a low risk of progression to cancer. However, many patients do opt for therapy of LSIL to relieve symptoms such as itching, burning, or psychological discomfort, associated with the lesions. The treatment of LSIL lesions is similar to that of HSIL.

For HIV-positive patients who have a reasonably life expectancy and have good functional status, surgical excision or ablation in an ambulatory setting is the primary form of treatment. Patients are sedated, and a field block or light general anesthetic is used. HRA with a colposcope is performed in the operating room using both acetic acid and Lugol's solution. High-grade lesions are excised and sent for pathology, and the area surrounding them is then fulgurated. Some clinicians have used laser ablation. Except for significant pain during the first 7 to 10 days, most patients tolerate this procedure well without significant complications. For some patients, severe pain may last up to three weeks. Data on the recurrence rate of anal HSIL after surgery, or the efficacy of this approach to prevent anal cancer have not yet been reported.

Likewise there have not yet been any reported studies of nonsurgical therapies for treatment of anal HSIL. Occasionally lesions may be small enough (i.e., less than one square centimeter at the base) that they might respond to local therapy that can be applied in the office setting. Such lesions can be treated with 80% trichloroacetic acid. Most lesions will require multiple applications over time, typically at intervals of one to two weeks, for complete resolution. Other treatment modalities, such as cryotherapy or infrared thermocoagulation, may be considered as well. New modalities such as therapeutic vaccination against HPV and immune-response modifiers (e.g., imiquimod) are being tested in clinical trials.

It is hoped that with the institution of anal cytology screening, a higher proportion of patients would be referred with anal lesions that are earlier in their natural history and thus smaller and more amenable to nonsurgical approaches to therapy. At the other end of the spectrum, some individuals have such extensive disease at the time of referral that both surgical and medical treatment may be futile. In such cases, patients still benefit from screening, since they can be examined at regular intervals to monitor for progression to invasive anal cancer. As with cervical cancer, treatment for invasive anal cancer is more successful at earlier stages, and it is hoped that if these individuals do develop anal cancer, regular monitoring would at least allow it to be detected as early as possible.

Following therapy a substantial number of patients will experience a recurrence or persistence of HSIL. In addition, patients who have extensive circumferential lesions should not have the entire lesions removed in one surgical procedure due to the risk of complications such as anal stenosis. Options for these patients include sequential procedures and/or close follow-up with biopsy of suspicious lesions.

If on biopsy the patient is diagnosed with LSIL, he or she should also continue to be monitored, probably at 6 to 12 month intervals, for progression to HSIL. If a patient having HSIL remains untreated, he or she should probably be monitored every 3 to 4 months for progression to invasive cancer.

Cost-Effectiveness of Anal Cytology Screening

To assess the clinical effectiveness and cost-effectiveness of such an anal cytology screening program, Goldie and colleagues [36] have modeled anal cytology screening under a variety of conditions. As described above, the elements of an anal screening program were assumed to be similar to those of the cervical program (Figure 10.1). Thus, if an abnormal anal cytology was found at screening, it would trigger HRA and biopsy of lesions suspicious for HSIL or cancer. Data from the literature support the use of anal cytology as a screening test for detection of ASIL [4], as well as the use

of HRA to detect HSIL [35]. The model assumed that surgical ablation by anal surgeons would be used for treatment of HSIL and that LSIL would be followed without treatment.

The results of this analysis are shown in Tables 10.3 through 10.6 [39]. Goldie et al. used a combination of data from the literature and a range of assumptions in areas for which there are no data in the literature. Among these assumptions were the rate of progression from HSIL to invasive cancer and the efficacy of treatment of HSIL to prevent anal cancer. The considered screening strategies included no screening, annual or semiannual anal cytology, and annual or semiannual anoscopies as screening tests. A state transition-modified Markov model was used to explore life expectancy, quality-adjusted life expectancy, lifetime costs, and incremental cost-effectiveness expressed as dollars per life–year saved. The model also included multiple assumptions biased against screening. In this analysis, the most cost-effective strategy in HIV-positive men with CD4+ greater than 500/mm^3 was an annual anal cytology smear (Table 10.3). At a cost of $11,100 per year of life saved (YLS), anal cytology screening in this high-risk group was very cost-effective. Overall, annual anal screening was found to be cost-effective for all HIV-positive men regardless of CD4+ level (Table 10.4, 10.5) [39].

Goldie et al. also analyzed the cost-effectiveness of anal cytology screening in HIV-negative MSM [40] (Table 10.6). In this analysis, the incremental cost-effectiveness of anal

TABLE 10.3. Discounted costs, life expectancy, quality-adjusted life expectancy, and incremental cost-effectiveness of screening for anal squamous intraepithelial lesions and squamous cell cancer in HIV-infected men (initiating screening early in HIV disease with CD4+ > 0.500 × 10^9/L)[1].

Screening strategy	Costs ($)	Life-expectancy (months)	C/E Ratio[2] ($/YLS)[3]	QALYs[4] (months)	C/E Ratio ($/QALY)
No screening	69,960	109.49		102.25	
Triennial anal Papanicolaou	72,620	112.17	Dominated	104.67	Dominated
Biennial anal Papanicolaou	72,900	112.49	11,800	104.97	13,000
Annual anal Papanicolaou	73,240	112.76	15,200	105.22	16,600
Semiannual anal Papanicolaou	73,600	112.85	45,600	105.30	49,600

[1] *Source*: Goldie et al., *JAMA* 1999; 281:1822–9 [38], with permission.
[2] C/E, cost-effectiveness; [3] YLS, years of life saved; [4] QALYs, quality-adjusted life years.

TABLE 10.4. Discounted costs, life expectancy, quality-adjusted life expectancy, and incremental cost-effectiveness of screening for anal squamous intraepithelial lesions and squamous cell cancer in HIV-infected men (initiating screening later in HIV disease with CD4+ $0.200 \times 10^9/L$–$0.500 \times 10^9 L$)[1].

Screening strategy	Costs ($)	Life-expectancy (months)	C/E Ratio ($/YLS)	QALYs (months)	C/E Ratio ($/QALY)
No screening	71,640	70.42		63.97	
Triennial anal Papanicolaou	73,360	71.38	Dominated	64.81	Dominated
Biennial anal Papanicolaou	73,630	71.56	21,000	64.97	Dominated
Annual anal Papanicolaou	73,920	71.73	21,100	65.12	23,800
Semiannual anal Papanicolaou	74,160	71.79	48,500	65.17	54,300

[1] *Source*: Goldie et al., *JAMA* 1999; 281:1822–9 [38], with permission.
C/E, cost-effectiveness; YLS, years of life saved; QALYs, quality-adjusted life years.

TABLE 10.5. Discounted costs, life expectancy, quality-adjusted life expectancy, and incremental cost-effectiveness of screening for anal squamous intraepithelial lesions and squamous cell cancer in HIV-infected men (initiating screening in late HIV disease with CD4+ $< 0.200 \times 10^9/L$)[1].

Screening strategy	Cost ($)	Life-expectancy (months)	C/E Ratio ($/YLS)	QALYs (months)	C/E Ratio ($/QALY)
No screening	75,540	38.52		33.13	
Triennial anal Papanicolaou	76,290	38.74	42,400	33.31	49,300
Biennial anal Papanicolaou	76,520	38.80	44,200	33.37	51,400
Annual anal Papanicolaou	76,790	38.86	49,100	33.42	57,100
Semiannual anal Papanicolaou	76,990	38.89	78,300	33.45	91,100

[1] *Source*: Goldie et al., *JAMA* 1999; 281:1822–9 [38], with permission.
C/E, cost-effectiveness; YLS, years of life saved; QALYs, quality-adjusted life years.

TABLE 10.6. Discounted costs, life expectancy, quality-adjusted life expectancy, and incremental cost-effectiveness of screening for anal squamous intraepithelial lesions and squamous cell cancer in homosexual and bisexual men[1].

Screening strategy	Costs ($)	Life-expectancy (months)	C/E Ratio ($/YLS)	QALYs (months)	C/E Ratio ($/QALY)
No screening	4,130	302.46		290.99	
Triennial anal Papanicolaou	5,178	304.07	7,800	292.78	7,000
Biennial anal Papanicolaou	5,583	304.36	16,700	293.10	15,100
Annual anal Papanicolaou	6,676	304.70	38,700	293.48	34,800
Semiannual anal Papanicolaou	8,744	304.85	159,600	293.65	143,500

[1] *Source*: Goldie et al., *JAMA* 1999; 281:1822–9 [38], with permission.
C/E, cost-effectiveness; YLS, years of life saved; QALYs, quality-adjusted life years.

cytology screening was $38,700 per YLS for annual screening, $16,700 per YLS for biennial screening, and $7,800 per YLS for triennial screening. These data indicate that optimal screening intervals for HIV-negative MSM would be 2 to 3 years, as long as their cytology remains normal. Once abnormal cytology is detected, the work-up of HIV-negative MSM is similar to that of HIV-positive MSM. At this time, there are insufficient data to recommend a screening program for HIV-positive women or high-risk HIV-negative women. However, studies to define the natural history of ASIL in these women are in progress and recommendations of this nature may be made in the next few years.

Barriers to Implementation of Screening for Anal HSIL

Despite the theoretical cost-effectiveness of anal cytology screening in high-risk populations, there are several barriers to immediate implementation of an anal cytology screening program. The first barrier is a lack of clinicians trained to perform adequate anal cytology. Although the required procedures are relatively simple to perform, care must be taken to obtain a sample containing enough cells and to avoid air-drying of the sample, which can cause artifacts [1]. A second barrier is a lack of clinicians trained to perform HRA and anal biopsies. There are currently no formal training or certification programs for HRA similar to those that exist for cervical colposcopy. A third barrier is that most anal surgeons are not trained in HRA; thus they may miss subtle HSIL lesions at the time of surgery, and such lesions could potentially remain untreated. Fourth, more data are needed on both the efficacy of surgical therapy and nonsurgical alternatives. Surgical therapy is currently painful and costly and is also associated with a potential for morbidity (e.g., infection, bleeding, or anal stenosis). New medical approaches are needed, particularly systemic approaches permiting treatment of widespread internal and external lesions. Fifth, there are no data on the actual efficacy of an anal cytology screening

program to prevent anal cancer. However, it is unlikely that these data will be available by the time a screening program is ready for implementation.

Conclusions—Anal Cancer: To Screen or Not to Screen?

Prevention of cervical cancer through cervical cytology screening depends on identification and treatment of cervical HSIL before it progresses to cancer. Like cervical cancer, anal cancer may be preventable through identification and treatment of anal HSIL. The data described in this chapter clearly document the high risk of anal cancer in select population groups and strongly point to the need for an anal cytology screening program, even in the era of HAART. As described previously the incidence of HSIL and anal cancer in high-risk populations is sufficiently high to justify screening in those groups, as demonstrated by cost-effectiveness analyses.

A series of reasons have been presented for why anal screening has not to date been implemented in MSM. While the issues of training are real, they can be resolved. The question of the efficacy of an anal screening program to prevent cancer cannot be definitely answered until a large group of high-risk individuals with HSIL has been followed for many years. Follow-up would ideally be performed in the context of a randomized trial comparing screening approaches, frequencies of screening, and treatment modalities. Such a study has both ethical and practical limitations. Since this question is unlikely to inform the decision regarding implementation of a screening program, it may be that the optimal course would be to establish screening and treatment programs in high-risk populations and study the incidence of anal cancer over time. This approach is similar to that used for cervical cytology screening. The lack of convenient, safe, and efficacious therapies for anal HSIL is a real problem, but progress is being made. Even in the absence of adequate treatment, it may be worthwhile to identify individuals with

HSIL, since they can be followed over time and observed for progression to invasive anal cancer. This approach, although as yet untested, may well save lives.

References

1. Palefsky J. Anal cancer in HIV-positive individuals: an emerging problem. *AIDS* 1994; 8:283–95.
2. Richart RM, Barron BA. A follow-up study of patients with cervical dysplasia. *Am J Obstet Gynecol* 1969; 105:383–93.
3. Kurman RJ, Solomon D. *The Bethesda system for reporting cervical/vaginal cytologic diagnoses: definitions, criteria and explanatory notes for terminology and specimen adequacy*. New York: Springer-Verlag, 1994.
4. Palefsky JM, Holly EA, Hogeboom CJ, et al. Anal cytology as a screening tool for anal squamous intraepithelial lesions. *J Acquir Immune Defic Syndr* 1997; 14:415–22.
5. Zaki SR, Judd R, Coffield LM, et al. Human papillomavirus infection and anal carcinoma. Retrospective analysis by in situ hybridization and the polymerase chain reaction. *Am J Pathol* 1992; 140:1345–55.
6. Frisch M, Glimelius B, van den Brule AJ, et al. Sexually transmitted infection as a cause of anal cancer. *N Engl J Med* 1997; 337:1350–8.
7. Walboomers JM, Jacobs MV, Manos MM, et al. Human papillomavirus is a necessary cause of invasive cervical cancer worldwide. *J Pathol* 1999; 189:12–9.
8. Bosch FX, Manos MM, Munoz N, et al. Prevalence of human papillomavirus in cervical cancer: a worldwide perspective. International Biological Study on Cervical Cancer (IBSCC) Study Group. *J Natl Cancer Inst* 1995; 87: 796–802.
9. Palefsky JM, Holly EA, Gonzales J, et al. Detection of human papillomavirus DNA in anal intraepithelial neoplasia and anal cancer. *Cancer Res* 1991; 51:1014–9.
10. Qualters JR, Lee NC, Smith RA, et al. Breast and cervical cancer surveillance, United States, 1973–1987. *MMWR* 1992; 41:1–15.
11. Melbye M, Rabkin C, Frisch M, et al. Changing patterns of anal cancer incidence in the United States, 1940–1989. *Am J Epidemiol* 1994; 139: 772–80.
12. Daling JR, Weiss NS, Hislop TG, et al. Sexual practices, sexually transmitted diseases, and the incidence of anal cancer. *N Engl J Med* 1987; 317:973–7.
13. Daling JR, Weiss NS, Klopfenstein LL, et al. Correlates of homosexual behavior and the incidence of anal cancer. *JAMA* 1982; 247:1988–90.
14. Holly EA, Whittemore AS, Aston DA, et al. Anal cancer incidence: genital warts, anal fissure or fistula, hemorrhoids, and smoking. *J Natl Cancer Inst* 1989; 81:1726–31.
15. Ogunbiyi OA, Scholefield JH, Robertson G, et al. Anal human papillomavirus infection and squamous neoplasia in patients with invasive vulvar cancer. *Obstet Gynecol* 1994; 83:212–6.
16. Melbye M, Sprogel P. Aetiological parallel between anal cancer and cervical cancer. *Lancet* 1991; 338:657–9.
17. Goedert JJ, Cote TR, Virgo P, et al. Spectrum of AIDS-associated malignant disorders. *Lancet* 1998; 351:1833–9.
18. Serraino D, Carrieri P, Pradie C, et al. Risk of invasive cervical cancer among women with, or at risk for, HIV infection, *Int J Cancer* 1999; 82:334–7.
19. Frisch M. Fourth International AIDS Malignancy Conference, Bethesda, MD, May 15–18, 2000.
20. Critchlow CW, Holmes KK, Wood R, et al. Association of human immunodeficiency virus and anal human papillomavirus infection among homosexual men. *Arch Intern Med* 1992; 152:1673–6.
21. Palefsky JM, Holly EA, Ralston ML, et al. Prevalence and risk factors for human papillomavirus infection of the anal canal in human immunodeficiency virus (HIV)-positive and HIV-negative homosexual men. *J Infect Dis* 1998; 177:361–7.
22. Palefsky JM, Holly EA, Ralston ML, et al. Anal squamous intraepithelial lesions in HIV-positive and HIV-negative homosexual and bisexual men: prevalence and risk factors. *J Acquir Immune Defic Syndr* 1998; 17:320–6.
23. Critchlow CW, Surawicz CM, Holmes KK, et al. Prospective study of high grade anal squamous intraepithelial neoplasia in a cohort of homosexual men: influence of HIV infection, immunosuppression and human papillomavirus infection. *AIDS* 1995; 9:1255–62.
24. Palefsky JM, Holly EA, Ralston ML, et al. High incidence of anal high-grade squamous intraepithelial lesions among HIV-positive and HIV-negative homosexual and bisexual men. *AIDS* 1998; 12:495–503.

25. Palefsky JM, Holly EA, Hogeboom CJ, et al. Virologic, immunologic, and clinical parameters in the incidence and progression of anal squamous intraepithelial lesions in HIV-positive and HIV-negative homosexual men. *J Acquir Immune Defic Syndr* 1998; 17:314–9.

26. Xi LF, Koutsky LA, Galloway DA, et al. Genomic variation of human papillomavirus type 16 and risk for high grade cervical intraepithelial neoplasia. *J Natl Cancer Inst* 1997; 89:796–802.

27. Xi LF, Critchlow CW, Wheeler CM, et al. Risk of anal carcinoma in situ in relation to human papillomavirus type 16 variants. *Cancer Res* 1998; 58:3839–44.

28. Williams AB, Darragh TM, Vranizan K, et al. Anal and cervical human papillomavirus infection and risk of anal and cervical epithelial abnormalities in human immunodeficiency virus-infected women. *Obstet Gynecol* 1994; 83:205–11.

29. Melbye M, Smith E, Wohlfahrt J, et al. Anal and cervical abnormality in women—prediction by human papillomavirus tests. *Int J Cancer* 1996; 68:559–64.

30. Palefsky JM, Holly EA, Ralston ML, et al. Prevalence and risk factors for anal human papillomavirus infection in human immunodeficiency virus (HIV)-positive and high-risk HIV-negative women. *J Infec Dis* 2001; 183:383–391.

31. Moscicki AB, Shiboski S, Broering J, et al. The natural history of human papillomavirus infection as measured by repeated DNA testing in adolescent and young women. *J Pediatr* 1998; 132:277–84.

32. Holly EA, Ralston ML, Darragh TM, et al. Prevalence and risk factors for anal squamous intraepithelial lesions in women. *J Natl Cancer Inst* 2001; 93:843–9.

33. Palefsky JM. Human papillomavirus infection and anogenital neoplasia in human immunodeficiency virus-positive men and women. *J Natl Cancer Inst Monogr* 1998; 23:15–20.

34. Heard I, Schmitz V, Costagliola D, et al. Early regression of cervical lesions in HIV-seropositive women receiving highly active antiretroviral therapy. *AIDS* 1998; 12:1459–64.

35. Minkoff H, Ahdieh L, Massad S, et al. The effect of highly active antiretroviral therapy on cervical cytologic changes associated with oncogenic HPV among HIV-infected women [abstr.]. 18th International Papillomavirus Conference; 2000 July 23–28; Barcelona, Spain.

36. Uberti-Foppa C, Lillo F, Ferari D. Longitudinal study on the effect of highly active antiretroviral therapy on the clinical outcome of HPV-related lesions in HIV-positive women [abstr.]. XIII International AIDS Conference, 2000 July 9–14; Durban, South Africa.

37. Carpenter CCJ, Cooper DA, Fischl MA, et al. Antiretroviral therapy in adults. updated recommendations of the International AIDS Society—USA Panel. *JAMA* 2000; 283:381–90.

38. Jay N, Holly EA, Berry M, et al. Colposcopic correlates of anal squamous intraepithelial lesions. *Dis Colon Rectum* 1997; 40:919–28.

39. Goldie SJ, Kuntz KM, Weinstein MW, et al. The clinical-effectiveness and cost-effectiveness of screening for anal squamous intraepithelial lesions in homosexual and bisexual HIV positive men. *JAMA* 1999; 281:1822–9.

40. Goldie SJ, Kuntz KM, Weinstein MC, et al. Cost-effectiveness of screening for anal squamous intraepithelial lesions and anal cancer in human immunodeficiency virus-negative homosexual and bisexual men. *Am J Med* 2000; 8:634–41.

11
Liver

Morris Sherman and Ian Wanless

Hepatocellular carcinoma (HCC) is the fifth most common cancer in the world [1,2]. In most countries, the cancer is diagnosed with the onset of symptoms, at a stage when the disease is usually advanced and incurable. Over the last 10 years the incidence of HCC has increased in many countries [3–8]. In Western countries and in Japan, this has prompted a search for methods for early detection of HCC. This in turn has led to the identification of putative preneoplastic lesions, which have been identified histologically as well as radiologically. Several distinct lesions have been identified, but in most cases the relationship between the putative preneoplastic lesion and the ultimate cancer is still uncertain. Radiological detection of these putative preneoplastic lesions raises the possibility of screening at-risk subjects for pre-HCC and offering treatment. In this chapter, we will discuss the epidemiology and pathogenesis of HCC, the histological and radiological identification of preneoplastic HCC lesions in the liver, and the identification and management of at-risk subjects.

The other primary cancer of the liver that occurs with appreciable frequency is cholangiocarcinoma (CC), which accounts for about 15% of all liver cancers [9]. Pre-existing bile duct disease is a recognized predisposing condition, which frequently arises in patients with no apparent risk factors. In particular, infestations with the liver flukes *Clonorchis sinensis* or *Opisthorchis viverrini* are associated with the development of CC [10,11]. These parasites are prevalent in Thailand and neighboring parts of South East Asia, and consequently, CC is relatively frequent in those areas. Elsewhere, the common predisposing biliary disease is primary sclerosing cholangitis [12,13]. In patients with this condition the lifetime incidence of CC is about 10% to 20% [12]. Very little is known about early lesions in the pathogenesis of CC, and apart from the predisposing conditions, no other clinical, histological, or radiological condition allows one to predict that CC will develop. No lesions that are definitely accepted as cancer precursors have been described. Dysplasia of biliary epithelium has been described in the presence of established cholangiocarcinoma, in sclerosing cholangitis, and in Caroli's disease, but its significance is unknown [14–16]. This dearth of information is partly due to the difficulty of sampling the biliary epithelium, and partly due to the lack of any reliable serological markers which can be used for cancer surveillance. Precursor lesions to CC will therefore not be discussed further.

Epidemiology of HCC

Unlike many cancers, the underlying causes of HCC are usually identifiable. The most common risk factor and predisposing condition worldwide is chronic infection with the hepatitis B virus (HBV), which accounts for about 52% of all HCC [2]. Chronic infection with the hepatitis C virus is the second most common cause, accounting for about 20% of all HCC [2]. Chronic liver disease and cirrhosis due to alcohol, genetic hemochromatosis, α-1-antitrypsin deficiency, and other uncommon or rare metabolic diseases are also recognized causes, although worldwide they each only account for a small fraction of all HCC.

The evidence linking chronic HBV infection with HCC has been developed in many prospective and retrospective studies. For example, Beasley et al. [17,18], in a now classic study, followed 3,454 male hepatitis B carriers and 19,253 uninfected male controls. They found the relative risk (RR) of HCC to be about 100 in HBV carriers versus noncarriers. The yearly incidence of HCC in the HBV surface antigen (HBsAg)-positive group was 0.5%, increasing to 1% by age 70. In cirrhotic HBV carriers, the RR was 961 compared to uninfected controls. The incidence of HCC in cirrhotics was 2.5%/yr. Sakuma et al. [19] found the RR of HCC associated with HBsAg carrier status in male Japanese railway workers to be 50. The incidence of HCC was 0.4%/yr.

Prospective and retrospective studies in cohorts of hepatitis B carriers (without an unexposed control group) have indicated that the incidence of HCC in HBV carriers varies widely [20–23]. Villeneuve et al. [20] found no tumors in a cohort infected with HBV and followed for 16 years. McMahon et al. [21] reported an annual incidence of HCC of 0.26% in a study of HBV-infected individuals in Alaska. Sherman et al. [22] described an annual incidence of 0.46% in their cohort. Fattovich et al. [23] found that the incidence of HCC in a cohort of hepatitis B carriers with cirrhosis was about 2% per year. Such widely differing results may be explained by the characteristics of the cohorts studied. The cohort reported by Villeneuve et al. [20] was relatively young, with a mean age of only 46, compared to the older age of the cohorts reported by the other authors [21–23].

The association between chronic hepatitis C and HCC has also been determined in both retrospective and prospective cohort analyses of hepatitis C carriers. Almost all the studies come to the same conclusion, namely, that there is a considerably increased risk of HCC, although the reported RRs vary considerably [24–27]. In chronic hepatitis C, cirrhosis is almost a neces-sary precondition for the development of HCC. Studies suggest that HCC is between 20 and 200 times more common in hepatitis C cirrhosis than in the noninfected. The incidence in these populations ranges from 1.3%/year to about 5%/year [24–27]. It should be noted that these are all clinic-based studies.

Two prospective studies from Japan showed that, in patients with cirrhosis due to viral hepatitis, the RR of developing HCC was higher in patients with hepatitis C infection compared with that in patients with hepatitis B infection [28,29]. The risk of HCC was also higher in cirrhotic patients co-infected with HBV and HCV compared with those infected with HBV or HCV alone [30].

The presence of cirrhosis of any cause increases the risk of HCC. Among hepatitis B patients the presence of cirrhosis substantially increases the risk of HCC, compared with that of noncirrhotic subjects. Sixty to eighty per cent of patients who develop HCC have underlying cirrhosis [31,32, M. Sherman (submitted)]. The annual risk of developing HCC among patients with cirrhosis is between 1% and 6% [28,30,33–39]. Again, the wide range in reported incidence rates of HCC among patients with cirrhosis reflects differences in age, gender, etiology, and duration of cirrhosis in the groups studied. Several studies have shown that the risk of HCC is higher in patients with cirrhosis due to viral infection compared with that in patients with cirrhosis due to nonviral causes [38,39], although a high rate of HCC has also been reported in patients with cirrhosis due to genetic hemochromatosis [40]. In contrast, low incidence rates are seen in biliary cirrhosis [41].

Increasing age and male sex are also independent risk factors for HCC in the presence of cirrhosis [39,41]. The increased incidence of HCC with age in HBsAg carriers shown by Beasley et al. [18] has also been confirmed in several surveillance studies of HBV-positive individuals [21,42–44]. The higher incidence of HCC in older age groups is likely a function of longer duration of infection, although an effect of age *per se* cannot be excluded. In the Alaska study, HCC was detected at a rate of 0.2%/year in asymptomatic HBsAg positive male carriers less than 20 years of age, increasing to 1.1% in males aged over 50 years at the start of screening [21]. Similarly, the positive correlation between age and HCC incidence is also seen in patients with known HBV chronic hepatitis as opposed to HBV carriers with uncharacterized liver disease [43] and with HBV cirrhosis [44].

The incidence of HCC in different countries varies depending on the prevalence of the major causes, namely, chronic liver disease due to chronic viral hepatitis. Similarly, the proportion of cases attributable to hepatitis B or hepatitis C varies in different geographic areas. Thus, for example, in Southeast Asia, hepatitis B is the most common underlying cause, whereas in Southern Europe, it is chronic hepatitis C. The highest overall incidence of HCC is in Asia, which accounts for about 76% of all cases worldwide [2]. In parts of China, the age-adjusted incidence rate (AAIR) exceeds 30/100,000/year [2]. Africa also carries a large burden of all HCC's, accounting for slightly less than 10% of all cases. The AAIR in parts of Africa exceeds 16/100,000/year [2]. In contrast, in Northern Europe and North America the AAIR is less than 5/100,000/yr. The AAIR in Southern Europe is in the intermediate range, at about 12/100,000/year [2].

In all areas the incidence rate of HCC increases with age, although the peak incidence occurs at different ages in different parts of the world. For example, in Asia the incidence increases progressively until an age of greater than 70 years [18], whereas in Africa the peak incidence is about age 55 [2]. In the highest risk areas, where HBV is the major cause of HCC, there is a relatively greater incidence in children and young adults. On the other hand, childhood HCC is rare when chronic hepatitis C is the predominant cause.

The incidence of HCC is rising in many countries, including Japan, Israel, Canada, Australia, Italy, and Spain, as well as in the United States and France [3–8]. This is closely tied to the epidemiology of viral hepatitis in these countries. In Japan, Italy and probably Eastern Europe, epidemics of chronic hepatitis C are related to mass vaccination of children in the 1940s to late 1950s, and possibly to inadequate sterilization of nondisposable needles and syringes up to the mid-1970s. Those infected with hepatitis C during this period have now been infected for more than 30 years and therefore have a significantly increased risk of having established cirrhosis. Thus the silent hepatitis C epidemic from that era is the likely cause of the increase in HCC incidence in those parts of the world [45,46].

In countries where hepatitis B is highly prevalent, vaccine campaigns have yet to have a significant impact on the overall HCC rate, although the rate of childhood HCC has been dramatically reduced [47]. In Northern Europe and North America, the increase in HCC is likely due to several factors. These include high levels of immigration from parts of the world where hepatitis B and hepatitis C are common, as well as the epidemic of intravenous drug use which began in the 1960s, which has continued unabated since. For example, a recent analysis of our own cases showed that 80% of cases of HCC occurred in immigrants [M. Sherman (submitted)].

Epidemiology of Chronic Hepatitis B

The epidemiology of hepatitis-B infection is different in highly endemic areas of the world, compared with areas where the infection rates are low. In endemic areas, most infections occur in childhood [48,49], whereas in nonendemic areas, most infections occur in adulthood [50]. Prevalence rates of hepatitis B infection are highest in Southeast Asia and sub-Saharan Africa [2]. In Hong Kong, China, and Taiwan, the overall prevalence of chronic hepatitis B ranges between 5% and 15% of the population [2,49,51,52]. In sub-Saharan Africa, the prevalence ranges from 5% to 25% in different studies [2,44,53,54]. In endemic areas, transmission is either vertical in the perinatal period, or horizontal in early childhood. Transmission of HBV in the neonatal period and in early childhood is associated with a high risk of chronicity [55,56]. Beasley et al. [56] showed that more than 90% of infants infected by their carrier mothers became chronic carriers. In contrast, an infection acquired in young adulthood rarely leads to chronic infection. The corollary is that most hepatitis B carriers acquired their disease in infancy or early childhood. The long duration of infection in endemic areas is likely a contributing factor to the development of HCC. It has been estimated for example, that a male Asian hepatitis-B carrier has a 20% to 25% lifetime risk of developing HCC [57].

Epidemiology of Chronic Hepatitis C

The current high prevalence of chronic hepatitis-C infection has three causes. The first, and probably most important, is healthcare interventions, mainly vaccination, in the 1940s and 50s and later, in areas where disposable needles and syringes were not available. Thus for example, in a population study in a single village in Italy, more than 30% of the population over age 50 were infected with hepatitis C, whereas hepatitis C infection was rare [58] in those under 30. In Egypt, which has the highest prevalence of chronic hepatitis C in the world, many infections are tied to the use of nondisposable needles and syringes used to administer treatment for schistosomiasis [59].

The second commonest cause worldwide, and probably the most common cause in North America, is widespread intravenous drug use (IVDU), which began in the 1960s. Unlike HIV infection, which tended to occur late in the course of IVDU, hepatitis C infection frequently occurs early, so that even casual IV users are frequently infected. Both these populations, after more than 30 to 40 years of infection, have a high prevalence of cirrhosis and consequently a high risk of HCC.

Transfusion of contaminated blood and blood products prior to 1990 accounts for a relatively small proportion of all patients with hepatitis C. Patients at highest risk of acquiring hepatitis C via this route were those who had the highest number of transfusions. These were also the patients most likely to die from the disease which necessitated the transfusion in the first place. In addition, most patients receiving transfusions are elderly people, who, even if they survive the illness which necessitated the transfusion, have a high likelihood of dying of intercurrent illnesses. Thus the incidence of HCC in this population is probably not as high as in the hepatitis C population in general.

Other Causes of HCC

The evidence that other causes of chronic liver disease also cause HCC is less solid. In most liver diseases, other than chronic hepatitis B, cirrhosis is an almost invariable precursor to HCC [28,30–39]. This has led to the concept that cirrhosis is a preneoplastic lesion, or that cirrhosis is a common pathway by which different liver diseases result in HCC. However, in chronic hepatitis B, HCC frequently develops in the absence of cirrhosis, although lesser degrees of liver fibrosis are almost always present. This will be discussed later in more detail. An alternate hypothesis is that cirrhosis and HCC are independent consequences of the same process, and that HCC develops more slowly than cirrhosis, except in patients with chronic hepatitis B. The common factor linking all liver diseases with HCC would be the presence of repeated or persistent low-grade necrosis, followed by regeneration, predisposing to an increased possibility of oncogenic mutations developing actively dividing cells in damaged liver tissue.

Alanine aminotransferase (ALT) is an enzyme released by the injured liver. The ALT concentration is a rough estimate of the severity of liver injury. We hypothesize that the risk of developing HCC is proportional to the area under the lifelong ALT curve. There is some evidence to support this hypothesis. Beasley et al. showed that evidence of previous active liver disease in hepatitis-B carriers increased the risk of developing HCC [18]. Curley et al. [60] similarly found that patients who had active ongoing hepatic injury developed HCC at a much higher rate than those with inactive disease.

Histological and Molecular Definition

Genetics of HCC

Unlike colon or lung cancer, the genetics of HCC are largely unknown. The study of HCC genetics began with analysis of integrated HBV DNA in human HCC. The HBV is a DNA virus, but its life cycle includes a reverse transcription stage, in which viral RNA is transcribed into DNA. As a result, HBV DNA can frequently be found integrated into human cellular DNA [61–65]. The regions of the virus which may become integrated are not entirely random. There are preferred regions of the viral genome where integration takes place [63–65]. These are the overlapping repeats of the pregenomic RNA molecule located in the core gene region. Thus, integration usually disrupts the core gene. This mechanism of integration results in the hepatitis B X gene being frequently included in the integrated fragment, as is the surface antigen gene. However, the surface antigen region is relatively long and may therefore also be disrupted in the integration process [61–65].

Initially it was hypothesized that the integrated HBV DNA was itself oncogenic. There is evidence that the hepatitis B X gene is responsible for upregulating several cellular growth-regulating genes [66–69]. HBV-X-gene–containing cloned integrations have been shown to induce tumorigenicity in cell-culture and nude-mouse models [70,71]. In addition a mutated (truncated) surface antigen gene also exhibited transactivating activities [72–74]. However, expression of these regions in HCC is variable, so that if HBV-DNA–induced upregulation of transcription is important in the pathogenesis of HBV-induced HCC, there must also be other pathways that do not require the presence of the HBV DNA sequences. An alternative hypothesis is that integration of hepatitis-B virus DNA disrupts a tumour suppressor gene [75]. Since some HCCs in HBV carriers do not contain HBV DNA, the presence of an integration *per se* was clearly not necessary for the development of HCC [76]. Furthermore, there did not seem to be a specific site in the human genome which was a preferred site for integration. Thus it was unlikely that gene inactivation by insertional mutagenesis was a necessary contributing factor. For the same reason *cis*-activation of a host gene seems unlikely.

Altered expression of a number of growth-promoting or growth-suppressing genes has been described in human HCC. However, it is difficult to know whether the altered pattern of expression of these genes is important in the pathogenesis of HCC. In human HCC, no consistent pattern of altered expression has been identified, with one exception. Mutations in the *p53* gene have been frequently (but not universally) documented in HCC's from Africa and the Far East [77–79]. *p53* expression may be disrupted, or perhaps more commonly, there is overexpression of an abnormal p53 protein. The *p53* gene seems to be normal in dysplastic nodules and becomes more frequently abnormal as the degree of tumour differentiation moves from well-differentiated to poorly differentiated [80]. In parts of the world where the content of aflatoxin in food is high, the pattern of *p53* gene mutations is consistent with that expected from the genotoxic effects of aflatoxin (i.e., a (G–T) mutation, usually at position 249) [78,81]. This has been taken to be evidence of aflatoxin injury playing a role in the pathogenesis of HCC. However, the association remains controversial [82]. In areas where aflatoxin intake is uncommon, *p53* mutations have also been identified, but in these regions, the typical G–T mutation at position 249 is not seen [83].

Loss of heterozygosity (LOH) has also been frequently described in human HCC. Loci where this has been found include 4q, 5q, 8p, 10q, 11p, 13p and 13q, 16q, and 17p [84–90]. The 17p LOH is probably the *p53* gene. This seems to be the most consistent LOH described. The implication is that a tumour suppressor gene may have been located within the deleted segment, and consequently, a smaller somatic mutation in the other allele results in decreased or altered expression of that tumour suppressor gene. Apart from the 17p locus, there is little consistency in the loci at which LOH has been demonstrated.

Proliferative Lesions in the Liver

Anatomic Definitions

Several anatomic lesions have been identified that have an increased prevalence in livers containing hepatocellular carcinoma. These lesions, including cirrhosis, dysplastic foci, and dysplastic nodules, have therefore been considered as possible precursor lesions for malignancy [91,92]. However, the evidence that these are involved in the pathogenesis of HCC remains weak. Unlike for colon cancer, there is no experimental model in which the progression from normal to dysplasia to cancer has been demonstrated. Even in the woodchuck infected with woodchuck hepatitis virus (an animal model of chronic hepatitis B infection with progression to HCC) the association of dysplasia with HCC has not been studied as a sequential phenomenon.

Precursor lesions to HCC have really only been studied in any detail in patients with chronic hepatitis B or hepatitis-C infection. Thus there is no information about whether the etiology of precursor lesions differs at all from the etiology of HCC itself.

Cirrhosis

The term cirrhosis refers to the presence of nodules in the liver consisting of parenchymal cells surrounded by fibrous tissue. These nodules are formed as the result of a number of processes including cell death and regeneration, laying down of scar tissue (fibrosis), and remodelling of existing scars. Initially, regeneration is probably polyclonal; that is, hyperplasia rather than neoplasia. Most nodules are less than 1 cm in size, but sometimes cirrhotic nodules can be very large.

While the definition and appearance of cirrhosis are well known, it is not widely appreciated that cirrhosis remodels and regresses extensively after active disease has abated, especially after hepatitis B e antigen seroconversion of chronic hepatitis B and in reformed alcoholism. Fibrous bands in the liver regress. Thick bands of fibrous tissue probably never disappear completely, but the finer strands of fibrous tissue may become even more fine, and may even disappear completely. This remodeling process results in large cirrhotic nodules with delicate and perforated septa that are subtle. Needle biopsies may yield underestimates of the amount of fibrosis and the architectural distortion that accompanies cirrhosis. Thus, many patients with hepatocellular carcinoma who are considered to be noncirrhotic actually have regressed cirrhosis [93,94]. The hepatocytes within the nodule can be normal, or they may show a variety of changes. Such changes may be related to the pathogenesis of HCC or may simply be an unrelated phenomenon in a liver at risk for malignancy. There are a confusing plethora of names given to these nodules, including adenomatous hyperplasia, macroregenerative nodules, dysplastic nodules, among others.

Dysplastic Focus

A dysplastic focus is a recognizable cluster of hepatocytes with distinct but irregular margins. The cells within the focus are fairly uniform but differ from those of adjacent hepatocytes with respect to cytoplasmic staining, nuclear size, nuclear atypia, and often HBsAg deposition. The focal nature of the lesions gives them the appearance of clones. Nuclei may be normal in size or large and hyperchromatic. The cytoplasmic contents of fat or glycogen may be more or less than those of the surrounding liver. The cellular changes within the foci have often been subdivided into large-cell dysplasia [95] and small-cell dysplasia [96]. Large-cell dysplasia is identified by the presence of large cells with large polyploid nuclei. These cells have normal nucleus-to-cytoplasmic ratios. Small-cell dysplasia is identified by the presence of small cells with nuclei of normal size, giving an increased nucleus-to-cytoplasmic ratio. Small-cell dysplasia is associated with an increased proliferation rate. Dysplastic lesions are called foci if smaller than 1 mm in diameter and nodules if at least 1 mm in diameter.

Dysplastic Nodules

Dysplastic nodules are composed of hepatocytes that have benign but not normal features. They may be subdivided into low-grade and high-grade dysplastic nodules. Dysplastic nodules have often been called adenomatous hyperplasia or type II macroregenerative nodules [94], terms that are now obsolete.

Dysplastic nodules occur in a quarter of explanted cirrhotic livers, often coexisting with hepatocellular carcinoma [91]. Dysplastic nodules are commonly detected by ultrasound examination as nodules larger than the background cirrhotic nodules. As the size of a lesion increases, there is a greater likelihood that high-grade or malignant lesions are present; benign lesions are seldom greater than 20 mm in diameter. Grossly, dysplastic nodules often bulge above the cut surface and have a soft texture. Lesions may be either more bile-stained or paler than surrounding liver. Necrosis and hemorrhage are not seen.

Histologically, low-grade and high-grade dysplastic nodules represent parts of a spectrum. Low-grade dysplastic nodules are comprised of hepatocytes which are minimally abnormal, but high-grade lesions have more atypia and may be difficult to distinguish from carcinoma. Cytoplasm may be eosinophilic or contain fat. The liver cell plates are 1 to 2 cells wide. The nodules are supplied by portal tracts, but arteries outside of portal tracts become increasingly prevalent as the lesions approach malignancy [97].

Differential Diagnosis

The criteria used to distinguish various hepatocellular nodular lesions have been summarized by Hytiroglou et al. [91]. A dysplastic nodule should be diagnosed if there are some features suggestive of a neoplastic process, but these features do not meet the criteria for malignancy. The cells of large regenerative (cirrhotic) nodules have the same appearance as cells of adjacent parenchyma. Other lesions composed of hepatocytes that may enter the differential diagnosis include hepatocellular adenoma, focal nodular hyperplasia, nodular regenerative hyperplasia, and lobar or segmental hyperplasia.

Adenomas are benign neoplasms composed of hepatocytes occurring in a liver that is otherwise histologically normal or nearly normal. These lesions almost always occur in a setting of treatment with oral contraceptive or anabolic steroids or with abnormal carbohydrate metabolism, especially glycogen-storage disease. Adenomas may regress after withdrawal of the stimulus. Malignant progression has been reported but is rare [98]. Histologically, the tumor cells resemble normal hepatocytes that are arranged in normal or slightly widened plates. The lesions are supplied with arteries, so such portal elements as portal veins, ducts, and ductules are not seen. Cellular atypia is usually minimal or absent. Mitoses are almost never seen.

Focal nodular hyperplasia tends to occur in women and is often detected as an incidental finding. The lesions are composed of normal-appearing hepatocytes supplied by portal tracts with ductular proliferation and deficient ducts and portal veins.

In nodular regenerative hyperplasia, the entire liver is composed of 1 to 2 mm nodules separated by small regions of atrophy. Occasionally there are larger nodules (large regenerative nodules) that present as a mass lesion visible by imaging techniques. These larger nodules have been called partial nodular transformation. Because vascular obliteration is thought to be the primary alteration in this lesion, portal hypertension is often present.

Lobar and segmental hyperplasia represents histologically normal liver that has undergone hyperplasia after much of the rest of the liver has undergone an injury, usually after hepatic vein thrombosis or obliteration of major bile ducts as in primary sclerosing cholangitis or biliary atresia. Therefore, the diagnosis requires either gross examination of the liver or imaging studies. It can easily be differentiated from a large regenerative nodule, which is usually more spherical, is separated from the capsule by severely altered parenchyma, and often contains prominently enlarged arteries.

Putative Preneoplastic Lesions in Cirrhosis

Claims have been made that dysplasia found in the cirrhotic liver is preneoplastic, that is, that the dysplastic cells are involved in the pathogenesis of the HCC, as opposed to simply being a marker of an at-risk situation [97–99]. Cells exhibiting various markers of proliferation are also thought to be preneoplastic. Proliferation markers include an increased proliferating cell nuclear antigen (PCNA) labeling index, an increased labeling index for silver staining of the nucleolar organizing region (AgNOR), and expression of Ki-67. It is clear that all these markers occur in patients at risk for HCC, and their presence often precedes the development of HCC within a relatively short time period. However, it is also clear that HCC may equally well develop elsewhere in the liver in the absence of a documented precursor lesion. It is not certain whether the presence of any or all of these lesions is a necessary precursor to the development of full-fledged cancer.

One way of determining the malignant potential of these lesions is to determine whether the lesions exhibit evidence of increased proliferation. Based on a number of studies, the lesions can be ranked in ascending order of intensity of proliferation. Large cirrhotic nodules show the least evidence of proliferation, similar to that seen in smaller cirrhotic nodules. Lesions showing large-cell dysplasia also have low proliferation indices, whereas small-cell dysplasia showed proliferation markers similar to HCC [100]. Dysplastic nodules also show markers of proliferation not very different from established HCC [100].

The presence of dysplasia and proliferation markers has also been used to clinically predict the development of HCC. Increased PCNA labeling index [101], increased Ki-67 expression [102], increased AgNOR [103], and the presence of both large- and small-cell dysplasia [35,104,105] in lesions sampled at the start of the study period have all been shown to be more frequent in patients who develop HCC within the follow-up period than in those who do not. The relationship between large-cell dysplasia and HCC is controversial. One study found that large-cell dysplasia was not associated with HCC, whereas large cirrhotic nodules, dysplastic nodules, and small-cell dysplasia were associated with HCC [91].

Large-cell dysplasia carries few markers of proliferation [100,106]. When the prevalence of large-cell dysplasia is compared between patients with and without HCC, large cell dysplasia is more common in those with HCC, but pathology review does not suggest a transition between the two lesions, either morphologically, or histochemically [105]. Others have suggested that a change to large-cell dysplasia may be a reaction to prolonged local cholestasis

[107]. On the other hand, large cell dysplasia is associated with significant chromosomal abnormalities [108]. Copy numbers of chromosomes, as measured using centromeric nucleic acid probes and by in-situ hybridization, are increased. Small cell dysplasia, on the other hand, does not appear to be associated with detectable chromosomal abnormalities, when these same methods are used. Another study demonstrated that large-cell dysplasia was almost universally associated with aneuploid and hyperploid changes, but the results also suggested that the dysplastic cells were not clonal, in turn suggesting that they were unlikely to be HCC precursors [109].

Small-cell dysplasia has characteristics which suggest that this condition may be a true precursor to HCC. First, proliferation markers are highly expressed [102,103]. Second, transitions have been described between small cell dysplasia and HCC, with the so-called nodule-in-nodule appearance [99,110]. This is the appearance of a small focus of HCC within a larger dysplastic nodule.

Clonal Populations of Cells in Hepatitis and Cirrhosis

The so-called irregular regeneration lesion [111], also described in cirrhotic livers, seems to predict the development of HCC. This is defined as a maplike grouping of parenchymal hepatocytes with bulging, anisocytosis, and pleiomorphism. These findings have been described in patients with chronic hepatitis C, but may also be present in patients with cirrhosis of other etiologies. It is suspected, although not proven, that the maplike areas are clonal expansions of hepatocytes, which would account for the morphological distinction between the maplike area and the surrounding liver cells.

When the liver of a patient with cirrhosis or late stage quiescent chronic hepatitis B is stained for HBsAg, the stain is taken up by discrete clumps of cells [112]. In contrast, during actively replicating infection with hepatitis B, HBsAg staining is only found in occasional cells. The distribution of the stain in cirrhosis strongly suggests a clonal population of cells (maplike distribution). In this instance, it is likely that the expression of the HBsAg is derived from an integrated template rather than from episomal viral DNA.

The molecular equivalent of this phenomenon can clearly be shown by Southern transfer and molecular hybridization of cellular DNA, using HBV DNA as a probe [113]. In many cancers from HBV-infected individuals, discrete bands of integrated HBV DNA are seen, indicating that many cells in the original preparation contained the same HBV DNA sequences integrated into the same site in cellular DNA, a phenomenon which could only be found in a clone of cells. Similar clonal preparations of integrated HBV DNA can be isolated from nonmalignant liver, including dysplastic nodules in hepatitis-B carriers, once more indicating that these lesions are preneoplastic lesions [113].

More recently others have confirmed the presence of clonal populations of cells in the cirrhotic liver. The X-linked phosphoglycerokinase (PGK) gene undergoes random inactivation by methylation at one of three sites. Aihara et al. [114] demonstrated that dysplastic nodules and HCC both contained *PGK* genes inactivated at a uniform locus, once more indicating the presence of a clonal population. Perhaps more importantly, this work clearly shows that at least some dysplastic nodules are monoclonal in origin, and are therefore neoplastic, rather than hyperplastic.

Thus, although the development of cirrhosis *per se* is not an oncogenic process, many cirrhotic livers contain both hyperplastic (regenerative) and preneoplastic nodules. The challenge is to distinguish these two lesions histologically and radiologically.

Clinical Detection of Early HCC

As originally conceived, HCC surveillance (i.e., a regular schedule of monitoring over time) had as its objective identification of early small HCC. However, with experience, it became clear that in addition to detecting early HCC, surveillance was also detecting other nodular lesions in the liver, including putative preneoplastic lesions, as well as nonneoplastic proliferative lesions, such as large cirrhotic nodules. Distinguishing between these different lesions radiologically, and even on percutaneous biopsy, has proven to be difficult. As yet, there is insufficient information to assume that preneoplastic lesions will definitely become neoplastic, and therefore, there are insufficient data to warrant treatment of preneoplasia, as opposed to fully established neoplasia.

The commonly used screening/surveillance tools are α-fetoprotein (AFP) concentration and ultrasonography. A summary of the available markers of risk for HCC is shown in Table 11.1.

Objectives of Surveillance

Whether HCC surveillance can achieve the objective of decreased disease-specific mortality has still to be demonstrated. To prove this would require a prospective randomized controlled trial comparing surveillance to no surveillance. Such a study would require thousands of subjects and a follow-up of at least 5 years. Given the widespread use of surveil-

TABLE 11.1. Markers of high risk for HCC.

Serological	Histological	Radiological
AFP	Cirrhosis	US—Nodular liver
AFP-L3	Large-cell dysplasia	CT—Vascular nodules
PIVKA II	Small-cell dysplasia	MRI—Vascular nodules
α-Fucosidase	Ki-67 staining	
	High PCNA labeling index	
	High AgNOR labeling index	
	Clonal HBsAg staining	

lance in formal and informal programs, the risk of contamination of the nonsurveillance group is so high as to preclude the study from ever being completed. Uncontrolled or nonrandomized studies have been inconclusive. Several retrospective, uncontrolled, or nonrandomized studies show little or no benefit for surveillance [34,115]. However, these studies did not adequately differentiate between prevalent and incident cases. Few studies included an intention-to-treat analysis.

Studies on the outcome of treatment of HCC indicate that a cure is possible in patients who undergo resection [116–120], some form of local ablation [121–123], or liver transplantation [124]. However, at best, 5-year survival is only 30% to 40%. This is partly because of progressive liver disease and partly because of recurrence of HCC due to intrahepatic metastases from the primary lesion or the development of second primaries. Unfortunately, most studies have also included patients at different stages of disease, so that it is not possible to accurately differentiate outcomes in patients with early- versus late-stage disease. Indeed, the staging of HCC is highly controversial at present [125–127]. Until a widely accepted staging system is developed, this uncertainty about outcome will persist.

In the absence of data from randomized trials, modeling data have been used to determine whether surveillance is effective and cost-effective. There are several published models of HCC screening. Sarasin et al. [128] undertook a Markov decision analysis of screening a cohort of cirrhotic until the development of Child's B cirrhosis, when screening stopped. Kang et al. [129] performed a decision analysis of screening hepatitis B carriers with AFP and ultrasound. We have performed a Markov analysis of a hepatitis B cohort, aged 30 at the beginning of screening [130]. All these analyses found approximately similar results. Screening will prolong life in the cohort for about 3 months. This seems a trivial improvement in survival, but over a cohort of 1,000 subjects, it translates to 250 years of life saved. Both Markov analyses showed that screening was always more expensive than no screening, but that the costs per life year gained under basal assumptions were in the range considered cost effective (less than $50,000 per life–year gained). However, there were several critical factors which affected the cost efficacy. If the incidence of HCC in the HBV cohort was less than 0.2%, screening became cost-ineffective. In the cirrhotic cohort, if the annual incidence of HCC was less than about 1.3%, surveillance became ineffective. This difference is related to the effect of cirrhosis on the rate of resection and on post-operative survival. Similarly, if survival after therapy for HCC was less than about 50%, screening became cost inefficient. Other important factors were the proportion of patients with small HCC's who actually underwent screening, and in the hepatitis B cohort, the age at onset of screening.

Serological Markers

α-Fetoprotein

In evaluating the performance characteristics of tests used for cancer screening, it is important to distinguish between the performance characteristics of the same tests used for diagnosis, or used for screening/surveillance. For example, the sensitivity and specificity of AFP as a diagnostic test (that is, when it is used after there is already a suspicion of HCC) will be better than when AFP is used as a screening test (that is, when there is no *a priori* reason to suspect that HCC is present). In many reports of the performance characteristics of AFP and ultrasound, these tests are used as diagnostic tests or the exact setting is not specified, making it difficult to evaluate their performance as surveillance tests.

AFP levels are frequently elevated in patients with established HCC. Initially, before the advent of ultrasonography and CT scanning, elevated AFP levels were the only noninvasive way of diagnosing HCC. The initial descriptions came from parts of the world where HCC was common and from patients with late stage disease. Thus it was not unusual to record AFP levels of greater than 10,000 ng/ml, and even greater than 100,000 ng/ml. However, when the performance characteristics of AFP are carefully evaluated, it is clear that its role even as a diagnostic test has not been adequately assessed. In the appropriate clinical setting, when the AFP concentration is very high, the likelihood of a false-positive is negligible, but the false-negative rate is high, since up to 40% of large HCC's do not secrete AFP. In tumors which secrete AFP, the concentration is related to the size of the tumor. Thus when small HCCs are the object of surveillance, a diagnostically high AFP is unlikely.

The first surveillance studies used serum AFP as the only marker of HCC [131,132]. The reported sensitivity of AFP for detecting HCC varied widely in both HBV-positive and predominantly HBV-negative populations [22,35,37,39,131–134], possibly because of the confusion between diagnosis and screening. If the level of AFP triggering investigation for HCC is increased (e.g., from 20 ng/L to 100 ng/L), as expected, the sensitivity of the AFP test falls from 39% to 13% and the specificity increases [22]. However, AFP is not specific for HCC. Titers also rise with flares of active hepatitis. Out of 44 HBV carriers with elevated AFP levels detected during surveillance for HCC, only 6 were found to have HCC on further investigation, and in 18 (41%), the raised AFP was associated with an exacerbation of underlying liver disease or with changes in HBV replication status [131]. DiBisceglie et al. [133] found that 25 of 29 AFP elevations in patients with chronic HBV infection were due to flares of inflammatory activity, and only 2 of 29 were due to HCC. In a direct comparison of the specificity of AFP as a diagnostic test for detecting HCC in HBV-negative and -positive patients, the specificity was only 50% in HBV-positive patients compared to 78% in HBV-negative patients [134].

Performance characteristics of AFP as a screening test were reported in three studies [22,35,37]. In these studies, the screening methodology was well described, and it was clear that AFP was used for surveillance, that is, for follow-up and monitoring of patients with chronic hepatitis. These studies report a sensitivity of 39% to 64%, a specificity of 76% to 91% and a positive predictive value of 9% to 32%.

More recently, tumor-specific fractions of AFP have been described. The circulating AFP pool exists as different protein subspecies with different degrees of glycosylation. These can be separated by electrophoresis or by lectin affinity chromatography. There are several glycosylated fractions of AFP, which appear to be more specific for HCC. Studies have described an increased fraction of these glycosylated fractions in patients with HCC compared to those with chronic hepatitis or cirrhosis [135–138]. There are also reports of alterations in the normal AFP/lectin-bound–AFP ratio developing in patients before the clinical diagnosis of HCC [139–141]. However, the value of these assays for HCC surveillance has yet to be established.

Other Markers

Concentrations of other serological markers have been found to be elevated in patients with HCC. These include α-fucosidase (AF) [142,143], and des-γ-carboxyprothrombin (DGCP) [144,145]. However, the value of using these tests for diagnosis has not been established. Assays for these markers have also been evaluated as screening tests. Some patients with small HCC's do have elevated AF or DGCP, without elevated AFP. However, the studies were small, with relatively short follow-up. Additional studies are needed before these tests can be considered useful.

Radiological Tests

Ultrasonography (US) is a better surveillance tool than AFP. The performance characteristics of ultrasound as a screening test for HCC have been defined by Sherman et al. [22] in a surveillance study of healthy HBsAg carriers and by Pateron et al. [37] in a surveillance study of patients with cirrhosis. The reported sensitivity was 71% and 78% respectively. The specificity was 93% in both studies. The positive predictive value was 14% and 73%, respectively. It remains to be determined whether these performance characteristics make these tests efficient economical approaches for HCC surveillance. It is difficult to assess the reports of accuracy of ultrasonography, because in most instances, the gold standard has been another radiological test rather than histology. US is reasonably sensitive in the detection of liver masses. However, in a cirrhotic liver there are often multiple masses. Most are simply cirrhotic nodules. Ultrasound is unable to distinguish between neoplastic and non-neoplastic nodules if the lesions are small, usually less than 1 cm in size. Larger HCCs have characteristic US findings, usually a hyperechoic mass lesion, often with a hypoechoic halo. Doppler US shows arterial flow within the mass. These characteristics are seldom present in small (<1 cm) lesions. Thus, the finding of a nodule on ultrasound should invariably lead to additional investigations.

Follow-up radiology, including triphasic computerized tomography (CT) scan with an HCC protocol, or magnetic resonance imaging (MRI) may show convincing evidence of HCC. However, as with US, when the lesions are small they may not be identified by these tests, or if they are, their appearances may be once more nonspecific. Once a mass has been found on one or more imaging techniques, a negative result from another imaging technique may simply be due to lack of sensitivity, rather than a true negative. Thus a negative result following a positive always requires further follow-up, either additional radiology, or interval testing. The false-negative rate from such a series of investigations is unknown, as is the false-positive rate. Even if the false-positive rate is low, the consequences of a wrong diagnosis may be major surgery, or other invasive treatment modalities.

Newer techniques such as contrast-enhanced US are not suitable for surveillance. CT scanning has not been evaluated for surveillance. It is more expensive than US, and requires intravenous contrast agents, with the concomitant risk of allergic reactions and renal complications. Furthermore, evaluation of small lesions suspicious for HCC on CT scanning is no less problematical than on US.

Who Should Undergo Surveillance?

The question of whether surveillance for HCC should be instituted at all may legitimately be asked, given the lack of data on efficacy. There are good reasons for considering surveillance. First among these is that progress in treating HCC is only going to come from better treatment of small lesions, not from improved treatment of late-stage disease. Surveillance may not be highly effective at present but if surveillance methodology is to improve, we will need to identify the deficiencies of current methods. If we do not screen our patients, we cannot improve surveillance methodologies. If we don't find small lesions, we cannot test new forms of treatment or improve on existing methods of treatment.

Studies to date have focused on surveillance in patients with chronic hepatitis B and on patients with hepatitis C and cirrhosis. However, within these groups, there are several factors which affect HCC incidence. We have already discussed the effects of age and gender and inflammatory activity on HCC risk. In chronic hepatitis B, ethnicity may also be a factor affecting risk, in that Asian and African hepatitis B carriers are at particularly elevated risk relative to other ethnic groups. This may be simply related to age at acquisition of disease, although there may be genetic or environmental factors as well.

No study has directly addressed the question of whether surveillance for HCC should or could be restricted to individuals over a certain age limit—as is suggested for surveillance of colorectal carcinoma [146]—while maintaining maximum benefit. Many hepatologists involved in studying surveillance would start surveillance at about age 40 in male HBV carriers, and possibly somewhat older in women (personal communications). Clearly surveillance started at a younger age (e.g., age 30) would miss fewer tumors, but the ideal starting age balancing efficacy with cost has not been defined.

Another important risk factor in the hepatitis B population is a family history of HCC. This has now been demonstrated in several studies [57]. Once again, this may be related to intrafamilial spread of hepatitis B at a young age, but genetic factors cannot be discounted.

All these factors can be used to define a target population for screening and surveillance in the hepatitis-B population. However, since the medical literature cannot provide hard and fast rules, the choice of a target population is at the discretion of the physician. Clinical practice guidelines do not yet exist.

For hepatitis C infection, possible strategies could include screening all hepatitis C carriers, or screening only those hepatitis C carriers with evidence of some liver disease, even if cirrhosis cannot be diagnosed with certainty. A third strategy might be to restrict the target population to only those HCV carriers with diagnosed or suspected cirrhosis. This raises the questions of whether it is appropriate to biopsy hepatitis C carriers to determine if cirrhosis is present so that they can be entered into surveillance programs, and whether it is appropriate to repeat biopsies periodically for the same reason.

Thus cirrhosis may be used as a diagnosis to further identify and refine selection of a target population for surveillance. This presupposes that the diagnosis of cirrhosis has been made by clinical or other means. Unfortunately, undiagnosed cirrhosis is common in patients with viral hepatitis. An English study reported that 56% percent of 305 patients presenting with HCC between 1978 and 1988 had previously undiagnosed cirrhosis [147]. Similarly, a Japanese study found that 20% of 3821 patients studied had previously undiagnosed cirrhosis [148], and thus would not have been recruited into a surveillance program if the presence of cirrhosis had been used to define the target population. Furthermore, cirrhosis may develop during follow-up and may still not be clinically apparent. A study of 412 Japanese HCV carriers found that 56% of the cohort had chronic hepatitis without cirrhosis, and 44% had cirrhosis at the time of recruitment [149]. Seventeen percent of the 63 patients with tumors that were diagnosed by surveillance over a median follow-up of 5 years were not known to be cirrhotic at the time of entry into the study [150]. The overall reported annual detection rate of HCC in surveillance studies which included individuals with chronic hepatitis as well as patients with cirrhosis is 0.8% to 4.1% [33–39]. The variation in incidence rates of HCC in these studies is a reflection of the varying percentage of individuals with chronic hepatitis and of the different causal factors between studies.

Persistently elevated AFP concentration also indicates an increased risk of HCC, as does the presence of foci of dysplastic cells on biopsy [35,38,130]. We have already discussed how histological markers, such as PCNA or AgNOR, or irregular nodular regeneration may predict the development of HCC. However, with the exception of chronic hepatitis B, these markers are most often found in patients who have established cirrhosis. Thus many of these patients will already have been enrolled in screening programs. It has been suggested that the presence of these markers should lead to a shorter screening interval. However, there are no data to support this practice.

An alternative strategy has been proposed by Ganne-Carre et al. [104]. They have developed a scoring system to assess risk of HCC. The system has been validated prospectively by the same group, but there are no independent reports of the efficacy of the system. There are also questions about whether the system is appropriate for patients with cirrhosis due to causes other than hepatitis C or alcoholic liver disease.

Surveillance Interval

There is little information about the optimal surveillance interval. From reports in the literature the time taken for a tumour to grow from undetectable to 2 cm is about 4–12 months [151–153]. Thus a 6-month surveillance interval would seem to be appropriate. There is no information as to how the prognosis differs if the HCC is discovered and treated at 1 cm versus at 2 or 3 cm. Studies reporting survival following diagnosis are uncontrolled and do not take lead-time bias into account. Thus, the ideal screening interval, which combines optimal detection with lowest cost, cannot be determined.

Prevention

Primary Prevention of Chronic Hepatitis B

Preventive strategies for HCC are summarized in Table 11.2. HCC related to HBV is a completely eradicable disease. HBV has no animal

TABLE 11.2. Strategies for prevention of HCC.

Primary	Secondary	Tertiary
Hepatitis B vaccination	?Population screening for chronic viral hepatitis	Treatment of viral hepatitis
Prevention of hepatitis B and C infection	HCC surveillance using 6 monthly US examinations	Hepatitis B: α-Interferon, Lamivudine
	?Population screening for hemochromatosis	Hepatitis C: α-Interferon and ribavirin

reservoir. The hepatitis B vaccine is highly effective when given to children [154,155] and in all probability, booster doses are not necessary. Universal vaccination against HBV is an achievable objective that has been implemented in many countries. As an example of what can be achieved, in Taiwan the incidence of childhood HCC has dropped dramatically since the introduction of universal vaccination [47]. However, since universal vaccination is only about 10 to 15 years old, HCC secondary to HBV infection will still be with us for about 40 to 50 years.

Primary Prevention of Hepatitis C

There is no hepatitis C vaccine, nor are prospects good for development of a hepatitis C vaccine in the near future. Primary prevention of HCC related to hepatitis C infection must therefore rest in preventing exposure. In the West, new cases of chronic hepatitis C occur almost exclusively in intravenous drug users. Transfusion-related disease and disease related to mass vaccination or to improperly sterilized reusable equipment are also almost nonexistent. Intravenous drug users are a notoriously difficult group to reach. Since infection with hepatitis C occurs early in the course of IVDU, interventions should be directed toward at-risk individuals, rather than at established users.

Strategies to Reduce the Incidence of HCC

Treatment of Chronic Viral Hepatitis

If the hypothesis about the development of HCC in chronic liver disease in correct, then persistent inflammation is a major stimulus for

oncogenesis. Therefore, prevention or reduction of the amount of inflammation should be beneficial in preventing the development of HCC. Treatment is now available for both hepatitis-C and hepatitis-B infection.

Active hepatitis B infection can be treated with α-interferon [156–160], or with lamivudine [161,162], a nucleoside analogue. Long-term results following interferon therapy have been reported. A limited course of interferon therapy results in remission of active inflammation, but not eradication of infection in about 40% of patients. The remission is subsequently maintained by host immune mechanisms. In Europe and Asia, successful antiviral therapy with interferon is associated with a reduction in the incidence of HCC [163,164].

Lamivudine, a nucleoside analogue, suppresses hepatitis B viral replication. It is not yet clear whether optimum treatment should be time-limited as with interferon, or whether long-term suppression of viral replication is required. Lamivudine therapy has not been available long enough to determine whether the incidence of HCC is reduced in treated patients.

Chronic hepatitis C is a "curable" disease. Successful therapy is associated with clearance of virus from serum, and in most cases, from liver as well. Hepatic inflammation is reduced. Long-term follow-up suggests that there is no recurrence of disease without reinfection [165]. Most long-term follow-up studies suggest that the incidence of HCC is reduced [166,167]. However, not all studies agree on this point [26]. More controversial is whether incomplete responses to therapy are also associated with a reduced incidence of HCC. Studies provide conflicting results, with some claiming that the incidence is reduced in all subjects treated with interferon, whereas most studies suggest that the benefit is limited to those who respond to treatment [167]. Given the long duration of infection before therapy in most cases, it is hard to believe that temporary partial suppression of viral replication for a few months really makes a difference to the oncogenic process.

Treatment of HCC Cancer Precursors

Surveillance today is aimed at finding established small HCC's. Many physicians today treat these lesions with some form of loco-regional therapy such as alcohol injection or radiofrequency ablation, often without biopsy. Given the difficulty in differentiating preneoplastic and neoplastic lesions radiologically, it is likely that in the absence of a biopsy, some treated lesions will be preneoplastic rather than fully developed HCC. There are as yet no data to indicate that this practice has advantages over the standard practice of treating only established confirmed HCC. Theoretically, by analogy with other cancers, treatment of preneoplastic lesions is more likely to be effective than treatment of established cancer. Colon cancer and cervical cancer are two examples in which surveillance identifies preneoplastic lesions (see Chapters 9 and 16). In both sites, surveillance clearly reduces the risk of death from the cancer. In contrast, lung and prostate cancer screening, in which the target is established cancer, remain controversial and probably are not effective in reducing mortality. However, in HCC the relationship between the preneoplastic lesion and the subsequent HCC is not so clearly that of parent and child. In colon and cervical carcinoma screening, identification of a lesion leads to removal of all neoplastic and potentially neoplastic tissue (e.g., colonic polypectomy or cervical cone biopsy). A better analogy for HCC is with colonic polyposis syndromes, where removal of a single polyp will not prevent subsequent development of a cancer elsewhere. A cirrhotic liver with detectable preneoplastic lesions (even fully developed small HCC) is likely to have other preneoplastic lesions (or even fully developed HCC) elsewhere in the liver. HCC is frequently multifocal with second primary lesions being common [168,169]. Removal of the apparent lesion is unlikely to prevent cancer completely. Perhaps, as with colonic polyposis syndromes the answer is to remove/replace the whole offending organ.

Conclusion

Screening/surveillance for HCC is a subject of increasing importance as the cohort of patients with chronic viral hepatitis ages. The topic has been the subject of debate at several recent international conferences. In the absence of data, it is impossible to develop consensus guidelines, but some form of practice guideline is sorely needed. The lack of data also points to the need for randomized controlled trials of screening/surveillance or of therapy of small lesions, whether they be preneoplastic or neoplastic. Multicenter studies would be preferable to reduce the time needed to recruit the appropriate number of subjects. HCC has not yet received the attention it deserves from the oncology community nor from funding agencies. However, over the next decade or so, this will likely change as the incidence of and mortality from HCC increases. The next 10 years will hopefully be a "golden age" of HCC research.

References

1. Parkin DM, Muir CS, Whelan SL, et al. *Cancer incidence in five continents*, Vol. VI. Lyon: IARC Scientific Publications, 1992.
2. Bosch FX. Global epidemiology of hepatocellular carcinoma. In: Okuda K, Tabor E (eds) *Liver Cancer*. New York: Churchill Livingston, 1997, pp. 13–37.
3. Simonetti RG, Camma C, Fiorello F, et al. Hepatocellular carcinoma a worldwide problem and the major risk factor. *Dig Dis Sci* 1991; 36:962–72.
4. EI-Serag H, Mason AC. Rising incidence of hepatocellular carcinoma in the United States. *N Engl J Med* 1999; 340:745–50.
5. Okuda K, Fujimoto I, Hanai A, et al. Changing incidence of hepatocellular carcinoma in Japan. *Cancer Res* 1987; 47:4967–72.

6. Taylor-Robinson SD, Foster GR, et al. Increase in primary liver cancer in the UK 1979–1974. *Lancet* 1997; 350:1142–3.

7. Deuffic S, Poynard T, Buffat L, et al. Trends in primary liver cancer. *Lancet* 1998; 351:214–15.

8. Stroffolini T, Andreone P, Andriulli A, et al. Characteristics of hepatocellular carcinoma in Italy. *J Hepatol* 1998; 29:944–52.

9. Parkin DM, Ohshima H, Srivatanakul P, et al. Cholangiocarcinoma: epidemiology, mechanisms of carcinogenesis and prevention. *Cancer Epidemiol Biomarkers Prev* 1993; 2:537–44.

10. Shin HR, Lee CU, Park HJ, et al. Hepatitis B and C virus, *Clonorchis sinensis* for the risk of liver cancer: a case-control study in Pusan, Korea. *Int J Epidemiol* 1996; 25:933–40.

11. Haswell-Elkins MR, Mairiang E, Mairiang P, et al. Cross-sectional study of *Opisthorchis viverrini* infection and cholangiocarcinoma in communities within a high-risk area in northeast Thailand. *Int J Cancer* 1994; 59:505–9.

12. Bergquist A, Glaumann H, Persson B, et al. Risk factors and clinical presentation of hepatobiliary carcinoma in patients with primary sclerosing cholangitis: a case-control study. *Hepatology* 1998; 27:311–16.

13. Kornfeld D, Ekbom A, Ihre T. Survival and risk of cholangiocarcinoma in patients with primary sclerosing cholangitis. A population-based study. *Scand J Gastroenterol* 1997; 32:1042–5.

14. Davis RI, Sloan JM, Hood JM, et al. Carcinoma of the extrahepatic biliary tract: a clinicopathological and immunohistochemical study. *Histopathology* 1988; 12:623–31.

15. Martins EB, Fleming KA, Garrido MC, et al. Superficial thrombophlebitis, dysplasia, and cholangiocarcinoma in primary sclerosing cholangitis. *Gastroenterology* 1994; 107:537–42.

16. Fozard JB, Wyatt JI, Hall RI. Epithelial dysplasia in Caroli's disease. *Gut* 1989; 30:1150–3.

17. Beasley RP, Hwang LY, Lin CC, et al. Hepatocellular carcinoma and hepatitis B virus: a prospective study of 22,700 men in Taiwan. *Lancet* 1981; 2:1129–33.

18. Beasley RP, Hwang, LY, Epidemiology of hepatocellular carcinoma. In: Vyas GN, Dienstag JL, Hoofnagle JH (eds) *Viral Hepatitis and Liver Disease*. New York: Grune and Stratton, 1984, pp. 209–24.

19. Sakuma K, Saitoh N, Kasai M, et al. Relative risks of death due to liver disease among Japanese male adults having various statuses for hepatitis B s and e antigen/antibody in serum: a prospective study. *Hepatology* 1988; 8:1642–6.

20. Villeneuve JP, Desrochers M, Infante-Rivard C, et al. A long-term follow-up study of asymptomatic hepatitis B surface antigen-positive carriers in Montreal. *Gastroenterology* 1994; 106:1000–5.

21. McMahon BJ, Alberts SR, Wainwright RB, et al. Hepatitis B-related sequelae. Prospective study of 1,400 hepatitis B surface antigen-positive Alaska native carriers. *Arch Intern Med* 1990; 150:1051–4.

22. Sherman M, Peltekian KM, Lee C. Screening for hepatocellular carcinoma in chronic carriers of hepatitis B virus: incidence and prevalence of hepatocellular carcinoma in a North American urban population. *Hepatology* 1995; 22:432–8.

23. Fattovich G, Giustina G, Schalm SW, et al. Occurrence of hepatocellular carcinoma and decompensation in western European patients with cirrhosis type B. The EUROHEP Study Group on Hepatitis B Virus and Cirrhosis. *Hepatology* 1995; 21:77–82.

24. Fattovich G, Giustina G, Degos F, et al. Morbidity and mortality in compensated cirrhosis type C: a retrospective follow-up study of 384 patients. *Gastroenterology* 1997; 2:463–72.

25. Bruix J, Barrera JM, Calvert X, et al. Prevalence of antibodies to hepatitis C virus in Spanish patients with hepatocellular carcinoma and hepatitis cirrhosis. *Lancet* 1989; ii:1004–6.

26. Niederau C, Lange S, Heintges T, et al. Prognosis of chronic hepatitis C: results of a large, prospective cohort study. *Hepatology* 1998; 28:1687–95.

27. Tong MJ, Blatt LM, Kao VW. Surveillance for hepatocellular carcinoma in patients with chronic viral hepatitis in the United States of America. *J Gastroenterol Hepatol* 2001; 16:553–9.

28. Kato Y, Nakata K, Omagari K, et al. Risk of hepatocellular carcinoma in patients with cirrhosis in Japan. *Cancer* 1994; 74:2234–8.

29. Ikeda K, Saitoh S, Koida I, et al. A multivariate analysis of risk factors for hepatocellular carcinoma: a prospective observation of 795 patients with viral and alcoholic cirrhosis. *Hepatology* 1993; 18:47–53.

30. Benvegnu L, Fattovich G, Noventa F, et al. Concurrent hepatitis B and C virus infection and risk of hepatocellular carcinoma in cirrhosis. A prospective study. *Cancer* 1994; 74:2442–8.

31. Van Roey G, Fevery J, Van Steenbergen W. Hepatocellular carcinoma in Belgium: clinical and virological characteristics of 154

consecutive cirrhotic and non-cirrhotic patients. *Hepatology* 2000; 12:61–6.

32. Chiesa R, Donato F, Tagger A, et al. Etiology of hepatocellular carcinoma in Italian patients with and without cirrhosis. *Cancer Epidemiol Biomarkers Prev* 2000; 9:213.

33. Cottone M, Turri M, Caltagirone M, et al. Screening for hepatocellular carcinoma in patients with Childs A cirrhosis: an 8 year prospective study by ultrasound and alphafetoprotein. *J Hepatol* 1994; 21:1029–34.

34. Zoli M, Magalotti D, Bianchi G, et al. Efficacy of a surveillance program for early detection of hepatocellular carcinoma. *Cancer* 1996; 78:977–85.

35. Oka H, Tamori A, Kuroki T, et al. Prospective study of alpha-fetoprotein in cirrhotic patients monitored for development of hepatocellular carcinoma. *Hepatology* 1994; 19:61–6.

36. Borzio M, Bruno S, Roncalli M, et al. Liver cell dysplasia is a major risk factor for hepatocellular carcinoma in cirrhosis. A prospective study. *Gastroenterology* 1995; 108:812–17.

37. Pateron D, Ganne N, Trinchet JC, et al. Prospective study of screening for hepatocellular carcinoma in Caucasian patients with cirrhosis. *J Hepatol* 1994; 20:65–71.

38. Colombo M, De Franchis R, Del Ninno E, et al. Hepatocellular carcinoma in Italian patients with cirrhosis. *Lancet* 1991; 325:675–80.

39. Zaman SN, Melia WM, Johnson RD, et al. Risk factors in development of hepatocellular carcinoma in cirrhosis: Prospective study of 613 patients. *Lancet* 1985; I:1357–60.

40. Fargion S, Fracanzani AL, Piperno A, et al. Prognostic factors for hepatocellular carcinoma in genetic haemochromatosis. *Hepatology* 1994; 20:1426–31.

41. Farinati F, Floreani A, DeMaria N, et al. Hepatocellular carcinoma in primary biliary cirrhosis. *J Hepatol* 1994; 21:315–16.

42. Villa E, Baldini GM, Pasquinelli C, et al. Risk factors for hepatocellular carcinoma in Italy: male sex. hepatitis B virus, non-A non-B infection and alcohol. *Cancer* 1988; 62:611–15.

43. Liaw Y-F, Tai D-I, Chu C-M, et al. Early detection of hepatocellular carcinoma in patients with chronic type B hepatitis. *Gastroenterology* 1986; 90:263–6.

44. Fattovich G, Brollo L, Giustina G, et al. Natural history and prognostic factors for chronic hepatitis type B. *Gut* 1991; 32:294–8.

45. Stanta G, Croce LS, Bonin S, et al. Cohort effect of HCV infection in liver cirrhosis assessed by a 25 year study. *J Clin Virol* 2000; 17:51–6.

46. Comandini UV, Tossini G, Longo MA, et al. Sporadic hepatitis C virus infection: a case-control study of transmission routes in a selected hospital sample of the general population in Italy. *Scand J Infect Dis* 1998; 30:11–15.

47. Chang MH, Chen CJ, Lai MS, et al. Universal hepatitis B vaccination in Taiwan and the incidence of hepatocellular carcinoma in children. Taiwan Childhood Hepatoma Study Group. *N Engl J Med* 1997; 336:1855–9.

48. Prozesky OW, Szmuness W, Stevens CE, et al. Baseline epidemiological studies for a hepatitis B vaccine trial in Kangwane. *S Afr Med J* 1983; 64:891–3.

49. Hsu HY, Chang MH, Chen DS, et al. Baseline seroepidemiology of hepatitis B virus infection in children in Taipei, 1984: a study just before mass hepatitis B vaccination program in Taiwan. *J Med Virol* 1986; 18:301–7.

50. McQuillan GM, Townsend TR, Fields HA, et al. Seroepidemiology of hepatitis B virus infection in the United States. 1976 to 1980. *Am J Med* 1989; 87 (3A Suppl):5–10.

51. Shimbo S, Zhang ZW, Qu JB, et al. Urban-rural comparison of HBV and HCV infection prevalence among adult women in Shandong Province, China. *Southeast Asian J Trop Med Public Health* 1997; 28:500–6.

52. Kwan LC, Ho YY, Lee SS. The declining HBsAg carriage rate in pregnant women in Hong Kong. *Epidemiol Infect* 1997; 119:281–3.

53. Madzime S, Adem M, Mahomed K, et al. Hepatitis B virus infection among pregnant women delivering at Harare Maternity Hospital, Harare Zimbabwe, 1996 to 1997. *Cent Afr J Med* 1999; 45:195–8.

54. Ahmed SD, Cuevas LE, Brabin BJ, et al. Seroprevalence of hepatitis B and C and HIV in Malawian pregnant women. *J Infect* 1998; 37:248–51.

55. Anderson KE, Stevens CE, Tsuei JJ, et al. Hepatitis B antigen in infants born to mothers with chronic hepatitis B antigenemia in Taiwan. *Am J Dis Child* 1975; 129:1389–92.

56. Beasley RP, Trepo C, Stevens CE, et al. The antigen and vertical transmission of hepatitis B surface antigen. *Am J Epidemiol* 1977; 105:94–8.

57. Yu MW, Chang HC, Liaw YF, et al. Familial risk of hepatocellular carcinoma among chronic

hepatitis B carriers and their relatives. *J Natl Cancer Inst* 2000; 92:1159–64.

58. Guadagnino V, Stroffolini T, Rapicetta M, et al. Prevalence, risk factors, and genotype distribution of hepatitis C virus infection in the general population: a community-based survey in southern Italy. *Hepatology* 1997; 26:1006–11.

59. Abdel-Aziz F, Habib M, Mohamed MK, et al. Hepatitis C virus (HCV) infection in a community in the Nile Delta: population description and HCV prevalence. *Hepatology* 2000; 32:111–15.

60. Curley SA, Izzo F, Gallipoli A, et al. Identification and screening of 416 patients with chronic hepatitis at high risk to develop hepatocellular carcinoma. *Ann Surg* 1995; 222:375–83.

61. Rogler CE, Sherman M, Su CY, et al. Deletion in chromosome 11p associated with a hepatitis B integration site in hepatocellular carcinoma. *Science* 1985; 230:319–22.

62. Shaul Y, Garcia PD, Schonberg S, et al. Integration of hepatitis B virus DNA in chromosome-specific satellite sequences. *J Virol* 1986; 59:731–4.

63. Yaginuma K, Kobayashi M, Yoshida E, et al. Hepatitis B virus integration in hepatocellular carcinoma DNA: duplication of cellular flanking sequences at the integration site. *Proc Natl Acad Sci USA* 1985; 82:4458–62.

64. Dejean A, Sonigo P, Wain-Hobson S, et al. Hepatitis B virus integration in hepatocellular carcinoma DNA through an 11-base pair direct repeat. *Proc Natl Acad Sci USA* 1984; 81: 5350–4.

65. Koshy R, Koch S, Freytag von Loringhoven A, et al. Integration of hepatitis B virus DNA. Evidence for integration in the single-strand gap. *Cell* 1983; 34:215–23.

66. Yamamoto S, Mita E, Nakatake H, et al. Trans-activating function of integrated hepatitis B virus. *Biochem Biophys Res Commun* 1993; 197:1209–15.

67. Twu JS, Lai MY, Chen DS, et al. Activation of protooncogene c-*jun* by the X protein of hepatitis B virus. *Virol* 1993; 192:346–50.

68. Wollersheim M, Debelka U, Hofschneider PH. A transactivating function encoded in the hepatitis B virus *X* gene is conserved in the integrated state. *Oncogene* 1988; 3:545–52.

69. Takada S, Koike K. Trans-activation function of a 3′ truncated *X* gene–cell fusion product from integrated hepatitis B virus DNA in chronic hepatitis tissues. *Proc Natl Acad Sci USA* 1990; 87:5628–32.

70. Miyaki M, Sato C, Sakai K, et al. Malignant transformation and EGFR activation of immortalized mouse liver epithelial cells caused by HBV enhancer-X from a human hepatocellular carcinoma. *Int J Cancer* 2000; 85:518–22.

71. Luber B, Arnold N, Sturzl M, et al. Hepatoma-derived integrated HBV DNA causes multistage transformation in vitro. *Oncogene* 1996; 12:1597–608.

72. Schluter V, Meyer M, Hofschneider PH, et al. Integrated hepatitis B virus X and 3′ truncated preS/S sequences derived from human hepatomas encode functionally active transactivators. *Oncogene* 1994; 9:3335–44.

73. Caselmann WH, Meyer M, Kekule AS, et al. A trans-activator function is generated by integration of hepatitis B virus preS/S sequences in human hepatocellular carcinoma DNA. *Proc Natl Acad Sci USA* 1990; 87:2970–4.

74. Kekule AS, Lauer U, Meyer M, et al. The preS2/S region of integrated hepatitis B virus DNA encodes a transcriptional transactivator. *Nature* 1990; 343:457–61.

75. Slagle BL, Zhou YZ, Butel JS. Hepatitis B virus integration event in human chromosome 17p near the *p53* gene identifies the region of the chromosome commonly deleted in virus-positive hepatocellular carcinomas. *Cancer Res* 1991; 51:49–54.

76. Fowler MJ, Greenfield C, Chu CM, et al. Integration of HBV–DNA may not be a prerequisite for the maintenance of the state of malignant transformation. An analysis of 110 liver biopsies. *J Hepatol* 1986; 2:218–29.

77. Bressac B, Galvin KM, Liang TJ, et al. Abnormal structure and expression of *p53* gene in human hepatocellular carcinoma. *Proc Natl Acad Sci USA* 1990; 87:1973–7.

78. Bressac B, Kew M, Wands J, et al. Selective G to T mutations of *p53* gene in hepatocellular carcinoma from southern Africa. *Nature* 1991; 350:429–31.

79. Lunn RM, Zhang YJ, Wang LY, et al. *p53* Mutations, chronic hepatitis B virus infection, and aflatoxin exposure in hepatocellular carcinoma in Taiwan. *Cancer Res* 1997; 57:3471–7.

80. Itoh T, Shiro T, Seki T, et al. Relationship between *p53* overexpression and the proliferative activity in hepatocellular carcinoma. *Int J Mol Med* 2000; 6:137–42.

81. Shimizu Y, Zhu JJ, Han F, et al. Different frequencies of *p53* codon-249 hot-spot mutations in hepatocellular carcinomas in

Jiang-su province of China. *Int J Cancer* 1999; 82: 187–90.

82. Denissenko MF, Koudriakova TB, Smith L, et al. The *p53* codon 249 mutational hotspot in hepatocellular carcinoma is not related to selective formation or persistence of aflatoxin B1 adducts. *Oncogene* 1998; 17:3007–14.

83. Kazachkov Y, Khaoustov V, Yoffe B, et al. *p53* abnormalities in hepatocellular carcinoma from United States patients: analysis of all 11 exons. *Carcinogenesis* 1996; 17:2207–12.

84. Yumoto Y, Hanafusa T, Hada H, et al. Loss of heterozygosity and analysis of mutation of *p53* in hepatocellular carcinoma. *J Gastroenterol Hepatol* 1995; 10:179–85.

85. Nose H, Imazeki F, Ohto M, et al. *p53* Gene mutations and 17p allelic deletions in hepatocellular carcinoma from Japan. *Cancer* 1993; 72:355–60.

86. Emi M, Fujiwara Y, Ohata H, et al. Allelic loss at chromosome band 8p21.3-p22 is associated with progression of hepatocellular carcinoma. *Genes Chromosom Cancer* 1993; 7:152–7.

87. Sakai K, Nagahara H, Abe K, et al. Loss of heterozygosity on chromosome 16 in hepatocellular carcinoma. *J Gastroenterol Hepatol* 1992; 7:288–92.

88. Ding SF, Habib NA, Dooley J, et al. Loss of constitutional heterozygosity on chromosome 5q in hepatocellular carcinoma without cirrhosis. *Br J Cancer* 1991; 64:1083–7.

89. Buetow KH, Murray JC, Israel JL, et al. Loss of heterozygosity suggests tumor suppressor gene responsible for primary hepatocellular carcinoma. *Proc Natl Acad Sci USA* 1989; 86:8852–6.

90. Wang HP, Rogler CE. Deletions in human chromosome arms 11p and 13q in primary hepatocellular carcinomas. *Cytogenet Cell Genet* 1988; 48:72–8.

91. Hytiroglou P, Theise ND, Schwartz M, et al. Macroregenerative nodules in a series of adult cirrhotic liver explants: issues of classification and nomenclature. *Hepatology* 1995; 21:703–8.

92. International Working Party. Terminology of nodular hepatocellular lesions. *Hepatology* 1995; 22:983–93.

93. Wanless IR, Nakashima E, Sherman M. Regression of human cirrhosis. morphologic features and the genesis of incomplete septal cirrhosis. *Arch Pathol Lab Med* 2000; 124:1599–607.

94. Nakashima E, Wanless IR. Most non-cirrhotic livers with hepatocellular carcinoma (HCC) have evidence of fibrosis or regressed cirrhosis:

implications for the pathogenesis of HCC. *Hepatology* 1999; 30:257A.

95. Anthony PP. Liver cell dysplasia: what is its significance? *Hepatology* 1987; 7:394–5.

96. Watanabe S, Okita K, Harada T. Morphologic studies of the liver cell dysplasia. *Cancer* 1983; 51:2197–205.

97. Ueda K, Terada T, Nakanuma Y, et al. Vascular supply in adenomatous hyperplasia of the liver and hepatocellular carcinoma: A morphometric study. *Hum Pathol* 1992; 23:619–26.

98. Ferrell LD. Hepatocellular carcinoma arising in a focus of multilobular adenoma. A case report. *Am J Surg Pathol* 1993; 17:525–9.

99. Arakawa M, Kage M, Sugihara S, et al. Emergence of malignant lesions within an adenomatous hyperplastic nodule in a cirrhotic liver. Observations in five cases. *Gastroenterology* 1986; 91:198–208.

100. Tiniakos DG, Brunt EM. Proliferating cell nuclear antigen and Ki-67 labeling in hepatocellular nodules: a comparative study. *Liver* 1999; 19:58–68.

101. Ballardini G, Groff P, Zoli M, et al. Increased risk of hepatocellular carcinoma development in patients with cirrhosis and with high hepatocellular proliferation. *J Hepatol* 1994; 20:218–22.

102. Dutta U, Kench J, Byth K, et al. Hepatocellular proliferation and development of hepatocellular carcinoma: a case-control study in chronic hepatitis C. *Hum Pathol* 1998; 29:1279–84.

103. Borzio M, Trere D, Borzio F, et al. Hepatocyte proliferation rate is a powerful parameter for predicting hepatocellular carcinoma development in liver cirrhosis. *Mol Pathol* 1998; 510:96–101.

104. Ganne-Carrie N, Chastang C, Chapel F, et al. Predictive score for the development of hepatocellular carcinoma and additional value of liver large cell dysplasia in Western patients with cirrhosis. *Hepatology* 1996; 23:1112–18.

105. Lee RG, Tsamandas AC, Demetris AJ. Large cell change (liver cell dysplasia) and hepatocellular carcinoma in cirrhosis: matched case-control study, pathological analysis, and pathogenetic hypothesis. *Hepatology* 1997; 26:1415–22.

106. Theise ND, Marcelin K, Goldfischer M, et al. Low proliferative activity in macroregenerative nodules: evidence for an alternate hypothesis concerning human hepatocarcinogenesis. *Liver* 1996; 16:134–9.

107. Natarajan S, Theise ND, Thung SN, et al. Large-cell change of hepatocytes in cirrhosis may represent a reaction to prolonged cholestasis. *Am J Surg Pathol* 1997; 21:312–18.

108. Terris B, Ingster O, Rubbia L, et al. Interphase cytogenetic analysis reveals numerical chromosome aberrations in large liver cell dysplasia. *J Hepatol* 1997; 27:313–19.

109. Rubin EM, DeRose PB, Cohen C. Comparative image cytometric DNA ploidy of liver cell dysplasia and hepatocellular carcinoma. *Mod Pathol* 1994; 7:677–80.

110. Cameron RG, Greig PD, Farber E, et al. Small encapsulated hepatocellular carcinoma of the liver. Provisional ayalysis of pathogenic mechanisms. *Cancer* 1993; 72:2550–9.

111. Shibata M, Morizane T, Uchida T, et al. Irregular regeneration of hepatocytes and risk of hepatocellular carcinoma in chronic hepatitis and cirrhosis with hepatitis-C-virus infection. *Lancet* 1998; 351:1773–7.

112. Wee A, Yap I, Guan R. Hepatocyte hepatitis B surface antigen expression in chronic hepatitis B virus carriers in Singapore: correlation with viral replication and liver pathology. *J Gastroenterol Hepatol* 1991; 6:466–70.

113. Yasui H, Hino O, Ohtake K, et al. Clonal growth of hepatitis B virus-integrated hepatocytes in cirrhotic liver nodules. *Cancer Res* 1992; 52:6810–14.

114. Aihara T, Noguchi S, Sasaki Y, et al. Clonal analysis of precancerous lesion of hepatocellular carcinoma. *Gastroenterology* 1996; 111:455–61.

115. Colombo M, de Franchis R, Del Ninno E, et al. Hepatocellular carcinoma in Italian patients with cirrhosis. *N Engl J Med* 1991; 325:675–80.

116. Llovet JM, Fuster J, Bruix J. Intention-to-treat analysis of surgical treatment for early hepatocellular carcinoma: resection versus transplantation. *Hepatology* 1999; 30:1434–40.

117. Figueras J, Jaurrieta E, Valls C, et al. Survival after liver transplantation in cirrhotic patients with and without hepatocellular carcinoma: a comparative study. *Hepatology* 1997; 25:1485–9.

118. Poon RT, Fan ST, Lo CM, et al. Long-term prognosis after resection of hepatocellular carcinoma associated with hepatitis B-related cirrhosis. *J Clin Oncol* 2000; 18:1094–101.

119. Hanazaki K, Wakabayashi M, Sodeyama H, et al. Surgical outcomme in cirrhotic patients with hepatitis C-related hepatocellular carcinoma. *Hepatogastroenterology* 2000; 47:204–10.

120. Fong Y, Sun RL, Jarnagin W, et al. An analysis of 412 cases of hepatocellular carcinoma at a Western certer. *Ann Surg* 1999; 229:790–9.

121. Livraghi T, Benedini V, Lazzaroni S, et al. Long term results of single session percutaneous ethanol injection in patients with large hepatocellular carcinoma. *Cancer* 1998; 83:48–57.

122. Lencioni R, Pinto F, Armillotta N, et al. Long-term results of percutaneous ethanol injection therapy for hepatocellular carcinoma in cirrhosis: a European experience. *Eur Radiol* 1997; 7:514–19.

123. Livraghi T, Giorgio A, Marin G, et al. Hepatocellular carcinoma and cirrhosis in 746 patients: long term results of percutaneous ethanol injection. *Radiology* 1995; 197:101–8.

124. Mazzaferro V, Regalia E, Montalto F, Pulvirenti A, et al. Risk of HBV reinfection after liver transplantation in HBsAg-positive cirrhosis. Primary hepatocellular carcinoma is not a predictor for HBV recurrence. The European Cooperative Study Group on Liver Cancer and Transplantation. *Liver* 1996; 16:117–22.

125. Llovet JM, Bru C, Bruix J. Prognosis of hepatocellular carcinoma: the BCLC staging classification. *Semin Liver Dis* 1999; 19:329–38.

126. Chevret S, Trinchet JC, Mathieu D, et al. A new prognostic classification for predicting survival in patients with hepatocellular carcinoma. Groupe d'Etude et de Traitement du Carcinome Hepatocellulaire. *J Hepatol* 1999; 31:133–41.

127. The Cancer of the Liver Italian Program (CLIP) Investigators. A new prognostic system for hepatocellular carcinoma: a retrospective study of 435 patients. *Hepatology* 1998; 751–5.

128. Sarasin FP, Giostra E, Hadengue A. Cost-effectiveness of screening for detection of small hepatocellular carcinoma in western patients with Child-Pugh class A cirrhosis. *Am J Med* 1996; 101:422–34.

129. Kang JY, Lee TP, Yap I, et al. Analysis of cost-effectiveness of different strategies for hepatocellular carcinoma screening in hepatitis B virus carriers. *J Gastroenterol Hepatol* 1992; 7:463–8.

130. Collier J, Krahn M, Sherman M. A cost-benefit analysis of the benefit of screening for hepatocellular carcinoma in hepatitis B carriers. *Hepatology* 1999; 30:481A.

131. Lok ASF, Lai C-L. Alpha-fetoprotein monitoring in Chinese patients with chronic hepatitis B virus infection: Role in the early detection of

Hepatocellular carcinoma. *Hepatology* 1989; 9:110–15.

132. McMahon BJ, Wainwright RW, Lanier AP. The Alaska Native HCC screening program: A population-based screening program for hepatocellular carcinoma. In: Tabor E, Di Bisceglie AM, Purcell RH (eds) *Etiology, pathology and treatment of hepatocellular carcinoma in North America.* Gulf: Houston 1991, pp. 231–41.

133. Di Bisceglie AM, Hoofnagle JH. Elevations of serum alpha-fetoprotein levels in patients with chronic hepatitis B. *Cancer* 1989; 64:2117–20.

134. Lee H-S, Chung YH, Kim CY. Specificities of serum alpha-fetoprotein in HBsAg+ and HBsAg– patients in the diagnosis of hepatocellular carcinoma. *Hepatology* 1991; 14:68–72.

135. Yamashita F, Tanaka M, Satomura S, et al. Prognostic significance of *Lens culinaris* agglutinin A-reactive alpha-fetoprotein in small hepatocellular carcinomas. *Gastroenterology* 1996; 111:996–1001.

136. Hayashi K, Kumada T, Nakano S, et al. Usefulness of measurement of *Lens culinaris* agglutinin-reactive fraction of alpha-fetoprotein as a marker of prognosis and recurrence of small hepatocellular carcinoma. *Am J Gastroenterol* 1999; 94:3028–33.

137. Okuda K, Tanaka M, Kanazawa N, et al. Evaluation of curability and prediction of prognosis after surgical treatment for hepatocellular carcinoma by lens culinaris agglutinin-reactive alpha-fetoprotein. *Int J Oncol* 1999; 14:265–71.

138. Kumada T, Nakano S, Takeda I, et al. Clinical utility of *Lens culinaris* agglutinin-reactive alpha-fetoprotein in small hepatocellular carcinoma: special reference to imaging diagnosis. *J Hepatol* 1999; 30:125–30.

139. Sato Y, Nakata K, Kato Y, et al. Early recognition of hepatocellular carcinoma based on altered profiles of alpha-fetoprotein. *N Engl J Med* 1993; 328:1802–6.

140. Shiraki K, Takase K, Tameda Y, et al. A clinical study of lectin-reactive alpha-fetoprotein as an early indicator of hepatocellular carcinoma in the follow-up of cirrhotic patients. *Hepatology* 1995; 22:802–7.

141. Taketa K, Endo Y, Sekiya C, et al. A collaborative study for the evaluation of lectin-reactive alpha-fetoproteins in early detection of hepatocellular carcinoma. *Cancer Res* 1993; 53: 5419–23.

142. Ishizuka H, Nakayama T, Matsuoka S, et al. Prediction of the development of hepatocellular-

carcinoma in patients with liver cirrhosis by the serial determinations of serum alpha-L-fucosidase activity. *Intern Med* 1999; 38:927–31.

143. Giardina MG, Matarazzo M, Morante R, et al. Serum alpha-L-fucosidase activity and early detection of hepatocellular carcinoma: a prospective study of patients with cirrhosis. *Cancer* 1998; 83:2468–74.

144. Izuno K, Fujiyama S, Yamasaki K, et al. Early detection of hepatocellular carcinoma associated with cirrhosis by combined assay of des-gamma-carboxy prothrombin and alpha-fetoprotein: a prospective study. *Hepatogastroenterology* 1995; 42:387–93.

145. Tsai SL, Huang GT, Yang PM, et al. Plasma des-gamma-carboxyprothrombin in the early stage of hepatocellular carcinoma. *Hepatology* 1990; 11:481–8.

146. Levin B, Bond JH. Colorectal cancer screening: Recommendations of the US preventive services task force. *Gastroenterology* 1996; 111: 1381–4.

147. Zaman SN, Johnson PJ, Williams R. Silent cirrhosis in patients with hepatocellular carcinoma. implications for screening in high-incidence and low-incidence areas. *Cancer* 1990; 65:1607–10.

148. The Liver Cancer Study Group of Japan. Primary liver cancer in Japan. clinicopathologic features and results of surgical treatment. *Ann Surg* 1990; 211:277–87.

149. Chiba T, Matsuzaki Y, Abei M, et al. The role of previous hepatitis B virus infection and heavy smoking in hepatitis C virus-related hepatocellular carcinoma. *Am J Gastroenterol* 1996; 91:1195–211.

150. Tsukuma H, Hiyama T, Tanaka S, et al. Risk factors for hepatocellular carcinoma among patients with chronic liver disease. *N Engl J Med* 1993; 328:1797–1801.

151. Chen DS, Sung JL, Sheu JC, et al. Serum alpha fetoprotein in the early stage of human hepatocellular carcinoma. *Gastroenterology* 1984; 86:1404–1409.

152. Sheu JC, Sung JL, Chen DS, et al. Growth rate of asymptomatic hepatocellular carcinoma and its clinical implications. *Gastroenterology* 1985; 89:259–266.

153. Yoshino M. Growth kinetics of hepatocellular carcinoma. *Jpn J Clin Oncol* 1983; 13:45–52.

154. Prozesky OW, Stevens CE, Szmuness W, et al. Immune response to hepatitis B vaccine in newborns. *J Infect* 1983; 1(Suppl):53–5.

155. Hwang LY, Beasley RP, Stevens CE, et al. Immunogenicity of HBV vaccine in healthy Chinese children. *Vaccine* 1983; 1:10–12.

156. Krogsgaard K. The long-term effect of treatment with interferon-alpha 2a in chronic hepatitis B. The Long-Term Follow-Up Investigator Group. The European Study Group on Viral Hepatitis (EUROHEP). Executive Team on Anti-Viral Treatment. *J Viral Hepat* 1998; 5:389–97.

157. Wong DK, Yim C, Naylor CD, et al. Interferon alfa treatment of chronic hepatitis B: randomized trial in a predominantly homosexual male population. *Gastroenterology* 1995; 108:165–71.

158. Thomas HC, Lok AS, Carreno V, et al. Comparative study of three doses of interferon-alpha 2a in chronic active hepatitis B. The International Hepatitis Trial Group. *J Viral Hepat* 1994; 1:139–48.

159. Di Bisceglie AM, Fong TL, Fried MW, et al. A randomized, controlled trial of recombinant alpha-interferon therapy for chronic hepatitis B. *Am J Gastroenterol* 1993; 88:1887–92.

160. Perrillo RP, Schiff ER, Davis GL, et al. A randomized, controlled trial of interferon alfa-2b alone and after prednisone withdrawal for the treatment of chronic hepatitis B. The Hepatitis Interventional Therapy Group. *N Engl J Med* 1990; 323:295–301.

161. Schalm SW, Heathcote J, Cianciara J, et al. Lamivudine and alpha interferon combination treatment of patients with chronic hepatitis B infection: a randomised trial. *Gut* 2000; 46:562–8.

162. Liaw YF, Leung NW, Chang TT, et al. Effects of extended lamivudine therapy in Asian patients with chronic hepatitis B. Asia Hepatitis Lamivudine Study Group. *Gastroenterology* 2000; 119:172–80.

163. Niederau C, Heintges T, Lange S, et al. D Long-term follow-up of HBeAg-positive patients treated with interferon alfa for chronic hepatitis B. *N Engl J Med* 1996; 334:1422–7.

164. Lin SM, Sheen IS, Chien RN, et al. Long-term beneficial effect of interferon therapy in patients with chronic hepatitis B virus infection. *Hepatology* 1999; 29:971–5.

165. Marcellin P, Boyer N, Gervais A, et al. Patients with chronic hepatitis C and sustained response to interferon-alpha therapy. *Ann Intern Med* 1997; 127:875–81.

166. Tanaka H, Tsukuma H, Kasahara A, et al. Effect of interferon therapy on the incidence of hepatocellular carcinoma and mortality of patients with chronic hepatitis C: a retrospective cohort study of 738 patients. *Int J Cancer* 2000; 87:741–9.

167. Yoshida H, Shiratori Y, Moriyama M, et al. Interferon therapy reduces the risk for hepatocellular carcinoma: national surveillance program of cirrhotic and noncirrhotic patients with chronic hepatitis C in Japan. IHIT Study Group. Inhibition of hepatocarcinogenesis by Interferon Therapy. *Ann Intern Med* 1999; 131:174–81.

168. Sheu JC, Huang GT, Chou HC, et al. Multiple hepatocellular carcinomas at the early stage have different clonality. *Gastroenterology* 1993; 105:1471–6.

169. Sakamoto M, Hirohashi S, Tsuda H, et al. Multicentric independent development of hepatocellular carcinoma revealed by analysis of hepatitis B virus integration pattern. *Am J Surg Pathol* 1989; 13:1064–7.

12
Pancreas

Ralph H. Hruban, Christine Iacobuzio-Donahue, and Michael Goggins

Pancreatic cancer is the fifth leading cause of cancer death. This year, it is estimated that about 28,000 Americans will be diagnosed with pancreatic cancer, and about 28,000 will die from it [1]. The extraordinary mortality rate for patients with pancreatic cancer is due, at least in part, to the fact that most patients with pancreatic cancer do not develop clinical symptoms until late in the course of their disease, after the cancer has spread beyond the gland [2,3]. We believe that an improved understanding of the precursors of invasive pancreatic cancer will lead to novel methods to detect these cancers at an early, potentially curable, stage. This chapter will briefly outline the current state of our knowledge of the epidemiology of pancreatic cancer, the pathology of precursor lesions, and potential novel approaches to the early detection and prevention of pancreatic cancer.

Epidemiology

An important first step in developing a screening test for pancreatic cancer or in implementing a prevention program is to identify those at risk for developing the disease. In this regard, relatively little is known about the epidemiology of pancreatic cancer precursor lesions. However, if such lesions (as defined later) are true precursors, they would be expected to share at least some risk factors with pancreatic cancer. Given the paucity of knowledge concerning risk factors for precursor lesions, emphasis in the ensuing sections is placed on

describing the epidemiology of pancreatic cancer.

Age, Gender, and Race

Pancreatic cancer is primarily a disease of the elderly [4]. Incidence rates increase with increasing age, and most cases occur between the ages of 60 and 80 years [5]. Pancreatic cancer cases below the age of 40 are rare, but they do occur. Not only are invasive cancers more common in the elderly, but Kozuka et al. [6] have shown that the epithelial precursors to invasive pancreatic cancer [known as "pancreatic intraepithelial neoplasia" (PanIN)] also increase with age, and recently Lüttges and colleagues [7] have shown that k-ras oncogene mutations are more common in PanINs in patients older than the age of 40.

Pancreatic cancer also occurs more frequently in men than in women [4,5]. In developed countries, the reported annual age-adjusted incidence rates for men range from 8.0 to 12.0 per 100,000 and for women from 4.5 to 7.0 per 100,000 [2,4,5,8,9]. While pancreatic cancer incidence rates appear to be declining in white males, they appear to be on the increase in women. A slight gender difference has been reported in the incidence of PanINs (19.9% for males, 16.8% for females), however this difference is probably not significant [6].

Race may also play a role in the development of pancreatic cancer. In the United States, the incidence and mortality rates for pancreatic cancer in African-Americans of both genders are higher than in whites [4,10,11]. The reasons for this are not clear, but comparisons between African-Americans and Native Africans suggest that lifestyle or the environment may play a role [10,11]. No significant racial differences have been reported in the incidence of PanINs.

Smoking

Cigarette smoking is one of the strongest recognized risk factors for the development of pancreatic cancer [4,12–19]. The reported relative risk associated with cigarette smoking has ranged from 1.6 to 3.1 [4]. While this relative risk may, at first glance, seem small, it is not. Given the large numbers of smokers, the impact of cigarette smoking on pancreatic cancer is great. For example, Mulder and colleagues used a computer simulation to estimate that the cessation of cigarette smoking in Europe would save between 68,000 and 176,000 lives that would have otherwise been lost to pancreatic cancer by the year 2020 [20].

The association between cigarette smoking and pancreatic cancer is supported by animal models [21–23], and we and others have shown that pancreatic cancers which arise in cigarette smokers are more likely to harbor activating point mutations in the *k-ras* oncogene than are cancers which arise in nonsmokers [24,25]. Furthermore, among the carcinogens in tobacco smoke are nitrosamines, which can induce G to A transitions at the second G of a GG pair. This type of transition is the most common type of *k-ras* mutation found in pancreatic adenocarcinomas [24,26]. Therefore, it is reasonable to expect that cigarette smoking would be associated with the development of PanINs, and there is strong epidemiologic, animal model, and molecular evidence tying cigarette smoking with the development of pancreatic cancer, although this association has not been carefully studied.

Chronic Pancreatitis

The relationship between chronic pancreatitis and pancreatic cancer is complex. Pancreatic cancers can induce chronic pancreatitis by obstructing pancreatic ducts [27], and conversely, a growing body of evidence now suggests that chronic pancreatitis increases the risk of developing pancreatic cancer [28–33].

While most epidemiological analyses of the association between chronic pancreatitis and the subsequent development of pancreatic cancer are clouded by the possibility that small subclinical pancreatic cancers can cause pancreatitis [30], recent analyses of familial pancreatitis kindreds establish that repeated episodes of pancreatitis do, in fact, increase the risk of developing pancreatic cancer [31,32]. Hereditary pancreatitis is caused by germline (inherited) mutations in the cationic trypsinogen gene [34,35], and Lowenfels and colleagues [32] have recently shown that affected family members in these kindreds have as high as a 40% lifetime risk of developing pancreatic cancer.

The mechanism by which chronic pancreatitis causes pancreatic cancer has not been established, but Volkholz et al. [36] have reported that epithelial dysplasias (PanINs) occur in pancreata with chronic pancreatitis, and that these dysplasias are more prevalent in areas of the pancreas with scarring and obstruction of secretory outflow. Furthermore, Gansauge et al. [37] have reported that some of these dysplasias harbor *p53* mutations, and others have reported that these dysplasias also harbor activating point mutations in the *k-ras* gene [38–40].

Thus, chronic pancreatitis, like cigarette smoking, has been linked epidemiologically and at the molecular level to the development of pancreatic cancer.

Previous Gastrectomy

Tersmette and Offerhaus [41] have demonstrated that patients with a remote history of partial gastrectomy have an increased risk of developing pancreatic cancer. This increased risk appears many years (>20) after gastrectomy and has been reported to be in the range of a 1.65 to 5-fold increase [41], although not all studies have found a statistically significant increased risk [42].

Diabetes Mellitus

The relationship between diabetes mellitus and pancreatic cancer is complex. Not only has diabetes been implicated in the development of pancreatic cancer, but cancer of the pancreas can also destroy normal pancreatic tissue and thus cause diabetes mellitus. The mechanism by which pancreatic cancer causes diabetes is not clear, but some have suggested that amylin production by pancreatic cancer may contribute to the development of diabetes [42–44]. In an attempt to rule out diabetes occurring as a complication of pancreatic cancer, several studies have also demonstrated an increased relative risk of pancreatic cancer among patients who have been diabetic for greater than 5 years [43,45].

Family History

Although ignored for many years, a family history of pancreatic cancer is slowly being recognized as a significant risk factor of the development of pancreatic cancer [46–49]. Four lines of evidence suggest that a family history of pancreatic cancer increases one's risk of developing pancreatic cancer.

First, the literature contains numerous anecdotal case reports of kindreds in which there have been several family members with pancreatic cancer [48,50–56]. Perhaps the most famous of these is former President Jimmy Carter [57]. His mother and two of his sisters died of pancreatic cancer [57]. As dramatic as they are, reports of single families do not firmly establish a causal relationship. They could simply be due to chance.

The second line of evidence, careful epidemiologic studies, is therefore more convincing [12,42,58–60]. For example, Silverman and colleagues [42] conducted a population-based case-control study of pancreatic cancer in Atlanta, Detroit, and New Jersey. 484 cases and 2099 controls were interviewed and Silverman et al. [42] found significantly increased risks for subjects reporting a first-degree relative with pancreatic cancer (OR = 3.2). Interestingly, significantly increased risks were also observed for subjects reporting a first-degree relative with

cancer of the colon (OR = 1.7) or ovary (OR = 5.3) [42]. The basis for these latter associations will be discussed later in the sections on the *BRCA2* Syndrome and hereditary nonpolyposis colorectal cancer (HNPCC).

The third line of evidence comes from prospective analyses of kindreds in which there have been an aggregation of pancreatic cancer [61]. For example, the National Familiar Pancreas Tumor Registry (NFPTR) was established at Johns Hopkins in 1994 to learn more about the role of inheritance in the etiology of pancreas cancer[1]. This registry now contains over 220 kindreds with an aggregation of pancreatic cancer. We prospectively followed family members from the first 150 kindreds enrolled in the NFPTR. Remarkably, when followed prospectively, members of these kindreds developed pancreatic cancer at a rate 18-fold greater than expected based on United States population-based Surveillance, Epidemiology, and End Results (SEER) program data [61]. Even more dramatically, the risk rose to 57-fold in those kindreds with three or more affected family members at the time of enrollment [61]. These findings not only help to establish that family history of pancreatic cancer is a significant risk factor for the development of pancreatic cancer, but they also help to establish that familial pancreatic cancer kindreds are a high-risk group that might be appropriate for pancreatic cancer screening and chemoprevention programs, as will be discussed later.

The fourth line of evidence that a family history of pancreatic cancer increases one's risk for developing pancreatic cancer comes from careful molecular biology studies in which the genetic bases for this relationship have been defined. Germline (inherited) mutations in *BRCA2*, *p16*, *STK11/LKB1*, the cationic trypsinogen gene, and in one of the DNA mismatch repair genes have all been demonstrated to increase risk of pancreatic cancer [32,35,62–74]. It is extremely important to rec-

---

[1] National Familial Pancreas Tumor Registry: Johns Hopkins Hospital, 600 North Wolfe Street, Meyer 7-181, Baltimore, MD 21287; Phone: 410–955–9132; Fax: 410–955–0115.

ognize the syndromes associated with these inherited gene defects, because individuals at risk can now be tested, and those found to harbor a germline mutation could benefit from screening and/or prevention programs, while those found not to harbor a mutation would be relieved of their anxiety.

BRCA2

In addition to their increased risk of breast and ovarian cancer, affected family members in kindreds with the second breast cancer syndrome (BRCA2) have an increased risk of developing pancreatic cancer [62,63,65,66]. This syndrome is not uncommon. For example, about 1% of the Ashkenazi Jewish population carries a germline BRCA2 mutation (6174delT) because of a founder effect, and carriers of this mutation have about a 10-fold increased risk of developing pancreatic cancer [65]. Importantly, because of the low penetrance of this gene, many individuals with germline BRCA2 mutations come from kindreds recognized to harbor the syndrome [62].

p16

Germline mutations in the p16 tumor suppressor gene cause the Familial Atypical Multiple Mole Melanoma (FAMMM) Syndrome and, in addition to skin lesions, patients with the FAMMM syndrome have an estimated 20-fold increased risk of developing pancreatic cancer [46,47,63,71–75].

Peutz-Jeghers Syndrome

The Peutz-Jeghers Syndrome is characterized by pigmented macules on the lips and buccal mucosa and by the development of hamartomatous polyps in the gastrointestinal tract [76]. Individuals with the Peutz-Jeghers Syndrome have been shown to have a markedly increased risk of developing pancreatic cancer [70], and Su and colleagues have recently shown that this increased risk is associated with inactivation of the Peutz-Jeghers gene (STK11/LKB1) [69,77]. The degree of this risk is hard to estimate, but Giardello et al. [70]

followed 31 patients with the syndrome from 1973 to 1985, and 15 of them developed cancer. The mean interval between diagnosis of the syndrome and diagnosis of cancer was 25 years, and the observed development of cancer in the patients with the syndrome was 18 times greater than expected in the general population (p < 0.001). Remarkably, four of the 15 cancers were pancreatic cancers, representing a 100-fold excess of pancreatic carcinoma in patients with the Peutz-Jeghers Syndrome.

Hereditary Nonpolyposis Colorectal Cancer

The hereditary nonpolyposis colorectal cancer syndrome (HNPCC) accounts for 4% to 13% of colon cancers, but affected individuals may also have an increased risk of developing endometrial, ovarian, pancreatic, and gastric cancer [68,78–84]. HNPCC has been shown to be caused by germline mutations in one of the DNA mismatch repair genes [85–89], and the neoplasms which arise in these patients have a characteristic genetic alteration called "microsatellite instability" (MSI) [86]. We have recently reported four pancreatic cancers with MSI all four showing loss of the hMlh1 DNA mismatch repair gene [67]. One of these four arose in a young patient with a synchronous colonic cancer, suggesting that this patient had a germline mutation [67]. Thus, although pancreatic cancer is not the most common cancer to develop in patients with HNPCC, patients with this syndrome are at risk, and the association between HNPCC and pancreatic cancer may explain the previously noted epidemologic observations linking a family history of colon cancer with the development of pancreatic cancer [42].

Hereditary Pancreatitis

As discussed earlier, patients with hereditary pancreatitis have an increased risk of developing pancreatic cancer [32]. Hereditary pancreatitis is an autosomal dominant syndrome characterized by the early onset of attacks of acute pancreatitis [34]. This syndrome is caused by germline mutations in the cationic trypsinogen gene, and as discussed earlier, affected patients have as much as a 40% lifetime risk of developing pancreatic cancer [28,31,32,35]. This risk is so high that it may warrant prophylactic pancreatectomy in selected individuals.

Summary of Epidemiology

Thus, careful epidemiologic and molecular studies have defined populations that have an increased risk of developing pancreatic cancer. Because of their increased risk, these populations will potentially benefit most from screening and chemoprevention programs. Such programs might also find application in those with precursor lesions for pancreatic cancer. There is a clear need for studies of the etiology of such precursors.

Precursors to Invasive Cancer

The first step in screening for and developing new approaches to the prevention of early pancreatic cancer is recognizing and defining early pancreatic neoplasia. In this regard, three conditions are of interest: (PanIN), intraductal papillary mucinous neoplasm (IPMN), and mucinous cystic neoplasm (MCN).

PanIN

The precursor lesions which give rise to invasive ductal adenocarcinomas of the pancreas have recently been characterized, and it is now clear that ductal adenocarcinomas arise from histologically well-defined epithelial proliferations in the small ducts and ductules of the pancreas [90–92]. These proliferations were first described by Sommers et al. and subsequently characterized by Cubilla and Fitzgerald, and by Kozuka [6,93,94]. Morphologically, these lesions are characterized by papillary epithelial proliferations with both cytological and architectural atypia [90–92]. A large number of pancreata have been examined for PanINs, and most studies have demon-

strated that PanINs with cytological and architectural atypia are found more frequently in pancreata with an invasive cancer than they are in pancreata without an invasive cancer [6,94]. A classification system for PanINs was established at a National Cancer Institute (NCI) Sponsored Pancreatic Cancer Think Tank which was held in Park City, Utah, in September, 1999. The details of this classification system are presented on the Web (*http://pathology.jhu.edu/pancreas_panin*). Briefly, flat duct lesions with minimal cytologic atypia are designated PanIN-1A, papillary lesions with minimal cytologic atypia PanIN-1B, duct lesions with moderate cytological and architectural atypia PanIN-2, and duct poliferations with significant cytological and architectural atypia are designated PanIN-3. Clinically, PanINs have been shown to progress to infiltrating carcinoma [95,96], and at the molecular level, PanINs have been shown to overexpress the *Her-2/neu* oncogene [97], to harbor activating point mutations in the *k-ras* oncogene [98,99] and inactivating mutations in the *p53*, *BRCA2*, *p16*, and *DPC4* tumor suppressor genes (Figure 12.1) [98,100–104]. The identification of noninvasive precursors is critical, because it suggests that pancreatic neoplasia can be detected prior to the development of an invasive carcinoma, at a stage in which it is still curable. That being said, with the exception of a few case reports, there is little or no data currently available on the natural history of PanINs. Simply put, the rate and frequency at which PanINs progress to infiltrating carcinoma has not been established.

IPMN

Intraductal papillary mucinous neoplasms of the pancreas are rare neoplasms characterized by papillary growths of mucin-producing epithelium within the large pancreatic ducts [105–113]. These neoplasms have been shown to harbor a number of genetic alterations, including activating point mutations in codon 12 of the *k-ras* oncogene [113–115]. IPMNs often have a prominent noninvasive precursor component, and they therefore can serve as an easily studied model system for progression to

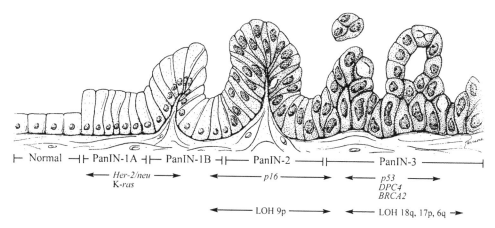

FIGURE 12.1. Progression model for infiltrating ductal carcinomas of the pancreas. Normal epithelium (far left) can progress through increasing grades of dysplasia (PanIN) to cancer-*in-situ* (far right) and then infiltrating carcinoma. This progression is associated with the accumulation of genetic alterations in specific genes. (Artwork by J. Parsons. *Source*: Hruban RH, 2000 [90], with permission).

cancer in the pancreas [113]. For example, Fujii and colleagues were able to separately microdissect the various components of a large number of IPMNs and demonstrate, at the molecular level, both genetic progression and genetic heterogeneity in these neoplasms [113]. Because they harbor many of the same genetic alterations and secrete many of the same proteins as ductal adenocarcinomas, IPMNs may be detected during screening for ductal cancers. It is however, important to distinguish IPMNs from ductal cancers because IPMNs have a much better prognosis [116].

MCN

Mucinous cystic neoplasms, like IPMNs, can have a prominent noninvasive component and are characterized by the proliferation of mucin-producing epithelium [117]. Unlike IPMNs, MCNs do not communicate with the main pancreatic duct. In addition, MCN often have a prominent stroma, reminiscent of the stroma seen in the normal ovary. The treatment of these neoplasms highlights the value of early detection. MCNs which are detected and resected before an invasive cancer develops are entirely curable, but patients with an invasive mucinous cystadenocarcinoma have only a 50% 5-year survival rate [117,118].

Early Detection

As discussed previously, there is an enormous need for a sensitive and specific screening test for the early detection of pancreatic cancer [119,120]. For example, patients with metastatic pancreatic cancer have a life expectancy of only a few short months [2], while patients who have their cancer surgically resected and who are found to have small tumors confined to the gland have a 5-year survival rate which approaches 25% [121]. A variety of approaches have therefore been explored to screen for pancreatic cancer, including the identification of biochemical and molecular markers and imaging.

Serum Markers

Carbohydrate antigen 19-9 (CA19-9) is the serum marker which has been most extensively evaluated as a screening test for pancreatic cancer [122]. Unfortunately, although CA19-9 is a useful marker for following response to treatment in patients known to have pancreatic cancer, it is not a useful screening test [122]. Some tumors do not secrete CA19-9 and, conversely, CA19-9 can be elevated in benign conditions. These limitations also apply to other serum markers such as CA-125, KAM17.1, CA2.2, CA-50 and CA-242.

Imaging Modalities

Among the imaging modalities currently used to diagnose pancreatic cancer, helical computerized tomography (CT), magnetic resonance imaging (MRI) and endoscopic ultrasound (EUS) have a sensitivity of about 90%. Endoscopic retrograde cholangiopancreatography (ERCP) is used less often for diagnosis of pancreatic cancer, given the risks associated with undergoing an ERCP (such as acute pancreatitis in about 5% of procedures). For all diagnostic modalities, cancers less than one to two centimeters in diameter, and those that cause diffuse enlargement of the pancreas, are the most difficult to diagnose. The skill and experience of the endosonographer is an important determinant in the accuracy of EUS. In expert hands, EUS is probably the imaging modality of choice for surveying the pancreases or at-risk individuals, because many pancreatic cancers that are not visualized on CT can be seen using endoscopic ultrasound (EUS). EUS also has an advantage over CT in that repeated fine needle aspirations can be performed painlessly and easily, compared with percutaneous biopsies obtained during CT.

There are limited data regarding the utility of screening for pancreatic cancer in at-risk individuals [123]. Brentnall and colleagues reported their experience screening high-risk families [124]. Of 14 patients from three families surveyed by EUS, seven were found to have EUS abnormalities suggestive of pancreatic ductal lesions. On ERCP, most of these seven had pancreatograms that were consistent with chronic pancreatitis, including some with unusually dilated ductal side branches. Most of those with abnormal findings were from a single large kindred with a dramatic phenotype wherein affected members develop pancreatic exocrine and/or endocrine insufficiency prior to the diagnosis of pancreatic cancer. All seven were referred for pancreatectomy, and all showed pancreatic dysplasia (high-grade PanINs) and chronic pancreatitis. Most families with a clustering of pancreatic cancer reported

to date do not present with such a phenotype, and therefore these screening results are probably not generalizable to most pancreatic cancer families [46,47].

It should be emphasized that PanINs are usually not large enough to be readily identifiable radiologically. Therefore, these lesions will have to be detected using some of the more novel screening approaches discussed in the sections which follow. On the other hand, early asymptomatic pancreatic cancers probably frequently distort local anatomy, and such distortions could be identifiable by EUS.

Telomerase

Telomerase is one of the more exciting new potential markers for pancreatic cancer [125–131]. Most normal cells lose their telomerase activity after embryologic development, while most pancreatic cancers express telomerase. Therefore, a number of groups have studied telomerase levels in pancreatic secretions, and most have found that high telomerase levels are associated with an invasive cancer. Remarkably, Suehara et al. [128] have reported that a patient with pancreatic cancer also had elevated telomerase activity in his pancreatic juice 19 months before a tumor was detected. This latter report is exciting because it demonstrates the potential for this novel approach to detect early neoplasms.

Genetic Alterations

A variety of genetic alterations have been identified in infiltrating pancreatic cancers and their precursors, and these alterations are potential new markers for early pancreatic cancer. For example, the majority of high-grade PanINs and 90% of infiltrating pancreatic cancers harbor activating point mutations in the *k-ras* oncogene, and a number of groups have demonstrated that altered *k-ras* genes can be detected in pancreatic juice, in duodenal fluid, and in stool samples from patients with pancreatic cancer [132,133]. In some cases, the mutations identified in the fluid or stool samples match the mutations in the patient's infiltrating carcinoma; in others, the mutations match those found in a PanIN [132,133]. Importantly, Berthélemy et al. [134] have reported that they were able to detect mutant *k-ras* genes in pancreatic juice samples from two patients months before these two patients developed a clinically recognizable cancer. *K-ras* oncogene mutations are, however, relatively common in low-grade PanINs, and mutant *k-ras* may therefore lack specificity as a marker for a lesion with a high risk of progressing on to invasive pancreatic cancer. Nonetheless, the studies performed to date provide an important "proof of principle"—mutant DNA shed from pancreatic cancer can be detected in secretions before a cancer is clinically detectable.

DNA methylation may be a more specific marker for pancreatic cancer [135–137]. Ueki and colleagues have recently characterized the methylation status of a series of pancreatic cancers, and they were able to demonstrate abnormal DNA methylation of at least one locus in 60% of the cancers [135]. This is an exciting finding because a variety of molecular techniques have been developed which can be used to detect rare methylated copies of DNA, even when the methylated DNA is admixed with many more nonmethylated copies of DNA [138]. To date, the DNA methylation status of PanINs has not been well studied.

New Approaches

Recently several new technologies have been developed which may lead to the development of new screening tests. These include serial analysis of gene expression (SAGE), gene chip arrays, and proteomics.

SAGE

SAGE was developed by Velculesco in Vogelstein and by Kinzler's laboratory [139]. This technique allows one to quantify gene expression in a tissue. Pancreatic cancer was one of the first tissues examined using SAGE [140], and when this was done, about 200 sequences ("tags") were identified that appear to be selectively highly expressed in pancreatic cancer [140]. Each of these tags has the potential for being a new marker for pancreatic cancer. For example, *TIMP-1* was one of the first genes found by SAGE to be preferentially expressed in pancreatic cancer, and Zhou et al. [141] have shown that patients with pancreatic cancer often have elevated serum TIMP-1 levels.

Gene Chip Array

Microarrays are a powerful tool for identifying genes that are overexpressed in cancers. Microarray approaches typically use several thousand oligonucleotide or cDNA clones arrayed on matrices such as glass slides [142]. Tissue arrays, in which many hundreds of tissues are arrayed and can be probed for evidence of gene amplification or loss [143], have also been used. Cells harboring overexpressed genes often produce their protein products in abundance, and these overexpressed genes are therefore good candidates for diagnostic assays [144,145].

Proteomics

Advances in protein chemistry technology have led to the development of the field of "proteomics". The term *proteome* was coined to describe the complete set of proteins present in a cell, and the term *proteomics* describes the large-scale characterization of proteins. Until recently, two-dimensional gel electrophoresis was the main separation technique for identifying differentially expressed proteins. Unfortunately, biological samples are simply too complex with respect to protein number for analysis on one protein chip. A novel protein chip approach has been used by Ciphergen (Palo Alto, CA) to decrease this complexity, and this approach is worth describing in greater detail. Multiple types of protein chips are used to resolve the proteins in a biological sample, each chip specific for the type of proteins that can be captured. The ProteinChip Array is placed into a ProteinChip Reader, and a laser is applied to the matrix of bound protein, ionizing and releasing it. The chip reader determines the molecular-weight profile of multiple proteins within a sample. By matching the experimental data with existing databases of protein mass data, it is possible to identify proteins that can then be confirmed using other techniques. By comparing normal and disease samples, using ProteinChip software, one can identify proteins which are present in one sample but not in the other [146].

Advances in protein chemistry technologies therefore have great potential for identifying novel proteins that could be used to design better screening tests for pancreatic and other cancers in biological samples. Thus, we believe that an improved understanding of the genetic alterations and gene expression patterns in PanINs and in infiltrating pancreatic cancers will lead to novel markers for early pancreatic cancer.

Impact of Screening

The benefit of pancreatic cancer screening is unknown, but estimates suggest modest benefits in keeping with other cancer surveillance strategies are possible. For example, a test with a sensitivity and specificity of 90% used on a target population with a 20% lifetime risk of pancreatic cancer would yield an average survival benefit of 1.5 years if screening commenced at age 50 (A. Lowenfels, personal communication). Because of the relatively low prevalence of the disease, screening the general population for pancreatic cancer will not be of value unless screening tests with extraordinary sensitivity and specificity can be developed.

Prevention

The absence of sensitive and specific screening tests for early pancreatic cancer heightens the importance of developing effective strategies to prevent the disease. Several approaches to preventing pancreatic cancer may seem obvious. For example, as discussed earlier, Mulder and colleagues have estimated that reasonable smoking reduction in Europe could save as many as 68,000 lives that would otherwise have been lost to pancreatic cancer by the year 2020 [20].

Chemoprevention strategies may also be around the corner. For example, most pancreatic cancers overexpress the enzyme Cox-2, and Cox-2 inhibitors have been shown to decrease the growth of pancreatic cancer in animal models [147–151]. Patients with a strong family history of pancreatic cancer, patients with a germline mutation in a gene known to predispose the carrier to pancreatic cancer, and patients with PanINs would all be reasonable candidates for inclusion in future chemoprevention trials.

Finally, prophylactic mastectomy has been shown to reduce the risk of dying from breast cancer and, although the morbidity and mortality of pancreas surgery is higher than that for breast surgery, prophylactic pancreatectomy might be a reasonable approach to cancer prevention in selected individuals at very high risk for developing pancreatic cancer [124,152]. For example, as discussed earlier, patients with familial pancreatitis have as high as a 40% lifetime risk of developing pancreatic cancer [32]. These patients lose most of their pancreatic function from the bouts of pancreatitis anyway, and they may benefit from prophylactic surgery, especially if it is performed at specialized centers with expertise in pancreatic surgery [121].

Conclusions

Pancreatic cancer is one of the deadliest of all of the cancers. New approaches to detect early pancreatic cancer and pancreatic cancer precursors, and to prevent pancreatic cancer in populations at risk, are urgently needed. We believe that the revolution in our understanding of the molecular genetics of pancreatic neoplasia which has occurred in the last 10 years will provide a basis for the development of these new approaches.

References

1. Greenlee RT, Murray T, Bolden S, et al. Cancer Statistics, 2000. *CA Cancer J Clin* 2000; 50:7–33.
2. Niederhuber JE, Brennan MF, Menck HR. The national cancer data base report on pancreatic cancer. *Cancer* 1995; 76:1671–7.
3. Warshaw AL, Castillo CFD. Pancreatic carcinoma. *N Engl J Med* 1992; 326:455–65.
4. Gold EB, Goldin SB. Epidemiology of and risk factor for pancreatic cancer. *Surg Oncol Clin N Am* 1998; 7:67–91.

5. Solcia E, Capella C, Klöppel G. *Atlas of tumor pathology: tumors of the pancreas*, 3rd Series ed. Washington, DC: Armed Forces Institute of Pathology, 1997.

6. Kozuka S, Sassa R, Taki T, et al. Relation of pancreatic duct hyperplasia to carcinoma. *Cancer* 1979; 43:1418–28.

7. Lüttges J, Reinecke-Lüthge A, Mollmann B, et al. Duct changes of *K-ras* mutations in the disease-free pancreas: analysis of type, age relation and spatial distribution. *Virchows Arch* 1999; 435:461–8.

8. Riela A, Zinsmeister AR, Melton LJI, et al. Increasing incidence of pancreatic cancer among women in Olmsted County, Minnesota, 1940 through 1988. *Mayo Clin Proc* 1992; 67: 839–45.

9. Levin DL, Connelly RR, Devesa SS. Demographic characteristics of cancer of the pancreas: mortality, incidence, and survival. *Cancer* 1981; 47 (Suppl):1456–68.

10. Kovi J, Heshmat MY. Incidence of cancer in negroes in Washington, D.C. and selected African cities. *Am J Epidemiol* 1972; 96:401–13.

11. Parkin DM, Pisani P, Ferlay J. Estimates of the worldwide incidence of eighteen major cancers in 1985. *Int J Cancer* 1993; 54:594–606.

12. Falk RT, Pickle LW, Fontham ET, et al. Life-style risk factors for pancreatic cancer in Louisana: a case-control study. *Am J Epidemiol* 1988; 128:324–36.

13. Fraumeni JF Jr. Cancers of the pancreas and biliary tract: epidemiological considerations. *Cancer Res* 1975; 35:3437–46.

14. Ghadirian P, Simard A, Baillargeon J. Tobacco, alcohol, and coffee and cancer of the pancreas. A population-based, case-control study in Quebec, Canada. *Cancer* 1991; 67:2664–70.

15. Howe GR, Jain M, Burch JD, et al. Cigarette smoking and cancer of the pancreas: evidence from a population-based case-control study in Toronto, Canada. *Int J Cancer* 1991; 47:323–8.

16. Mack TM, Yu MC, Hanisch R, et al. Pancreas cancer and smoking, beverage consumption, and past medical history. *J Natl Cancer Inst* 1986; 76:49–60.

17. Mills PK, Beeson WL, Abbey DE, et al. Dietary habits and past medical history as related to fatal pancreas cancer risk among adventists. *Cancer* 1988; 61:2578–85.

18. Stolzenberg-Solomon RZ, Albanes D, Nieto FJ, et al. Pancreatic cancer risk and nutrition-related methyl-group availability indicators in male smokers. *J Natl Cancer Inst* 1999; 91: 535–41.

19. Wynder EL, Mabuchi K, Maruchi N, et al. A case control study of cancer of the pancreas. *Cancer* 1973; 31:641–8.

20. Mulder I, van Genugten ML, Hoogenveen RT, et al. The impact of smoking on future pancreatic cancer: a computer simulation. *Ann Oncol* 1999; 10 (4 Suppl):74–8.

21. Fujii H, Egami H, Chaney W, et al. Pancreatic ductal adenocarcinomas induced in Syrian hamsters by N-nitrosobis(2-oxopropyl)amine contain a *c-Ki-ras* oncogene with a point-mutated codon 12. *Mol Carcinog* 1990; 3:296–301.

22. Schuller HM, Jorquera R, Reichert A, et al. Transplacental induction of pancreas tumors in hamsters by ethanol and the tobacco-specific nitrosamine 4-(methylnitorsamino)-1-(3 pyridyl)-1-butanonel. *Cancer Res* 1993; 53:2498–501.

23. Rivenson A, Hoffmann D, Prokopczyk B, et al. Induction of lung and exocrine pancreas tumors in F344 rats by tobacco-specific and *Areca*-derived *N*-nitrosamines. *Cancer Res* 1988; 48:6912–7.

24. Hruban RH, van Mansfeld ADM, Offerhaus GJA, et al. *K-ras* oncogene activation in adenocarcinoma of the human pancreas. A study of 82 carcinomas using a combination of mutant-enriched polymerase chain reaction analysis and allele-specific oligonucleotide hybridization. *Am J Pathol* 1993; 143:545–54.

25. Berger DH, Chang H, Wood M, et al. Mutational activation of *K-ras* in nonneoplastic exocrine pancreatic lesions in relation to cigarette smoking status. *Cancer* 1999; 85:326–32.

26. Topal MD. DNA repair, oncogenes and carcinogenesis. *Carcinogenesis* 1988; 9:691–6.

27. Gambill EE. Pancreatitis associated with pancreatic carcinoma: A study of 26 cases. *Mayo Clin Proc* 1971; 46:174–7.

28. Finch MD, Howes N, Ellis I, et al. Hereditary pancreatitis and familial pancreatic cancer. *Digestion* 1997; 58:564–9.

29. Chari ST, Mohan V, Pitchumoni CS, et al. Risk of pancreatic carcinoma in tropical calcifying pancreatitis: an epidemiologic study. *Pancreas* 1994; 9:62–6.

30. Gold EB, Cameron JL. Chronic pancreatitis and pancreatic cancer. *N Engl J Med* 1993; 328:1485–6.

31. Lerch MM, Ellis I, Whitcomb DC, et al. Maternal inheritance pattern of hereditary pancreati-

tis in patients with pancreatic carcinoma. *J Natl Cancer Inst* 1999; 91:723–4.

32. Lowenfels AB, Maisonneuve EP, Dimagno YE, et al. International Hereditary Pancreatitis Study Group. Hereditary pancreatitis and the risk of pancreatic cancer. *J Natl Cancer Inst* 1997; 89:442–6.

33. Lowenfels AB, Maisonneuve P, Cavallini G, et al. Pancreatitis and the risk of pancreatic cancer. *N Engl J Med* 1993; 328:1433–7.

34. Whitcomb DC. Hereditary pancreatitis: new insights into acute and chronic pancreatitis. *Gut* 1999; 45:317–22.

35. Whitcomb DC, Gorry MC, Preston RA, et al. Hereditary pancreatitis is caused by a mutation in the cationic trypsinogen gene. *Nat Genet* 1996; 14:141–5.

36. Volkholz H, Stolte M, Becker V. Epithelial dysplasias in chronic pancreatitis. *Virchows Arch [A] Pathol Anat Histol* 1982; 396:331–49.

37. Gansauge S, Schmid RM, Muller J, et al. Genetic alterations in chronic pancreatitis: evidence for early occurrence of *p53* but not *K-ras* mutations. *Br J Surg* 1998; 85:337–40.

38. Tabata T, Fujimori T, Maeda S, et al. The role of *Ras* mutation in pancreatic cancer, precancerous lesions, and chronic pancreatitis. *Int J Pancreatol* 1993; 14:237–44.

39. Orth M, Gansauge F, Gansauge S, et al. *K-ras* mutations at codon 12 are rare events in chronic pancreatitis. *Digestion* 1998; 59:120–4.

40. Tabata T, Fujimori T, Maeda S, et al. The role of *ras* mutation in pancreatic cancer, precancerous lesions, and chronic pancreatitis. *Int J Pancreatol* 1993; 14:237–44.

41. van Rees BP, Tascilar M, Hruban RH, et al. Remote partial gastrectomy as a risk factor for pancreatic cancer: potential for preventive strategies. *Ann Oncol* 1999; 10 (Suppl 4):204–7.

42. Silverman DT, Schiffman M, Everhart J, et al. Diabetes mellitus, other medical conditions and familial history of cancer as risk factors for pancreatic cancer. *Br J Cancer* 1999; 80:1830–7.

43. Chow W-H, Gridley G, Nyren O, et al. Risk of pancreatic cancer following diabetes mellitus: a nationwide cohort study in Sweden. *J Natl Cancer Inst* 1995; 87:1–2.

44. Everhart J, Wright D. Diabetes mellitus as a risk factor for pancreatic cancer. A meta-analysis. *JAMA* 1995; 273:1605–9.

45. Gapstur SM, Gann PH, Lowe W, et al. Abnormal glucose metabolism and pancreatic cancer mortality. *JAMA* 2000; 283:2552–8.

46. Hruban RH, Petersen GM, Ha PK, et al. Genetics of pancreatic cancer: from genes to families. *Surg Oncol Clin North Am* 1998; 7:1–23.

47. Hruban RH, Petersen GM, Goggins M, et al. Familial pancreatic cancer. *Ann Oncol* 1999; 10 (Suppl):69–73.

48. Lynch HT, Fitzsimmons ML, Smyrk TC, et al. Familial pancreatic cancer: clinicopathologic study of 18 nuclear families. *Am J Gastroenterol* 1990; 85:54–60.

49. Lynch HT, Smyrk T, Kern SE, et al. Familial pancreatic cancer: a review. *Semin Oncol* 1996; 23:251–75.

50. Dat NM, Sontag SJ. Pancreatic carcinoma in brothers. *Ann Intern Med* 1982; 97:282.

51. Ehrenthal D, Haeger L, Griffin T, et al. Familial pancreatic adenocarcinoma in three generations. *Cancer* 1987; 59:1661–4.

52. Grajower MM. Familial pancreatic cancer. *Ann Intern Med* 1983; 98:111.

53. Katkhouda N, Mouiel J. Pancreatic cancer in mother and daughter. *Lancet* 1986; 2:747.

54. Ghadirian P, Simard A, Baillargeon J. Cancer of the pancreas in two brothers and one sister. *Int J Pancreatol* 1987; 2:383–91.

55. MacDermott RP, Kramer P. Adenocarcinoma of the pancreas in four siblings. *Gastroenterology* 1973; 65:137–9.

56. Reimer RR, Fraumeni JF Jr, Ozols RF, et al. Pancreatic cancer in father and son. *Lancet* 1977; 1:911–12.

57. Brinkley D. *The Unfinished Presidency: Jimmy Carter's journey beyond the White House.* New York: Penguin Group, 1998.

58. Fernandez E, La Vecchia C, D'Avanzo B, et al. Family history and the risk of liver, gallbladder, and pancreatic cancer. *Cancer Epidemiol Biomarkers Prev* 1994; 3:209–12.

59. Ghadirian P, Boyle P, Simard A, et al. Reported family aggregation of pancreatic cancer within a population-based case-control study in the Francophone community in Montreal, Canada. *Int J Pancreatol* 1991; 10:183–96.

60. Price TF, Payne RL, Oberleitner MG. Familial pancreatic cancer in south Louisiana. *Cancer Nurs* 1996; 19:275–82.

61. Tersmette AC, Petersen GM, Offerhaus GJ, et al. Increased risk of incident pancreatic cancer among first-degree relatives of patients with familial pancreatic cancer. *Clin Cancer Res* 2001; 7:738–44.

62. Goggins M, Schutte M, Lu J, et al. Germline *BRCA2* gene mutations in patients with appar-

ently sporadic pancreatic carcinomas. *Cancer Res* 1996; 56:5360–4.

63. Lal G, Liu G, Schmocker B, et al. Inherited predisposition to pancreatic adenocarcinoma: role of family history and germ-line *p16*, *BRCA1*, and *BRCA2* mutations. *Cancer Res* 2000; 60: 409–16.

64. Sharan SK, Morimatsu M, Albrecht U, et al. Embryonic lethality and radiation hypersensitivity mediated by Rad51 in mice lacking *BRCA2*. *Nature* 1997; 386:804–10.

65. Ozcelik H, Schmocker B, DiNicola N, et al. Germline *BRCA2 6174delT* mutations in Ashkenazi Jewish pancreatic cancer patients. *Nat Genet* 1997; 16:17–8.

66. Tulinius H, Olafsdottir GH, Sigvaldason H, et al. Neoplastic diseases in families of breast cancer patients. *J Med Genet* 1994; 31:618–21.

67. Wilentz RE, Goggins M, Redston M, et al. Genetic, immunohistochemical, and clinical features of medullary carcinomas of the pancreas: a newly described and characterized entity. *Am J Pathol* 2000; 156:1641–51.

68. Lynch HT, Voorhees GJ, Lanspa S, et al. Pancreatic carcinoma and hereditary nonpolyposis colorectal cancer: a family study. *Br J Cancer* 1985; 52:271–3.

69. Su GH, Hruban RH, Bova GS, et al. Germline and somatic mutations of the *STKII/LKBI* Peutz-Jeghers gene in pancreatic and biliary cancers. *Am J Pathol* 1999; 154:1835–40.

70. Giardiello FM, Welsh SB, Hamilton SR, et al. Increased risk of cancer in the Peutz-Jeghers syndrome. *N Engl J Med* 1987; 316: 1511–4.

71. Bergman W, Watson P, de Jong J, et al. Systemic cancer and the FAMMM syndrome. *Br J Cancer* 1990; 61:932–6.

72. Ciotti P, Strigini P, Bianchi-Scarra G. Familial melanoma and pancreatic cancer. Ligurian Skin Tumor Study Group [letter; comment]. *N Engl J Med* 1996; 334:469–70.

73. Moskaluk CA, Hruban H, Lietman A, et al. Novel germline *p16* (*INK4*) allele (Asp145Cys) in a family with multiple pancreatic carcinomas. [Mutations in Brief No. 148 online.] *Hum Mutat* 1998; 12:70.

74. Goldstein AM, Fraser MC, Struewing JP, et al. Increased risk of pancreatic cancer in melanoma-prone kindreds with *p16 INK4* mutations. *N Engl J Med* 1995; 333:970–4.

75. Lynch HT, Fusaro RM. Pancreatic cancer and the familial atypical multiple mole melanoma (FAMMM) syndrome. *Pancreas* 1991; 6:127–31.

76. Jeghers HMD, McKusick VAMD, Katz KHMD. Generalized intestinal polyposis and melanin spots of the oral mucosa, lips and digits. *N Engl J Med* 1949; 241:992–1005.

77. Jenne DE, Reimann H, Nezu J, et al. Peutz-Jeghers syndrome is caused by mutations in a novel serine threonine kinase. *Nat Genet* 1998; 18:38–43.

78. Lynch HT, Smyrk TC, Watson P, et al. Genetics, natural history, tumor spectrum, and pathology of hereditary nonpolyposis colorectal cancer: an updated review. *Gastroenterology* 1993; 104: 1535–49.

79. Fitzgibbons RJ Jr, Lynch HT, Stanislav GV, et al. Recognition and treatment of patients with hereditary nonpolyposis colon cancer (Lynch Syndromes I and II). *Ann Surg* 1987; 206: 289–95.

80. Lynch HT, Lanspa S, Smyrk T, et al. Hereditary nonpolyposis colorectal cancer (Lynch Syndromes I & II). Genetics, pathology, natural history, and cancer control, part 1. *Cancer Genet Cytogenet* 1991; 53:143–60.

81. Lynch HT, Krush AJ,. Heredity and adenocarcinoma of the colon. *Gastroenterology* 1967; 53: 517–27.

82. Lynch HT, Smyrk T, Lynch JF. Overview of natural history, pathology, molecular genetics and management of HNPCC (Lynch Syndrome). *Int J Cancer* 1996; 69:38–43.

83. Goggins M, Offerhaus GJA, Hilgers W, et al. Pancreatic adenocarcinomas with DNA replication errors (RER+) are associated with wild-type *K-ras* and characteristic histopathology: Poor differentiation, a syncytial growth pattern, and pushing borders suggest RER+. *Am J Pathol* 1998; 152:1501–7.

84. Watson P, Lynch HT. Extracolonic cancer in hereditary nonpolyposis colorectal cancer. *Cancer* 1993; 71:677–85.

85. Liu B, Parsons R, Papadopoulos N, et al. Analysis of mismatch repair genes in hereditary nonpolyposis colorectal cancer patients. *Nat Med* 1996; 2:169–74.

86. Parsons R, Li G-M, Longley MJ, et al. Hypermutability and mismatch repair deficiency in RER+ tumor cells. *Cell* 1993; 75:1227–36.

87. Leach FS, Nicolaides NC, Papadopoulos N, et al. Mutations of a mutS homolog in hereditary nonpolyposis colorectal cancer. *Cell* 1993; 75: 1215–36.

88. Kunkel TA. Slippery DNA and diseases. *Nature* 1993; 365:207–8.

89. Fishel R, Lescoe MK, Rao MRS, et al. The human mutator gene homolog *MSH2* and its association with hereditary nonpolyposis colon cancer. *Cell* 1993; 75:1027–38.

90. Hruban RH, Wilentz RE, Kern SE. Genetic progression in the pancreatic ducts. *Am J Pathol* 2000; 156:1821–5.

91. Hruban RH, Wilentz RE, Goggins M, et al. Pathology of incipient pancreatic cancer. *Ann Oncol* 1999; 10 (Suppl):9–11.

92. Hruban RH, Goggins M, Parsons J, et al. Progression model for pancreatic cancer. *Clin Cancer Res* 2000; 6:2969–72.

93. Sommers SC, Murphy SA, Warren S. Pancreatic duct hyperplasia and cancer. *Gastroenterology* 1954; 27:629–40.

94. Cubilla AL, Fitzgerald PJ. Morphological lesions associated with human primary invasive nonendocrine pancreas cancer. *Cancer Res* 1976; 36:2690–8.

95. Brat DJ, Lillemoe KD, Yeo CJ, et al. Progression of pancreatic intraductal neoplasias to infiltrating adenocarcinoma of the pancreas. *Am J Surg Pathol* 1998; 22:163–9.

96. Brockie E, Anand A, Albores-Saavedra J. Progression of atypical ductal hyperplasia/carcinoma in situ of the pancreas to invasive adenocarcinoma. *Ann Diagn Pathol* 1998; 2: 286–92.

97. Day JD, DiGiuseppe JA, Yeo CJ, et al. Immunohistochemical evaluation of *HER-2/neu* oncogene expression in pancreatic adenocarcinoma and pancreatic intraepithelial neoplasms. *Hum Pathol* 1996; 27:119–24.

98. Moskaluk CA, Hruban RH, Kern SE. *p16* and *K-ras* gene mutations in the intraductal precursors of human pancreatic adenocarcinoma. *Cancer Res* 1997; 57:2140–3.

99. DiGiuseppe JA, Hruban RH, Offerhaus GJA, et al. Detection of *K-ras* mutations in mucinous pancreatic duct hyperplasia from a patient with a family history of pancreatic carcinoma. *Am J Pathol* 1994; 144:889–95.

100. Yamano M, Fujii H, Takagaki T, et al. Genetic progression and divergence in pancreatic carcinoma. *Am J Pathol* 2000; 156:2123–33.

101. Wilentz RE, Iacobuzio-Donahue CA, Argani P, et al. Loss of expression of *Dpc4* in pancreatic intraepithelial neoplasia: evidence that *DPC4* inactivation occurs late in neoplastic progression. *Cancer Res* 2000; 60:2002–6.

102. Wilentz RE, Geradts J, Maynard R, et al. Inactivation of the *p16* (*INK4A*) tumor-suppressor gene in pancreatic duct lesions: loss of intranuclear expression. *Cancer Res* 1998; 58: 4740–4.

103. Goggins M, Hruban RH, Kern SE. *BRCA2* is inactivated late in the development of pancreatic intraepithelial neoplasia: evidence and implications. *Am J Pathol* 2000; 156:1767–71.

104. DiGiuseppe JA, Hruban RH, Goodman SN, et al. Overexpression of p53 protein in adenocarcinoma of the pancreas. *Am J Clin Pathol* 1994; 101:684–8.

105. Iacobuzio-Donahue CA, Klimstra D, Adsay NV, et al. Dpc-4 protein is expressed in virtually all human intraductal papillary mucinous neoplasms of the pancreas: comparison with conventional ductal carcinomas. *Am J Pathol* 2000; 157:755–61.

106. Azar C, Van de Stadt J, Rickaert F, et al. Intraductal papillary mucinous tumours of the pancreas. Clinical and therapeutic issues in 32 patients. *Gut* 1996; 39:457–64.

107. Loftus EV, Olivares-Pakzad BA, Batts KP, et al. Intraductal papillary-mucinous tumors of the pancreas: clinicopathologic features, outcome and nomenclature. *Gastroenterol* 1996; 110:1909–18.

108. Morohoshi T, Kanda M, Asanuma K, et al. Intraductal papillary neoplasms of the pancreas. A clinicopathologic study of six patients. *Cancer* 1989; 64:1329–35.

109. Nagai E, Ueki T, Chijiiwa K, et al. Intraductal papillary mucinous neoplasms of the pancreas associated with so-called "mucinous ductal ectasia." Histochemical and immunohistochemical analysis of 29 cases. *Am J Surg Pathol* 1995; 19:576–89.

110. Paal E, Thompson LD, Przygodzki RM, et al. A clinicopathologic and immunohistochemical study of 22 intraductal papillary mucinous neoplasms of the pancreas, with a review of the literature. *Mod Pathol* 1999; 12:518–28.

111. Shyr Y-M, Su CH, Tsay SH, et al. Mucin producing neoplasms of the pancreas: intraductal papillary and mucinous cystic neoplasms. *Ann Surg* 1996; 223:141–6.

112. Tian F, Myles J, Howard JM. Mucinous pancreatic ductal ectasia of latent malignancy: an emerging clinicopathologic entity. *Surgery* 1992; 111:109–13.

113. Fujii H, Inagaki M, Kasai S, et al. Genetic progression and heterogeneity in intraductal papillary-mucinous neoplasms of the pancreas. *Am J Pathol* 1997; 151:1447–54.

114. Tada M, Omata M, Ohto M. *Ras* gene mutations in intraductal papillary neoplasms of the

pancreas. Analysis in five cases. *Cancer* 1991; 67:634–7.

115. Z'graggen K, Rivera JA, Compton CC, et al. Prevalence of activating *K-ras* mutations in the evolutionary stages of neoplasia in intraductal papillary mucinous tumors of the pancreas. *Ann Surg* 1997; 226:491–8.

116. Paye F, Sauvanet A, Terris B, et al. Intraductal papillary mucinous tumors of the pancreas: pancreatic resections guided by preoperative morphological assessment and intraoperative frozen section examination. *Surgery* 2000; 127: 536–44.

117. Wilentz RE, Albores-Saavedra J, Zahurak M, et al. Pathologic examination accurately predicts prognosis in mucinous cystic neoplasms of the pancreas. *Am J Surg Pathol* 1999; 23:1320–7.

118. Zamboni G, Scarpa A, Bogina G, et al. Mucinous cystic tumors of the pancreas: clinicopathological features, prognosis, and relationship to other mucious cystic tumors. *Am J Surg Pathol* 1999; 23:410–22.

119. Wilentz RE, Slebos RJC, Hruban RH. Screening for pancreatic cancer using techniques to detect altered gene products. In: Reber HA (ed) *Pancreatic cancer: pathogenesis, diagnosis, and treatment.* Totowa: Humana Press, Inc, 1997, pp. 113–36.

120. Hruban RH, Yeo CJ, Kern SE. Screening for pancreatic cancer. In: Kramer B, Provok P, Gohagan J (ed) *Screening theory and practice.* New York: Dekker Publishing, 1999, pp. 441–59.

121. Yeo CJ, Cameron JL, Lillemoe KD, et al. Pancreaticoduodenectomy for cancer of the head of the pancreas. 201 patients. *Ann Surg* 1995; 221:721–33.

122. Ritts RE, Pitt HA. CA 19-9 in pancreatic cancer. *Surg Oncol Clin North Am* 1998; 7:93–101.

123. Goggins M, Canto M, Hruban RH. Can we screen high-risk individuals to detect early pancreatic carcinoma? *J Surg Oncol* 2000; 74: 243–8.

124. Brentnall TA, Bronner MP, Byrd DR, et al. Early diagnosis and treatment of pancreatic dysplasia in patients with a family history of pancreatic cancer. *Ann Intern Med* 1999; 131: 247–55.

125. Hiyama E, Kodama T, Shinbara K, et al. Telomerase activity is detected in pancreatic cancer but not in benign tumors. *Cancer Res* 1997; 57:326–31.

126. Iwao T, Hiyama E, Yokoyama T, et al. Telomerase activity for the preoperative diagnosis of pancreatic cancer. *J Natl Cancer Inst* 1997; 89:1621–3.

127. Morales CP, Burdick JS, Saboorian MH, et al. In situ hybridization for telomerase RNA in routine cytologic brushings for the diagnosis of pancreaticobiliary malignancies. *Gastrointest Endosc* 1998; 48:402–5.

128. Suehara N, Mizumoto K, Kusumoto M, et al. Telomerase activity detected in pancreatic juice 19 months before a tumor is detected in a patient with pancreatic cancer. *Am J Gastroenterol* 1997; 93:1967–71.

129. Suehara N, Mizumoto K, Tanaka M, et al. Telomerase activity in pancreatic juice differentiates ductal carcinoma from adenoma and pancreatitis. *Clin Cancer Res* 1997; 3(12 Pt 1):2479–83.

130. Tsutsumi M, Tsujiuchi T, Ishikawa O, et al. Increased telomerase activities in human pancreatic duct adenocarcinomas. *Jpn J Cancer Res* 1997; 88:971–6.

131. Uehara H, Nakaizumi A, Tatsuta M, et al. Diagnosis of pancreatic cancer by detecting telomerase activity in pancreatic juice: comparison with *K-ras* mutations. *Am J Gastroenterol* 1999; 94:2513–18.

132. Caldas C, Hahn SA, Hruban RH, et al. Detection of *K-ras* mutations in the stool of patients with pancreatic adenocarcinoma and pancreatic ductal hyperplasia. *Cancer Res* 1994; 54: 3568–73.

133. Wilentz RE, Chung CH, Sturm PDJ, et al. *K-ras* mutations in the duodenal fluid of patients with pancreatic carcinoma. *Cancer* 1998; 82:96–103.

134. Berthélemy P, Bouisson M, Escourrou J, et al. Identification of *K-ras* mutations in pancreatic juice in the early diagnosis of pancreatic cancer. *Ann Intern Med* 1995; 123:188–91.

135. Ueki T, Toyota M, Sohn TA, et al. Hypermethylation of multiple genes in pancreatic carcinoma. *Cancer Res* 2000; 60:1835–9.

136. Baylin SB, Herman JG, Graff JR, et al. Alterations in DNA methylation: a fundamental aspect of neoplasia. *Adv Cancer Res* 1998; 72:141–96.

137. Merlo A, Herman JG, Mao L, et al. 5′ CpG island methylation is associated with transcriptional silencing of the tumor-suppressor *p16/CDKN2/MTS1* in human cancers. *Nat Med* 1995; 1:686–92.

138. Belinsky SA, Nikula KJ, Palmisano WA, et al. Aberrant methylation of *p16(INK4a)* is an

early event in lung cancer and a potential bio-marker for early diagnosis. *Proc Natl Acad Sci USA* 1998; 95:11891–6.

139. Velculescu VE, Zhang L, Vogelstein B, et al. Serial analysis of gene expression. *Science* 1995; 270:484–7.

140. Zhang L, Zhou W, Velculescu VE, et al. Gene expression profiles in normal and cancer cells. *Science* 1997; 276:1268–72.

141. Zhou W, Sokoll LJ, Bruzek DJ, et al. Identifying markers for pancreatic cancer by gene expression analysis. *Cancer Epidemiol Biomarkers Prev* 1998; 7:109–12.

142. Schena M, Shalon D, Davis RW, et al. Quantitative monitoring of gene expression patterns with a complementary DNA microarray [comments]. *Science* 1995; 270:467–70.

143. Schraml P, Kononen J, Bubendorf L, et al. Tissue microarrays for gene amplification surveys in many different tumor types. *Clin Cancer Res* 1999; 5:1966–75.

144. Xu J, Stolk JA, Zhang X, et al. Identification of differentially expressed genes in human prostate cancer using subtraction and microarray. *Cancer Res* 2000; 60:1677–82.

145. Ross DT, Scherf U, Eisen MB, et al. Systematic variation in gene expression patterns in human cancer cell lines [comments]. *Nat Genet* 2000; 24:227–35.

146. Merchant M, Weinberger SR. Recent advancements in surface-enhanced laser desorption/ionization-time of flight-mass spectrometry. *Electrophoresis* 2000; 21:1164–77.

147. Molina MA, Sitja-Arnau M, Lemoine MG, et al. Increased cyclooxygenase-2 expression in human pancreatic carcinomas and cell lines: growth inhibition by nonsteroidal anti-inflammatory drugs. *Cancer Res* 1999; 59:4356–62.

148. Yip-Schneider MT, Barnard DS, Billings SD, et al. Cyclooxygenase-2 expression in human pancreatic adenocarcinomas. *Carcinogenesis* 2000; 21:139–46.

149. Koshiba T, Hosotani R, Miyamoto Y, et al. Immunohistochemical analysis of cyclooxygenase-2 expression in pancreatic tumors. *Int J Pancreatol* 1999; 26:69–76.

150. Okami J, Yamamoto H, Fujiwara Y, et al. Overexpression of cyclooxygenase-2 in carcinoma of the pancreas. *Clin Cancer Res* 1999; 5:2018–24.

151. Tucker ON, Dannenberg AJ, Yang EK, et al. Cyclooxygenase-2 expression is up-regulated in human pancreatic cancer. *Cancer Res* 1999; 59:987–90.

152. Evans JP, Burke W, Chen R, et al. Familial pancreatic adenocarcinoma: association with diabetes and early molecular diagnosis. *J Med Genet* 1995; 32:330–5.

13
Lung

Pamela M. Marcus and William D. Travis

The chapter begins with a brief discussion of the epidemiology, detection, and prevention of lung cancer lesions, that is, those lesions with malignant morphology. An understanding of these issues and related topics is helpful when addressing lung cancer precursor lesions, as many of the issues surrounding invasive lesions also apply to the precursors.

Lung Cancer: Epidemiology, Detection, and Prevention

The epidemiology of lung cancer has been discussed in great detail elsewhere (See [1], for example). Lung cancer is a public health problem in most developed countries [1], and is likely to become a problem in many developing nations as the popularity of cigarette smoking increases [8].

In the United States, lung cancer is the second most common cancer in terms of incidence and the leading cause of cancer-related death [2]. About 164,000 persons in the United States were expected to be newly diagnosed with lung cancer in 2000, and 157,000 were expected to die of the disease [2]. Both incidence and mortality rates are higher for males than for females [9]. While incidence and mortality rates for United States males appear to be decreasing, rates for females, on the other hand, appear to be either increasing (mortality) or stabilizing (incidence) [9].

Because most lung cancers are diagnosed after onset of symptoms and at an advanced stage, survival after diagnosis is poor [10]. The 5-year relative survival rate is estimated to be about 14%, although the figure varies by stage at diagnosis (localized: 48.5%; distant: 2.3%) [10].

Most lung cancers fall into one of four histologic subtypes: adenocarcinoma, squamous cell carcinoma, small-cell carcinoma, and large-cell carcinoma [11]. Adenocarcinoma is the most frequent histologic type (about 29%), followed by squamous cell carcinoma (about 24%), small-cell carcinoma (about 15%), and large-cell carcinoma (about 7%) [6,12]. The pathogenesis of squamous cell carcinoma has been well described [7]; the pathogenesis of other cell types has not.

The most important risk factor for lung cancer is tobacco smoking. About 85% of lung cancer is attributable to cigarette smoking [13]. Relative to persons who have never smoked, persons who smoke experience at least a 10-fold elevation in risk of squamous cell, large-cell, and small-cell carcinoma [1]. Cigarette smoking also is associated with adenocarcinoma, but to a lesser degree, on the order of about a 2-fold elevation in risk [1]. Other suspected or established risk factors for lung cancer include environmental tobacco smoke, air pollution, indoor radon, asbestos and other occupational exposures, and previous non-neoplastic lung disease [1]. Dietary and nutritional factors also have been considered: some studies have shown a reduction in lung cancer risk with consumption of fresh fruits and vegetables (especially those high in β-carotene), while others have shown an elevation in risk with intake of foods rich in fat and cholesterol [1]. With the exception of asbestos and certain aspects of tobacco exposure, risk factors for specific lung cancer histologies have not been studied or elucidated.

If it were possible, the most effective way to reduce the lung cancer burden in the US and other developed nations would be to eliminate cigarette smoking and other avenues of tobacco exposure. Smoking cessation programs have had limited success, however [14], and rates of smoking initiation among adolescents are alarmingly high [15]. Furthermore, it is likely that lung cancer risk remains elevated in former smokers for at least 10 years after cessation [1]. Some researchers believe that these individuals never achieve the lung cancer risk of a person who has never smoked [13].

Early detection of asymptomatic lung cancer through screening is appealing, but to date, no reduction in lung cancer mortality has been observed with routine chest X-ray or sputum cytology [16]. The Prostate, Lung, Colorectal, and Ovarian Cancer Screening Trial (PLCO) is currently evaluating the usefulness of an annual chest X-ray and has ample statistical power to identify a small (on the order of 10–20%) reduction in lung cancer mortality, but findings are likely to be years away [17]. Spiral computerized tomography (CT) may prove to be an effective screening modality, given its excellent resolution [4], but no definitive data regarding its ability to reduce lung cancer mortality are available at this time [18].

The molecular biology of lung cancer has been extensively studied, and as a result, many genetic abnormalities that are characteristic of the disease have been documented [19]. Abnormalities have been found in numerous chromosomal regions, including 3p (multiple regions, including the *FHIT* gene site), 5q (*APC*, *MCC* loci), 9p (*CDKN2*), 13q (*RB*), and 17p (*p53*). Additionally, abnormal expression has been observed for the *HER-2/neu* (*ERBB2*) gene as well as genes in the *ras* and *myc* families. Because certain abnormalities are observed in the very early stages of lung carcinogenesis (both neoplastic and preneo-

plastic), they may ultimately serve to identify individuals with preneoplastic changes or very small invasive lesions. Although many suggestions for "molecular marker" lung cancer screening tests have been made, research is currently in its preliminary stages and has not progressed to the point that any test has been shown to provide a clinical benefit.

Chemoprevention of lung cancer is another attractive option, but to date has not proved fruitful: three large randomized controlled trials found no reduction in lung cancer incidence with regimens of supplemental β-carotene either alone (Physician's Health Study) or in conjunction with α-tocopherol (ATBC) or retinol (CARET) [20–22]; disturbingly, two of the trials (CARET and ATBC β-carotene arm) observed a significant increase in lung cancer incidence and mortality [21,22].

Precursor Lung Cancer Lesions

Precursor lung cancer lesions were first formally recognized in 1981 with the inclusion of squamous dysplasia and CIS in the second edition of the WHO's Histologic Typing of Lung Tumors [23]. The third edition, published in 1999, included another two lesions, atypical adenomatous hyperplasia (AAH) and difuse idiopathic pulmonary neuroendocrine hyperplasia (DIPNECH) [6]. Atypical mesothelial hyperplasia has been proposed as a precursor pleural lesion [24,25]; it was considered but ultimately not included as a precursor lesion in the 1999 classification because of the difficulty in separating the mesothelial hyperplasia that occurs in a reactive setting from that which occurs in a preneoplastic setting [7]. Clinical settings that appear to increase risk of lung cancer but are not thought to reside explicitly in the pathogenetic pathway (e.g., interstitial fibrosis, bronchiectasis, squamous papillomatosis, and cystic lung lesions [7]) will not be discussed in this chapter.

A summary of pathologic and clinical characteristics of squamous dysplasia/CIS, AAH, and DIPNECH is found in Table 13.1.

TABLE 13.1. Characteristics of squamous dysplasia/CIS, AAH, and DIPNECH.

	Squamous dysplasia/CIS (precursor bronchial squamous lesions)	AAH	DIPNECH
Corresponding invasive lesion	Squamous cell carcinoma	Adenocarcinoma, including bronchioloalveolar carcinoma	Carcinoid tumor
Location	Bronchial epithelium	Alveoli and respiratory bronchioles	Bronchiolar epithelium
Lesion size	Variable	Usually less than 5 mm; cases reported up to 10 mm	Less than 5 mm
Microscopic characteristics	Thickening of the squamous epithelium, due to cytologic atypia Increased nuclear to cytoplasmic ratio Presence of mitosis Continuum from mild, moderate, severe dysplasia to CIS	Bronchioloalveolar proliferation Bronchioles line by monotonous, slightly atypical cuboidal to low-column epithelial cells Papillary growth pattern may be present but not dominant feature Nuclear cytoplasmic inclusions may be seen	Neuroendocrine (NE) cell proliferation Scattered NE cells, NE bodies (small nodules), or linear proliferations of NE cells within bronchiolar epithelium Airway fibrosis
Presentation	Discovered in lung cancer resection specimens; also detected by sputum cytology and bronchial biopsy	Most often incidentally discovered in patients with adenocarcinoma, in particular BAC	Obstructive airways disease, including asthma and bronchitis
Differential diagnoses	Atypical squamous metaplasia; radiation/ chemotherapy induced atypia	Nonmucinous bronchioloaveolar carcinoma; type II pneumocyte hyperplasia with interstitial inflammation and/or fibrosis	Reactive secondary lesion to airway inflammation/ fibrosis

Squamous Dysplasia/CIS (Precursor Bronchial Squamous Lesions)

Squamous dysplasia and CIS are considered to be precursor lesions for squamous cell carcinoma [7]. Basal cell hyperplasia, goblet cell hyperplasia, and squamous metaplasia, generally accepted to be earlier phases in the pathogenesis of squamous cell carcinoma, were not considered to be precursor lesions by the 1999 WHO/IASLC panel [6], perhaps due to the lack of cellular atypia and frequency of spontaneous regression. Because squamous dysplasia and CIS are precursors of the same invasive lesion, they are usually grouped together as "preinvasive bronchial squamous lesions" or, in this chapter, "precursor bronchial squamous lesions".

Squamous dysplasia and CIS are both characterized by cellular atypia and thickening of the squamous epithelium. The 1999 WHO/IASLC classification [6] includes three subclassifications of squamous dysplasia (mild, moderate, and severe), defined by the degree of atypia and thickening [6]. CIS is characterized by replacement of the entire thickness of the bronchial epithelium by cytologic abnormalities suggestive of carcinoma, and is differentiated from invasive squamous cell carcinoma by the presence of an intact basement membrane [6]. Genetic abnormalities observed in squamous dysplasia and carcinoma-in-situ include loss of heterozygosity (LOH) at chromosome 3p (including the *FHIT* region), 5q (*APC-MCC* region), 9p21 (*CDKN2*), 13q14 (*RB*), and 17p13 (*p53*), all of which have been observed in either equal or greater degrees in invasive squamous cell carcinoma of the lung as well [19,26,27]. In data of Wistuba et al., LOH at 3p was the most frequently observed abnormality in squamous dysplasia; LOH at 9p21 and 17p3 were also frequently observed in CIS [27].

Epidemiology (Etiology, Prevalence)

Epidemiologic data on precursor squamous lesions are limited. No reports of etiologic research are available, although it seems fair to assume that the risk factors for invasive squamous bronchial lesions would also be associated with precursor lesions. Therefore, it is likely that older age and cigarette smoking strongly increase the risk of these precursor lesions [13]; certain occupational exposures may increase risk also [28].

Prevalence estimates of precursor bronchial squamous lesions are available from randomized controlled clinical trials of mass screening as well as other types of studies (Table 13.2). For the identified studies, prevalence is available primarily for individuals at elevated risk of lung cancer. This means, unfortunately, that the majority of estimates presented in Table 13.2 overestimate prevalence in the general population.

Prevalence estimates are available from three studies of mass screening conducted as part of NCI's Early Lung Cancer Detection Program (Table 13.2, Part A) [29–31]. The 30,000 or so participants were male and smoked at least one pack of cigarettes a day at study entry. Among participants who received sputum cytology and chest X-ray on their first screen, the prevalence of cellular atypia ranged from 0.1% to 4%, and the prevalence of CIS ranged from 0.05% to 0.1%.

Prevalence data for cellular atypia, squamous dysplasia, and CIS are available from five studies [32–36] that did not assess the efficacy of mass screening (Table 13.2, Part B). Two examined occupational cohorts exposed to uranium or chromium, two examined individuals with severe respiratory difficulties, and one examined persons who were known or suspected to have lung cancer and persons whose lung cancer status was unknown at study entry.

The range of prevalence estimates across these five studies is quite wide, perhaps due to differences in extent of exposure, method of detection, and small sample sizes. The prevalence of squamous dysplasia ranged from a low of 0.05% in a series of former heavy smokers undergoing lung reduction surgery [35] to a high of 73% in a series of chronic obstructive pulmonary disorder (COPD) patients who smoked for at least 40 years [33]. The prevalence of CIS in these studies was lower and less variable. Prevalence among series of nonsmokers included in two of the studies was observed to be 0% [34,36]. Among smokers, the prevalence of CIS ranged from a low of 0% in the series undergoing lung reduction surgery [35] to a high of 15% among the series of individuals who were known or suspected to have lung cancer and underwent fluorescence bronchoscopy [34].

Four additional reports included information on detection of precursor bronchial squamous lesions using white-light or LIFE (light-induced fluorescent endoscopy) bronchoscopy [37–40], but these reports did not provide sufficient data from which to calculate a reasonable estimate of prevalence.

Detection

Squamous dysplasia and CIS can present symptomatically, although it is more likely for such lesions to be asymptomatic and to be detected through screening or during work-up for invasive lung lesions. The manner in which these lesions are detected has changed over time. Thirty years ago, many precursor bronchial squamous lesions were initially identified on screening sputum cytology and then confirmed using a bronchoscopic or surgical procedure. These lesions usually were not observable on chest X-ray and, as such, were termed "roentgenographically occult lung cancer". Characteristics of these lesions have been well documented [41–44].

After three large randomized controlled clinical trials failed to show a reduction in lung cancer mortality with intense screening regimens that included sputum cytology [16,45,46], the practice of using sputum cytology diminished. In recent years, fluorescence bronchoscopy, in particular white-light and laser-induced bronchoscopy (LIFE), have become useful tools for the detection of precursor bronchial squamous lesions [5,37,38,40]. LIFE was approved by the US Federal Drug Administration (FDA) in 1996 as an adjunct to white-light bronchoscopy for the purpose of "localization of high-grade preinvasive bronchial lesions (moderate/severe dysplasia and CIS) that are of prognostic significance" [5]. Findings of Kurie et al. [38], however, question whether the use of LIFE provides additional detection benefit over and above that of white-light bronchoscopy [5,38].

Prevention

As is the case with invasive lung cancer, prevention of the majority of precursor bronchial squamous lesions undoubtedly would be best accomplished by elimination of tobacco exposure. However, the large number of former smokers who remain at elevated risk, as well as the large number of current smokers who are unsuccessful at quitting, indicates that other methods are necessary. Epidemiologic studies of diet and lung cancer, which showed an inverse association between lung cancer incidence and certain dietary factors (including dietary β-carotene), suggested that chemoprevention using dietary supplementation or derivatives of dietary factors might be a useful alternative [47].

The first clinical trials of lung cancer chemoprevention considered reversal of premalignancy as endpoints. In these trials, patients identified as having squamous metaplasia, squamous dysplasia, or other cellular abnormalities, either through biopsy or sputum cytology, were given dietary supplements or pharmaceuticals. These trials are summarized in Table 13.3.

In the early 1980's, Mathe et al., using their "metaplasia index (MI)" (a semiquantitative measure of squamous metaplasia in bronchial biopsies), observed a significant reduction in the MI of 30 heavy smokers after a 6-month regimen of 25 mg of etretinate daily [48]. Results were promising, although the lack of a

control arm (i.e., placebo-controlled) limited conclusions. Since then, two placebo-controlled randomized trials have shown a reduction in the occurrence of precursor lesions in association with administration of a chemopreventive regimen: Van Poppel et al. observed a significant reduction in micronuclei counts with a daily regimen of 20 mg β-carotene for 14 weeks [49], and Heimburger et al. observed a significant reversal in squamous metaplasia with a daily regimen of 10 mg folate plus 500 μg of hydroxocobalamin for four months [50]. However, four placebo-controlled randomized clinical trials resulted in no benefit: Arnold et al. observed similar reductions in sputum atypia with a 6-month course of 25 mg of etretinate daily or placebo [51]; Lee et al. observed similar reductions in the MI for persons receiving 1 mg/kg of isotrentinoin a day for 6 months or placebo [52]; McLarty et al. observed no significant reduction in sputum atypia after a regimen of 50 mg of β-carotene and 25,000 IU of retinol on alternating days for a minimum of 3 years [53]; and Kurie et al. observed no significant reversal of squamous metaplasia or dysplasia after a daily regimen of 200 mg N-(4-hydroxyphenyl)retinamide (4-HPR) for 6 months [54].

Of interest here is that ATBC and CARET, the large chemoprevention trials that examined regimens of β-carotene in conjunction with α-tocopherol and retinol respectively, observed on significant reduction in the incidence of squamous cell carcinoma [55,56].

Atypical Adenomatous Hyperplasia (AAH)

AAH is considered to be a precursor lesion for adenocarcinoma, including bronchioloalveolar carcinoma (BAC) [57]. Lesions that are characterized by bronchioalveolar proliferation but do not meet the criteria for bronchioloalveolar carcinoma are considered to be AAH, although it is often difficult to distinguish AAH from nonmucinous BAC [57]. The term "atypical adenomatous hyperplasia" was adopted by the WHO/IASLC panel in 1999 to end widespread variation in nomenclature [6]. Previously, names such as "alveolar atypical hyperplasia",

TABLE 13.2. Prevalence of cellular atypia, squamous dysplasia, and CIS and additional characteristics in selected studies. Part A: Mass screening programs utilizing sputum cytology. Participants were males at elevated risk of lung cancer but were not suspected of having the disease. Part B: Studies other than those of mass screening.

A:

First author, year	Country	Dates	Description of subjects	Subjects, n	Prevalence of AT/SD/CIS, %	Characteristics of subjects
Frost, 1984 [29]	US	1973–1978	Early Lung Cancer Detection Program – Johns Hopkins. Initial screen. Dual-screen arm received chest X-ray and sputum cytology; control arm received chest X-ray only	Dual-screen: 5,226 Control: 5,161	Dual-screen: AT: 4% CIS: 0.1% Control: AT: not applicable CIS: 0%	Median age: 53 y/o Smoked ≥1 pack/day 25% in dual-screen had potential occupational exposure to lung carcinogens
Flehinger, 1984 [30]	US	1974–1978	Early Lung Cancer Detection Program – Memorial Sloan-Kettering. Initial screen. Dual-screen arm received chest X-ray and sputum cytology; control arm received chest X-ray only	Dual-screen: 4,968 Control: 5,072	Dual-screen: AT: 0.1% CIS: 0.1% Control: AT: not applicable CIS: 0%	Median age: 48 y/o Smoked ≥1 pack/day 11% in dual-screen had potential occupational exposure to lung carcinogens
Fontana, 1984 [31]	US	1971–1976	Early Lung Cancer Detection Program – Mayo Lung Project. Initial screen. All participants received chest X-ray and sputum cytology	10,933	AT: 0.3% CIS: 0.05%	Median age: 55 y/o Smoked ≥1 pack/day 9% had potential occupational exposure to lung carcinogens

B.

First author, year	Country	Dates	Description of subjects; detection method	Subjects, n	Prevalence of AT/SD/CIS, n, %	Characteristics of subjects
Saccamanno, 1974 [36]	US	1957–?	Uranium workers (M: miner; NM: not miner; S: smoker; NS: nonsmoker) Sputum cytology	M/S: 2,349 M/NS: 1,208 NM/S: 1,569 NM/NS: 432	M/S: marked AT 12%; CIS 1% M/NS: marked AT 5%; CIS 0% N/M/S: marked At 7%; CIS 1% NM/NS: marked AT 2%, CIS 0%	No additional characteristics available
Lam, 1993 [34]	Canada	?	Two groups of subjects: 1. known or suspected to have lung cancer 2. not known to have lung cancer Fluorescence bronchoscopy	Group 1: 53 Group 2: 41	Group 1: SD: 23% CIS: 15% Group 2: Current smokers: SD: 69% CIS: 0% Exsmokers: SD: 37% CIS: 13% Nonsmokers: SD: 12% CIS: 0%	No additional characteristics available
Ishikawa, 1994 [32]	Japan	1975–1993	Chromium workers Autopsy	13	(percents are approximate) 1 had presence of CIS (8%); 2 had history of SD while alive (15%)	All males; All three with precursor lesions had lung cancer also; 9 were smokers
Kennedy, 1996 [33]	US	1993–1995	Subjects had COPD and 40+ years of smoking history Persons with diagnosis of cancer within 5 years and recent exposure to chemopreventive agents were excluded Sputum cytology	553	Mild SD: 258, 47% Moderate SD: 133, 25% Severe SD: 4, 1% CIS: 5, 1%	Mean years of smoking cessation: Mild SD: 8.3 Moderate SD: 8.4 Severe SD: 5.5 CIS: 2.5
Pigula, 1996 [35]	US	?	Subjects undergoing lung reduction surgery for severe diffuse emphysema Many possible detection methods, including chest X-ray, CT, and surgery	210	SD: 1, 0.05% CIS: 0	Former heavy smoker

AT, moderate or marked atypia on sputum cytology; SD, squamous dysplasia; CIS, carcinoma in situ; ROLC, roentgenographically occult lung cancer.

TABLE 13.3. Clinical trails of lung cancer chemoprevention utilizing intermediate endpoints.

First author, year	Study design	Regimen	Participants, n	Participant characteristics	Findings (study end)
Mathe, 1982 [48]	Intervention only—no control group	25 mg etretinate daily; 6 months	30	Males and females; 15+ pack-years; MI > 15%	Positive (?)—metaplasia index (MI) significantly reduced after treatment, but no control group for comparison
Heimburger, 1988 [50]	RCT	10 mg folate plus 500 µg of hydroxocobalamin daily versus placebo; 4 months	73 (36 to intervention; 37 to placebo)	Males; 20+ pack-years; current smokers; metaplasia on at least 1 of 3 sputum samples	Positive—significant reversal of squamous metaplasia observed with use of a categorical "cytology score" (levels: normal cytology, squamous metaplasia without atypia, squamous metaplasia with atypia). Reversal based on observed versus expected change in cytology score category.
Arnold, 1992 [51]	RCT	25 mg etretinate daily versus placebo; 6 months	150 (75 to intervention; 75 to placebo)	Males and females; 15+ pack-years; current smokers; mild atypia on 2/3 sputum samples or moderate/severe atypia on 1/3 sputum samples	Negative—similar degree of atypia improvement in both arms
Van Poppel, 1992 [49]	RCT	20 mg β-carotene daily versus placebo; 14 weeks	114 (53 to intervention; 61 to placebo)	Males; 15+ cigarettes per day for 2+ years	Positive—% reduction in micronuclei significant for intervention arm but not placebo arm; % reduction significantly better in treatment arm versus placebo arm.
Lee, 1994 [52]	RCT	1 mg/kg isotetinoin daily versus placebo	86 (44 to intervention; 47 to placebo)	Males and females; 15+ pack-years; current smokers or former smokers who quit within last 6 months; MI > 15% and/or dysplasia	Negative—similar reductions in mean MI for both intervention and placebo arm. Number of complete reversals the same in both arms.
McLarty, 1995 [53]	RCT	50 mg β-carotene and 25,000 IU retinol on alternating days versus placebo; minimum of 3 years	755 (378 to intervention; 377 to placebo)	Males and females; former asbestos workers with documented exposure	Negative—similar distribution of pathology (normal, metaplasia, atypia, malignancy) in both arms
Kurie, 2000 [54]	RCT	200 mg 4-HPR daily versus placebo; 6 months	70 (34 to intervention; 36 to placebo)	Males and females; 20+ pack-years; metaplasia or dysplasia at baseline	Negative—greater % reduction in squamous metaplasia in intervention but not statistically significant; authors conclude that the intervention had "no detectable effect" on squamous metaplasia or dysplasia.

RCT, randomized controlled trial; patients blinded to regimen.

"alveolar cell hyperplasia", "atypical alveolar hyperplasia", "atypical bronchioloalveolar cell hyperplasia", "alveolar epithelial hyperplasia", "bronchioloalveolar adenoma", "bronchioloalveolar cell adenoma", and "early stage lesions of bronchioloalveolar carcinoma" had all been used to describe this lesion [7].

The pathogenesis of adenocarcinoma of the lung is not as clearly defined as that of squamous cell carcinoma [58]. In addition to AAH, pulmonary scars had been proposed as precursor lesions, but that notion is no longer favored [59]. There also have been suggestions of an adenoma–carcinoma sequence similar to that observed in colonic cancer pathogenesis [59] (see Chapter 9). The recognition of AAH as a precursor lesion for adenocarcinoma represents an important first step in the clarification of the natural history of adenocarcinoma of the lung.

AAH lesions are small (usually less than 5 mm) and are found in the alveoli, particularly those near respiratory bronchioles [57]. They are characterized by ill-defined proliferation, consisting of monotonous, slightly atypical, cuboidal to low-column, epithelial cells. Papillary growth patterns and nuclear cytoplasmic inclusions may be seen. Genetic abnormalities observed in AAH include LOH at chromosomes 3p (including the *FHIT* region), 9p, and 17p (*p53*), as well as *K-ras* (at codon 12) and *HER-2/neu* mutations [19,26,60–63]. These same abnormalities also are observed in adenocarcinomas [60,62,64].

Epidemiology (Etiology, Prevalence)

As for precursor bronchial squamous lesions, few epidemiologic data are available for AAH. No reports of etiologic research are available, although risk factors for adenocarcinoma of the lung are likely to be risk factors for AAH also. These include older age, cigarette smoking, and possibly, certain occupational exposures and previous respiratory illnesses [1,28]. Because adenocarcinoma has been observed in a greater proportion of nonsmoking females than nonsmoking males, hormonal factors may also influence risk of AAH [1]. Many of the reports listed in Table 13.4, which presents estimates of

the prevalence of AAH, provide data on characteristics of persons with AAH, supporting the notion that older age and heavy smoking are likely to be risk factors. Prevalence of AAH seems to be a bit higher in Japanese patient series as compared to those in other countries, suggesting that certain factors (perhaps genetic) that are more common among Japanese persons may increase risk. Alternatively, Japanese investigators may be more attentive to searching for this lesion than those in other countries. The small number of studies conducted in other countries does not make for a good comparison, and therefore does not provide compelling data for an elevated risk of AAH among Japanese persons. Omitted from Table 13.4 are two reports written in Japanese [65,66] and four studies that provided very limited epidemiologic data [61,67–69].

Prevalence estimates are available from reports of incidental detection of AAH in lung cancer resection tissue and from two autopsy studies. Prevalence estimates based on incidental detection are biased in that they overestimate prevalence in the general population (because they are calculated using persons at elevated risk). One of the two autopsy studies was conducted among decedents known to have had lung cancer, thus posing the same problem; the other autopsy study, however, was conducted among decedents known not to have lung cancer, and therefore it slightly underestimates prevalence in the general population.

Of the seven lung resection studies, five examined patients undergoing resection for any histologic type of lung cancer [59,70–73], and two examined patients undergoing resection for adenocarcinoma [58,74]. In the former group, overall prevalence of AAH ranged from a low of 5% [59] to a high of 21% [72] (Table 13.4, Part A), but the prevalence of AAH in patients with adenocarcinoma or BAC alone ranged from about 17% [73,74] to 35% [72]. In the two reports restricted to resection of adenocarcinoma, AAH prevalences were 6% [58] and 19% [74]. As would be expected, the prevalence of AAH among patients with nonadenocarcinoma subtypes is lower, but at the same time it is not trivial. For patients with squamous cell, large- and small-cell carcinomas, AAH

TABLE 13.4. Prevalence of atypical adenomatous hyperplasia (AAH) and additional characteristics in selected studies. Part A: Lung resection studies. Part B: Autopsy studies.

A:

First author, year	Country	Dates	Source; nomenclature	Pts, n	Prevalence of AAH, n (%)	Characteristics of pts with AAH	AAH prevalence by dominant primary lesion (number with invasive lesion, number with AAH)*	Multiplicity of AAH lesions
Miller, 1990 [71]	Canada	1986–1989	Consecutive lung resections for lung cancer; bronchioloalveolar cell adenoma	247	23 (9%)	Not available	SQ (100,3): 3% AtCd (23,2): 9% AA (64,8): 13% BAC (45,9): 20% NEC (21,1): 5% LCA (10,0): 0%	41 AAH in total 14 patients: 1 lesion 9 pateints: >1 lesion
Nakanishi, 1990 [72]	Japan	1979–1985	Lung resections for lung cancer; alveolar epithelial hyperplasia	70	15 (21%)	73% male Mean age: 63 y/o All smokers 53% > 20+ pack–years	SQ (29,2): 6.9% AC (29,10): 35% LCC (10,1): 10% (2 carcinomas with no histology info—both had AAH)	30 AAH in total 9 patients: 1 lesion 6 patients: >1 lesion
Carey, 1992 [58]	Scotland	1986–1990	Consecutive lung resections for lung adenocarcinoma; alveolar atypical hyperplasia	175	10 (6%)	30% male All current smokers or former smokers who quit within 2 years prior to surgery	All AC—no finer breakdown available	Not available

Study	Country	Years	Indication	N	AAH (%)	Demographics	Histology	Lesions
Weng, 1992 [73]	Japan	1984–1987	Lung resections for lung cancer; atypical bronchioloalveolar cell hyperplasia	165	27 (16%); Males: 22 (20%, n = 110); Females: 5 (9%, n = 55)	81% male Mean age Males: 67 y/o Females: 63 y/o Mean pack–years: Males: 41 Females: 20	Males: SQ (38,4): 11% SCC (4,1): 25% AC (51,13): 26% LCC (12,3): 25% ASQ (5,1): 20% Females: SQ (5,1): 20% SCC (1,0): 0% AC (48,4): 8% LCC (1,0): 0%	Males: 103: 1 lesion 7: >1 lesion Females: 51: 1 lesion 4: >1 lesion
Noguchi, 1994 [59]	Japan	1965–1989	Lung resections for lung cancer; AAH	2,098	108 (5%)	Not available	AC (1118,87): 8% SCC (766,7): 1% LCC (152,10): 7% SCC (62,4): 7%	Not available
Takigawa, 1999 [74]	Japan	1983–1998	Lung resections for lung adenocarcinoma, AAH	137	26 (19%);	46% male Median age: 65 y/o 50% nonsmokers 19% had family history of lung cancer 19% had history of respiratory disease	All patients: BAC (52,9): 17% Non-BAC: (85,17): 20% Nonsmokers: BAC (35,4): 11% Non-BAC (42,9): 21%	Not available
Chapman, 2000 [70]	Scotland	1989–1998	Lung resections for lung cancer; AAH	582	70 (12%)	53% male Mean age: 62 years	SQ (214,7): 3% AC (224,52): 23% LCC (24,3): 13% Other mal (115,7): 6% Benign (5,1): 20%	Total AAH lesions unavailable 24: 1 lesion 46: >1 lesion

TABLE 13.4. *Continued*
B:

First author, year	Country	Dates	Source, nomenclature	Pts, n	Prevalence of AAH, n (%)	Characteristics of pts with AAH	AAH prevalence by dominant primary lesion (number with invasive lesion, number with AAH)[1]	Multiplicity of AAH lesions
Sterner, 1997 [75]	US	1993–1994	Lung specimens from consecutive autopsies. Excluded cases with history of primary or metastatic lung cancer. Not restricted to elderly; atyical alveolar cell hyperplasia	100	2 (2%)	Not applicable	Not applicable	All had 1 lesion
Yokose, 2000 [76]	Japan	1986–1990	Lung specimens from consecutive autopsy studies. Restricted to elderly (60 and older), AAH	241	16 (7%)	38% male Median age: Males: 78 Females: 79 75% had cancer 7% (n = 2) had lung cancer	All patients with lung cancer: SQ (10,0): 0% AC (13,2): 15% LCC: (1,0): 0% SCC (4,0): 0%	19 AAH in total No additional information available

[1] SQ, squamous; AtCd, atypical carcinoid; AA, acinar adenocarcinoma; BAC, bronchioloalveolar carcinoma; NEC, neuroendocrine carcinoma; LCA, large cell anaplastic carcinoma; AC, adenocarcinoma; LCC, large cell carcinoma; SCC, small cell carcinoma; ASQ, adenosquamous carcinoma.

prevalence is on the order of 10% or greater. In the autopsy studies, AAH prevalence was 2% in a study in which no individuals with lung cancer were included [75] and 7% in a study including only persons with lung cancer [76]. In the study with only lung cancer patients [76], AAH was identified only in persons with adenocarcinoma.

Detection and Prevention

AAH is rarely, if ever, detected symptomatically; instead, AAH is usually incidentally identified in lung cancer resection tissue [57]. The typical AAH lesion is unlikely to be detected on chest X-ray. Detection of AAH using low-dose screening spiral CT has been reported [77,78], but the ability of CT to detect AAH is probably strongly dependent on lesion size and CT slice thickness.

Prevention of AAH has not been formally studied, but once again, elimination of tobacco exposure and other lung adenocarcinoma risk factors is likely to reduce the prevalence of the lesion. No significant reduction in adenocarcinoma incidence was observed in either the ATBC or CARET trials [55,56].

Diffuse Idiopathic Pulmonary Neuroendocrine Hyperplasia (DIPNECH)

DIPNECH is considered to be a precursor lesion for carcinoid tumors, and is characterized by an increased number of neuroendocrine cells, small nodules, or linear proliferations of neuroendocrine cells within the peripheral bronchiolar epithelium [57]. Neuroendocrine cell hyperplasia is a relatively common phenomenon, occurring in response to nonspecific reactions secondary to airway or interstitial inflammation and/or fibrosis. For such a condition to be classified as DIPNECH, however, the proliferation must be considered to be a primary condition [57].

Epidemiology (Etiology, Prevalence)

DIPNECH was formally described in 1992 by Aguayo et al. [79]. The authors described a case series of six patients with diffuse hyperplasia of pulmonary neuroendocrine cells, but with no history of cigarette smoking and no concomitant lung disease. Since that publication, a few additional case reports have been published using the nomenclature DIPNECH or a variation thereof [80–83]. Case reports of pulmonary neuroendocrine cell hyperplasia published before the work of Aguayo et al. [84–89], and two published after [64,90], describe patients with conditions that may very well have been DIPNECH. DIPNECH appears to be an early stage of a pathologic process that may proceed from neuroendocrine cell hyperplasia to carcinoid tumorlets, and may finally proceed to carcinoid tumors [57].

Table 13.5 displays characteristics of the patients decribed in case reports of DIPNECH. Judging from these reports, DIPNECH appears to preferentially affect older women and non-smokers. Therefore, it is likely that cigarette smoking is not a meaningful risk factor for DIPNECH. Because women constitute nearly all case reports of DIPNECH, an hormonal etiology comes to mind, although no supporting evidence is available. The absence of etiologic research on carcinoid tumors precludes suggestion of other risk factors for DIPNECH.

DIPNECH is quite rare, and, as such, no population-based prevalence estimates are available. Considering all definite, probable, and possible DIPNECH case reports, it appears that no more than 50 cases of DIPNECH have been documented. Miller et al. [64] report eight possible cases of DIPNECH in a series of 25 patients undergoing lung resection for peripheral carcinoid tumors, suggesting that the prevalence of DIPNECH among individuals with carcinoid tumors could be as high as 32%.

Detection and Prevention

Patients with DIPNECH generally present with serious idiopathic respiratory difficulties that resemble asthma or bronchitis. DIPNECH can be viewed on chest X-ray and spiral CT, but is usually confirmed on open-lung biopsy or lung transplantation because of the necessity of treatment. It appears that no research regarding DIPNECH or carcinoid prevention has been undertaken. Given the rarity of the con-

TABLE 13.5. Reports of DIPNECH: patient characteristics.

First author, year	Country	Source	Pts, n	Patient characteristics	Presence of carcinoid tumors

Aguayo, 1992 [79]	US	Clinical presentation; open-lung biopsy	6	2 males, 4 females
				Ages
				  Males: 22, 48 y/o
				  Females: 61, 67, 68, 76 y/o
				All nonsmokers
					All females had carcinoid tumors; 48 y/o male had carcinoid tumorlets

Armas, 1995 [80]	US	Clinical presentation; bronchoscopy; open-lung biopsy	1	Female 70 y/o Nonsmoker	No mention of carcinoid tumors
Sheerin, 1995 [83]	England	Clinical presentation; complete lung resection and transplantation	1	Female First clinical presentation at 42 y/o; lung removed at 53 y/o 5 pack–years of smoking	No mention of carcinoid tumors
Brown, 1997 [81]	Canada	Clincal presentation; complete lung resection and transplantation	1	Female 65 y/o 18 pack–years of smoking	No mention of carcinoid tumors
Cohen, 1998 [82]	US	Clinical presentation; open-lung biopsy	3	Female Age range: 49–62 Two nonsmokers; 1 former smoker	No mention of carcinoid tumors

dition, it is unlikely that DIPNECH prevention will ever be formally undertaken in preventive medicine.

Atypical Mesothelial Hyperplasia

Atypical mesothelial hyperplasia may be a precursor lesion for malignant mesothelioma [7], a malignancy arising in the pleura of the lung. The nomenclature "mesothelioma-in-situ" and "malignant mesothelioma-in-situ" also have been used to describe mesothelial precursor lesions [7,25], although the recently formed International Mesothelioma Panel recommended against the use of these terms [7]. The fact that no pecursor lesion for malignant mesothelioma is officially recognized underlines our lack of understanding of its pathogenetic process.

Atypical mesothelial hyperplasia, which is characterized by marked atypical mesothelial proliferation that is highly suspicious of malig-

nancy, is troublesome in that such proliferation can develop in a reactive manner as well as (hypothetically) developing as part of the carcinogenic process leading to malignant mesothelioma [7]. Some researchers, therefore, have suggested that diagnosis of a mesothelial precursor lesion should occur only if malignant mesothelioma is present. They have suggested the nomenclature "malignant mesothelioma-in-situ" to reflect that situation [7,25].

Epidemiology (Etiology, Prevalence)

No epidemiologic research has been conducted on atypical mesothelial hyperplasia as a precursor lesion rather than a reactive condition, since they are histologically indistinguishable. However, the epidemiology of malignant mesothelioma has been well described [1], and therefore inferences can be made. Asbestos, the principal cause of mesothelioma, would almost certainly be a risk factor of atypical mesothelial hyperplasia if such lesions were truly meso-thelial precursor lesions. Whitaker et al. present a case series of seven patients, diagnosed between 1975 and 1989 at two Australian medical centers, who fulfilled the authors' criteria for mesothelioma-in-situ; of the seven, six were known to have extensive asbestos exposure [25]. With the exception of exposure to naturally occurring zeolite (erionite) fibers and high doses of ionizing radiation, no other established or strongly suspected causes of malignant mesothelioma are known [1], and therefore no other risk factors for mesothelial precursor lesions can be suggested.

Two reports provide information on the prevalence of in-situ lesions accompanying malignant mesotheliomas: Henderson et al. report a prevalence of 1% (22 out of more than 1,500 [24]), but Cury et al. report a prevalence of 23% (7 out of 31) in a much smaller case series [91].

Detection and Prevention

Little information is available on the detection of atypical mesothelial hyperplasia independent of malignant mesothelioma detection, although it is likely that these lesions are detected symptomatically. In the presence of malignant mesothelioma, the precursor lesion appears to be detected incidentally in biopsy samples [25]. Prevention of atypical mesothelial hyperplasia has not been studied, but given the association with mesothelioma, elimination of asbestos exposure, as well as exposure to zeolite fibers, would probably prevent most lesions. No reduction in malignant mesothelioma was observed in CARET (whose study population included a large number of individuals with occupational exposure to asbestos) with a daily regimen of 20 mg of β-carotene and 25,000 IU of retinol for an average of four years [21].

Conclusion

Current understanding of the epidemiology of precursor lung cancer lesions is limited. Much of what is assumed regarding precursor lung cancer lesions has been inferred from knowledge of invasive lung cancer lesions, and although it is likely that most inferences are correct, more directed studies could prove to be very fruitful. Recent technological advances have already improved our understanding and will undoubtedly improve detection of precursor lesions in years to come. Easier detection of these lesions hopefully will spark new and expanded research programs that will allow for a better understanding of the epidemiologic aspects of lung cancer precursor lesions.

References

1. Blot WJ, Fraumeni JF Jr. Cancers of the lung and pleura. In: Schottenfeld D, Fraumeni JF Jr (eds) *Cancer epidemiology and prevention.* New York: Oxford University Press, 1996, pp. 637–65.
2. Ginsberg RJ, Vokes EE, Raben A. Non-small cell lung cancer. In: DeVita VT Jr, Hellman S, Rosenberg SA (eds) *Cancer: principles and practice of oncology.* Philadelphia: Lippincott-Raven, 1997, pp. 858–911.
3. Ihde DC, Gladstein E, Pass HI. Small Cell Lung Cancer. In: DeVita VT Jr, Hellman S, Rosenberg SA (eds) *Cancer: principles and practice of oncology.* Philadelphia: Lippincott-Raven, 1997, pp. 911–49.
4. Henschke CI, McCauley DI, Yankelevitz DF, et al. Early Lung Cancer Action Project: overall design and findings from baseline screening. *Lancet* 1999; 354:99–105.
5. Lam S, Kennedy T, Unger M, et al. Localization of bronchial intraepithelial neoplastic lesions by fluorescence bronchoscopy. *Chest* 1998; 113:696–702.
6. Travis WD, Colby TB, Corrin B, et al. *Histologic typing of lung and pleural tumors*, 3rd ed. Berlin: Springer, 1999.
7. Travis WD. Pathology of pulmonary incipient neoplasia. In: Henson DE, Albores-Saavedra J (eds) *Pathology of incipient neoplasia.* New York: Oxford University Press, 2001, pp. 295–318.
8. Baron JA, Rohan TE. Tobacco. In: Schottenfeld D, Fraumeni JF (eds) *Cancer epidemiology and prevention.* New York: Oxford University Press, 1996, pp. 269–89.
9. Reis LAG, Eisner MP, Kosary CL, et al. *SEER Cancer Statistics Review, 1973–1997.* Bethesda, MD: National Cancer Institute, 2000.

10. Greenlee RT, Murray T, Bolden S, et al. Cancer statistics, 2000. *CA Cancer J Clin* 2000; 50:7–33.

11. Travis WD, Travis LB, Devesa SS. Lung cancer. *Cancer* 1995; 75:191–202.

12. *Surveillance, epidemiology and end results cancer incidence. Public-use database, 1973–1997.* Bethesda, MD: National Cancer Institute, 2000.

13. Schottenfeld D. Etiology and epidemiology of lung cancer. In: Pass HI, Mitchell JB, Johnson DH, et al. (eds) *Lung cancer: principles and practice.* Philadelphia: Lippincott Williams and Wilkins, 2000, pp. 368–88.

14. Hughes JR. New treatments for smoking cessation. *CA Cancer J Clin* 2000; 50:143–51.

15. Tobacco use among high school students—United States, 1997 *MMWR* 1998; 47:229–33.

16. Wolpaw DR. Early detection in lung cancer. Case finding and screening. *Med Clin North Am* 1996; 80:63–82.

17. Gohagan JK, Levin DL, Prorok PC, et al. eds. The Prostate, Lung, Colorectal and Ovarian (PLCO) Cancer Screening Trial. *Controlled Clin Trials* 2001; 21 Supp:249S–406S.

18. Marcus PM, Prorok PC. Reanalysis of the Mayo Lung Project data: the impact of confounding and effect modification. *J Med Screen* 1999; 6:47–9.

19. Minna JD, Sekido Y, Fong KM, et al. Molecular biology of lung cancer. In DeVita VT, Hellman S, Rosenberg SA (eds) *Cancer: principles and practice of oncology.* Philadelphia: Lippincott-Raven, 1997; 849–67.

20. Hennekens CH, Buring JE, Manson JE, et al. Lack of effect of long-term supplementation with beta carotene on the incidence of malignant neoplasms and cardiovascular disease. *N Engl J Med* 1996; 334:1145–9.

21. Omenn GS, Goodman GE, Thornquist MD, et al. Effects of a combination of beta carotene and vitamin A on lung cancer and cardiovascular disease. *N Engl J Med* 1996; 334:1150–5.

22. The Alpha-Tocopherol Beta Carotene Cancer Prevention Study Group. The effect of vitamin E and beta carotene on the incidence of lung cancer and other cancers in male smokers. *N Engl J Med* 1994; 330:1029–35.

23. *Histologic typing of lung tumors,* 2nd ed. Geneva: World Health Organization, 1981.

24. Henderson DW, Shilkin KB, Whitaker D. Reactive mesothelial hyperplasia vs mesothelioma, including mesothelioma in situ: a brief review. *Am J Clin Pathol* 1998; 110:397–404.

25. Whitaker D, Henderson DW, Shilkin KB. The concept of mesothelioma in situ: implications for diagnosis and histogenesis. *Semin Diagn Pathol* 1992; 9:151–61.

26. Gazdar AF, Lam S, Wistuba II. Molecular and cytologic techniques of early detection. In: Pass HI, Mitchell JB, Johnson DH, et al. (eds) *Lung cancer: principles and practice.* Philadelphia: Lippincott Williams and Wilkins, 2000, pp. 407–24.

27. Wistuba II, Behrens C, Milchgrub S, et al. Sequential molecular abnormalities are involved in the multistage development of squamous cell lung carcinoma. *Oncogene* 1999; 18: 643–50.

28. Zahm SH, Brownson RC, Chang JC, et al. Study of lung cancer histologic types, occupation, and smoking in Missouri. *Am J Ind Med* 1989; 15:565–78.

29. Frost JK, Ball WCJ, Levin ML, et al. Early lung cancer detection: results of the initial (prevalence) radiologic and cytologic screening in the Johns Hopkins study. *Am Rev Respir Dis* 1984; 130:549–54.

30. Flehinger BJ, Melamed MR, Zaman MB, et al. Early lung cancer detection: results of the initial (prevalence) radiologic and cytologic screening in the Memorial Sloan-Kettering study. *Am Rev Respir Dis* 1984; 130:555–60.

31. Fontana RS, Sanderson DR, Taylor WF, et al. Early lung cancer detection: results of the initial (prevalence) radiologic and cytologic screening in the Mayo Clinic study. *Am Rev Respir Dis* 1984; 130:561–5.

32. Ishikawa Y, Nakagawa K, Satoh Y, et al. Characteristics of chromate workers' cancers, chromium lung deposition and precancerous bronchial lesions: an autopsy study. *Br J Cancer* 1994; 70:160–6.

33. Kennedy TC, Proudfoot SP, Franklin WA, et al. Cytopathological analysis of sputum in patients with airflow obstruction and significant smoking histories. *Cancer Res* 1996; 56:4673–8.

34. Lam S, MacAulay C, Hung J, et al. Detection of dysplasia and carcinoma in situ with a lung imaging fluorescence endoscope device. *J Thorac Cardiovasc Surg* 1993; 105:1035–40.

35. Pigula FA, Keenan RJ, Ferson PF, et al. Unsuspected lung cancer found in work-up for lung reduction operation. *Ann Thorac Surg* 1996; 61:174–6.

36. Saccomanno G, Archer VE, Auerbach O, et al. Development of carcinoma of the lung as reflected in exfoliated cells. *Cancer* 1974; 33:256–70.

37. Keith RL, Miller YE, Gemmill RM, et al. Angiogenic squamous dysplasia in bronchi of individuals at high risk for lung cancer. *Clin Cancer Res* 2000; 6:1616–25.

38. Kurie JM, Lee JS, Morice RC, et al. Autofluorescence bronchoscopy in the detection of squamous metaplasia and dysplasia in current and former smokers. *J Natal Cancer Inst* 1998; 90:991–5.

39. Lam S, Kennedy T, Unger M, et al. Localization of bronchial intraepithelial neoplastic lesions by fluorescence bronchoscopy. *Chest* 1998; 113:696–702.

40. Venmans BJ, van Boxem TJ, Smit EF, et al. Outcome of bronchial carcinoma in situ. *Chest* 2000; 117:1572–6.

41. Cortese DA, Pairolero PC, Bergstralh EJ, et al. Roentgenographically occult lung cancer. A ten-year experience. *J Thorac Cardiovasc Surg* 1983; 86:373–80.

42. Melamed MR, Zaman MB, Flehinger BJ, et al. Radiologically occult in situ and incipient invasive epidermoid lung cancer: detection by sputum cytology in a survey of asymptomatic cigarette smokers. *Am J Surg Pathol* 1977; 1:5–16.

43. Pierard P, Vermylen P, Bosschaerts T, et al. Synchronous roentgenographically occult lung carcinoma in patients with resectable primary lung cancer. *Chest* 2000; 117:779–85.

44. Woolner LB, Fontana RS, Cortese DA, et al. Roentgenographically occult lung cancer: pathologic findings and frequency of multicentricity during a 10-year period. *Mayo Clin Proc* 1984; 59:453–66.

45. Fontana RS, Sanderson DR, Woolner LB, et al. Screening for lung cancer. A critique of the Mayo Lung Project. *Cancer* 1991; 67:1155–64.

46. Melamed MR, Flehinger BJ, Zaman MB, et al. Screening for early lung cancer. Results of the Memorial Sloan-Kettering study in New York. *Chest* 1984; 86:44–53.

47. Herbst RS, Khuri FR, Hong WK. Chemoprevention: scientific rationale and clinical studies. In: Pass HI, Mitchell JB, Johnson DH, et al. (eds) *Lung cancer*. Philadelphia: Lippincott Williams and Wilkins, 2000, pp. 438–50.

48. Mathe G, Gouveia J, Hercend T, et al. Correlation between precancerous bronchial metaplasia and cigarette consumption, and preliminary results of retinoid treatment. *Cancer Detect Prev* 1982; 5:461–6.

49. van Poppel G, Kok FJ, Hermus RJ. Beta-carotene supplementation in smokers reduces the frequency of micronuclei in sputum. *Br J Cancer* 1992; 66:1164–8.

50. Heimburger DC, Alexander CB, Birch R, et al. Improvement in bronchial squamous metaplasia in smokers treated with folate and vitamin B12. Report of a preliminary randomized, double-blind intervention trial. *JAMA* 1988; 259:1525–30.

51. Arnold AM, Browman GP, Levine MN, et al. The effect of the synthetic retinoid etretinate on sputum cytology: results from a randomised trial. *Br J Cancer* 1992; 64:737–43.

52. Lee JS, Lippman SM, Benner SE, et al. Randomized placebo-controlled trial of isotretinoin in chemoprevention of bronchial squamous metaplasia. *J Clin Oncol* 1994; 12:937–45.

53. McLarty JW, Holiday DB, Girard WM, et al. Beta-carotene, vitamin A, and lung cancer chemoprevention: results of an intermediate endpoint study. *Am J Clin Nutr* 1995; 62 (Suppl):1431–8.

54. Kurie JM, Lee JS, Khuri FR, et al. N-(4-hydroxyphenyl)retinamide in the chemoprevention of squamous metaplasia and dysplasia of the bronchial epithelium. *Clin Cancer Res* 2000; 6:2973–9.

55. Albanes D, Heinonen OP, Taylor PR, et al. Alpha-tocopherol and beta-carotene supplements and lung cancer incidence in the alpha-tocopherol, beta-carotene cancer prevention study: effects of base-line characteristics and study compliance. *J Natl Cancer Inst* 1996; 88:1560–70.

56. Omenn GS, Goodman GE, Thornquist MD, et al. Risk factors for lung cancer and for intervention effects in CARET, the Beta-Carotene and Retinol Efficacy Trial. *J Natl Cancer Inst* 1996; 88:1550–9.

57. Travis WD, Linder J, Mackay B. Classification, histology, cytology, and elctron miscroscopy. In: Pass HI, Mitchell JB, Johnson DH, et al. (eds) *Lung cancer: principles and practice*. Philadelphia: Lippincott Williams and Wilkins, 2000, pp. 453–95.

58. Carey FA, Wallace WA, Fergusson RJ, et al. Alveolar atypical hyperplasia in association with primary pulmonary adenocarcinoma: a clinicopathological study of 10 cases. *Thorax* 1992; 47:1041–3.

59. Noguchi M, Shimosato Y. The development and progression of adenocarcinoma of the lung. In: Hansen HH (ed) *Lung cancer: advances in basic and clinical research*. Norwell, MA: Kluwer Academic Publishers, 1995, pp. 131–42.

60. Carey FA. Pulmonary adenocarcinoma: classification and molecular biology [editorial]. *J Pathol* 1998; 184:229–30.

61. Kerr KM, Carey FA, King G, et al. Atypical alveolar hyperplasia: relationship with pulmonary adenocarcinoma, *p53*, and *c-erbB-2* expression. *J Pathol* 1994; 174:249–56.

62. Kitaguchi S, Takeshima Y, Nishisaka T, et al. Proliferative activity, *p53* expression and loss of heterozygosity on 3p, 9p and 17p in atypical adenomatous hyperplasia of the lung. *Hiroshima J Med Sci* 1998; 47:17–25.

63. Westra WH, Baas IO, Hruban RH, et al. *K-ras* oncogene activation in atypical alveolar hyperplasias of the human lung. *Cancer Res* 1996; 56:2224–8.

64. Miller RR, Muller NL. Neuroendocrine cell hyperplasia and obliterative bronchiolitis in patients with peripheral carcinoid tumors. *Am J Surg Pathol* 1995; 19:653–8.

65. Kodama T, Nishiyama H, Nishiwaki Y, et al. Histopathological study of adenocarcinoma and hyperplastic epithelial lesions of the lung. *Lung Cancer (Haigan)* 1988; 8:325–33.

66. Morinaga S, Shimosato Y. Pathology of the microadenocarcinoma in the periphery of the lung. *Pathol Clin Med Jpn* 1987; 5:74–80.

67. Niho S, Yokose T, Suzuki K, et al. Monoclonality of atypical adenomatous hyperplasia of the lung. *Am J Pathol* 1999; 154:249–54.

68. Rao SK, Fraire AE. Alveolar cell hyperplasia in association with adenocarcinoma of lung. *Mod Pathol* 1995; 8:165–9.

69. Suzuki K, Ogura T, Yokose T, et al. Loss of heterozygosity in the tuberous sclerosis gene associated regions in adenocarcinoma of the lung accompanied by multiple atypical adenomatous hyperplasia. *Int J Cancer* 1998; 79:384–9.

70. Chapman AD, Kerr KM. The association between atypical adenomatous hyperplasia and primary lung cancer. *Br J Cancer* 2000; 83:632–6.

71. Miller RR. Bronchioloalveolar cell adenomas. *Am J Surg Pathol* 1990; 14:904–12.

72. Nakanishi K. Alveolar epithelial hyperplasia and adenocarcinoma of the lung. *Arch Pathol Lab Med* 1990; 114:363–8.

73. Weng SY, Tsuchiya E, Kasuga T, et al. Incidence of atypical bronchioloalveolar cell hyperplasia of the lung: relation to histological subtypes of lung cancer. *Virchows Arch A Pathol Anat Histopathol* 1992; 420:463–71.

74. Takigawa N, Segawa Y, Nakata M, et al. Clinical investigation of atypical adenomatous hyperplasia of the lung. *Lung Cancer* 1999; 25:115–21.

75. Sterner DJ, Mori M, Roggli VL, et al. Prevalence of pulmonary atypical alveolar cell hyperplasia in an autopsy population: a study of 100 cases. *Mod Pathol* 1997; 10:469–73.

76. Yokose T, Ito Y, Ochiai A. High prevalence of atypical adenomatous hyperplasia of the lung in autopsy specimens from elderly patients with malignant neoplasms. *Lung Cancer* 2000; 29: 125–30.

77. Kaneko M, Kusumoto M, Kobayashi T, et al. Computed tomography screening for lung carcinoma in Japan. *Cancer* 2000; 89:2485–8.

78. Sone S, Takashima S, Li F, et al. Mass screening of lung cancer with mobile spiral computed tomography scanner. *Lancet* 1998; 351:1242–5.

79. Aguayo SM, Miller YE, Waldron JAJ, et al. Brief report: idiopathic diffuse hyperplasia of pulmonary neuroendocrine cells and airways disease. *N Engl J Med* 1992; 327:1285–8.

80. Armas OA, White DA, Erlandson RA, et al. Diffuse idiopathic pulmonary neuroendocrine cell proliferation presenting as interstitial lung disease. *Am J Surg Pathol* 1995; 19:963–70.

81. Brown MJ, English J, Muller NL. Bronchiolitis obliterans due to neuroendocrine hyperplasia: high-resolution CT—pathologic correlation. *Am J Roentgenol* 1997; 168:1561–2.

82. Cohen AJ, King TEJ, Gilman LB, et al. High expression of neutral endopeptidase in idiopathic diffuse hyperplasia of pulmonary neuroendocrine cells. *Am J Respir Crit Care Med* 1998; 158:1593–9.

83. Sheerin N, Harrison NK, Sheppard MN, et al. Obliterative bronchiolitis caused by multiple tumourlets and microcarcinoids successfully treated by single lung transplantation. *Thorax* 1995; 50:207–9.

84. Anonymous. Case records of the Massachusetts General Hospital. Weekly clinicopathological exercises. Case 50—1978. *N Engl J Med* 1978; 299:1402–8.

85. Churg A, Warnock ML. Pulmonary tumorlet. A form of peripheral carcinoid. *Cancer* 1976; 37:1469–77.

86. Miller MA, Mark GJ, Kanarek D. Multiple peripheral pulmonary carcinoids and tumorlets of carcinoid type, with restrictive and obstructive lung disease. *Am J Med* 1978; 65:373–8.

87. Ranchod M. The histogenesis and development of pulmonary tumorlets. *Cancer* 1977; 39: 1135–45.

88. Ranchod M, Levine GD. Spindle-cell carcinoid tumors of the lung: a clinicopathologic study of 35 cases. *Am J Surg Pathol* 1980; 4:315–31.

89. Salyer DC, Salyer WR, Eggleston JC. Bronchial carcinoid tumors. *Cancer* 1975; 36:1522–37.

90. Jessurun J, Manivel JC, Simpson R. Idiopathic diffuse hyperplasia of pulmonary neuroendocrine cells (IDHPNC): a consequence of diffuse bronchiolitis. *Lab Invest* 1994; 706:151a.

91. Cury PM, Butcher DN, Corrin B, et al. The use of histological and immunohistochemical markers to distinguish pleural malignant mesothelioma and in situ mesothelioma from reactive mesothelial hyperplasia and reactive pleural fibrosis. *J Pathol* 1999; 189:251–7.

14
Skin

Richard P. Gallagher and Tim K. Lee

Incidence rates for all types of skin cancer, cutaneous malignant melanoma (CMM), squamous cell carcinoma (SCC), and basal cell carcinoma (BCC) increased markedly in the last half of the twentieth century in white populations throughout the world [1–4], although mortality has recently fallen [5], at least for melanoma in younger age groups. Skin cancer is now a major public health problem in Western countries, with increasing resources being devoted to treatment and prevention programs.

Over the past 20 years, a great deal has been learned about risk factors for skin cancers, and in general, the factors fall into three categories. The first category consists of host susceptibility factors and includes light skin and hair color and sun-sensitivity [6–11]. The most important of the environmental factors (the second category) is ultraviolet (UV) radiation, whether from solar or artificial sources [9,12–15]. UV radiation is causally related to all types of skin cancer. The third group of factors include freckling and nevi; these appear to be related both to host susceptibility and sunlight [6–11].

Much of the data on the relationship between UV radiation and CMM, the most dangerous form of skin cancer, has indicated a long lag period between the relevant solar exposure and appearance of a frank malignancy. In fact the strongest associations between solar UV and melanoma, appear to occur for childhood [16–17] and early life exposure [18].

Similarly, data on age at diagnosis of squamous cell carcinoma indicate that a great deal of accumulated exposure was necessary for the appearance of SCC. Recent case-control studies have proved this assumption correct [19]. This late appearance of frank malignancy, coupled with the need to devise appropriate prevention recommendations, has generated an interest in the study of precursor lesions for skin cancers, particularly acquired melanocytic nevi and actinic keratoses.

Melanocytic Nevi

Clinical Definition of Nevi, and Descriptive Data

Melanocytic nevi are benign neoplasms of the skin, arising as clusters of melanocytes. The initial studies of nevi by Pack et al. [20–21] mentioned no clear clinical criteria by which nevi were enumerated, and none were evaluated pathologically. Because of the potential difficulties in determining whether pigmented lesions are, in fact, nevi, investigators began to elaborate clinical criteria to make counts more reliable or repeatable.

Nicholls [22], in the first cross-sectional study representative of a population (Australian), counted only pigmented lesions greater than 2 mm in diameter and "either palpable or seen to deform the surface architecture of the skin when viewed tangentially". The intent was to minimize the probability of including freckles, and perhaps some solar keratoses. Of course the criteria would probably also have excluded some legitimate macular nevi.

The International Agency for Research on Cancer (IARC) has developed a detailed protocol in an attempt to standardize methods for counting nevi [23], and this protocol is now commonly used in studies. Countable lesions are defined as "brown to black pigmented macules or papules which are reasonably well defined and are darker in colour than the surrounding skin". Use of standard methods should make counts across studies more comparable. Within studies, up to 10% of variation in full body counts may be attributable to interobserver variation if more than one counter is used, even with standardized methods.

Notwithstanding these problems, a great deal has been learned about risk factors for nevi. The earliest studies of nevi indicated greater densites in whites with very fair and "light brown" skin than in with whites with darker skin or in blacks [20]. Nevi were also more common on sun-exposed sites than on sites not exposed [21].

Nicholls [22] showed that nevus density increases with age in both males and females, and that sun-exposed sites reach their peak nevus counts at a younger age than sites which are not commonly exposed. Further, males appear to develop more nevi than females, perhaps because they spend more time in the sun than females. Nicholls also observed that nevus counts drop in individuals above age 40.

Although some 1 to 2% of the population are born with one or more nevi (congenital nevi), most melanocytic nevi develop after birth [24]. Acquired melanocytic nevi begin to become clinically apparent in the first year or two of life [25]. Nevus density appears to peak in teenage years [26–27]. As noted above, cross-sectional data suggest that nevus density decreases with age [26–27], however because no true longitudinal studies have been conducted, it is impossible to say with certainty that this phenomenon is not due to more recent cohorts having more nevi due to sun exposure.

Nevi as Risk Markers for Melanoma

Nevus density is the strongest predictor of melanoma risk, whether the variable is measured using nevus counts on the arm [6,28] or whole-body counts [29]. Furthermore, about 50% of melanomas have traces of pre-existing nevi on pathologic examination [30], indicating that the malignancies arose from the nevi. The different anatomic site distribution of nevi and melanomas, however, also suggests that a proportion of melanomas arise *de novo* [31].

Risk Factors for Nevi in Adults

Analytic studies of nevi among adults have been conducted to try to evaluate factors associated with high nevus density. The investigation of Armstrong et al. [32] analyzed data from control subjects collected during an investigation of melanoma, and demonstrated higher palpable nevus counts among those with intermediate skin color, southern European grandparents, and sunburns up to age 10. The latter factor, however, was confounded by the number of sunburns in the 10 years prior to the study. Presence of palpable nevi on the forearms appeared also to be associated with increased alcohol intake and with increased retinol intake, although no other studies have attempted to replicate these dietary findings.

Augustsson et al. [33] analyzed site distribution of nevi among 310 adult subjects of ages 30 to 50 and found higher nevus density on sites which are intermittently exposed to sunlight. This study also yielded higher counts on subjects with a history of sunburn, although the difference was not statistically significant. An American investigation [34] showed similar findings for sunburn history and also demonstrated a higher nevus density in sun-sensitive subjects. As nevi arise mainly during the first 2 decades of life, the major potential difficulty with studies of nevi among adults is that it is not clear that the outcome measure, nevi, occurs after the exposures in question.

Risk Factors for Nevi in Children

More recently, a series of analytic cross-sectional studies conducted predominantly among white children has dramatically increased our knowledge of risk factors for nevi (Table 14.1.). Rampen et al. [35] examined 116 children, of ages 6 to 9, as well as 133 students, of ages 18

TABLE 14.1. Studies of acquired melanocytic nevi in children to age 18.

Reference	Study location/date	No. of subjects	Trends in nevus prevalence with:					
			Light versus dark skin color	Light versus dark hair color	Sun sensitivity/ propensity to burn	Freckling	Sunburns	Increasing solar exposure
Rampen, et al. [35]	Netherlands, 1985	116	↑		↑			
Sigg & Pelloni [36]	Switzerland	939	↑			↑		
Green, et al. [37]	Australia, 1986	211	↑	↑	↑		↑	↑
Sorahan, et al. [38]	UK	187	↑		No assoc.			
Gallagher, et al. [39,40]	Canada, 1987	1,146	↑	No assoc.	↑	↑	↑	No assoc.
Pope, et al. [41]	UK	1,953 white children	↑	→	↑	↑	↑	↑
Coombs, et al. [42]	New Zealand, 1987	349	↑	No assoc.	↑	↑	No assoc.	↑
English & Armstrong [44]	Australia, 1985	2,376	↑	Irregular[1]	Irregular[2]	Irregular[2]		
Kelly, et al. [45]	Australia	1,123	↑		↑	↑		↑
Harrison, et al. [25]	Australia	506	↑	Irregular[1]	↑	↑	↑	↑
Green, et al. [47]	Australia, 1990–1993	102	↑	↑	↑	↑		
Luther, et al. [48]	Germany, 1988–1993	357	↑	Irregular[1]	↑	↑	↑	↑

[1] Irregular: higher counts in subjects with blonde and light brown hair than in black hair; low counts in red heads.
[2] Highest counts in intermediate sun sensitivity and intermediate levels of freckling.

to 30. Nevi were more frequent in males and increased with increasing age. Nevus density was higher in subjects who were sun sensitive.

Sigg and Pelloni [36] examined 939 Swiss schoolchildren of ages 6 to 16, and again noted higher counts in boys, as well as in subjects with fair skin. They also noted higher nevus counts in children with freckles.

Green and colleagues [37], in a study of 211 Australian children of ages 7 to 11, found that light skin, hair, and eye color and sun sensitivity were associated with elevated nevus counts. Boys had higher counts than girls of the same age, and a history of melanoma in a first or second degree relative was also associated with elevated counts. Finally, children with higher nevus counts also reported more sun exposure. Sorahan et al. [38] examined 187 British children of ages 8 and 9 and also found higher counts in those with light skin color and a family history of cancer, although no association with sun sensitivity was detected.

Gallagher et al. [39] evaluated nevus density in 913 Canadian school children 6 to 18 years of age and found that nevus density increased with age, was higher in boys than girls of the same age, and was elevated on intermittently sun-exposed sites compared to minimally or maximally sun-exposed sites. Higher nevus density was seen in those with sun-sensitive skin, those who freckled easily, and those with a history of severe or frequent sunburn [40].

Pope et al. [41] examined 2,140 English children and reported increased nevus prevalence with sun sensitivity, a history of sunburn, a tendency to freckle, and increased sun exposure.

Coombs et al. [42], in New Zealand, found higher nevus counts in male students, ages 14 to 15, than in female students, and an increased nevus prevalence in those who reported sunbathing relative to those who did not engage in this activity.

The first major investigation of nevi in a Mediterranean population was conducted by Richard et al. [43] among male students of ages 17 to 24. Although Richard's subjects were older than those in previous studies, his results are included here because of the unique population examined. Nevus counts were higher on sun-exposed sites. The density of small nevi (those ≤ 2mm) was highest on constantly sun-exposed sites, but the density of large nevi (≤ 5 mm) was highest on intermittently exposed sites. The authors also noted that the density of large nevi was highest on subjects reporting sun-sensitivity and high levels of beach-related high-sun-exposure activities.

Two studies of Australian school children and one of preschool children were reported in 1994. English and Armstrong [44] found higher counts in boys of ages 5 to 14 than in girls of the same age. Children with red hair had few nevi, but those with fair skin had generally higher counts than those with darker skin. Numbers of nevi were positively associated with the degree of freckling until freckling became moderate to heavy, after which, nevi decreased.

Kelly and colleagues [45] showed a relationship between latitude of residence (in Australia) and nevus counts in children age 6, 9, 12, and 15; this relationship persisted after adjustment for phenotype factors. Those children who lived closer to the equator had higher counts, suggesting a relationship between nevus density and sun exposure in childhood.

Harrison et al. [25] examined 506 Australian children of ages 1 to 6 and found that nevus prevalence increased with age. Counts were higher in children with light skin, freckles, and a history of sunburn. Very high counts (upper quartile) were associated with elevated sun exposure.

Green et al. [46] examined a group of adolescents of ages 11 to 12 in 1990 and demonstrated higher nevus counts in those with light eye and skin color, and sun sensitivity. A relationship with freckling similar to that shown by English and Armstrong [44] was seen, that is, an increase in nevi in children with moderate freckling compared with children with no freckling, followed by a decrease in nevus prevalence in very heavily freckled subjects. A reduced nevus count was seen in children with red hair, compared to those with blond, brown, or black hair.

Green et al. [47] followed 102 Australian school children of ages 11 to 13 for a period of 3 years to determine factors contributing to new nevi. Increases were greatest for those with blonde or red hair, sun sensitivity, and heavy facial freckling.

A German study of factors related to nevi in children examined at age 7 and again at age 12 indicated that the largest increases tended to be seen in sun-sensitive, freckled children who had had intense sun exposure [48].

In summary, the available data show a strong similarity in host susceptibility factors among subjects at risk for high nevus density in childhood and those at risk for melanoma as adults. These include light skin, light hair, and sun sensitivity. Factors indicative of both host susceptibility and heavy solar exposure, such as freckling and sunburn history, also show a relationship with both nevi and melanoma. Finally, the major environmental factor implicated in risk of melanoma, sunlight exposure, particularly in childhood also appears to be key in generating high nevus counts.

To date, no long-term cohort studies of subjects with nevi have been undertaken to observe directly whether those with high nevus density as children have elevated risk of melanoma as adults. Because sunlight plays an important role in childhood nevus density and in melanoma risk among adults, nevi assume increasing importance as an intermediate endpoint in programs to prevent malignant melanoma.

Prevention

As nevi are known to be precursors of at least some melanomas, prevention or attenuation of new nevi has been explored in several recent studies. These primarily are designed to evaluate whether sunscreens might prevent the development of nevi in children, and by extension, reduce later risk of melanoma. The previously noted study of Luther et al. [48] enumerated nevi in 866 children prior to age 7 and then re-examined a subset of 357 of the same children 5 years later, retrospectively collecting information on host factors, sun exposure, and sunscreen use. On univariate analysis, children who used sunscreen regularly developed significantly more new nevi than those who did not use sunscreen. However, after

adjustment for other variables, including host susceptibility and sunlight exposure, this relationship was no longer significant.

A cross-sectional study by Autier et al. [49] of nevi among European children indicated that sunscreen use does not protect children against development of nevi, although use of protective clothing is effective. In both the German [48] and the European study, a potential explanation for the higher nevus counts in sunscreen users is found in further data collected by Autier et al. [50]. In this randomized trial, subjects going on vacation were randomized to receive either SPF-10 or SPF-30 sunscreens. The products were identical in appearance and were identically packaged. Subjects kept diaries of sun exposure, and at the end of the vacation, those using high SPF sunscreen had spent more time in the sun. The results indicate that the use of high-potency sunscreens may encourage greater solar exposure than would be the case if low-potency sunscreens or no sunscreen at all were utilized.

Only one randomized trial of sunscreen use and nevi has been reported to date [51]. This study followed 309 white children, ages 6 to 7 and 9 to 10 at enrollment, who had their nevi counted and host susceptibility factors assessed. The children were then randomized to receive (through their parents) SPF-30 sunscreen or to receive no sunscreen (ambient use only). Parents of children in the sunscreen group were instructed to apply the sunscreen anytime the child was expected to be in the sun for 30 minutes or more. Parents of children randomized to receiving no sunscreen were given no instructions. After close follow-up for a 3-year period, nevi were counted again. Children in the sunscreen group developed fewer new nevi than those in the no-sunscreen group. The difference was most pronounced among children who freckled. The data showed overall sunlight exposure to be similar in the two study groups, although the proportion of episodes in which exposed body sites were not protected by sunscreen was higher in the no-sunscreen group.

The major advantage of a randomized trial of sunscreens and nevi, compared with a cross-sectional retrospective study, is that uncontrolled confounding due to sun sensitivity and other host susceptibility factors is minimized. In addition, during the time of follow-up, a more accurate estimate of solar exposure is possible than would be the case in a retrospective study. Finally, quantitative data can be obtained (from the sunscreen group at least) on sunscreen use during the trial.

While this study requires replication, the results indicate that sunscreens may be active in attenuating the precursor lesion for a substantial proportion of melanomas.

Atypical or Dysplastic Nevi

Reports of an association between nevi with atypical clinical appearance and melanoma risk date back over a century [52], but it was not until 1978 that the terms *B-K mole syndrome* [53] and *familial atypical multiple mole–melanoma syndrome* [54] were applied to the clinical picture seen in patients with these nevi. The studies establishing these terms outlined the elevated risk of melanoma in patients with multiple atypical nevi among sets of families which had markedly elevated risk for melanoma. Familial melanoma associated with heritable atypical or dysplastic nevi is rare, however, and probably accounts for fewer than 5% of melanomas in North America. However, for some members of the families with this condition, melanoma risk can be very high, 56% between the ages of 20 and 59 [55], approaching 100% over a lifetime.

Families with atypical nevus syndrome are usually recognized clinically when a family member presents with a dermatological complaint and they are placed under surveillance. Recently mutations have been found in the *CDKN2A* gene on the short arm of chromosome 9 (9p21). This tumour suppressor gene, which regulates cell cycling, is thought to account for much of the cutaneous melanoma in high-risk families [56].

Atypical or dysplastic nevi are present, however, not only in members of families with heritable elevated risk of melanoma [57], but also in cases of sporadic melanoma [28,58]. In a very well-conducted study of 716 melanoma cases and 1,014 age- and sex-matched controls,

a total of 104 (10.3%) of the controls had at least one clinically dysplastic nevus, and 285 (43.3%) had one [59]. The nevi were defined as dysplastic if they were 5mm or more in diameter, had a flat component, and satisfied two or more of the following criteria: variable pigmentation, irregular asymmetric outline, and indistinct borders. The presence of one clinically dysplastic nevus was associated with a relative risk for melanoma of 2.3 (95% CI: 1.4–3.6), and the presence of 10 or more with a relative risk of 12 (95% CI: 4.4–31). This elevated risk is substantially greater than that seen for banal nevi, where the presence of 25 to 49 nevi conferred a relative risk of 1.8 (95% CI: 1.3–2.5), and the presence of 100 or more nevi conferred a relative risk of 3.4 (95% CI: 2.0–5.7), by comparison with subjects with fewer than 25. A continuing challenge to the concept of the dysplastic nevus as a risk factor for melanoma, however, is the difficulty in agreeing on criteria for clinical diagnosis. In the study of Tucker et al. [59], 10.9% of cases and 12.6% of the controls had one or more "indeterminate" lesions. A melanocytic lesion was considered "indeterminate" when examiners could not agree on whether it was atypical or not. Agreement on diagnostic criteria has been problematic for pathologic definition of dysplastic nevi as well.

A recent study evaluated risk factors for the presence of one or more clinically atypical nevi in a Swedish female population [60]. The study found that the risk of having an atypical nevus increased with the number of banal nevi, with a relative risk of 26.0 (95% CI: 11.4–59.6) in subjects with 100 or more such nevi. For subjects with fewer than 50 banal nevi, risk factors for having an atypical nevus also included the presence of freckling and a history of beach vacations between the ages of 10 and 19. In women with 50 or more banal nevi, inability to tan appeared to be associated with an increased risk of atypical nevi, but this did not reach statistical significance.

While the dysplastic or clinically atypical nevus is certainly a risk factor for malignant melanoma, it is of limited use as a research or screening tool simply because it is hard to recognize without special training. The presence of greater than 100 normal nevi is likely to be more useful in detecting those at high risk of melanoma, at least on a screening basis.

Actinic Keratoses

Actinic or solar keratoses (AK) are dysplastic premalignant lesions of the epidermis, which are thought to be precursors of squamous cell carcinoma [61,62]. Relatively few detailed studies of AK have been conducted specifically to evaluate these lesions. Most have been run as adjuncts to studies of nonmelanocytic skin cancer, particularly SCC.

Descriptive Data

Prevalence of AKs is very high in individuals among white populations exposed to strong sunlight. They are more common in subjects with fair skin, those who are sun sensitive, and those with a history of childhood sunburn [63]. In an Australian study, 1,040 men and women, age 40 and greater, had sunlight-exposed body sites examined by either a dermatologist or dermatologic trainee, and 59.2% had one or more AK [61]. Other studies in tropical areas [64] have found slightly lower prevalence rates (43%). However, even in areas of low sunlight such as the UK, the solar keratosis prevalence rate among subjects over age 60 was shown to be at least 23% [65]. Prevalence rates are higher in males than in females [61,64,65].

Sunlight Exposure and Actinic Keratoses

Prevalence of AKs is strongly related to sunlight exposure. The rate has been shown to be higher in outdoor workers in Maryborough, Australia, a town of high UV exposure, than in outdoor workers in Melbourne, which has lower ambient UV values [66].

Skin damage due to solar exposure, as measured by cutaneous microtopography, is also related to AK; an increasing risk of AKs is seen with increasing sun damage [67]. Reported occupational sun exposure appears to have a stronger association with AK prevalence than

childhood or intermittent recreational sunlight, suggesting that chronic accumulated solar exposure is more important in accounting for AKs [64]. To date, the most quantitative study assessing the relationship between AKs and sunlight was conducted on a group of traditional fishermen called the Maryland watermen. A sun exposure history was taken from the seamen, and a skin examination which enumerated skin cancers and actinic keratoses [68,69], was performed by a dermatologist. Men whose average annual solar exposure was greater than the median had a 50% greater chance of having one or more AKs than those whose solar exposure was below the median.

Squamous cell carcinoma risk is elevated among those with immune compromise and especially among transplant patients [70]. A study aimed at finding whether there is an increase in AKs in renal transplant patients [71] is difficult to interpret because no actual overall prevalence figures are given, and no comparison is made with a nontransplant population.

AK as a Risk Marker for Skin Cancers

The presence of actinic keratoses on the skin is an indicator of elevated risk for both basal cell carcinoma and squamous cell carcinoma of the skin. Marks et al. [72] examined the head and neck, forearms and hands of 6,416 Australian subjects, age 40 and over, for the presence of AKs, BCCs, and SCCs. The presence of AKs was associated with increased risks of both types of nonmelanocytic skin cancer.

A case-control study conducted in a cohort of Australian subjects of ages 40 to 64 found a relative risk of BCC of 10.4 among subjects with 40 or more solar keratoses [8], and a relative risk of 34.3 for SCC. A similar relationship between solar keratoses and BCC has also been reported in a Mediterranean population; the presence of one or more AKs puts subjects at a 2.8-fold risk of the disease compared to those without evidence of these lesions [73].

A further study has examined the potential for actinic keratoses to act as a risk marker for melanoma [74]. The investigation, conducted on 258 cases and 281 controls, found a 5.5 fold increased risk for melanoma in subjects with 10 or more AKs on the left forearm, after controlling for age, sex, and hair color. This study also indicated that the presence of both a large number of nevi and many AKs was associated with a melanoma risk greater than that seen in the presence of only one of these factors. It is of interest, however, to note that these investigators did not, in general, find the presence of AKs to be correlated with high nevus density. Probably, this is because AKs increase with age, while nevi appear to decline with age after the fourth decade. Other investigations have also indicated that the presence of AKs may indicate increased risk of melanoma [75,76].

Prevention

Despite evidence of their association, the rate of transformation of AKs to SCCs is very low, and there is good evidence that many AKs appear to regress spontaneously, particularly in the absence of sun exposure [61]. Most research to date has focused on the use of sun avoidance and daily sunscreen use as means of attenuating new lesions and causing regression of existing AKs.

Two randomized trials and one cross-sectional study have been conducted to evaluate the use of sunscreens in reducing actinic keratoses. Thompson et al. [77] conducted a randomized trial to evaluate daily application of broad-spectrum high-SPF sunscreen on the head and neck, forearms, and hands as a means to prevent new AKs on these sites. Subjects were 588 individuals, age 40 or over, with 1 to 30 existing AKs. The subjects were randomized to either daily sunscreen use or daily use of the base cream without active ingredients. Subjects were followed from September, 1991, to March, 1992, and 431 completed the trial. At the end of the trial, subjects in the sunscreen group had fewer new AKs and more remissions of prevalent AKs than those in the group receiving the cream base.

Naylor et al. [78] conducted a randomized trial in Lubbock, Texas, to evaluate broad-spectrum sunscreens as chemopreventive agents against AKs. Fifty-three subjects with prior evidence of AKs or a nonmelanocytic skin

cancer were enrolled in the trial. All prevalent nonmelanocytic skin cancers were surgically removed, and all AKs were removed with liquid nitrogen. Subjects were then randomized to receive SPF-29 sunscreen or the cream base without active ingredients. Subjects were instructed to apply sunscreen to all sun-exposed parts of the body, and to avoid over-exposure to the sun. Individuals were followed at 1 month, 3 months, and every 3 months afterward, for a total of 2 years. At follow-up sessions, lesions identified as AKs were removed with liquid nitrogen, and all suspected malignancies were biopsied and removed surgically. At the end of the study, all AKs clinically diagnosed on sun-exposed areas and removed during the course of the study were aggregated, and comparisons were made between the two groups. The results showed that a significantly lower mean number of AKs developed annually in the sunscreen arm of the study in comparison with the nonsunscreen arm (13.6 versus 27.9). The analysis also revealed, however, an imbalance in risk factors between the two groups, and after adjustment, the authors concluded that use of the sunscreen accounted for a 36% reduction in new nevi in the sunscreen group.

Harvey et al. (1996) [65] conducted a cross-sectional study of AKs among a random sample of 560 males and females, age 60 and over, living in South Glamorgan, UK. Subjects were seen in their homes, and 137 confirmed AKs were recorded and photographed by the study registrar. On univariate analysis, subjects who used no sunscreen had an elevated risk (RR = 1.8; 95% CI: 1.2–2.9). However, the relationship between sunscreen use and AK prevalence was confounded by age. Those subjects who were oldest were also least likely to use sunscreen and were most likely to have an AK. Thus the study was uninformative about whether sunscreens protect against AKs.

Freckles and Lentigos

Freckles are increased areas of melanin pigmentation thought to be a result of functionally overactive melanocytes [79,80]. They occur on areas which are heavily sun-exposed, such as the face and forearms and sometimes the shoulders, and are most pronounced in the summer. They fade markedly in the winter, when UV exposure is low. Histologically, these overactive melanocytes are no different from melanocytes in individuals without freckling.

Lentigos are similar to freckles, but on histologic examination the lesions appear to contain an increased concentration of melanocytes, although no proliferation takes place. Clinically, they tend to fade less in the winter months than do freckles.

Subjects with a substantial degree of freckling are at higher risk of cutaneous melanoma than those without freckles [7,28,81]. Freckles and nevi appear to increase risk for melanoma in an additive way, suggesting that they may be independent risk factors for the disease [28].

Freckles are clearly a risk factor for melanoma, and perhaps, for other skin cancers, but they cannot be considered precursor lesions for skin cancers as there is no evidence that skin cancers arise from these lesions.

Conclusions

The study of precursor lesions has provided a great deal of information on the factors which eventually increase risk of skin cancer. Prevention studies suggest that precursor lesions, such as actinic keratoses and melanocytic nevi, can be utilized as endpoints in chemoprevention trials aimed at evaluating the usefulness of sunscreens in the prevention of squamous cell carcinoma and perhaps cutaneous malignant melanoma. These lesions are also apt to be ideal intermediate endpoints for use in community trials which seek to alter susceptible childrens' outdoor behavior. More use will be made of them as we move toward prevention rather than treatment of cancer.

References

1. Horn-Ross PL, Holly EA, Brown SR, et al. Temporal trends of cutaneous malignant melanoma among Caucasians in the San Francisco–Oakland SMSA. *Cancer Causes Control* 1991; 2:299–305.

2. Gallagher RP, Ma B, McLean DI, et al. Trends in basal cell carcinoma, squamous cell carcinoma, and melanoma of the skin, from 1973 through 1987. *J Am Acad Dermatol* 1990; 23:413–21.

3. MacLennan R, Green A, McLeod GRC, et al. Increasing incidence of cutaneous melanoma in Queensland Australia. *J Natl Cancer Inst* 1992; 84:1427–32.

4. Kaldor J, Shugg D, Young B, et al. Non-melanoma skin cancer: ten years of cancer registry based surveillance. *Int J Cancer* 1993; 53:886–91.

5. LaVecchia C, Lucchini F, Negri E, et al. Recent declines in worldwide mortality from cutaneous melanoma in youth and middle age. *Int J Cancer* 1999; 81:62–6.

6. Holman CDJ, Armstrong BK. Pigmentary traits, ethnic origin, benign nevi, and family history as risk factors for cutaneous malignant melanoma. *J Natl Cancer Inst* 1984; 72:257–66.

7. Elwood JM, Gallagher RP, Hill GB, et al. Pigmentation and skin reaction to sun as risk factors for cutaneous melanoma: the Western Canada melanoma study. *Brit Med J* 1984; 288:99–102.

8. Kricker A, Armstrong BK, English DR, et al. Pigmentary and cutaneous risk factors for non-melanocytic skin cancer—a case-control study. *Int J Cancer* 1991; 48:650–62.

9. Gallagher RP, Hill GB, Bajdik CD, et al. Sunlight exposure, pigmentary factors, and risk of non-melanocytic skin cancer. I. Basal cell carcinoma. *Arch Dermatol* 1995; 131:157–63.

10. Gallagher RP, Hill GB, Bajdik CD, et al. Sunlight exposure, pigmentation factors, and risk of nonmelanocytic skin cancer. II. Squamous cell carcinoma. *Arch Dermatol* 1995; 131:164–9.

11. Zanetti R, Rosso S, Martinez C, et al. The multicentre south European study "Helios" I: skin characteristics and sunburns in basal cell and squamous cell carcinoma of the skin. *Br J Cancer* 1996; 73:1440–6.

12. Van Dam RM, Huang Z, Rimm E, et al. Risk factors for basal cell carcinoma of the skin in men: results from the Health Professionals Follow-up Study. *Am J Epidemiol* 1999; 150: 459–68.

13. Elwood JM, Jopson J. Melanoma and sun exposure: an overview of published studies. *Int J Cancer* 1997; 73:198–203.

14. English DR, Armstrong BK, Kricker A, et al. Case-control study of sun exposure and squamous cell carcinoma of the skin. *Int J Cancer* 1998; 77:347–53.

15. Kricker A, Armstrong BK, English DR, et al. Does intermittent sun exposure cause basal cell carcinoma? A case-control study. *Int J Cancer* 1995; 60:489–94.

16. Holman CDJ, Armstrong BK. Cutaneous malignant melanoma and indicators of total accumulated exposure to the sun: an analysis separating histogenetic types. *J Natl Cancer Inst* 1984; 73:75–82.

17. Khlat M, Vail A, Parkin M, et al. Mortality from melanoma in migrants to Australia by age at arrival and duration of stay. *Am J Epidemiol* 1992; 135:1103–13.

18. Mack TM, Floderus B. Malignant melanoma risk by nativity, place of residence at diagnosis, and age at migration. *Cancer Causes Control* 1991; 2:401–11.

19. Rosso S, Zanetti R, Martinez C, et al. The multi-centre south European study "Helios" II: different sun exposure patterns in the aetiology of basal cell and squamous cell carcinoma of the skin. *Br J Cancer* 1996; 73:1447–54.

20. Pack GT, Davis J. The relation of race and complexion to the incidence of moles and melanomas. *Ann NY Acad Sci* 1963; 100:719–42.

21. Pack GT, Lenson N, Gerber DM. Regional distribution of moles and melanomas. *Arch Surg* 1952; 65:862–70.

22. Nicholls EM. Development and elimination of pigmented moles, and the anatomical distribution of primary malignant melanoma. *Cancer* 1973; 32:191–5.

23. English DR, MacLennan R, Rivers JK, et al. *Epidemiological studies of melanocytic naevi: protocol for identifying and recording naevi. IARC Internal Report No. 90/002.* Lyon: International Agency for Research on Cancer, 1990; 1–22.

24. Rivers JK, Frederiksen PC, Dibdin C. A prevalence survey of dermatoses in the Australian neonate. *J Am Acad Dermatol* 1990; 23:77–81.

25. Harrison SL, MacLennan R, Speare R, et al. Sun exposure and melanocytic naevi in young Australian children. *Lancet* 1994; 344:1529–32.

26. Cooke KR, Spears GF, Skegg DC. Frequency of moles in a defined population. *J Epidemiol Community Health* 1985; 39:48–52.

27. MacKie RM, English J, Aitchison TC, et al. The number and distribution of benign pigmented moles in an English population. *Br J Dermatol* 1985; 113:167–74.

28. Osterlind A, Tucker MA, Hou-Jensen K, et al. The Danish case-control study of cutaneous malignant melanoma. I. Importance of host factors. *Int J Cancer* 1988; 42:200–6.

29. Holly EA, Kelly JW, Shpall SN, et al. Number of melanocytic nevi as a major risk factor for malignant melanoma. *J Am Acad Dermatol* 1987; 17:459–68.

30. Skendar-Kalenas TM, English DR, Heenan PJ. Benign melanocytic lesions: risk markers or precursors of malignant melanoma? *J Am Acad Dermatol* 1995; 33:1000–7.

31. Weinstock MA, Colditz GA, Willett WC, et al. Moles and site-specific risk of cutaneous malignant melanoma in women. *J Natl Cancer Inst* 1989; 81:948–52.

32. Armstrong BK, deKlerk NH, Holman CDJ. Etiology of common acquired melanocytic nevi: constitutional variables, sun exposure and diet. *J Natl Cancer Inst* 1986; 77:329–35.

33. Augustsson A, Stierner U, Rosdahl I, et al. Regional distribution of melanocytic naevi in relation to sun exposure and site-specific counts predicting total number of naevi. *Acta Derm Venereol* 1992; 72:123–7.

34. Dennis LK, White E, Lee JAH, et al. Constitutional factors and sun exposure in relation to nevi: a population based, cross-sectional study. *Am J Epidemiol* 1996; 143:248–56.

35. Rampen F, ven den Meeren H, Boezeman J. Frequency of moles as a key to melanoma incidence? *J Am Acad Dermatol* 1986; 15:1200–3.

36. Sigg C, Pelloni F. Frequency of acquired melanonevocytic nevi and their relationship to skin complexion in 939 schoolchildren. *Dermatologica* 1989; 179:123–8.

37. Green A, Siskind V, Hansen ME, et al. Melanocytic nevi in school children in Queensland. *J Am Acad Dermatol* 1989; 20:1054–60.

38. Sorahan T, Ball P, Grimley R, et al. Benign pigmented nevi in children from Kidderminster, England: prevalence and associated factors. *J Am Acad Dermatol* 1990; 22:747–50.

39. Gallagher RP, McLean DI, Yang CP, et al. Anatomic distribution of acquired melanocytic nevi in white school children. *Arch Dermatol* 1990; 126:466–71.

40. Gallagher RP, McLean DI, Yang CP, et al. Suntan, sunburn, and pigmentation factors and the frequency of acquired melanocytic nevi in children. *Arch Dermatol* 1990; 126:770–6.

41. Pope DJ, Sorahan T, Marsden JR, et al. Benign pigmented nevi in children. *Arch Dermatol* 1992; 128:1201–6.

42. Coombs BD, Sharples KJ, Cooke KR, et al. Variation and covariates of the number of benign nevi in adolescents. *Am J Epidemiol* 1992; 136:344–55.

43. Richard MA, Grob JJ, Gouvernet J, et al. Role of sun exposure on nevus; first study in age-sex phenotype-controlled populations. *Arch Dermatol* 1993; 129:1280–5.

44. English DR, Armstrong BK. Melanocytic nevi in children. I. Anatomic sites and demographic and host factors. *Am J Epidemiol* 1994; 139:390–401.

45. Kelly JW, Rivers JK, MacLennan R, et al. Sunlight: a major factor associated with the development of nevocytic nevi in Australian schoolchildren. *J Am Acad Dermatol* 1994; 30:40–8.

46. Green A, Siskind V, Hansen M-E, et al. Melanocytic nevi in schoolchildren in Queensland. *J Am Acad Dermatol* 1989; 20:1054–60.

47. Green A, Siskind V, Green L. The incidence of melanocytic naevi in adolescent children in Queensland Australia. *Melanoma Res* 1995; 5:155–60.

48. Luther H, Altmeyer P, Garbe K, et al. Increase of melanocytic nevus counts in children during 5 years of follow-up and analysis of associated factors. *Arch Dermatol* 1996; 132:1473–8.

49. Autier P, Dore J-F, Cattaruzza MS, et al. Sunscreen use, wearing clothes, and nevi in 6 and 7 year old European children. *J Natl Cancer Inst* 1998; 90:1873–80.

50. Autier P, Dore J-F, Negrier S, et al. Sunscreen use and duration of sun exposure: a double blind randomized trial. *J Natl Cancer Inst* 1999; 91: 1304–9.

51. Gallagher RP, Rivers JK, Lee TK, et al. Broad-spectrum sunscreen use and the development of new nevi in white children a randomized controlled trial. *JAMA* 2000; 283:2955–60.

52. Cawley EP. Genetic aspects of malignant melanoma. *Arch Dermatol* 1952; 65:440–50.

53. Clark WH, Reimer RR, Greene M, et al. Origin of familial malignant melanomas from heritable melanocytic lesions. "The B-K mole syndrome." *Arch Dermatol* 1978; 114:732–8.

54. Lynch HT, Frichot BC, Lynch JF. Familial atypical multiple mole-melanoma syndrome. *J Med Genetics* 1978; 15:352–6.

55. Greene MH, Clark WH Jr, Tucker MA, et al. High risk of malignant melanoma in melanoma-prone families with dysplastic nevi. *Ann Intern Med* 1985; 102:458–65.

56. Goldstein AM, Tucker MA. Screening for *CDK-N2A* mutations in hereditary melanoma. *J Natl Cancer Inst* 1997; 89:676–8.

57. Tucker MA, Fraser MC, Goldstein AM, et al. The risk of melanoma and other cancers in melanoma prone families. *J Invest Dermatol* 1993; 100 (Suppl):350–5.

58. Augustsson A, Stierner U, Rosdahl I, et al. Common and dysplastic naevi as risk factors for cutaneous melanoma in a Swedish population. *Acta Dermatol Venereol* 1990; 71:518–24.

59. Tucker MA, Halpern A, Holly EA, et al. Clinically recognized dysplastic nevi, a central risk factor for cutaneous melanoma. *JAMA* 1997; 277:1439–44.

60. Titus-Ernstoff L, Mansson-Brahme E, Thorn M, et al. Factors associated with atypical nevi: a population-based study. *Cancer Epidemiol Biomarkers and Prev* 1998; 7:207–10.

61. Marks R, Foley P, Goodman G, et al. Spontaneous remission of solar keratoses: the case for conservative management. *Br J Dermatol* 1986; 115:649–55.

62. Bendl BJ, Graham JH. New concepts on the origin of squamous cell carcinoma of the skin: solar (senile) keratosis with squamous cell carcinoma-a clinicopathologic and histochemical study. *Proc Natl Cancer Conf* 1970; 6:471–88.

63. Marks R, Ponsford MW, Selwood TS, et al. Non-melanocytic skin cancer and solar keratoses in Victoria. *Med J Aust* 1983; 2:619–22.

64. Frost CA, Green AC, Williams GM. The prevalence and determinants of solar keratoses at a tropical latitude (Queensland, Australia). *Br J Dermatol* 1998; 139:1033–9.

65. Harvey I, Frankel S, Marks R, et al. Non-melanoma skin cancer and solar keratosis. II. Analytic results of the South Wales skin cancer study. *Br J Cancer* 1996; 74:1308–12.

66. Marks R, Selwood TS. Solar keratoses, the association with erythemal ultraviolet radiation in Australia. *Cancer* 1985; 56:2332–6.

67. Holman CDJ, Armstrong BK, Evans PR, et al. Relationship of solar keratosis and history of skin damage to objective measures of actinic skin damage. *Br J Dermatol* 1984; 110:129–138.

68. Strickland PT, Vitasa BC, West SK, et al. Quantitative carcinogenesis in man: ultraviolet B dose dependence of skin cancer in Maryland watermen. *J Natl Cancer Inst* 1989; 81:1910–13.

69. Vitasa BC, Taylor HR, Strickland PT, et al. Association of nonmelanoma skin cancer and actinic keratoses with cumulative solar ultraviolet exposure in Maryland watermen. *Cancer* 1990; 6:2811–17

70. Boyle J, Mackie RM, Briggs JD, et al. Cancer, warts, and sunshine in renal transplant patients. *Lancet* 1984; I:702–5.

71. Bouwes Bavinck JN, De Boer AD, Vermeer BJ, et al. Sunlight, keratotic skin lesions and skin cancer in renal transplant recipients. *Br J Dermatol* 1993; 129:242–9.

72. Marks R, Rennie G, Selwood T. The relationship of basal cell carcinomas and squamous cell carcinomas to solar keratoses. *Arch Dermatol* 1988; 124:1039–42.

73. Naldi L, DiLandro A, D'Avanzo B, et al. Host-related and environmental risk factors for cutaneous basal cell carcinoma: evidence from an Italian case-control study. *J Am Acad Dermatol* 2000; 42:446–52.

74. Bataille V, Sasieni P, Grulich A, et al. Solar keratoses: a risk factor for melanoma but negative association with melanocytic naevi. *Int J Cancer* 1998; 78:8–12.

75. Green A, O'Rourke M. Cutaneous melanoma in association with other skin cancers. *J Natl Cancer Inst* 1985; 74:977–80.

76. Dubin N, Moseson M, Pasternack BS. Epidemiology of malignant melanoma: pigmentary traits, ultraviolet radiation, and identification of high-risk populations. *Recent Res Cancer Res* 1986; 102:56–75.

77. Thompson SC, Jolley D, Marks R. Reduction of solar keratoses by regular sunscreen use. *N Engl J Med* 1983; 329:1147–51.

78. Naylor MF, Boyd A, Smith DW, et al. High sun protection factor sunscreens in the suppression of actinic neoplasia. *Arch Dermatol* 1995; 131: 170–5.

79. MacKie RM. Melanocytic naevi and malignant melanoma. In: Champion RH, Burton JL, Burns DA, et al. (eds) *Textbook of Dermatology*, 6th ed., Vol. II. Oxford: Blackwell Science, 1998, pp. 1717–21.

80. Halpern AC. Precursor melanocytic lesions. In: Miller SJ, Maloney ME (eds) *Cutaneous Oncology*. Oxford: Blackwell Scientific, 1998, pp. 224–34.

81. Marrett LD, King WD, Walter SD, et al. Use of host factors to identify people at high risk of cutaneous malignant melanoma. *Can Med Assoc J* 1992; 147:445–53.

15
Breast

Thomas E. Rohan and Rita A. Kandel

Benign breast disease causes considerable morbidity. Indeed, it has been estimated that up to 17% of women undergo a biopsy for benign breast disease by the age of 50 [1], and that, on a population basis, biopsies for benign breast disease are about four times as common as those for breast cancer [2]. However, these figures probably overestimate the current situation with respect to biopsied benign breast disease, given the increasing use of fine needle aspiration as a diagnostic modality. Nevertheless, the true extent of the condition is unknown, since those women who are biopsied for benign breast disease represent an unknown proportion of all women with this condition [2].

Women with benign breast disease are at increased risk of developing subsequent breast cancer [3]. However, benign breast disease is a heterogeneous condition, consisting of many histological entities [4,5], and risk varies by histological subcategory [3]. One model of the natural history of breast cancer posits that it develops as a result of the progression of breast tissue through specific histological forms of benign breast disease. Essentially, according to this model, nonatypical proliferative changes and proliferative disease with atypia represent successive steps preceding the development of in-situ cancer and then invasive carcinoma. This model is supported by experimental and epidemiological evidence. Experimentally, xenografts of MCF10AneoT cells (these cells are derived from MCF10A, an immortal human breast epithelial cell line originating from a breast with benign fibrocystic disease, and they

have lost anchorage independence in vitro) have been shown to progress from intraductal proliferative changes to lesions resembling atypical hyperplasia of the human breast, and ultimately to lesions resembling carcinoma in situ [6]. Transgenic rat [7] and mouse [8] models have also demonstrated the stepwise development of breast cancer. Epidemiologic studies have shown that the risk of subsequent breast cancer is increased in women with proliferative epithelial disorders affecting the small ducts and the terminal ductal lobular units of the breast, particularly (in some studies) when the epithelial proliferation is accompanied by atypical features (following section) [3]. The higher risk associated with atypia is consistent with the notion that it is more proximal to carcinoma than proliferative disease without atypia. As a result of such findings, benign proliferative epithelial disorders of the breast are considered to have malignant potential [9].

Given the relative commonness of benign breast disease, and given that some forms of benign breast disease are associated with increased risk of subsequent breast cancer, efforts to understand its etiology, to diagnose it expeditiously, and to prevent it, are obviously warranted.

Histological Definition

The human breast contains both structural elements (connective tissue, fat, blood vessels, and lymphatic tissue) and functional elements (the mammary gland, composed of lobules and ducts lined by epithelial cells) [3]. Although many histological entities are included in the rubric benign breast disease, the relevant lesions with respect to the risk of subsequent breast cancer (see following section) are those which are of epithelial origin; these lesions include fibroadenoma, sclerosing adenosis, solitary papilloma, and hyperplasia with or without atypia [3,4,10]. The fundamental feature of epithelial hyperplasia is an increased number of cells (three or more) relative to the number normally found (one to two) above the basement membrane [4,5,11] (Figure 15.1). The cells tend to protrude into or fill and distend the duct lumina. Ductal epithelial hyperplasias display a spectrum of changes ranging from mild to florid. They are classified further as proliferative disease without atypia or atypical ductal hyperplasia, depending on the architectural patterns and the cytologic appearance of the cells (Figure 15.1). Another type of epithelial hyperplasia, micropapillary apocrine change, is not associated with increased breast cancer risk [12] in the absence of other forms of epithelial hyperplasia. Lobular hyperplasia can also develop, but only the atypical form is associated with increased risk of invasive carcinoma [13,14].

Ductal carcinoma in situ (DCIS) is a spectrum of diseases characterized by noninvasive epithelial proliferation. Although DCIS is the penultimate step in the progression from normal breast tissue to invasive cancer, its status as a precursor is somewhat ambiguous. This is because when it is low grade and small in extent, DCIS is considered to be a risk factor for the development of invasive breast cancer, but when it is high grade, it is considered to be a localized stage of cancer with invasive potential [10].

Benign Breast Disease: Relationship to Breast Cancer

Although there has been much debate about the relationship between benign breast disease and risk of subsequent breast cancer [3,15], it is now generally accepted that breast cancer risk is increased in women with a history of benign breast disease, and in particular, in women with specific histological types of benign breast disease [3]. The association between benign breast disease and risk of breast cancer has been investigated in many studies [16–39], the vast majority of which have shown positive associations [16–18,20–25,27–39]. However, interpretation of the findings of the early studies [16,18,19–21,23] is difficult because diverse terminologies (namely, cystic disease, chronic mastitis, fibrocystic disease) were used to embrace a wide variety of histological entities (e.g., cysts, duct ectasia, sclerosing adenosis, ductal hyperplasia with varying degrees of atypia, and lobular hyperplasia), and there may have been differences between studies in the composition of their study groups by histological subcategory.

The study by Page et al. [28] was the first to show the predictive importance of atypical hyperplasia (and in particular, atypical lobular hyperplasia), and since then, several prospective studies have demonstrated that the proliferative epithelial disorders affecting the small ducts and the terminal duct lobular units of the breast are most strongly associated with increased risk of breast cancer. Indeed, the results of these studies have been remarkably consistent (despite some variability in the magnitude of the relative risks for breast cancer) in showing the gradation in risk from nonproliferative forms of benign breast disease, to proliferative disease without atypia, to atypical hyperplasia (Table 15.1). The majority of these studies [28,31,36,38,39] used either the histological classification system of Dupont and Page [28] or a closely related system [37]. The results of two studies [22,38] suggested that the risk of breast cancer associated with atypical lobular hyperplasia is greater than that associated with atypical ductal hyperplasia, but another study [40] found no difference in risk by location of the atypical hyperplasia. Currently, both types of atypical hyperplasias are considered to confer a 4 to 5 fold increase in risk [10].

There is also some evidence that the risk of subsequent breast cancer is increased in

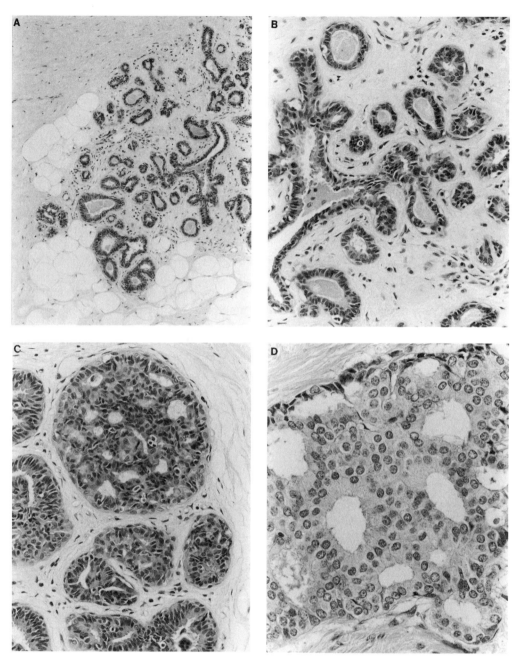

FIGURE 15.1. Terminal duct-lobular unit of breast at low (A) and at higher magnifications (B). The ductules are lined by a single layer of epithelial cells and the myoepithelial cells are flattened cells present around the periphery of the ductules. (C) Terminal duct-lobular unit showing florid epithelial hyperplasia without atypia. (D) Terminal duct-lobular unit showing atypical duct hyperplasia. (Original magnification ×100 (A), ×250 (B,C), and ×400 (D).)

TABLE 15.1. Summary of cohort studies of subsequent breast cancer risk in women with biopsy-determined benign proliferative epithelial disorders of the breast.

Reference	No. in cohort	Number of breast cancers	Median length of follow-up (years)	Reference group	RR (95% CI)[1]		
					Nonproliferative disease	Proliferative disease without atypia	Atypical hyperplasia
Hutchinson, et al. [25]	1,441	66	12.9[2]	Second and Third National Cancer Surveys	Not presented	2.8 (1.9–4.1)	2.9 (0.3–10.3)
Dupont and Page [40]	3,303	134	17	Nonproliferative lesions	1	1.9 (1.2–2.9)	5.3 (3.1–8.8)
Carter, et al. [29]	16,692	431	8.3	Screened, no biopsy	1.5 (1.1–2.0)	1.9 (1.5–2.4)	3.0 (2.1–4.1)
				Other benign breast lesions	1.3 (0.9–1.9)	1.6 (1.2–2.3)	2.5 (1.7–3.8)
Palli, et al. [31]	~6,000	62	Not presented	Nonproliferative lesions	1	1.3 (0.5–3.5)	13.0 (4.1–41.7)
Dupont, et al. [36]	15,161	95	Not presented	Nonproliferative lesions	1	1.3 (0.8–2.2)	4.3 (1.7–11.0)
Bodian, et al. [3]	1,799	157	20.6[2]	Connecticut Tumor Registry	1.6 (1.0–2.6)	2.1 (1.7–2.6)	3.0 (1.5–6.0)[3]
Marshall, et al. [38]	Not presented	174	~8.4[4]	Nonproliferative lesions	1	1.7 (1.2–2.6)	3.4 (2.0–5.9)
Minami, et al. [39]	1,826[5]	11	7.6[2]	Screened, no biopsy	0.9 (0.1–7.7)	7.3 (2.2–24.3)	16.0 (3.3–76.9)

[1] Relative risk (95% confidence interval).
[2] Mean.
[3] Moderate or severe atypia; for mild atypia the RR (95% CI) was 2.3 (1.6–3.4).
[4] Weighted average for cases and controls.
[5] 373 subjects with biopsy-defined benign breast disease and 1,453 subjects screened but with no biopsy.

women with a history of fibroadenoma [21,25, 29,33,34,41–43]. However, assessment of this relationship is complicated by the fact that the breast tissue surrounding a fibroadenoma may also contain histological changes that influence breast cancer risk. Only three studies have accounted for this possibility [25,33,42], and of these, two [33,42] found an increased risk in those with fibroadenomas and no proliferative disease in the adjacent parenchyma, and the other [25] found no association in such individuals.

Several studies have elaborated further on various aspects of the relationship between benign breast disease and breast cancer risk. Risk associated with atypical hyperplasia appears to be higher in relatively young women than in older women [29,32], in premenopausal women than in postmenopausal women [36,38], and in those with a family history of breast cancer than in those without such a history [28,32,36,40]. Findings regarding the relationship between risk of breast cancer and time since biopsy for benign breast disease have been rather variable. One study [44] found that the risk following diagnosis of either proliferative disease without atypia or atypical hyperplasia is greatest in the first 10 years after diagnosis of the benign lesion; another study [32] found no variation in risk associated with atypical hyperplasia in connection to the time since biopsy for that lesion; and an expanded version of the latter study [38] found no variation in risk of breast cancer with time since biopsy for either proliferative disease without atypia or atypical lobular hyperplasia (and atypical hyperplasia overall), but an increase in risk with time since biopsy for atypical ductal hyperplasia. Finally, subsequent breast cancers appear to arise equally as often in the ipsilateral as in the contralateral breast [31,38,40,45]. This observation has been interpreted to suggest that hyperplasia is simply a marker of risk [38] rather than a precursor. However, it does not preclude the possibility that hyperplasia is indeed a precursor (especially given that the peak incidence rate for benign breast disease occurs 15 to 20 years before that for breast cancer [2]). It also does not preclude the possibility that the presence of hyperplasia in one breast is indicative of a generalized disease process affecting both breasts, and that progression is as likely to occur first in the contralateral breast as in the ipsilateral breast.

Molecular Changes

Cancer arises from the accumulation of multiple genetic events [46]. Attempts have been made to determine whether genetic changes occur in normal breast or breast tissue with benign breast disease and whether such changes are associated with the development of breast cancer. In this regard, evidence for loss-of-heterozygosity (LOH) has been sought in several studies [47–52].

LOH has been detected in normal breast tissue adjacent to breast cancer [47]. Although it is possible that the normal tissue contained isolated cancer cells, it is more likely that genetic changes can precede phenotypic alterations. O'Connell et al. [48], in a study of 399 cases of benign breast disease, discovered LOH in at least one locus in 37% of breast tissues exhibiting hyperplasia without atypia and in 42% of breast tissues with atypical hyperplasia. When the breast tissue contained several foci of hyperplasia without atypia, only 15% of lesions showed similar LOH phenotypes [48]. Two other studies of breast tissue with epithelial hyperplasia reported that about 8% [49] and at least 13% [50] of the samples examined showed LOH. Lizard-Nacol et al. [51] reported that no LOH was detected in any of the 8 loci examined in 50 cases of benign breast tissue. However, 37 of these were phylloides tumors, which are circumscribed nodules composed of hypercellular stroma and a proliferation of ductal structures, and there were no cases with epithelial hyperplasia. LOH has also been detected in breast papillomas [52]. These contradictory findings may reflect, in part, differences in the DNA loci examined, in the methods of evaluation used, and in the underlying pathological lesions examined.

Other molecular changes have also been detected in benign breast disease. Microsatellite sequence alterations were detected in 5 of 12 cases of atypical hyperplasia [53] but in only 1 of 112 informative cases of epithelial hyperplasia without atypia [49]. However, Larson et al. [54] found that 22% of normal breast tissues showed microsatellite changes. Using comparative genomic hybridization, Aubele et al. [55] demonstrated the presence of allelic imbalances in benign breast disease and showed that the number of allelic imbalances increased with the severity of the histological changes which ranged from ductal hyperplasia without atypia to invasive breast cancer. Aneuploidy occurs in both nonproliferative and proliferative forms of benign breast disease [56–58], and simple chromosomal changes have been detected in benign phylloides tumors [59]. Alterations in single genes have also been described in benign breast disease. For example, *p53* mutations and protein accumulation occur in benign breast tissue [60–62] as does *cyclin D1* gene amplification [63].

It has only recently been appreciated that alterations in the tumor suppressor genes *BRCA1* or *BRCA2* can occur in sporadic breast cancer. One study has provided indirect evidence of changes in the *BRCA1* gene in benign breast disease in individuals with family histories of either breast cancer or of cancer syndromes. Lalle et al. [64] showed that three of nine benign breast lesions of these women had allele losses near the 17q12–q21 locus. To our knowledge there have been no reports of changes in the *BRCA* genes in benign breast disease in the absence of a family history of breast cancer. However, two recent immunhistochemical studies showed normal distribution of the BRCA1 protein in nonmalignant breast tissues, suggesting that BRCA1 may not be altered in benign breast disease in the absence of a family history of cancer [2,3].

Although there have been numerous studies describing genetic abnormalities in DCIS, it is only recently that we have begun to appreciate that there are two forms of DCIS, one with little risk for recurrence or invasion and the other with increased invasive potential [13]. Evalua-

tion of genetic alterations in relationship to the clinical course of DCIS might shed more light on the role of such alterations in breast cancer development.

Clearly, genetic changes can occur in normal tissue and in benign breast disease, but their association with genetic changes in breast cancer as well as with risk of subsequent breast cancer has just begun to be investigated. In this regard, one study that examined the correlation between the LOH pattern in benign breast tissue and the LOH pattern in the corresponding breast cancer in the same specimen found that 37% of breast tissues containing hyperplasia without atypia and 45% of those with atypical hyperplasia shared at least one locus of LOH with the adjacent cancer tissue [48]. Kasami et al. [65] reported on the case of a woman who had breast papillomas and epithelial hyperplasia with focal atypia and who also had LOH. No breast cancer developed within 25 years of follow-up, suggesting that these changes do not always give rise to malignancy [65]. Micale et al. [56] found aneuploidy in 9 cases of benign breast disease and detected similar changes in the corresponding cancer in the same specimen, suggesting that this type of change might contribute to carcinogenesis. Cummings et al. [66] showed that the copy number of chromosome 1 in breast tissue increased as the severity of the associated histological changes increased from hyperplasia to atypical ductal hyperplasia to DCIS. Two prospective studies have suggested that molecular alterations may be indicators of increased breast cancer risk. In a case-control study nested in a cohort of women with benign breast disease, Rohan et al. [67] showed that the accumulation of immunohistochemically detected p53 protein in breast epithelium was associated with a 2.5-fold increase in subsequent breast cancer risk. Recently, another nested case-control study showed *c-erbB-2/neu* amplification, in association with either typical or atypical proliferative disease, to be associated with a 7.2-fold increase in breast cancer risk [68]. The association between genetic alterations and breast cancer risk requires further study.

Descriptive Epidemiology

Frequency of Occurrence of Benign Proliferative Epithelial Disorders of the Breast

On a population basis, difficulties arise in attempting to estimate the frequency of occurrence of benign breast lesions in general, and of benign proliferative epithelial disorders in particular, since an unknown proportion of women with benign breast disease comes to clinical attention and proceed to biopsy [69]. Therefore, histopathological confirmation of the presence of benign proliferative epithelial disorders of the breast is obtained in only a proportion of cases, and these cases represent an unknown proportion of cases present in the general population [11]. Nevertheless, estimates of the frequency of occurrence of benign proliferative epithelial disorders can be obtained from autopsy and epidemiological studies.

Autopsy Studies

Autopsy studies can provide estimates of the prevalence of a condition at death, particularly when the condition of interest is nonfatal, and the included subjects form an unselected series of individuals [11]. In this regard, several autopsy studies have yielded data on the prevalence of benign proliferative epithelial disorders of the breast [70–80]. Although direct comparison of their results is compromised by differences between studies in histopathological terminology, these studies do indicate that benign proliferative epithelial disorders of the breast are relatively common at death, with prevalence estimates ranging from around 5% to 15% [70,72] to as high as 64% [79]. Furthermore, in most of these series, the prevalence of proliferative epithelial disorders was considerably greater than that of occult carcinoma of the breast discovered at autopsy. This suggests that even if benign proliferative epithelial disorders of the breast are precursors of breast cancer, the latter is not an inevitable consequence of the former, and that factors other than those responsible for the development of the precursor lesion are responsible for its progression to carcinoma.

Epidemiological Studies

There appear to be no published estimates of the incidence rates of benign proliferative epithelial disorders of the breast. However, several studies have yielded estimates of the incidence rates of broader groupings of benign breast disease [2,81–84]. These studies are very consistent in showing that the incidence rates of benign breast disease (variously referred to in these reports as fibrocystic disease or benign mammary dysplasia) increase rapidly with age until about 40 to 44 years, with peak incidence rates being somewhere between 200 and 400/100,000 per annum. Although incidence rates decrease rapidly thereafter (with commencement of the decline corresponding approximately to the onset of menopause), the disease remains relatively common, with estimates of the annual incidence rate ranging from about 100/100,000 women in the early postmenopausal years to 20 to 30/100,000 women in the later postmenopausal years [11].

Etiology

If benign breast lesions (or certain types thereof) are precursors of breast cancer, then risk factors for the former should be a subset of those for the latter (the same argument applies to in situ breast cancer). Therefore, investigation of the etiology of putative precursor lesions has focussed largely on factors which have been studied in relation to the etiology of breast cancer (i.e., menstrual and reproductive history, use of oral contraceptives and hormone replacement therapy, cigarette smoking, obesity, and, more recently, diet).

Although some studies have found that, as with risk of breast cancer [85], risk of benign breast disease is increased in association with early age at menarche, late age at menopause, and nulliparity or low parity, these associations have not been observed consistently [11,86]. Discrepancies between the associations of these (and other) factors with risk of benign breast disease and breast cancer might partly reflect the fact that most studies of benign breast disease have not focussed on proliferative epithelial disorders (with or without atypia). However, several case-control [84, 87–89,90–98] and cohort studies [99–102] have either reported on associations of various factors (menstrual, reproductive, anthropometric, and sociodemographic) with risk of proliferative disorders [84,87–89,91–98] or have graded the biopsies of women with so-called fibrocystic disease according to the degree of epithelial proliferation and cytological atypia which they displayed and then examined variation in risk by degree of atypia [90,91,99]. Of these studies, none of those which examined age at menarche found evidence of an association with risk [84,88,90,91,96–98,100]; most [84,90,91,97,99] observed no association with age at first pregnancy, but two [87,88] observed positive associations; one [98] of those studies which examined risk associated with parity [83,88,90–92,96–101] observed an inverse association, and the remainder observed no association; several [93,96,100] showed that risk was increased in those with a family history of breast cancer, but several others [90–92,97] showed no association; three [93,95,100] provided some evidence for an inverse association with body mass index [weight (kg)/height (m)^2], and three others [90–92] did not; and none of those [89–91,93,101] which examined risk in association with cigarette smoking observed an association.

Other variables which have been studied in relation to risk of benign breast disease include use of oral contraceptives (OCs) and hormone replacement therapy (HRT) and diet. Of the many cohort [83,103–105] and case-control studies [106–118] of OCs and benign breast disease, a majority [83,101,104,106–110,112, 113,115–117] have provided evidence suggestive of an inverse association between duration of use and risk of all histological types of benign breast disease combined. Two studies [101,117], presented results for the association between OC use and risk of benign proliferative epithelial disorders of the breast, and several studies (all case-control) examined the association

between oral contraceptive use and risk of benign breast disease by degree of histological atypia [114,117,119–122]. Of the former [101,117], one [101] indicated reduced risk of benign proliferative epithelial disorders in association with OC use, but the other [117] indicated no association. Of the latter, two [120,122] found reduced risk of all grades of atypia (that is, no variation in the magnitude of the protective effect by degree of atypia); one [117] found no association overall or by degree of atypia; one [119] found reduced risk of benign breast disease when atypia was absent or minimal but not when it was marked; one [121] found reduced risk of benign breast disease with low- and intermediate-grade atypia, but not with high grade atypia; and one [114] found that in premenopausal women, use of oral contraceptives was associated with increased risk of benign breast disease with either minimal or severe atypia and with a slight decrease in risk of intermediate grades of atypia.

Several studies have found increased risk of benign breast disease for women who have ever used HRT [123–127], while others have found either no association [115,118,128,129] or decreased risk [89,130]. Of those studies which have examined the risk of benign breast disease in association with duration of use [113,123, 125–127,131], only one [113] failed to find evidence of a positive association. In general, studies have examined risk for all histological types of benign breast disease combined rather than for those histological types which are associated with increased risk of breast cancer. In this regard, one recent prospective study [101] observed increased risk of benign proliferative epithelial disorders in association with HRT use of more than 8 years, but an earlier case-control study, in which the association between HRT use and risk of benign breast disease was examined by degree of cytological atypia, found no evidence for a linear relationship between degree of atypia and risk [132].

Several case-control studies [96,133–136] and one cohort study [137] have examined the association between diet and risk of benign proliferative epithelial disorders of the breast. Two of these studies [133,134] indicated positive associations between saturated fat intake (or indices thereof) and risk of atypical [133] or proliferative forms [134] of benign breast disease, but the remaining four studies [96,135–137] provided little support for a role for dietary fat in the etiology of proliferative forms of benign breast disease. With respect to other nutrients, one study provided some evidence for inverse associations between retinol and β-carotene intake and risk [135] and also found strong inverse associations between dietary fiber and its components (soluble and insoluble non-starch polysaccharides and cellulose) and risk [138]. These findings were supported to some extent by those of another study [96] in which risk of benign epithelial hyperplasia was reduced in association with consumption of fruit and leafy orange-red vegetables, both of which contain fiber and micronutrients such as β-carotene. However, in another study [139] carotene and retinol intake were not associated with risk of atypical or nonatypical forms of benign proliferative epithelial disorders of the breast. One study [137] found no association between dietary calcium intake and risk of benign proliferative epithelial disorders of the breast.

There have been relatively few investigations of risk factors for carcinoma-in-situ of the breast. In a recent population-based case-control study [140], women with a family history of breast cancer and those with a history of biopsied benign breast disease had a 2-fold greater risk of carcinoma-in-situ. There was also some evidence for an increase in risk with age at first giving birth and for a decrease in risk with increasing parity. Previous studies have mostly indicated greater risks of in-situ breast cancer in association with a family history of breast cancer [141–144], a history of benign breast disease [141–145], age at first giving birth [142–146], nulliparity [141,143], and HRT use [142,147–149], and inverse associations of risk with body mass index [141,142] and age at menarche [142]. However, some studies have not found associations with age at first birth [141], body mass index [145], age at menarche [141,143–145], and HRT use [144,150,151].

In general, the available epidemiological evidence suggests that there are similarities between the epidemiology of benign proliferative epithelial disorders of the breast, in-situ cancer, and invasive breast cancer, consistent with but not proving the hypothesis that benign lesions progress to in-situ disease and then to breast cancer. However, it is evident that there are some inconsistencies between the results of the various studies of benign proliferative epithelial disorders of the breast, and similarly, between the results of studies of in-situ breast cancer. For benign breast disease (in particular), those inconsistencies which have been observed may reflect differences between studies in the distribution of the case groups by histological subcategory of benign breast disease and in the method of classifying benign breast disease [11]. They may also reflect the fact that studies of biopsy-confirmed benign breast disease (like studies of other potentially premalignant conditions) are prone to selection bias. For these reasons, there is a need for studies in which histological classification is based upon a standard well-accepted classification scheme, and in which the problem of selection bias is minimised. The latter might be accomplished by conducting studies within screened populations [152].

Etiologically, the constellation of risk factors for the putative precursor lesions suggests that, as with breast cancer, endogenous hormones play a critical role in their development. However, endocrinological studies of benign lesions have not yielded a clear picture of the specific hormonal perturbations which are associated with such lesions [9], perhaps reflecting the methodological issues referred to above.

Detection

For some cancer sites (for example, the cervix), the purpose of screening is to detect either histologic precursors of carcinoma or early carcinoma [153]. However, for the breast, the objective of screening is to detect invasive cancer at an early stage, prior to metastasis, and thereby to improve the survival rate for women with the disease. Nevertheless, mammographic screening for breast cancer might also result in the detection of ductal carcinoma-in-situ, as discussed further in the chapter on screening (see chapter 22). Currently, there is no evidence concerning the value (in relation to subsequent mortality) of detecting and treating atypical hyperplastic lesions of the breast.

Prevention

There has been relatively little investigation of methods for the prevention of benign breast disease (including benign proliferative epithelial disorders of the breast) in women. However, a number of experimental studies have examined the effect of various chemopreventive agents on mammary epithelial proliferation rates or the development of proliferative lesions. Specifically, retinoids have been shown to inhibit cell proliferation, and to induce differentiation and apoptosis [154]. Recently, 4-(hydroxyphenyl) retinamide, a synthetic retinoid which can inhibit mammary carcinogenesis in animal models, has been shown to inhibit the development and progression of hyperplastic lesions in the terminal end buds of rat mammary glands [155]. Retinoic acid, and the synthetic peroxisome proliferator-activated receptor γ ligand troglitazne, both inhibited the development of 7,12-dimethylbenz[a]anthracene-induced preneoplastic lesions in a mouse mammary gland organ culture model [156]. Conjugated linoleic acid has been shown to reduce by 50% the formation of premalignant lesions (intraductal proliferation) in the rat mammary gland and to increase apoptosis [157]. The latter phenomenon was accompanied by a decrease in bcl-2 expression. Diets deficient in vitamin D and calcium induce hyperplasia and hyperproliferation in the mouse mammary gland, and these changes can be inhibited by calcium supplementation [158]. Selenium, when administered as Se-methylselenocysteine, has been shown to reduce the number of intraductal proliferations (cancer precursors) in the mammary glands of methylnitrosourea-treated rats, and when administered as triphenylselenonium, selenium inhibits the clonal growth of such lesions [159]. Exposure of noncancerous human mammary epithelial cells to benzo(α)pyrene induces aberrant proliferation and down-regulation of apoptosis, but these changes can be counteracted to some extent by administration of the phytochemicals indole-3-carbinol, genistein, and epigallo catechin gallate [160]. In contrast, a recent study in women showed that short-term dietary supplementation with soy protein (which contains isoflavones) had no effect on mammary epithelial proliferation rates [161]. The findings described here raise the possibility of testing (at least some of) these agents for potential anti-carcinogenic effects in humans by conducting randomized trials using benign proliferative epithelial disorders of the breast as intermediate endpoints.

Vitamin E administration and methylxanthine restriction might also have preventive value, although evidence in support of their preventive roles is limited. Two small randomized studies showed that administration of vitamin E did not ameliorate the symptoms of benign breast disease [162,163], whereas two nonrandomized studies showed that restriction of methylxanthines (including caffeine) resulted in resolution or improvement of the symptoms of benign breast disease in a substantial proportion of cases [164,165].

Conclusions

Experimental and epidemiological evidence supports the notion that benign proliferative epithelial disorders of the breast are precursors of breast cancer: experimental models have shown that proliferative lesions progress to breast cancer, and epidemiological studies have shown that the peak incidence rate for benign breast disease occurs 15 to 20 years before that for breast cancer [2], and that women with proliferative forms of benign breast disease are at increased risk of breast cancer. Nevertheless, the precise nature of the relationship between the two conditions remains uncertain. From the available evidence, it would appear that there are two possibilities: either benign proliferative epithelial disorders of the breast progress to breast cancer, or the benign lesions and breast cancer might be independent outcomes resulting from the action on breast tissue of (at least partially) overlapping sets of etiological factors [166]. In either case, as indicated earlier, risk factors for benign proliferative epithelial disorders of the breast should be a subset of those for breast cancer. The currently available epidemiological evidence provides some support for the notion that benign proliferative epithelial disorders and breast cancer do share risk factors, but further study of risk factors for benign proliferative epithelial disorders of the breast, although important in elucidating the etiology of these conditions, seems unlikely to resolve the issue of whether or not they truly are precursors of breast cancer. In this regard, recent and ongoing molecular studies might help if they can demonstrate that breast cancers represent clonal outgrowths of pre-existing benign lesions. However, such studies are still in their infancy. Finally, if risk factors for benign proliferative epithelial disorders of the breast are indeed a subset of those for breast cancer, and if these benign conditions do progress to breast cancer, then factors other than those responsible for the development of the benign conditions should influence their progression to breast cancer. Hence, it may be of interest to study risk factors for breast cancer in women with benign proliferative epithelial disorders of the breast.

Acknowledgment. The authors thank Alfredo Morabia for his helpful comments on this chapter.

References

1. Hislop TG, Elwood MJ. Risk factors for benign breast disease: a 30-year cohort study. *Can Med Assoc J* 1981; 124:283–91.
2. Fleming NT, Armstrong BK, Sheiner HJ. The comparative epidemiology of benign breast lumps and breast cancer in Western Australia. *Int J Cancer* 1982; 30:147–51.
3. Bodian CA. Benign breast diseases, carcinoma in situ, and breast cancer risk. *Epidemiol Rev* 1993; 15:177–87.
4. Page DL, Anderson TJ. *Diagnostic histopathology of the breast.* Edinburgh: Churchill Livingstone, 1987.
5. Schwartz GF, Lagios MD, Carter D, et al. Consensus conference on the classification of ductal carcinoma in situ. *Hum Pathol* 1997; 28:1221–4.
6. Miller FR, Soule HD, Tait L, et al. Xenograft model of progressive human proliferative breast disease. *J Natl Cancer Inst* 1993; 85: 1725–32.
7. Davies BR, Platt-Higgins AM, Schmidt G, et al. Development of hyperplasias, preneoplasias, and mammary tumors in MMTV-*c-erbB-2* and MMTV-*TFF* transgenic rats. *Am J Pathol* 1999; 155:303–14.
8. Li Y, Hively WP, Varmus HE. Use of MMTV-*Wnt-1* transgenic mice for studying the genetic basis of breast cancer. *Oncogene* 2000; 19:1002–9.
9. Wang DY, Fentiman IS. Epidemiology and endocrinology of benign breast disease. *Breast Cancer Res Treat* 1985; 6:5–36.
10. Fitzgibbons PL, Henson DE, Hutter RVP. Benign breast changes and risk for subsequent breast cancer: an update of the 1985 consensus statement. Cancer Committee of the College of American Pathologists. *Arch Pathol Lab Med* 1998; 122:1053–5.
11. Cook MG, Rohan TE. The patho-epidemiology of benign proliferative epithelial disorders of the female breast. *J Pathol* 1985; 146:1–15.
12. Page DL, Dupont WD, Jensen RA. Papillary apocrine change of the breast: associations with atypical hyperplasia and risk of breast cancer. *Cancer Epidemiol Biomark Prev* 1996; 5:29–32.
13. Page DL, Jensen RA, Simpson JF. Premalignant and malignant disease of the breast: the role of the pathologist. *Mod Pathol* 1998; 11: 120–8.
14. Page DL, Kidd TE, Dupont WD, et al. Lobular neoplasia of the breast. *Hum Pathol* 1991; 22: 1232–9.
15. Webber W, Boyd N. A critique of the methodology of studies of benign breast disease and breast cancer risk. *J Natl Cancer Inst* 1986; 77:397–404.
16. Davis HH, Simons M, Davis JB. Cystic disease of the breast: relationship to carcinoma. *Cancer* 1964; 17:957–78.
17. Black MM, Barclay THC, Cutler SJ, et al. Association of atypical characteristics of benign breast lesion with subsequent risk of breast cancer. *Cancer* 1972; 29:338–43.
18. Donnelly PK, Baker KW, Carney JA, et al. Benign breast lesions and subsequent breast carcinoma in Rochester, Minnesota. *Mayo Clin Proc* 1975; 50:650–6.

19. Devitt JE. Breast cancer and preceding clinical benign breast disorders. A chance association. *Lancet* 1976; i:793–5.

20. Monson RR, Yen S, MacMahon B, et al. Chronic mastitis and carcinoma of the breast. *Lancet* 1976; ii:224–6.

21. Kodlin D, Winger EE, Morgenstern NL, et al. Chronic mastopathy and breast cancer: a follow-up study. *Cancer* 1977; 39:2603–7.

22. Page DL, Vander Zwag R, Rogers LW, et al. Relation between component parts of fibrocystic disease complex and breast cancer. *J Natl Cancer Inst* 1978; 61:1055–63.

23. Coombs LJ, Lilienfeld AM, Bross ID, et al. A prospective study of the relationship between benign breast diseases and breast carcinoma. *Prev Med* 1979; 8:40–52.

24. Moskowitz M, Gartside P, Wirman JA, et al. Proliferative disorders of the breast as risk factors for breast cancer in a self-selected population: pathologic markers. *Radiology* 1980; 134:289–91.

25. Hutchinson WB, Thomas DB, Hamlin WB, et al. Risk of breast cancer in women with benign breast disease. *J Natl Cancer Inst* 1980; 65:13–20.

26. Devitt JE. Clinical benign disorders of the breast and carcinoma of the breast. *Surg Gynecol Obstet* 1981; 152:437–40.

27. Roberts MM, Jones V, Elton RA, et al. Risk of breast cancer in women with history of benign disease of the breast. *Br Med J* 1984; 288: 275–8.

28. Dupont WD, Page DL. Risk factors for breast cancer in women with proliferative breast disease. *N Engl J Med* 1985; 312:146–51.

29. Carter CL, Corle DK, Micozzi MS, et al. A prospective study of the development of breast cancer in 16,692 women with benign breast disease. *Am J Epidemiol* 1988; 128:467–77.

30. Ris H-B, Niederer U, Stirnemann H, et al. Long-term follow-up of patients with biopsy proven benign breast disease. *Ann Surg* 1988; 207:404–9.

31. Palli D, del Turco MR, Simoncini R, et al. Benign breast disease and breast cancer: a case-control study in a cohort in Italy. *Int J Cancer* 1991; 47:703–6.

32. London SJ, Connolly JL, Schnitt SJ, et al. A prospective study of benign breast disease and the risk of breast cancer. *JAMA* 1992; 267: 941–4.

33. McDivitt RW, Stevens JA, Lee NC, et al. Histologic types of benign breast disease and the

risk for breast cancer. *Cancer* 1992; 69:1408–14.

34. Krieger N, Hiatt RA. Risk of breast cancer after benign breast diseases. *Am J Epidemiol* 1992; 135:619–31.

35. Nomura Y, Tashiro H, Katsuda Y. Benign breast disease as a breast cancer risk in Japanese women. *Jpn J Cancer Res* 1993; 84:938–44.

36. Dupont WD, Parl FF, Hartmann WH, et al. Breast cancer risk associated with proliferative breast disease and atypical hyperplasia. *Cancer* 1993; 71:128–65.

37. Bodian CA, Perzin KH, Lattes R, et al. Prognostic significance of benign proliferative breast disease. *Cancer* 1993; 71:3896–907.

38. Marshall LM, Hunter DJ, Connolly JL, et al. Risk of breast cancer associated with atypical hyperplasia of lobular and ductal types. *Cancer Epidemiol Biomarkers Prev* 1997; 6:297–301.

39. Minami Y, Ohuchi N, Taeda Y, et al. Risk of breast cancer in Japanese women with benign breast disease. *Jpn J Cancer Res* 1999; 90:600–6.

40. Page DL, Dupont WD, Rogers LW, et al. Atypical hyperplastic lesions of the female breast. A long-term follow-up study. *Cancer* 1985; 55:2698–708.

41. Levi F, Randimbison L, Te V-C, et al. Incidence of breast cancer in women with fibroadenoma. *Int J Cancer* 1994; 57:681–3.

42. Dupont WD, Page DL, Parl FF, et al. Long-term risk of breast cancer in women with fibroadenoma. *N Engl J Med* 1994; 331:10–15.

43. Ciatto S, Bonardi R, Zappa M, et al. Risk of breast cancer subsequent to histological or clinical diagnosis of fibroadenoma—retrospective longitudinal study of 3938 cases. *Ann Oncol* 1997; 8:297–300.

44. Dupont WD, Page DL. Relative risk of breast cancer varies with time since diagnosis of atypical hyperplasia. *Hum Pathol* 1989; 20: 723–5.

45. Connolly J, Schnitt S, London S, et al. Both atypical lobular hyperplasia (ALH) and atypical ductal hyperplasia (ADH) predict for bilateral breast cancer risk. *Lab Invest* 1992; 66:13A.

46. Vogelstein B, Kinzler KW. The multistep nature of cancer. *Trends Genet* 1993; 9:138–41.

47. Deng G, Lu Y, Zlotnikov G, et al. Loss of heterozygosity in normal tissue adjacent to breast carcinomas. *Science* 1996; 274:2057–9.

48. O'Connell P, Pekkel V, Fuqua SAW, et al. Analysis of loss of heterozygosity in 399 premalignant breast lesions at 15 genetic loci. *J Natl Cancer Inst* 1998; 90:697–703.

49. Dillon EK, de Boer WB, Papadimitriou JM, et al. Microsatellite instability and loss of heterozygosity in mammary carcinoma and its probable precursors. *Br J Cancer* 1997; 76:156–62.

50. Lakhani SR, Slack DN, Hamoudi RA, et al. Detection of allelic imbalance indicates that a proportion of mammary hyperplasia of usual type are clonal, neoplastic proliferations. *Lab Invest* 1996; 74:129–35.

51. Lizard-Nacol S, Lidereau R, Collin F, et al. Benign breast disease: absence of genetic alterations at several loci implicated in breast cancer malignancy. *Cancer Res* 1995; 55:4416–19.

52. Lininger RA, Park W-S, Man Y-G, et al. LOH at 16p13 is a novel chromosomal alteration detected in benign and malignant microdissected papillary neoplasms of the breast. *Hum Pathol* 1998; 29:1113–18.

53. Rosenberg CL, Larson PS, Romo JD, et al. Microsatellite alterations indicating monoclonality in atypical hyperplasias associated with breast cancer. *Hum Pathol* 1997; 28:214–19.

54. Larson PS, de las Morenas A, Cupples LA, et al. Genetically abnormal clones in histologically normal breast tissue. *Am J Pathol* 1998; 152:1591–8.

55. Aubele MM, Cummings MC, Mattis AE, et al. Accumulation of chromosomal imbalances from intraductal proliferative lesions to adjacent in situ and invasive ductal breast cancer. *Diagn Mol Pathol* 2000; 9:14–19.

56. Micale MA, Wisscher DW, Gulino SE, et al. Chromosomal aneuploidy in proliferative breast disease. *Hum Pathol* 1994; 25:29–35.

57. Sneige N, Sahin A, Dinh M, et al. Interphase cytogenetics in mammographically detected breast lesions. *Hum Pathol* 1996; 27:330–5.

58. Lundin C, Mertens F. Cytogenetics of benign breast lesions. *Breast Cancer Res Treat* 1998; 51:1–15.

59. Dietrich CU, Pandis N, Rizou H, et al. Cytogenetic findings in phyllodes tumors of the breast: karyotypic complexity differentiates between malignant and benign tumours. *Hum Pathol* 1997; 28:1379–82.

60. Millikan R, Hulka B, Thor A, et al. *p53* mutations in benign breast disease. *J Clin Oncol* 1995; 13:2293–300.

61. Kandel RA, Li S-Q, Ozcelik H, et al. p53 protein accumulation and mutations in normal and benign breast tissue. *Int J Cancer* 2000; 87:73–8.

62. Gudlaugsdottir S, Sigurdardottir V, Snorradottir M, et al. *p53* mutations analysis in benign and malignant breast lesions: using needle rinses from fine-needle aspirations. *Diagn Cytopathol* 2000; 22:268–74.

63. Zhu XL, Hartwick W, Rohan T, et al. Cyclin *D1* gene amplification and protein expression in benign breast disease and breast carcinoma. *Modern Path* 1998; 11:1082–8.

64. Lalle P, De Latour M, Rio P, et al. Detection of allelic losses on 17q12-q21 chromosomal region in benign lesions and malignant tumors occurring in a familial context *Oncogene* 1994; 9:437–42.

65. Kasami M, Vnencak-Jones CL, Manning S, et al. Loss of heterozygosity and microsatellite instability in breast hyperplasia. No obligate correlation of these genetic alterations with subsequent malignancy. *Am J Pathol* 1997; 150:1925–32.

66. Cummings MC, Aubele M, Mattis A, et al. Increasing chromosome 1 copy number parallels histological progression in breast carcinogenesis. *Br J Cancer* 2000; 82:1204–10.

67. Rohan TE, Hartwick W, Miller AB, et al. Immunohistochemical detection of c-erbB-2 and p53 in benign breast disease and breast cancer risk. *J Natl Cancer Inst* 1998; 90:1262–9.

68. Stark A, Hulka BS, Joens S, et al. *HER-2/neu* amplification in benign breast disease and the risk of subsequent breast cancer. *J Clin Oncol* 2000; 18:267–74.

69. Rohan TE, Jain M, Miller AB. A case-cohort study of diet and risk of benign proliferative epithelial disorders of the breast (Canada). *Cancer Causes Control* 1998; 9:19–27.

70. Frantz VK, Pickren JW, Melcher GW, et al. Incidence of chronic cystic disease in so-called normal breasts. *Cancer* 1951; 4:762–83.

71. Sloss PT, Bennett WA, Clagett OT. Incidence in normal breasts of features associated with chronic cystic mastitis. *Am J Pathol* 1957; 33:1181–91.

72. Sandison AT. *An autopsy study of the adult human breast. National Cancer Institute Monograph 8, DHEW PHS*. Washington, DC: US GPO, 1962.

73. Humphrey LJ, Swerdlow M. Histologic changes in clinically normal breasts at postmortem examination. *Arch Surg* 1966; 92:192–3.

74. Kramer WM, Rush BF Jr. Mammary duct proliferation in the elderly. A histopathologic study. *Cancer* 1973; 31:130–7.

75. Sasano N, Tateno H, Stemmerman GN. Volume and hyperplastic lesions of breasts of Japanese women in Hawaii and Japan. *Prev Med* 1978; 7:196–204.

76. Nielsen M, Jensen J, Andersen J. Precancerous and cancerous breast lesions during lifetime and at autopsy. A study of 83 women. *Cancer* 1984; 54:612–15.

77. Alpers CE, Wellings SR. The prevalence of carcinoma in situ in normal and cancer-associated breasts. *Hum Pathol* 1985; 16:796–807.

78. Bhathal PS, Brown RW, Lesueur GC, et al. Frequency of benign and malignant breast lesions in 207 consecutive autopsies in Australian women. *Br J Cancer* 1985; 51:271–8.

79. Nielsen M, Thomsen JL, Primdahl S, et al. Breast cancer and atypia among young and middle aged women: a study of 110 medicolegal autopsies. *Br J Cancer* 1987; 56:814–19.

80. Sarnelli R, Squartini F. Fibrocystic condition and "at risk" lesions in asymptomatic breasts: a morphologic study of postmenopausal women. *Clin Exp Obstet Gynecol* 1991; 18:271–9.

81. Ory H, Cole P, MacMahon B, et al. Oral contraceptives and reduced risk of benign breast disease. *N Engl J Med* 1976; 249:419–22.

82. Cole P, Elwood JM, Kaplan SD. Incidence rates and risk factors of benign breast neoplasms. *Am J Epidemiol* 1978; 108:112–20.

83. Brinton LA, Vessey MP, Flavel R, et al. Risk factors for benign breast disease. *Am J Epidemiol* 1981; 113:203–14.

84. Soini I, Aine R, Laushlati K, et al. Independent risk factors of benign and malignant breast lesions. *Am J Epidemiol* 1981; 114:507–14.

85. Kelsey JL. Breast cancer epidemiology: summary and future directions. *Epidemiol Rev* 1993; 15:256–63.

86. Goehring C, Morabia A. Epidemiology of benign breast disease, with special attention to histologic types. *Epidemiol Rev* 1997; 19:310–27.

87. Lance LL. Risk factors for benign breast disease. *Am J Epidemiol* 1981; 114:606–7.

88. Parazzini F, La Vecchia C, Franceschi S, et al. Risk factors for pathologically confirmed benign breast disease. *Am J Epidemiol* 1984; 120:115–22.

89. Parazzini F, Ferraroni M, La Vecchia C, et al. Smoking habits and risk of benign breast disease. *Int J Epidemiol* 1991; 20:430–4.

90. Berkowitz GS, Kelsey JL, LiVolsi VA, et al. Risk factors for fibrocystic disease and its histopathologic components. *J Natl Cancer Inst* 1985; 75:43–50.

91. Pastides H, Kelsey JL, Holford TR, et al. An epidemiologic study of fibrocystic breast disease with reference to ductal epithelial atypia. *Am J Epidemiol* 1985; 121:440–7.

92. Bright RA, Morrison AS, Brisson J, et al. Histologic and mammographic specificity of risk factors for benign breast disease. *Cancer* 1989; 64:653–7.

93. Rohan TE, Cook MG. Alcohol consumption and risk of benign proliferative epithelial disorders of the breast in women. *Int J Cancer* 1989; 43:631–6.

94. Rohan TE, Cook MG, Baron JA. Cigarette smoking and benign proliferative epithelial disorders of the breast in women: a case-control study. *J Epidemiol Community Health* 1989; 43:362–8.

95. Ingram D, Nottage E, Ng S, et al. Obesity and breast disease: the role of female sex hormones. *Cancer* 1989; 64:1049–53.

96. Ingram DM, Nottage E, Roberts T. The role of diet in the development of breast cancer: a case-control study of patients with breast cancer, benign epithelial hyperplasia and fibrocystic disease of the breast. *Br J Cancer* 1991; 64:187–91.

97. London SJ, Stein EA, Henderson IC, et al. Carotenoids, retinol, and vitamin E and risk of proliferative benign breast disease and breast cancer. *Cancer Causes Control* 1992; 3:503–12.

98. Minami Y, Ohuchi N, Taeda Y, et al. Risk factors for benign breast disease according to histopathological type: comparisons with risk factors for breast cancer. *Jpn J Cancer Res* 1998; 89:116–23.

99. Hsieh C, Walker AM, Trapido EJ, et al. Age at first birth and breast atypia. *Int J Cancer* 1984; 33:309–12.

100. Rohan TE, Jain M, Miller AB. Alcohol consumption and risk of benign proliferative epithelial disorders of the breast: a case-control study. *Public Health Nutr* 1998; 1:139–45.

101. Rohan TE. Cigarette smoking and risk of benign proliferative epithelial disorders of the female breast. *Eur J Epidemiol* 1999; 15:529–35.

102. Friedenreich C, Bryant H, Alexander F, et al. Risk factors for benign proliferative breast disease. *Int J Epidemiol* 2000; 29:637–44.

103. Royal College of General Practitioners. *Oral contraceptives and health*. London: Pitman Medical, 1974, pp. 25–6.

104. Ory H, Cole P, MacMahon B, et al. Oral contraceptives and reduced risk of benign breast diseases. *N Engl J Med* 1976; 294:419–22.

105. Rohan TE, Miller AB. A cohort study of oral contraceptives and risk of benign breast disease. *Int J Cancer* 1999; 82:191–6.

106. Vessey MP, Doll R, Sutton PM. Investigation of the possible relationship between oral contraceptives and benign and malignant breast disease. *Cancer* 1971; 28:1395–9.

107. Sartwell PE, Arthes FG, Tonascia JA. Epidemiology of benign breast lesions: lack of association with oral contraceptive use. *N Engl J Med* 1973; 288:551–4.

108. Kelsey JL, Lindfors KK, White C. Case-control study of the epidemiology of benign breast diseases with reference to oral contraceptive use. *Int J Epidemiol* 1974; 3:333–40.

109. Kelsey JL, Holford TR, White C, et al. Oral contraceptives and breast disease. *Am J Epidemiol* 1978; 107:236–44.

110. Fasal E, Paffenbarger RS. Oral contraceptives as related to cancer and benign lesions of the breast. *J Natl Cancer Inst* 1975; 55:767–73.

111. Nomura A, Comstock GW. Benign breast tumor and estrogenic hormones: a population-based retrospective study. *Am J Epidemiol* 1976; 103:439–44.

112. Lees AW, Burns PE, Grace M. Oral contraceptives and breast disease in premenopausal northern Albertan women. *Int J Cancer* 1978; 22:700–7.

113. Ravnihar B, Seigel DG, Lindtner J. An epidemiologic study of breast cancer and benign breast neoplasias in relation to the oral contraceptive and estrogen use. *Eur J Cancer* 1979; 15:395–405.

114. Berkowitz GS, Kelsey JL, LiVolsi VA, et al. Oral contraceptive use and fibrocystic breast disease among pre- and postmenopausal women. *Am J Epidemiol* 1984; 120:87–96.

115. Parazzini F, La Vecchia C, Franceschi S, et al. Risk factors for pathologically confirmed benign breast disease. *Am J Epidemiol* 1984; 120:115–22.

116. Franceschi S, La Vecchia C, Parazzini F, et al. Oral contraceptives and benign breast disease: a case-control study. *Am J Obstet Gynecol* 1984; 149:602–6.

117. Rohan TE, L'Abbé KA, Cook MG. Oral contraceptives and risk of benign proliferative epithelial disorders of the breast. *Int J Cancer* 1992; 50:891–4.

118. Rautalahti M, Albanes D, Haukka J, et al. Risk factors for histologically confirmed benign breast tumors. *Eur J Epidemiol* 1994; 10:259–65.

119. LiVolsi VA, Stadel BV, Kelsey JL, et al. Fibrocystic disease in oral-contraceptive users. *N Engl J Med* 1978; 299:381–5.

120. Kampert JB, Wood DA, Paffenbarger RS. Oral contraceptives and breast disease. In: Feig SA, McLelland R (eds) *Breast carcinoma. Current diagnosis and treatment.* Chicago: Masson, 1983, pp. 597–607.

121. Pastides H, Kelsey JL, LiVolsi VA, et al. Oral contraceptive use and fibrocystic breast disease with special reference to its histopathology. *J Natl Cancer Inst* 1983; 71:5–9.

122. Hsieh C-C, Crosson AW, Walker AM, et al. Oral contraceptive use and fibrocystic breast disease of different histologic classifications. *J Natl Cancer Inst* 1984; 72:285–90.

123. Jick SS, Walker AM, Jick H. Conjugated estrogens and fibrocystic disease. *Am J Epidemiol* 1986; 124:746–51.

124. Nomura A, Comstock GW. Benign breast tumor and estrogenic hormones: a population-based retrospective study. *Am J Epidemiol* 1976; 103:439–44.

125. Trapido EJ, Brinton LA, Schairer C, et al. Estrogen replacement therapy and benign breast disease. *J Natl Cancer Inst* 1984; 73: 1101–5.

126. Berkowitz GS, Kelsey JL, Holford TR, et al. Estrogen replacement therapy and fibrocystic breast disease in postmenopausal women. *Am J Epidemiol* 1985; 121:238–45.

127. Pastides H, Najjar MA, Kelsey JL. Estrogen replacement therapy and fibrocystic breast disease. *Am J Prev Med* 1987; 3:282–6.

128. Sartwell PE, Arthes FG, Tonascia JA. Epidemiology of benign breast lesions: lack of association with oral contraceptive use. *N Engl J Med* 1973; 288:551–4.

129. Boston Collaborative Drug Surveillance Program. Surgically confirmed gallbladder disease, venous thromboembolism, and breast tumors in relation to postmenopausal estrogen therapy. *N Engl J Med* 1974; 290:15–19.

130. Tzigounis V, Cardamakis E, Ginopoulos P, et al. Incidence of benign and malignant breast disorders in women taking hormones (contraceptive pill or hormone replacement therapy). *Anticancer Res* 1996; 16:3997–4000.

131. Rohan TE, Miller AB. Hormone replacement therapy and risk of benign proliferative epithe-

lial disorders of the breast. *Eur J Cancer Prev* 1999; 8:123–30.

132. Berkowitz GS, Kelsey JL, Li Volsi VA, et al. Exogenous hormone use and fibrocystic disease by histopathologic component. *Int J Cancer* 1984; 34:43–9.

133. Lubin F, Wax Y, Ron E, et al. Nutritional factors associated with benign breast disease etiology: a case-control study. *Am J Clin Nutr* 1989; 50:551–6.

134. Hislop TG, Band PR, Deschamps M, et al. Diet and histologic types of benign breast disease defined by subsequent risk of breast cancer. *Am J Epidemiol* 1990; 131:263–70.

135. Rohan TE, Cook MG, Potter JD, et al. A case-control study of diet and benign proliferative epithelial disorders of the breast. *Cancer Res* 1990; 50:3176–81.

136. London SJ, Sacks FM, Stampfer MJ, et al. Fatty acid composition of the subcutaneous adipose tissue and risk of proliferative benign breast disease and breast cancer. *J Natl Cancer Inst* 1993; 85:785–93.

137. Rohan TE, Jain M, Miller AB. A case-cohort study of diet and risk of benign proliferative epithelial disorders of the breast (Canada). *Cancer Causes Control* 1998; 9:19–27.

138. Baghurst PA, Rohan TE. Dietary fibre and risk of benign proliferative epithelial disorders of the breast. *Int J Cancer* 1995; 63:481–5.

139. London SJ, Stein EA, Henderson IC, et al. Carotenoids, retinol, and vitamin E and risk of proliferative benign breast disease and breast cancer. *Cancer Causes Control* 1992; 3:503–12.

140. Trentham-Dietz A, Newcomb P, Storer BE, et al. Risk factors for carcinoma *in situ* of the breast. *Cancer Epidemiol Biomarkers Prev* 2000; 9:697–703.

141. Weiss HA, Brinton LA, Brogan D, et al. Epidemiology of *in situ* and invasive breast cancer in women aged under 45. *Br J Cancer* 1996; 73:1298–305.

142. Longnecker MP, Bernstein L, Paganini-Hill A, et al. Risk factors for *in situ* breast cancer. *Cancer Epidemiol Biomark Prev* 1996; 5:961–5.

143. Kerlikowske K, Barclay J, Grady D, et al. Comparison of risk factors for ductal carcinoma in situ and invasive breast cancer. *J Natl Cancer Inst* 1997; 89:77–82.

144. Gapstur SM, Morrow M, Sellers TA. Hormone replacement therapy and risk of breast cancer with a favorable histology: results of the Iowa Women's Health Study. *J Am Med Assoc* 1999; 281:2091–7.

145. Brinton LA, Hoover R, Fraumeni JF Jr. Epidemiology of minimal breast cancer. *J Am Med Assoc* 1983; 249:483–7.

146. Lambe M, Hsieh C-C, Tsaih S-W, et al. Parity, age at first birth and the risk of carcinoma *in situ* of the breast. *Int J Cancer* 1998; 88:330–2.

147. Brinton LA, Hoover R, Fraumeni JF Jr. Menopausal oestrogens and breast cancer risk: an expanded case-control study. *Br J Cancer* 1986; 54:825–32.

148. Schairer C, Byrne C, Keyl PM, et al. Menopausal estrogen and estrogen–progestin replacement therapy and risk of breast cancer (United States). *Cancer Causes Control* 1994; 5:491–500.

149. Colditz GA, Hankinson SE, Hunter DJ, et al. Use of estrogens and progestins and the risk of breast cancer in postmenopausal women. *N Engl J Med* 1995; 332:1589–93.

150. Stanford JL, Weiss NS, Voigt LF, et al. Combined estrogen and progestin hormone replacement therapy in relation to risk of breast cancer in middle-aged women. *J Am Med Assoc* 1995; 274:137–42.

151. Henrich JB, Kornguth PJ, Viscoli CM, et al. Postmenopausal estrogen use and invasive versus *in situ* breast cancer risk. *J Clin Epidemiol* 1998; 51:1277–83.

152. Dubin N, Pasternack BS. Breast cancer screening data in case-control studies. *Am J Epidemiol* 1984; 120:8–16.

153. Helvie MA, Hessler C, Frank TS, et al. Atypical hyperplasia of the breast: mammographic appearance and histologic correlation. *Radiology* 1991; 179:759–64.

154. Gottardis MM, Lamph WW, Shalinsky DR, et al. The efficacy of 9-*cis* retionoic acid in experimental models of cancer. *Breast Cancer Res Treat* 1996; 38:85–96.

155. Green A, Shilkaitis A, Christov K. 4-(Hydroxyphenyl)retinamide selectively inhibits the development and progression of ductal hyperplastic lesions and carcinoma in situ in mammary gland. *Carcinogenesis* 1999; 20:1535-40.

156. Mehta RG, Williamson E, Patel MK, et al. A ligand of peroxisome proliferator-activated receptor γ, retinoids, and prevention of preneoplastic mammary lesions. *J Natl Cancer Inst* 2000; 92:418–23.

157. Ip C, Ip MM, Loftus T, et al. Induction of apoptosis by conjugated linoleic acid in cultured mammary tumor cells and premalignant lesions

of the rat mammary gland. *Cancer Epidemiol Biomarkers Prev* 2000; 9:689–96.

158. Lipkin M, Newmark HL. Vitamin D, calcium and prevention of breast cancer: a review. *J Amer Coll Nutr* 1999; 18 (Suppl):392–7.

159. Ip C, Thompson HJ, Ganther HE. Selenium modulation of cell proliferation and cell cycle biomarkers in normal and premalignant cells of the rat mammary gland. *Cancer Epidemiol Biomark Prev* 2000; 9:49–54.

160. Katdare M, Osborne MP, Telang NT. Inhibition of aberrant proliferation and induction of apoptosis in pre-neoplastic human mammary epithelial cells by natural phytochemicals. *Oncol Res* 1998; 5:311–15.

161. Hargreaves DF, Potten CS, Harding C, et al. Two-week dietary soy supplementation has an estrogenic effect on normal premenopausal breast. *J Clin Endocrinol Metab* 1999; 84: 4017–24.

162. Ernster VL, Goodson WH, Hunt TK, et al. Vitamin E and benign breast "disease": a double-blind, randomized clinical trial. *Surgery* 1985; 97:490–4.

163. London RS, Sundaram GS, Murphy L, et al. The effect of vitamin E on mammary dysplasia: a double-blind study. *Obstet Gynecol* 1985; 65: 104–6.

164. Minton JP, Abou-Issa H, Reiches N, et al. Clinical and biochemical studies on methylxanthine-related fibrocystic breast disease. *Surgery* 1981; 90:299–304.

165. Brooks PG, Gart S, Heldfond AJ, et al. Measuring the effect of caffeine restriction on fibrocystic breast disease. *J Reprod Med* 1981; 26:279–82.

166. Thomas DB. Epidemiologic and related studies of breast cancer etiology. In: Lilienfeld AM (ed) *Reviews in cancer epidemiology*, Vol. I. North Holland: Elsevier, 1980, pp. 153–217.

16
Cervix

Eduardo L. Franco and Alex Ferenczy

Cervical cancer and its precursors are basically of two main histological lineages depending on whether they originate in squamous or in glandular cervical epithelium. There are important differences between these two types in terms of the etiology, natural history, detection, and prevention of the resulting lesions that require that the information be described separately. The first section of this chapter deals with preinvasive squamous lesions. Glandular precursor lesions of adenocarcinoma of the cervix will be covered later in this chapter as a separate section.

Squamous Intraepithelial Lesions

Introduction

Descriptive Epidemiology of Invasive Cervical Cancer

Cervical cancer is one of the most common malignant diseases of women. In the U.S. each year there are approximately 12,800 new cases of invasive cervical cancer with 4,600 deaths due to this disease [1]. During the last decade, an estimated 371,000 new cases of invasive cervical carcinoma were diagnosed annually worldwide, representing nearly 10% of all female cancers. Its incidence is seventh overall among all cancer sites, regardless of gender, and is third among women, after breast and colorectal cancer [2]. In developing countries, cervical cancer was the most frequent neoplastic disease of women until the early 1990s, when the breast became the predominant cancer site [3,4]. The highest risk areas for cervical cancer are in Central and South America, Southern and Eastern Africa, and the Caribbean, with average incidence rates of approximately 40 per 100,000 women per year. Though risk in Western Europe and North America is considered relatively low, at less than 10 new cases annually per 100,000 women, rates are 10 times higher in some parts of Northeastern Brazil, where the cumulative lifetime risk can approach 10% [5].

Every year, an estimated 190,000 deaths from cervical cancer occur worldwide, with over three-fourths of them in developing countries, where mortality from this disease is the highest among deaths caused by neoplasms [6]. In general, there is a correlation between incidence and mortality across all regions, but some areas, such as Africa, seem to have a disproportionately higher mortality. Less than 50% of women in developing countries who contract cervical cancer survive longer than 5 years whereas the 5-year survival rate in developed countries is about 66% [6]. Moreover, cervical cancer generally affects multiparous women in the early postmenopausal years. In high-fertility developing countries, these women are the primary source of moral and educational values for their school-age children. The premature loss of these mothers has important social consequences for the community.

Cervical Cancer Precursors

The natural history of cervical cancer begins as a slow process of disruption of the normal maturation of the transformation zone epithelium of the uterine cervix near its squamo-columnar junction. Initially, this process of abnormal changes is limited to the cervical epithelium and does not involve the adjacent connective tissue. This preinvasive phase is known variably as dysplasia, under the traditional nomenclature, as cervical intraepithelial neoplasia (CIN), according to the classification scheme of the World Health Organization (WHO), or as squamous intraepithelial lesion (SIL), as per the more recent Bethesda classification system (see later discussion on the correspondence among classification schemes). Preinvasive lesions are invariably asymptomatic and can only be discovered through cytological examination using the Papanicolaou technique (the Pap test), and their presence is confirmed via magnification by colposcopic examination and biopsy. If left untreated, early morphologically low-grade lesions may eventually extend to the full thickness of the cervical epithelium. Such a high-grade lesion used to be called cervical carcinoma-*in-situ* (CIS). Subsequently, the disease may traverse the lining formed by the basement membrane that separates the epithelium from the underlying connective tissue and become invasive. This process may take a decade or longer but will eventually occur in a substantial proportion of CIS patients. As an invasive cancer, the lesion will grow unconstrained and reach small blood and lymphatic vessels which will be the ports of entry for cervical cancer to become metastatic in nearby pelvic lymph nodes, and eventually in distant lymph nodes and other body sites. Most women with clinically invasive cancer present with symptoms and signs such as postcoital bleeding, recurrent cystitis, and exophytic, ulcerated cervical lesions, respectively. The original, primary lesion typically infiltrates the parametrium and obstructs the ureters, leading to renal failure and uremia. Pressure against nerve trunks and the sacral plexus produces persistent pain. As soon as invasion of pelvic lymph nodes occur, the disease becomes considerably worse clinically.

In the US, for each new case of invasive cancer found by Pap cytology screening there are approximately 50 other cases of abnormal smears consistent with precursor lesions. The women harboring these lesions need close monitoring by cytology and, if results persist, also by colposcopy and biopsy [7]. To this triage burden, one must add twice as many cases of equivocal or borderline atypias, also known as "atypical squamous cells of undetermined significance" (ASCUS). These women are either followed by repeat cytology or sent for colposcopic examination. Altogether, ASCUS and SIL findings account for over 10% of all Pap smears that are processed in screening programs [7], which imposes a great burden on the health care system. For convenience, the terms CIN and SIL will be used interchangeably throughout this section.

Cytopathology of Cervical Squamous Cell Cancer Precursors

Classification

Table 16.1 summarizes the various classifications systems for cervical cytopathology showing the equivalence of terms used to define preinvasive lesions. The original class system proposed by Papanicolaou was exclusively for cervico-vaginal cytology (not histology) and consisted of five numeric designations as follows: I, benign; II, minor abnormalities considered benign; III, cellular abnormalities suggestive of but not diagnostic of malignancy; IV, abnormalities strongly suggestive of malignancy; and V, changes consistent with cancer [8]. This system was widely adopted during the 30 years that followed its publication, but was modified to suit the preferences of different laboratories internationally, and to accommodate more complex subgroupings. As the field of diagnostic cytopathology evolved, and a better understanding of how cytologic changes correlate with tissue structure was acquired, refined classification schemes were proposed to replace the original Papanicolaou classes. The dysplasia designation evolved from work on the histopathology of lesions primarily by Reagan et al. [9] and quickly became adopted in practice

TABLE 16.1. Correspondence among reporting terminologies for cervical cytology and pathology reports.

Papanicolaou class system	Dysplasia terminology	Original CIN terminology	Modified CIN terminology	Bethesda system (SIL terminology)
I	Normal	Normal	Normal	Within normal limits
II	Atypia (multiple qualifiers)			Benign cellular changes (infection or repair)
II	Atypia (epithelial cell abnormalities)			ASCUS/AGCUS with qualifier[1]
II or III		Koilocytotic atypia, flat condyloma, without epithelial changes	Low grade CIN	LSIL
III	Mild dysplasia or dyskaryosis	CIN grade 1	Low grade CIN	LSIL
III or IV	Moderate dysplasia or dyskaryosis	CIN grade 2	High grade CIN	HSIL
IV	Severe dysplasia or dyskaryosis	CIN grade 3	High grade CIN	HSIL
IV or V	Carcinoma in situ	CIN grade 3	High grade CIN	HSIL
V	Invasive carcinoma	Invasive carcinoma	Invasive carcinoma	Invasive carcinoma

[1] Whether a reactive or premalignant/malignant process is favored.

Abbreviations: CIN, cervical intraepithelial neoplasia; ASCUS, atypical squamous cells of undetermined significance; AGCUS, atypical glandular cells of undetermined significance; LSIL, low grade squamous intraepithelial lesion; HSIL, high grade squamous intraepithelial lesion.

to denote lesions that were less extensive than those of carcinoma-*in-situ*. This scheme is also widely recognized as the WHO classification.

In 1968, Richart coined the term CIN to denote and grade the extent of precancerous epithelial changes in histopathology specimens in approximate one-to-one correspondence with the three degrees of dysplasia (mild, moderate, and severe) that were in use at the time. He also combined severe dysplasia and carcinoma-*in-situ* as one histological entity (CIN 3) [10]. This scheme has been in widespread use since then. In the 1980s, the realization that the pathologic changes in the cervical epithelium possibly reflected the etiologic role of human papillomavirus (HPV) infection led to the proposal of a simplified two-grade histological system that combined the abnormalities consistent with presence of the virus (koilocytotic or condylomatous atypia) with mild dysplasia to create a low-grade lesion category and assigned a high-grade CIN category to more extensive squamous changes [11].

The state of confusion caused by the existence of multiple classification schemes and their modified variants in use by different laboratories in the late 1980s led the US National Cancer Institute (NCI) to convene a workshop in 1988 to propose a new uniform system for cervico-vaginal cytology reporting. The recommendations from this workshop, and their subsequent revisions, became known as the Bethesda system [12–14]. The main feature of the new system was the creation of the term SIL as a two-tiered scheme consisting of low-grade (LSIL) and high-grade SIL (HSIL), where HPV-associated changes in the absence of other squamous abnormalities are classified as LSIL and more advanced degrees of dysplasia and carcinoma-in-situ (corresponding to CIN 2 and 3) are combined into HSIL as a single lesion grade. The rationale behind the SIL terminology was to create a uniform nomenclature of cytologic reporting which is based on the current understanding of the natural history of cervical cancer precursors. LSIL is unstable and may regress as often as it may persist (hence the term "lesion" rather than neoplasia). Because it is impossible to distinguish CIN 2 from CIN 3 and carcinoma-in-situ morphologically, and in a reproducible fashion, and because the biologic behavior of these three lesions is essentially the same, they were grouped under the name of HSIL. The Bethesda system also created ASCUS as a new category for equivocal atypias, in an attempt to resolve the ambiguity of the class II of the old Papanicolaou scheme. Unfortunately, the adoption of ASCUS created more confusion than improvement in the classification scheme, leading many laboratories to misuse this category to include also lesser abnormalities of a benign nature. In North America, the Bethesda system is largely used, but in Europe many laboratories still favor the dysplasia/CIS classification (i.e., mild, moderate and severe dysplasia, and CIS). Because of these problems and other issues with its implementation, the Bethesda system was reassessed in April 2001, after 10 years of continuous use in the US.

Morphologic Changes

The morphologic hallmark of mild dysplasia (CIN 1 or LSIL) is koilocytotic atypia (Figure 16.1). This is manifest in otherwise mature superficial or intermediate cells by enlarged, irregular nuclei with hyperchromasia and perinuclear halo ("koilos" in Greek). Other features include a slightly convoluted nuclear membrane, occasional binucleation, and a moderately increased nuclear:cytoplasimic ratio. Sometimes, the cytoplasm around the halo stains densely eosinophilic. These changes are pathognomonic of HPV infection as no other known pathogens produce these changes. Malignant basal/parabasal cells are usually not seen in LSIL Pap smears.

Moderate and severe dysplasia and CIS (CIN 2 and 3, respectively, or HSIL) (Figure 16.2) contain malignant basal/parabasal cells of different numbers (on Pap test) or levels of epithelial involvement in histology. The cytoplasm is scarce and the nuclei are large, hyperchromatic, and irregular (anisokaryosis), producing a nuclear/cytoplasmic ratio in favor of the nuclei. Nucleoli can be seen, and the chromatin is reticular or granular, with irregular bands and chromocenters. Cellular cohesion

and organization are impaired, and mitotic figures often have abnormal forms [15].

Overall, LSIL is best viewed as a well-differentiated, clinically unstable lesion that is characterized morphologically by the cytopathic effects of a productive HPV infection. HSIL, on the other hand, shows a variable degree of transepithelial disorganization with malignant basal/parabasal cells.

Descriptive Epidemiology

Sources of Data

Most epidemiologic studies of pre-invasive cervical lesions refer to prevalence data from cytopathology series, few of which are population-based. Only a fraction of the low-grade lesions found on Pap screening end up being assessed by histology. As a result, the only universal source of information is the distribution of lesion grades based on cytology, which is not a diagnostic, confirmatory test. On the other hand, a high-grade lesion found on cytology is more often than not reassessed via colposcopy/biopsy, at least in most industrialized countries. This, if it leads to a histological diagnosis of CIS, is considered the "strongest" endpoint for the purposes of epidemiologic surveillance. Few population-based tumor registries collect data on pre-invasive or *in situ* cancers; this permits only a limited assessment of the incidence of such lesions. Natural history studies represent a third source of data that is useful for epidemiologic purposes. These investigations obtain baseline cytologic information on specific population groups and are able to measure incident lesions among those who were free of abnormalities at enrolment.

Prevalence of Lesions

In compliance with specific legislation enacted in 1990, the US Centers of Disease Control and Prevention (CDC) established the National Breast and Cervical Cancer Early Detection Program (NBCCEDP), which provides grants to state health agencies to undertake screening among underserved or ethnic minority women. Although not population-based, the NBCCEDP is possibly the largest cytopathol-

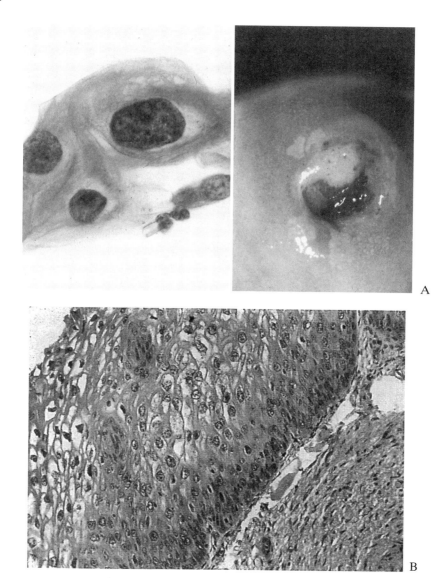

FIGURE 16.1. A: Low-grade squamous intraepithelial lesion (LSIL): On the left is the cytologic appearance of a koilocyte, pathognomonic of productive HPV infection. In contrast to adjacent normal intermediate cells, it is characterized by nuclear enlargement and irregular nuclear membrane. The perinuclear halo is not specific for HPV infection (Papanicolaou stain, magnification: 400×). On the right is the colposcopic appearance of a small acetowhite LSIL (at 12 o'clock), located near the external os of the cervix (magnification: 25×). B: Histology of LSIL: The upper two-thirds of the epithelium contains koilocytes; cell cohesion and maturation are maintained; the parabasal cells and basal layer are intact (H&E stain, magnification: 250×).

ogy database in existence that is entirely based on the Bethesda classification system and that meets very high quality control standards [7]. Given the variety of health care delivery settings providing information nationwide, the NBCCEDP provides an adequate portrait of the situation with respect to cervical cytology screening in the US today and can therefore be used as a source of prevalence data.

From October 1991 through June 1995, approximately 313,000 women had baseline Pap smears in the NBCCEDP with the follow-

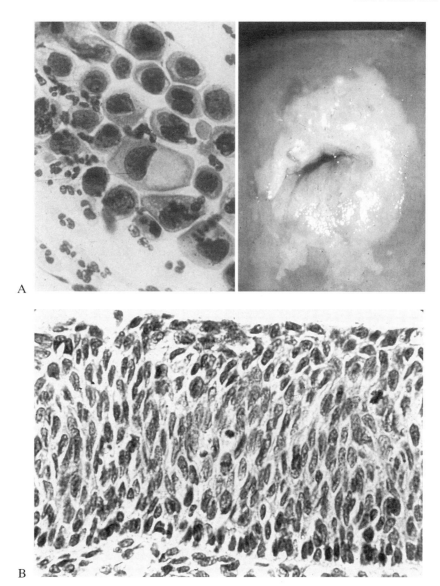

FIGURE 16.2. A: High-grade squamous intraepithelial lesion (HSIL): On the left is the cytology of malignant basal/parabasal cells with irregular nuclei and scant cytoplasm. The cells are consistent with HSIL (Papanicolaou stain, magnification: 350×). On the right is the colposcopic appearance of an acetograyish HSIL with sharp margin. Note differential color tone with the normal, immature squamous metaplastic transformation zone on the posterior lip of the cervix at the 12 o'clock location (magnification: 25×). B: Histology of HSIL: There is transepithelial replacement by malignant basal/parabasal cells, and cell cohesion and maturation are lost. An abnormal mitotic figure is seen in the upper one-third layer at the 2 o'clock position. The overall cytologic alterations are consistent with nuclear aneuploidy and high oncogenic risk, nonproductive HPV infection (H&E stain, magnification: 250×).

ing distribution of results: 81.4% normal, 7.9% benign cellular changes consistent with either infection or reactive atypia, 5.2% ASCUS, 2.9% LSIL, 0.8% HSIL, and <0.1% invasive cancer. Unsatisfactory and other diagnoses comprised 1.7% of all smears [16]. There was a marked variation in the distribution of lesion grades by age. The proportion of ASCUS smears was highest (7.6%) among women younger than 30 years of age and fell gradually to 2.7% among those 65 years of age or older. The variation was even more pronounced for LSIL diagnoses with the following prevalences by age: 6.8%, 3.1%, 1.6%, 0.9%, and 0.6%, for the age groups less than 30, 30 to 39, 40 to 49, 50 to 64, and 65 years or greater, respectively. HSIL rates also decreased with age albeit less pronouncedly than for LSIL (range 1.4%–0.3% as per the latter age groups). 13,019 women were referred for histological verification by colposcopy with or without biopsy because of the degree of abnormality shown on the screen smear. The frequencies of histologically verified lesions by grade were: CIN 1, 27.3%; CIN 2 or CIN 3/CIS, 21.9%; and invasive cancer, 0.8% [16].

Other large-scale screening programs indicate somewhat different detection rates of preinvasive lesions. For example, the cervical cancer mass screening program underway in Norway since 1990 has processed in excess of 500,000 Pap smears annually. First screen results in 1991–92 had the following prevalence figures: condylomatous changes (HPV cytopathic effects), 1.2%; mild dysplasia, 0.5% moderate dysplasia, 0.5%; severe dysplasia and CIS, 0.6%. Recording these results using the Bethesda classification (HPV effects combined with mild dysplasia and reassigned to LSIL, moderate and severe dysplasia/CIS combined as HSIL) would yield 1.7% LSIL and 1.1% HSIL [17]. A strong correlation with the woman's age was also seen—the proportion of LSIL was highest (3.2%) among women of less than 20 years of age and fell gradually to 0.1% among women of 70 years of age and older. On the other hand, the HSIL detection rate peaked at age 30 to 39, at 1.7%, and fell to 0.6% in the latter older age group [17].

Overall, the comparability among detection rates of CIN/SIL in different populations is affected by several factors including screening practices, coverage of the program, quality of the cytopathology information, cytomorphologic criteria used, and target groups. In addition to the age distribution of screenees, screening era is the single most important variable determining the relative prevalence of cervical cancer precursors in different populations. Most series indicate an increase in the detection rates of cervical dysplasia and CIS occurring throughout the 1970s and 1980s, particularly among young women [18–21]. There are probably two related reasons for the increases: a cohort effect caused by the increasingly greater proportion of women at higher risk of lesion development in successive age cohorts—that is, those with multiple sexual partners and an early sexual debut—and the intensification of screening efforts in the last 25 years in Western countries, leading to more aggressive case findings of treatable precursors.

Incidence of SIL

Despite the difficulty associated with obtaining valid estimates of the incidence rates of CIN/SIL several studies have undertaken such measurements in specific populations. Table 16.2 summarizes the published results with respect to the type of lesion outcome and the method for ascertaining lesion outcome and other study characteristics. Most publications refer to cohorts of women participating in screening programs [22–24,26–30,32–34,36, 37,39], while others present compilations from tumor registry data [25,35] or analyze specific cohorts of women assembled as a part of trials of therapy or disease-monitoring studies [31,38, 40]. Several studies were able to measure incidence rates among women who were deemed cytologically normal at enrollment [22,24,27,29–33,39,40], a critical prerequisite to remove prevalent cases from the incidence rate calculations.

Incidence rates of all grades of dysplasia/SIL are distributed within a 1,000-fold range from 4 to over 4,000 per 100,000 women–years. Study era or screening coverage period and method for ascertaining outcome are the most important factors influencing variability. Earlier studies and those reporting results for screen-

TABLE 16.2. Summary of published studies providing information on incidence rates of preinvasive cervical malignant lesions and associated abnormalities.

Study (first author, year) [reference]	Population	Ascertainment of outcome	Outcome, study period	Incidence rate (×100,000 woman-years)	Observations
Stern, 1964 [22]	US, Los Angeles	Histology	Dysplasia, 1955–64 CIS	110 (crude) 4	Screening population, all ages, Pap-negative at enrollment
Peritz, 1977 [23]	US, San Francisco	Histology	Dysplasia CIS	83 (crude) 91	Health maintenance plan cohort, N = 17,942
Parkin, 1982 [24]	England, Leeds and Wakefield	Histology or persistent abnormality on follow-up smear	Dysplasia, 1976–77 CIS	239 (crude) 69	Screening population, all ages, N = 81,890, Pap-negative at enrollment, estimates corrected for unconfirmed diagnoses
Chow, 1986 [25]	US, Atlanta	Histology	CIS, 1975–77, white CIS, 1978–80 CIS, 1981–83 CIS, 1975–77, black CIS, 1978–80 CIS, 1981–83	62 (age-adjusted) 53 40 118 82 52	Tumor registry data
Anderson, 1988 [26]	Canada, British Columbia	Histology	CIS, 1955–65 CIS, 1966–75 CIS, 1976–85	4–80 (age-adjusted) 80–140 140–220	Screening program, all ages, N = 462,000 in 1985
Miller, 1991 [27]	Canada, Toronto	Cytology	Dysplasia, 1962–81 CIS	4,292 (crude) 24	Retrospective cohort within a cytopathology database, all ages, 16,053 woman–years, Pap-negative at enrollment
Miller, 1991 [27]	Canada, British Columbia	Histology	Dysplasia, 1981–85	90 (crude), cohort 1 200, cohort 2 300, cohort 3	Screening program cohorts, N = 215,000
Friedell, 1992 [28]	US, Kentucky	Histology	All dysplasias, 1986–87: Mild Moderate Severe CIS	195 (age-adjusted) 90 59 46 38	Screening population, all ages, N = 420,000

Study	Location	Method	Outcome	Rate	Population
Gram, 1992 [29]	Norway, Troms and Finnmark	Histology	CIN 3, 1980–89	238 (crude)[1]	Screening population, N = 43,016, ages 23–72, Pap-negative at enrollment
Kainz, 1995 [30]	Austria, Vienna	Cytology	CIN, 1980–84 CIN, 1985–89	433 (crude)[1] 864	Screening population, N = 12,604, all ages, Pap-negative at enrollment
Liggins, 1995 [31]	New Zealand	Cytology followed by histology or DNA ploidy	Dysplasia or worse lesions, 1980–86	890 (crude)	Cohort using contraception, N = 7,200, ages 20–39, Pap-negative at enrollment in 2 tests
Morrison, 1996 [32]	Canada, British Columbia	Histology	CIS + invasive, 1949–92	60 (crude), cohort 1 90, cohort 2	Screening program cohorts, N = 119,000, Pap-negative at enrollment
Bos, 1997 [33]	Denmark, Maribo	Histology	CIN, 1966–82	190 (crude)	Screening population, all ages, 106,000 woman-years, Pap-negative at enrollment
Forsmo, 1997 [34]	Norway, Sor-Trondelag	Histology	CIS, 1988–92	47 (crude) 51 (age-adjusted)	Screening population, N = 127,000, all ages
Bergström, 1999 [35]	Sweden	Histology	CIN 3 + CIS, 1958–59 CIN 3 + CIS, 1968–70 CIN 3 + CIS, 1980–85	5 (age-adjusted) 100 90	Tumor registry data
Blohmer, 1999 [36]	Germany, Berlin	Histology	CIN 1–3, 1980–81 CIN 1–3, 1988–89	100 (crude) 390	Screening population, all ages
Quinn, 1999 [37]	England	Histology	CIN 3 + CIS, 1995	80 (age-adjusted)	Screening population, all ages
Kibur, 2000 [38]	Finland, Helsinki	Histology	CIN 3 + CIS + invasive, 1983–94	33 (crude)[1]	Primiparous women, all ages, N = 72,791; 221,342 woman-years
Sawaya, 2000 [39]	US, NBCCEDP	Cytology	LSIL, 1991–98 HSIL ASCUS	677 (crude)[1] 161 2,630	Screening population, N = 128,805, 15.7 mos follow-up, all ages, Pap-negative at enrollment
Sawaya, 2000 [40]	US, multicenter	Cytology, colposcopy, and histology	SIL (Pap) SIL (colpo/histology) ASCUS/AGCUS (Pap)	266 (crude)[1] 163 1,982	Hormone replacement trial of postmenopausal women, N = 2,561; 4,895 woman-years, Pap-negative at enrollment

[1] Calculated from data given in the article.

Abbreviations: CIN, cervical intraepithelial neoplasia; CIS, carcinoma in situ; SIL, squamous intraepithelial lesion; LSIL, low grade SIL; HSIL, high grade SIL; ASCUS, atypical squamous cells of undetermined significance; AGCUS, atypical glandular cells of undetermined significance; NBCCEDP, National Breast and Cervical Cancer Early Detection Program.

ing periods in the 1950s through the 1970s had the lowest rates, most likely because of the reasons mentioned above for prevalence data. With one important exception [25], studies spanning multiple periods tended to corroborate this observation [26,30,35,36]. Studies using cytology as the primary method for detecting lesions [27,30,31,39,40] tended to yield higher incidence rates (range: 400–4,000/100,000 woman–years) than those based on histological ascertainment of cytological findings (range: 4–300/100,000 woman–years). Although the sensitivity of Pap cytology is much lower than its specificity, the low prevalence of precursor lesions in screening conditions makes the false positive rate become a more critical element in the extent and direction of the measurement error than the false negative rate. Thus, the resulting rate via cytological detection is an overestimate of the true rate (see Chapter 5).

Incidence of CIS

The NCI's Surveillance, Epidemiology, and End Results (SEER) program coordinates population-based tumor registration in the states of Connecticut, Hawaii, Iowa, New Mexico, and Utah, and in the metropolitan areas of Detroit, Atlanta, San Francisco–Oakland, and Seattle–Puget Sound. Since 1973, the SEER program has systematically collected information on all cases of both invasive cancer and CIS for various anatomical sites of cancer, thus providing an adequate epidemiologic surveillance mechanism to identify time trends and risk differentials with respect to sociodemographic variables. SEER program data are available via a publicly available CD–ROM [41]. The program's stringent quality control ensures very high rates of histopathological verification for registered cases.

Figure 16.3 shows trends in the incidence rates of cervical CIS in selected SEER registration areas. On average, for most areas, rates slowly increased from 1980 to 1990 and then began to rise more markedly from 1990. Figure 16.4 shows the incidence rates of cervical CIS separately for white and black women in all SEER registration areas. The trend among white women followed the latter pattern of a more pronounced increase in rates since the late 1980s. On the other hand, rates of CIS among black women, which were twice as high as those for white women in the 1970s, declined until 1989 and then began to increase in parallel with

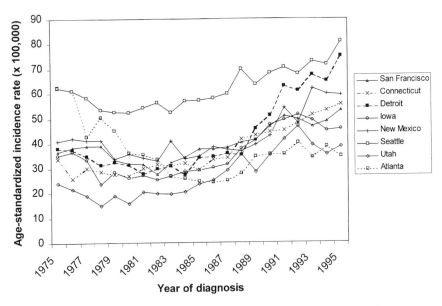

FIGURE 16.3. Incidence rates of cervical CIS in selected SEER registration areas. Rates are standardized according to the age structure of the 1970 US population and expressed per 100,000 women.

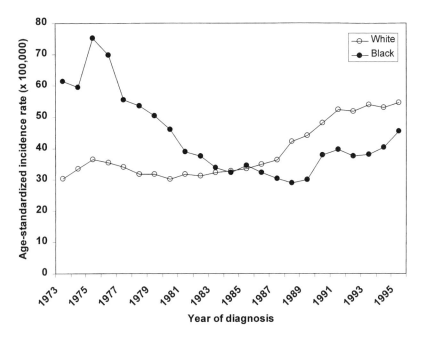

FIGURE 16.4. Incidence rates of cervical CIS by race in all SEER registration areas. Rates are standardized according to the age structure of the 1970 US population and expressed per 100,000 women.

rates in whites. Reasons for the increase in incidence in the last decade may include the intensification of screening efforts and cohort effect as described above—with screening possibly benefiting a relatively larger proportion of white women than of black women at first—but also the adoption of the Bethesda classification in the early 90s, which may have led to a more liberal interpretation of a CIS diagnosis to include moderate and severe dysplasias, lesion grades that are encompassed under the HSIL category.

Differences between precursor and invasive lesions with respect to the age when incidence rates peak provide important clues as to the duration of the preclinical phase of the natural history of cervical cancer. Figure 16.5 shows age-specific incidence rates of both CIS and invasive cervical cancer in all SEER areas averaged over the 1991 to 1995 period. The CIS incidence rate increased more steeply with age than that for invasive cancers, reaching a peak at ages 25 to 29 years (191 new cases per 100,000 woman–years), and then declined gradually at older ages. The incidence of invasive cancers leveled off after ages 40 to 44 (15–18 new cases per 100,000 woman–years), leav-

ing a gap between peak incidence rates for CIS and invasive cancer of approximately 15 years. However, considering the historical changes in screening practices and lesion classification one must consider the peak incidence rate of CIS in previous registration periods. By considering five successive calendar periods, namely 1973 to 1975, 1976 to 1980, 1981 to 1985, 1986 to 1990, and 1991 to 1995, and taking the age-specific rate at age 25 to 29 as the baseline or reference risk, the relative rates for the age group 30 to 34 years are 1.04, 0.99, 0.89, 0.83, and 0.73, for each of the latter periods, respectively, indicating a gradual shift in the peak incidence rate from 30 to 34 years to 25 to 29 years since 1973. This has been accompanied by a gradual increase in the relative rates by period for the 20 to 24 age group: 0.42, 0.51, 0.60, 0.66, and 0.80, respectively. In the last period (1991–95), the incidence rate at age 20 to 24, at 80% of that at age 25 to 29, was already greater than that at age 30 to 34, which was 73% of the magnitude of the peak incidence rate at age 25 to 29. If this trends continues, the peak incidence of CIS may eventually shift to the age group 20 to 24 years. Interestingly, however, a

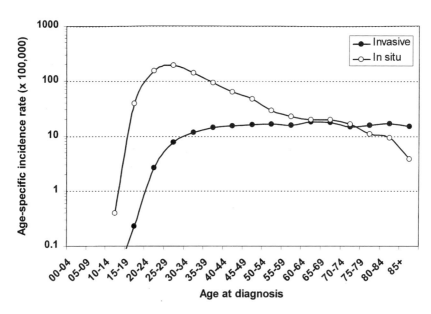

FIGURE 16.5. Age-specific incidence rates of cervical CIS and invasive carcinoma in all SEER registration areas during 1991–95. Rates are standardized according to the age structure of the 1970 US population and expressed per 100,000 women.

similar trend is not seen for invasive cervical cancer using SEER data.

Rates of Progression and Regression

Several natural history studies have analyzed risks of progression in the continuum of pre-invasive lesions stages. For the most part, these studies are plagued by the following main problems: (i) small sample size, highly selected study population, or insufficient follow-up time; (ii) reporting of crude rates of progression and regression without regard to a proper actuarial analysis of cumulative risk over time; (iii) variable methods for detecting lesion development during follow-up, that is, those using cytology cannot provide reliable estimates of lesion rates, and those using histology may have altered the course of the natural history of the disease because frequent cervical biopsies may remove the entire lesion. In sum, these problems tend to affect the comparability of results across studies. These drawbacks notwithstanding, natural history studies have been consistent at least in providing a few basic tenets: the vast majority of LSILs are transient, regressing to normal within relatively short periods.

However, some may progress to HSIL or to cancer over variable periods of time. HSIL, on the other hand, carries a much greater probability of progressing to invasion, albeit most such lesions will eventually regress. A few review and meta-analytical studies have attempted to summarize rates of progression and regression along the continuum of cervical dysplastic changes using different criteria for selecting investigations and for combining natural history data [42–46].

Östor conducted a pooled analysis of studies published from 1950 to 1993 to derive average estimates of regression and progression by grade of CIN [42]. The average probabilities of regression were 57% for CIN 1, 43% for CIN 2, and 32% for CIN 3. The equivalent probabilities of progression to CIS were 11% for CIN 1 and 22% for CIN 2, and of progression to invasion were 1% for CIN 1, 5% for CIN 2, and 12% for CIN 3. A substantial proportion of lesions were biopsied, including cone biopsy, and classified as persistent without further qualification as to the duration of the sojourn time within each grade. The percentages classified as persistent were 32%, 35%, and 56%, for grades 1, 2, and 3, respectively [42].

Mitchell et al. conducted similar overviews but considered the method for ascertaining lesions during follow-up to stratify the estimates [43,44]. Considering only studies with cytological follow-up, and all grades of CIN combined, the probabilities of regression, persistence, and progression to any higher grade lesion were 34%, 41% and 25%, respectively, and 10% of the lesions progressed to CIS, 1% to invasive cancer. The equivalent cumulative probabilities for all grades of CIN that had been followed by both cytology and biopsy were 45%, 31%, and 23%, for regression, persistence, and progression, respectively. Within the latter probability, progression to CIS was 14% and to invasive cancer 1.4%. Progression rates to invasive cancer for studies following up only CIS patients by biopsy ranged from 29% to 36% [43,44].

In a meta-analysis of studies published since 1970 involving over 27,000 patients followed without treatment, Melnikow et al. [45] calculated the following weighted average rates of progression to HSIL at 24 months according to baseline cytological abnormality: ASCUS, 7.1%, LSIL, 20.8%, and HSIL (persistence), 23.4%. Cumulative progression rates to invasive cancer at 24 months by cytological abnormality were 0.3% for ASCUS, 0.2% for LSIL, and 1.4% for HSIL. The following average rates of regression to a normal Pap smear were estimated: 68.2% for ASCUS, 47.4% for LSIL, and 35.0% for HSIL [45].

Holowaty et al. calculated relative risks (RR) of progression and regression by follow-up time for moderate and severe dysplasias, with mild dysplasia taken as referent [46]. Within a 2-year period, RRs of CIS were 8.1 for moderate dysplasia and 22.7 for severe dysplasia. The equivalent RRs of invasive cancer were 4.5 and 20.7 for the latter lesion grades, respectively [46].

Etiology

Epidemiologic research conducted during the past 30 years has been fairly consistent in demonstrating similar risk factors for cervical cancer and for its precursor CIN/SIL stages, although the strength of the epidemiologic associations seems to be somewhat lower for precursor lesions than for invasive cancer. In fact, the similarity of risk factor profiles has lent credibility to the natural history model specifying that the abnormal changes seen in the cervical epithelium in reality follow a continuum leading to invasive cervical carcinoma.

Sexual Behavior

Prominent among the risk factors is the role of two measures of sexual activity, namely number of sexual partners and age at first intercourse [47–53], and also the sexual behavior of the woman's male partners [51]. The consistency of the sexually-transmitted-disease model for cervical neoplasia led much of the laboratory and epidemiologic research designed to identify the putative microbial agent or agents acting as the intermediate cause of cervical cancer. Research conducted during the late 1960s and 1970s was focused on the possibility of an etiologic role for the Herpes simplex viruses (HSV). Although HSV was proven to be carcinogenic in vitro and in vivo, clinical studies eventually demonstrated that only a fraction of cervical carcinomas contained traces (viral DNA) of HSV infection, and epidemiologic studies failed to demonstrate an association between HSV and cervical cancer [reviewed in 54].

Role of HPV Infection

In the 1980s, a solid research base emerged implicating HPV infection as the sexually transmitted cause of cervical cancer and its precursors. HPVs are small, double-stranded DNA viruses of approximately 55 nm with an icosahedral protein capsid containing 72 capsomers. The genome is circular and contains 7,500–8,000 base pairs. Taxonomically, papillomaviruses are a subfamily in the Papoviridae family. As infectious agents, papillomaviruses are highly specific to their respective hosts. Different HPVs are classified as types on the basis of DNA sequence homology in the *E6*, *E7*, and *L1* genes. More than 120 different HPV types have been catalogued so far [55].

Clinical, subclinical, and latent HPV infections are the most common sexually transmitted viral diseases today [56]. Latent genital HPV infection can be detected in 5% to 40%

of sexually active women of reproductive age [57]. In most cases, genital HPV infection is transient or intermittent [58–62]; the prevalence is highest among young women soon after the onset of sexual activity and falls gradually with age, possibly as a reflection of accrued immunity and decrease in sexual activity (decrease in number of sexual partners) [56,63].

Table 16.3 shows the RRs for the association between HPV infection via viral DNA detection and risk of CIN/SIL as estimated in several epidemiologic studies conducted during the past 10 years [64–81]. In general, the associations are all of high magnitude—in some studies RRs greater than 100 have been observed [75,76,80]. The magnitude of the association with HSIL (CIN 2/3) is greater than that for LSIL (CIN 1). In addition, associations tend also to be stronger when viral exposure definition is restricted to HPV 16 [76,81], the main viral genotype found in cervical cancers worldwide [82]. Some studies in Table 16.3 ascer-

TABLE 16.3. Epidemiologic studies[1] of the association between cervical HPV infection and cervical cancer precursor lesions.

Study: first author, year [reference]	Method of HPV DNA detection	Lesion grade outcome and method of ascertainment	OR or RR (95% confidence interval)	Observations
Morrison, 1991 [64]	PCR	SIL on histology	10.4 (3.6–30.4)	HPVs 16, 18, 33
VandenBrule, 1991 [65]	PCR	Mild/severe dysplasia and CIS on cytology	68.1 (45.4–102.4)	HPVs 16, 18, 31, 33; cross-sectional study
Kadish, 1992 [66]	NAH	SIL on cytology or histology	17.3 (6.1–52.9)	All types; cross-sectional study
Koutsky, 1992 [67]	NAH	CIN 2/3 on histology	11.0 (4.6–26.0)	HPVs 16, 18; cohort study
Levine, 1993 [68]	NAH	HSIL on cytology	10.3 (3.3–32.0)	All types
Schiffman, 1993 [69]	PCR	CIN on cytology	18.2 (13.6–24.3)	All types
Bosch, 1993 [70]	PCR	CIN 3 on histology	56.9 (24.8–130.6) 15.5 (8.2–29.4)	All types; Spain All types; Colombia
Becker, 1993 [71]	PCR	CIN on cytology	4.7 (1.6–14.1)	All types
Coker, 1993 [72]	PCR	CIN 1 on cytology CIN 2/3	11.7 (4.3–32.0) 21.9 (6.4–74.5)	HPVs 16, 18, 33
Becker, 1994 [73]	NAH PCR	CIN 2/3 on histology	12.8 (8.2–20.0) 20.8 (10.8–40.2)	All types
Brisson, 1994 [74]	NAH	CIN 2/3 on histology	8.7 (5.1–15.0)	HPV 16
Liaw, 1995 [75]	PCR	CIN 1 on histology CIN 2/3	14.0 (6.1–32.0) 122.3 (38.5–388.9)	All types
Olsen, 1995 [76]	PCR	CIN 2/3 on histology	72.8 (27.6–191.9) 182.4 (54.0–616.1)	All types HPV 16
Sasagawa, 1997 [77]	PCR	LSIL on histology HSIL	9.4 (4.5–19.0) 77.0 (28.0–217.0)	HPVs 16, 18, 31, 33, 35, 45, 52, 58, 59
Liaw, 1999 [78]	PCR	LSIL on cytology or histology HSIL	3.8 (2.6–5.5) 12.7 (6.2–25.9)	All types; cohort study
MacLehose, 1999 [79]	PCR	CIN 2/3 on histology	8.4 (2.9–29.4)	All types
Herrero, 2000 [80]	PCR	LSIL on cytology or histology HSIL	29.0 (8.4–100.0) 320.0 (97.0–1000.0)	HPV 16
Schiff, 2000 [81]	PCR	CIN 2/3 on histology	7.9 (4.7–13.2) 41.7 (12.0–144.6)	All types HPV 16

[1] Case-control studies except as noted.

Abbreviations: PCR, polymerase chain reaction; NAH, nucleic acid hybridization; CIN, cervical intraepithelial neoplasia; CIS, carcinoma-in-situ; SIL, squamous intraepithelial lesion; LSIL, low-grade SIL; HSIL, high-grade SIL.

tained exposure to a broad spectrum of HPVs, whereas others restricted detection to only a few of the so-called oncogenic types (to be discussed later). In all, the associations are very strong; no other risk factor for cervical neoplasia is of comparable magnitude. In fact, few associations in cancer research tend to be as strong as that between HPV and cervical neoplasia—those of heavy smoking in lung cancer and chronic hepatitis B infection in liver carcinoma being notable exceptions [83].

The WHO's International Agency for Research on Cancer (IARC), in its monograph series on carcinogenicity evaluation, has classified HPV types 16 and 18 as carcinogenic to humans, HPV types 31 and 33 as probably carcinogenic, and other HPV types (except 6 and 11) as possibly carcinogenic [57]. This classification was made conservatively on the basis of the available published evidence up to 1994, which targeted primarily the aforementioned HPV types. These types were targeted because they are among the most common and because their genome sequences were published before those of other HPVs (thus facilitating widespread availability of DNA probes). However, the epithelial lining of the anogenital tract is the target for infection by over 40 different mucosotropic HPV types. Genital types are typically divided into groups based on the presumed oncogenic potential. HPV types 16, 18, 31, 33, 35, 39, 45, 51, 52, 56, 58, 59, and 68 are considered to be of high oncogenic risk because of their frequent association with cervical cancer and CIN. The remaining genital types, for example, HPV types 6, 11, 42–44, and some rarer types, are considered of low or no oncogenic risk [82,84,85]. These may cause subclinical and clinically visible benign lesions known as flat and acuminate condylomata, respectively.

Today, it is well established that infection with high oncogenic risk HPV types is the central causal factor in cervical cancer [57,63,86,87]. It may even be a necessary cause of this disease and of its precursors [88–90]. HPV infection should be considered as a risk exposure, however, since most women who engage in sexual activity will probably acquire HPV infection over a lifetime. As mentioned above, the vast majority of these infections will be transient; only a small proportion will become persistent [58–62,91,92]. A substantial increase in risk of CIN exists for women who develop persistent, long-term infections with oncogenic HPV types, as defined above [59,67,78,92–97].

Smoking

Tobacco smoking is a well-known risk factor for cervical cancer and dysplasia [reviewed in 98]. A direct carcinogenic action of cigarette smoking on the cervix is conceivable since nicotine metabolites can be found in the cervical mucus of smokers [99]. Another plausible mechanism for involvement of smoking in cervical carcinogenesis is suppression of local immune response to HPV infection [56,100]. However, proper assessment of the association is affected by confounding by other variables. Since smoking is associated with sexual behavior (women who smoke tend to have an early sexual debut and to have more partners than nonsmokers), it cannot be easily determined whether the association with cervical neoplasia is genuine or spurious because it is impossible to effectively eliminate confounding by adjusting for variables of sexual activity. Studies that attempted to control for the confounding effect of age at first intercourse and number of sexual partners (or other surrogate variables for sexual behavior) generally found an independent role for tobacco smoking in CIN with RRs for current versus never smokers in the range of 1.5–4.5 [48–51,74,101–105]. Some of these studies also found a positive trend with the number of cigarettes smoked and the duration of smoking along with lower risks for former smokers [48,74,101–105]. A few studies have failed to find any association with cigarette smoking [67,76,77,81].

One possible explanation for the variability in results may be differences in the distribution of the CIN/SIL grades in the composition of the case groups included in epidemiologic investigations. Smoking seems to be a more important risk factor for HSIL/CIN 2 or HSIL/CIN 3 than for LSIL/CIN 1 [49,50,69,74,106], suggesting that this variable acts at a later stage during the preinvasive phase of the natural history of cervical neoplasia. The variability in results can also be explained under the assumption that smoking per se may not be a risk factor (or perhaps not a strong one) and that the appearance that it is may be the result of confounding by sexual activity and its intermediate endpoint, HPV infection [107]. Under this assumption, incomplete control of confounding could account for the presumed risk elevations attributable to smoking. Some empirical evidence to that effect comes from studies that showed that the association with smoking disappears after adjustment for both sexual activity markers and HPV infection [76,77]. On the other hand, one study reported that smoking seems to be a key risk factor in progression from low-grade to high-grade lesions (particularly CIN 3) among HPV positive women with CIN, even after further adjustment for the type of HPV found in the specimen [106]. Curiously, smoking seems to exert a protective effect against the development of persistent HPV infection [58,59], a critical intermediate endpoint in the genesis of cervical lesions. The biologic rationale for this finding is not clear.

Parity

The number of live births is a consistent risk factor for cervical cancer, as demonstrated by epidemiologic studies. There is a linear trend in the parity–risk relationship association, as seen in large studies in North America and in Latin America [108,109]. An association with parity is plausible in the sense that multiple pregnancies may have a cumulative traumatic or immunosuppressive effect on the cervix thereby facilitating the acquisition of HPV infection [110]. Another mechanism that is not mutually exclusive with the above is the pregnancy-induced hormonal effect on the cervix, which could affect HPV genome elements that are responsive to progesterone [111]. Nutritional deficiencies that may develop during pregnancy may also mediate risk of cervical neoplasia (the role of nutrients will be discussed later). In analogy with smoking, epidemiologic studies must carefully control for

the potential confounding effects of sexual activity to obtain unbiased estimates of the association with parity.

The association between parity and CIN has been less consistent than that for invasive carcinoma. The association has been found in a few studies, most of which used multivariate control of confounding by sexual activity and other variables. RRs for multiple pregnancies were found to be in the range of 1.5–4.0 [49,51,69,112,113]. Parity emerged as a risk factor independent of HPV infection in some studies [50,68]. On the other hand, some investigations failed to find an association with parity either on crude or adjusted analyses [47,50,71,76,77,79,114].

As noted above for smoking, the variability in results may be related to the relative distribution of lesion grades in case series included in the epidemiologic studies. Cuzick et al. found that risk elevations trending upward with the number of pregnancies existed for CIN 3 but not for CIN 2 or CIN 1 [49].

Oral Contraceptive Use

An increased risk of cervical cancer among oral contraceptive (OC) users is found mainly among long-term users, after adjustment for most potential confounders. The association seems to be somewhat stronger for adenocarcinomas than for squamous cell carcinomas [reviewed in 115,116]. The plausibility of the association rests on the potential for hormonal effects in HPV-containing cervical cells, as it has been shown that steroid stimulation may trigger viral oncogene-related events that may culminate in integration of the virus into the host's genome [111]. Confounding is also likely to play a role, since women using contraception tend to be more sexually active than those abstaining from any method, barrier or hormonal. In addition, women using OC are less likely to use barrier methods of contraception, which has been shown in some studies to exert a protective effect against CIN [49,112–114] and cervical cancer [reviewed in 115]. It is also possible that the associations with recent OC use seen in some studies using CIN as endpoint (see later) may be due to detection bias because OC users undergo more frequent gynecological examinations than nonusers thereby enhancing detection of early disease [117]. Overall, the net effect of these biases is to confound the relation between OC use and CIN away from the null, towards a falsely inflated, positive association. Therefore, the association can only be properly assessed if variables such as sexual activity, use of barrier methods, and history of Pap smears (as an indicator of the differential surveillance of CIN between OC users and nonusers) are carefully measured and controlled for in the analysis.

OC use emerged as a risk factor for CIN in several studies with RRs mostly below 2.0 among women who had ever used OCs [47,49,74,113,114,117–120]. The excess risk was restricted to long-term users in some studies [47,49,74,114,119] and to current or recent users in others [113,117], the latter being particularly suggestive of a detection bias effect. Not all studies were able to control the analysis for the potential confounding effects mentioned above. Risk elevations seemed to be restricted to HSIL in some studies [47,49,74,119]. On the other hand, several other studies saw no increase in risk due to OC use [50,51,64,79,93,112,121], regardless of how OC use was analyzed (ever/never, duration, or time since last use). Interestingly, some of the latter studies found RRs for ever use that were below unity [50,79,112,121], sometimes consistent with a significant protective effect [112].

Dietary Factors

Much attention has been given to the role of dietary factors and serum micronutrients in the etiology of cervical cancer. The weight of the evidence for an effect of diet on risk of cervical cancer indicates that high intake of foods containing carotenoids and vitamin C and, to a lesser extent, of vitamins A and E may reduce the risk of cervical cancer [reviewed in 115,116,122]. There is ample biological plausibility for a protective effect of diet in the genesis of cervical neoplasia. Carotenoids, tocopherols, and ascorbic acid are potent antioxi-

dants that can quench intracellular reactive radicals, thus potentially preventing DNA damage. β-Carotene, in particular, may have an additional favorable property as a metabolic precursor to retinoic acid, which acts by modulating epithelial cell growth and differentiation. Dietary factors may also have a role in cervical immunity [56,122]. However, assessment of the effect of nutritional factors is complicated by methodological difficulties in measuring circulating micronutrients and in obtaining reasonably accurate diet intake information from interviews. Confounding is also an important concern because of the effects that some risk factors, such as smoking and OC use, may have on the levels of such micronutrients as folate, vitamin C, and β-carotene [123,124].

Epidemiologic studies that assessed the effects of dietary factors on CIN risk had mostly consistent results indicating protective effects for consumption of fruits and vegetables, β-carotene, and vitamins A, C, and E [122,125–129]. Two exceptions were of a well-conducted study that did not identify any associations [130] and another that found a positive, rather than an inverse, association with dietary β-carotene [131]. In general, the results based on assessment of dietary intake by food frequency questionnaires have been corroborated by assays of plasma micronutrient levels. Inverse associations have been found for carotenoids such as β-carotene [123,125,132] and lycopene [123,126], for tocopherols [132–134], and for folates [127,129,135]. Associations with retinol seemed to be less consistent or nonexistent [123,131,136]. In two studies, there seemed to be a consistent trend for the negative associations between the severity of CIN and carotenoids [132] and vitamin E [132,133]. On the basis of the strong rationale for a preventive mechanism and the empirical evidence from observational studies, a number of randomized controlled trials of chemoprevention have been conducted or recently initiated in different populations using dietary supplementation and CIN endpoints. Unfortunately, however, the results from these trials have not always corroborated those from observational studies [reviewed in 124].

Genetic Control of Immune Response

HPV infection does not always progress to neoplastic disease, and its prevalence declines with age in most populations. These facts suggest that the immune system must play a key role in the course of HPV infection. Moreover, immunocompromised individuals, including organ transplant recipients, have an increased incidence of HPV-associated diseases of the external genital skin and of CIN [137,138]. Such lines of evidence implicate immune function in the persistence of HPV infection and progression to cervical cancer. The human leukocyte antigen (HLA) genes, whose protein products are involved in antigen presentation to T cells, play a role in the regulation of the cell-mediated Th-1 immune response. Certain HLA alleles or haplotypes seem to have an influence on susceptibility to HPV infection and cervical neoplasia, probably by regulating the immune response against HPV infection and ultimately by interfering with the establishment of productive persistent infections and cervical lesions.

Several studies have reported on the role of HLA with respect to susceptibility to CIN and invasive cervical cancer, but results have not always been consistent. Both positive and negative associations have been observed for specific alleles and haplotypes, although results have varied across studies. This is likely to be due to ethnic variation in the frequency of the alleles as well as study limitations in terms of sample size and variability in typing assay performance. Another critical issue is the excessive number of combinations of alleles and their haplotypes that are analyzed in epidemiologic studies, typically in the hundreds. This inevitably leads to the discovery of some spurious associations, hence the need for consistency across studies before the validity of such HLA findings can be accepted.

The class II HLA alleles, which primarily mediate cell-mediated immune response to exogenous antigens are the best characterized. HLA class II genes are expressed in cell types that are considered to be specialized antigen-presenting cells. These include dendritic or Langerhans cells, present in the cervical epithe-lium, and macrophages, present in the subepithelial stroma. HLA class II molecules present viral peptides to naive T-helper cells via dendritic cells. T-helper cells are activated by interleukins to become cytotoxic lymphocytes (CTLs) which eventually migrate into the viral-infected epithelium producing cytolysis of HPV-infected keratinocytes.

The most consistent finding is an increased risk of HPV infection and cervical disease in individuals with the *DQB1*03* allele [137–142]. This association has been observed in European and American populations. An increased risk of CIN and invasive cervical cancer has also been associated with the *DRB1*15* allele and related *DRB1*1501–DQB1*0602* haplotype among Hispanic and Swedish patients [143–145]. Separate studies have also found an increased CIN risk among carriers of the haplotype *DQA1*0102–DQB1*0602* in Norwegian [146] and Swedish [145] populations. Conversely, protective effects have been observed for the *DRB1*13* alleles among German, American, and French populations [137,141]. Interestingly, in some studies the strength of the association for the alleles of interest was increased when the examination was restricted to HPV-16 positive cases. This suggests a genuine mediation effect for HLA control of viral exposure. Although numerous studies in geographically diverse populations have found associations with these alleles, inconsistencies nonetheless exist. A case in point is the *DRB1*1501–DQB1*0602* haplotype, mentioned above as positively associated with risk of CIN and cervical cancer. A well-conducted study in a United States population found this combination to be inversely associated with risk of HSIL [141].

Human Immunodeficiency Virus Infection

Patients infected with the human immunodeficiency virus (HIV) are prone to develop a variety of infections and health conditions in response to their debilitated immune system. HIV infection impairs cell-mediated immunity, thus increasing the risk of infections, such as HPV, that are placed in check by that arm of the immune system. HPV-associated diseases, such as genital warts and malignancies of the lower anogenital tract, and latent HPV infection per se are particularly common among HIV-infected women. In late 1992, because of the frequency of such coincidental findings, the CDC expanded the list of AIDS-defining conditions to include cervical cancer. It also included high-grade CIN among the clinical categories for surveillance of HIV-positive women [147].

Latent HPV infection and SIL are much more common among HIV-infected women than in HIV-negative women from the same populations [reviewed in 148,149]. HPV prevalence estimates among HIV-positive women in various studies since 1996 are in the range of 40% to 95%, whereas the equivalent range in HIV-negative women in the same studies is 23%–55%. The equivalent figures for SIL prevalence estimates are 10%–36% and 1%–12%, respectively [150–155]. Ancillary risk factors for SIL tend to be CD4 counts and age [148,149]. A meta-analysis of several studies published between 1986 and 1998 indicated that HPV and HIV infection seem to interact synergistically to increase risk of CIN, with some further mediation by the degree of immunosuppression [156]. With the successful adoption of antiretroviral therapy in the last few years, women are surviving longer with their HIV disease. Little is known, however, about the potential impact of HIV therapy on the natural history of SIL among HIV-infected women.

Detection and Screening

Pap Cytology

The Pap test is one of the first cancer screening tests and is undoubtedly the one with the best record of accomplishments in contemporary medical practice. Pap test screening targets mainly the detection of cervix cancer precursors, thereby allowing close monitoring of equivocal or low-grade abnormalities on repeat tests, or immediate referral for colposcopy, biopsy, and treatment of high-grade or more-severe lesions. Prevention of invasive cervical cancer is thus accomplished by arresting neo-plastic development within the cervical epithelium before it becomes invasive (see section on treatment to follow). There are two types of cervical cancer screening programs: opportunistic (or sporadic) and systematic (or organized). Opportunistic screening is carried out by suggestion from a physician or healthcare provider when a woman presents for consultation for other health reasons. Systematic screening occurs within a system that has mechanisms to identify the target population and invite all of its members to participate. There is widespread belief that systematic screening may be superior to opportunistic screening in terms of cost-effectiveness [157], but this contention has been challenged [158].

Pap-test screening guidelines vary widely. The WHO recommends at a minimum that every woman should have a Pap test between ages 35 and 40 years. If health delivery resources are available, the frequency of screening should be increased to every 10 years starting at 35 years of age, and then to every 5 years for women aged 35 to 55. The WHO best-case target is to have the frequency increased to every 3 years among sexually-active women aged 25 to 60 years [159]. The latter guideline is similar to the one recommended by the Union Internationale Contre le Cancer (UICC) [160]. More conservative variations of the UICC norm include extending the age range to 18–69 years and adopting the triennial frequency only after two consecutively negative annual Pap tests. Variations of the more conservative guidelines have been adopted by agencies such as the US Preventive Services Task Force [161], the American Cancer Society [162], the Canadian Task Force on the Periodic Health Examination [163], and other consensus workshops [164].

There have been no prospective controlled trials of Pap screening efficacy, either randomized or not. The evidence for the efficacy of Pap smear screening in cervical cancer comes mainly from three sources (see Chapters 22 and 24): (i) epidemiologic studies that indicate that the risk of invasive cervical cancer is 2 to 10 times greater in women who have not been screened, and that risk increases with time since last normal smear or with lower frequency of screening [165,166]; (ii) population surveillance, which indicates that cervical cancer incidence and mortality rates have decreased sharply following the introduction of cytology screening in Scandinavian countries, in Canada, and in the US [160,164,167], and that moreover, reductions in incidence and mortality seem to be proportional to the intensity of screening efforts, that is, the proportion of the population covered [168]; and (iii) multiple national and international consensus panels worldwide.

In spite of its success, Pap cytology has important limitations. A recent meta-analysis including only studies unaffected by verification bias indicated that the average sensitivity of Pap cytology to detect CIN or invasive cervical cancer was 51% (95% CI: 37%–66%) and its average specificity was 98% (95% CI: 97%–99%) [169]. The Pap test's high false-negative rate is thus its most critical limitation. About one-third of false-negative diagnoses are attributable to slide interpretation errors and two-thirds to poor sample collection and slide preparation [170]. False-negative diagnoses have important medical, financial, and legal implications, the latter being a particularly acute problem in North America where false-negative smears are among the most frequent reasons for medical malpractice litigation. Pap cytology is based on highly subjective interpretation of morphologic alterations and is also dependent on optimally collected samples. Also, the highly repetitive nature of the work of screening many Pap smears leads to fatigue, which invariably causes errors in interpretation. Conversely, despite the test's relatively high specificity, false-positive results will be particularly common in populations with low prevalence of CIN and cancer. False-positive cytology results lead to unnecessary and frequently invasive procedures in a fairly large number of women, and these procedures in turn result in increased patient anxiety and costs. The solution to minimizing errors in cytology is to improve the quality of smear taking, slide processing, and overall diagnostic performance of cervical cytology, remedies which incur high costs for a screening program. In many settings, especially developing countries, cytology-based programs have failed to

reduce cervical cancer rates substantially [171,172]. This state of affairs has elicited interest from the medical technology industry in developing new tests with adequate sensitivity and specificity for detecting clinically significant cancer precursors.

Cytology Automation

The general requirements for an automated screening device include sensitivity and specificity at least equal to the conventional method, a relatively low cost compared to the conventional approach, and a relatively shorter time to obtain a diagnosis. There are several automated systems being tested and marketed, ranging from robotic devices that process the cervical cell suspensions and prepare standardized thin-layer slides to computer-assisted slide scanners that map the smear to detect abnormal cells, thereby separating any slides that contain suspect images for subsequent reading by a cytotechnologist. A key advantage is the potential to alleviate the shortage of qualified manpower in cytopathology. Comparative trials, mostly funded by the private sector, are ongoing in many laboratories in North America and in Europe to answer questions related to screening efficacy and cost effectiveness of automated devices.

At present, there is only one device approved by the Food and Drug Administration (FDA) for quality control of cytology and for primary screening for cervix cancer and its precursors in the US. This is the AutoPap Screening System (Tripath Imaging Inc., Burlington, NC), which scans close to 200 conventional Pap smears a day with a high speed video camera. Morphometric algorithms indicate for the cytotechnologists to manually screen slides that contain the most likely abnormal cells. Conversely, those without likely abnormalities (approximately 25% to 50%) are filed without the need for human review. The device outperforms human review of manually screened negative smears (for quality control) by a factor of 5 to 7, and in a primary screening mode for low-risk women, performs as well as humans with a sort rate (no review of smears needed) of up to 50%. On the other hand, the device is cumbersome and its large throughput and high cost per slide make it cost effective only for large-volume laboratories [173].

Thin-Layer Liquid-Based Cytology

The ThinPrep system (Cytyc, Inc., Boxborough, MA) and AutoCyte Prep System (Tripath Imaging Inc., NC) are liquid-based alternatives to the conventional method of Pap smear preparation. The sample recovered from the cervix is suspended in a cell-preserving solution rather than placed on a glass slide. As a result, virtually all cellular material is made available to the laboratory. With the conventional Pap smear, only 20% of the cervical cells harvested from the cervix are placed manually on the glass slide [174]. In the thin-layer samples, excess blood and inflammatory cells are lysed, and approximately 50,000 diagnostic cells are randomly machine-selected and transferred as a thin layer onto a glass slide by a robotic cell processor. The slides are stained and then read by cytotechnologists. Results from clinical and epidemiologic studies have shown that automating the production of thin-layer slides can improve detection of atypical cells, precursor lesions, and cancer by producing uniformly cleaner slides free of blood, inflammatory debris, and cell clumps, that interfere with microscopic reading [174,175]. One attractive feature of this system is the ability to save the supernatant of remaining cells in a standardized fashion for subsequent panel testing for HPV DNA and for *Chlamydia trachomatis* testing [170,174,175]. The US FDA approved the ThinPrep Pap test in 1996 as significantly superior and equivalent to the conventional Pap smear for the detection of CIN and cervical cancer [176], and in 1999 approved the AutoCyte Prep System as equivalent to the conventional Pap smear for the same purposes. Additional large-scale prospective studies, using histological verification of the results for low- and high-risk women who tested negative with liquid-based cytology are needed to allow estimation of its diagnostic performance, including specificity. The data will provide a better assessment of the impact of liquid-based cytology on cervical cancer screening as well as

answers to the perceived problems of additional costs and validity that currently are impeding its more-widespread use.

Cervicography

This is a technique in which a photograph of the cervix is obtained after application of 5% acetic acid and evaluated by a specialist at a remote site for the presence of lesions. Cervicography was proposed as a cervical cancer screening tool by Stafl [177] and offers potential as a screening test in developing countries or in remote areas where well-trained cytotechnologists and colposcopists cannot be easily recruited [178]. The major drawback of cervicography in most studies is its low specificity leading to a very high rate of colposcopy referrals [reviewed in 179], a situation which might overburden healthcare resources if the technique were to be used in developing countries. A recent population-based study of 8,460 women in a high-risk area concluded that cervicography has lower sensitivity than Pap cytology for detecting HSIL but marginally better sensitivity for detecting cancers, with comparable levels of specificity [180].

Spectroscopy

This is an emerging technique under experimentation. It requires devices that use electrical and/or optical stimulation of the cervical tissue to distinguish between malignant and nonmalignant areas. The excited cervical epithelium (normal, precancerous, and cancerous) and underlying stroma reflect light or emit fluorescence, and the resulting voltage or wavelength characteristics are analyzed by a computer according to preprogrammed algorithms that distinguish normal from abnormal tissue. Limited studies with one of these devices, the polar probe, have shown promising results, but formal comparative trials confirming these results will be required before it can be recommended as a screening tool in cervical cancer [178].

Visual Inspection

Given the limited financial resources and the high prevalence of CIN and cancer in developing countries, low technology screening approaches may be attractive. Direct visual inspection (DVI) of the cervix after application of 3% to 5% acetic acid has shown great promise in such settings as a screening strategy, with performance comparable to that of conventional cytology [157,181]. In one large trial in Zimbabwe, DVI was more sensitive than Pap cytology (77% versus 44%, respectively) but had lower specificity than the latter (64% versus 91%, respectively) [182]. In another well-conducted study in South Africa, DVI had comparable sensitivity to cytology, but yielded substantially more false-positive results [183]. The high frequency of false-positive results may place a heavy demand on the limited resources of developing areas. Attempts to improve the specificity of DVI are now underway.

HPV Testing

The rationale for using HPV testing in primary screening of CIN and cancer in asymptomatic women stems from the now widely accepted tenet that virtually all cervical cancers arise from HPV infection with oncogenic types [89]. There are two main varieties of nucleic-acid hybridization techniques used to detect specific sequences of HPV DNA in clinical samples, depending on whether there is amplification of the DNA target or of the reaction signal. Polymerase chain reaction (PCR) techniques are of the former variety and the Hybrid Capture (Digene Inc., Beltsville, MD) assay belongs to the latter type. There are several HPV type-specific and consensus PCR protocols available for HPV detection. The so-called consensus protocols detect a broad spectrum of HPV types. Two consensus PCR protocols [184,185] have been widely used in epidemiologic studies of the etiology and natural history of CIN and cancer. PCR techniques are able to detect very low concentrations of target molecules in clinical samples, which makes them particularly prone to false-positive results due to contamination if appropriate specimen processing measures and laboratory containment are not used. PCR has been largely used for research purposes due to its ability to differentiate among individual HPV types. This requirement is not essential for screening purposes, because detection of oncogenic HPVs in the sample, irrespective of the type, would form the basis for referral. The Hybrid Capture assay in its current formulation [Hybrid Capture II (HC-II)], detects the 13 oncogenic types described previously (section on etiology) as a combined probe. The commercially available HC-II is the only HPV test that has been approved by the FDA for clinical use. Cervical samples are obtained by a cone-shaped cytobrush which is placed in a transport-medium–containing tube and sent to a laboratory. Alternatively, the residual cell suspension in the liquid-based cytology collection vial may be used for HPV DNA testing.

A number of studies have assessed the efficacy of HPV testing, either alone or in combination with Pap cytology, for two main purposes: for use in the triage (management) of women with minor grade cytologic abnormalities (ASCUS or LSIL) in referral smears to decide whether or not immediate colposcopy referral is warranted, and for primary screening of asymptomatic women, either opportunistic or organized. For triage purposes, a condition which calls for high sensitivity, HPV testing can improve the predictive value of a repeat Pap smear or even replace it, helping to detect HSIL or invasive lesions that were erroneously classified as ASCUS or LSIL on smears [157,186,187]. The results of a large scale trial have indicated that HPV testing may be more appropriate in the triage of ASCUS findings than in LSIL [188].

For primary screening purposes, several large scale studies have shown that HPV testing generally yields sensitivity comparable to or higher than that of Pap cytology but with somewhat lower specificity [189–195]. This raises concerns about the excessive number of women who would have to be referred for colposcopy, particularly in populations with high HPV prevalence [157,196,197]. However, by redefining the positive HPV test threshold, some studies have been able to obtain adequate levels of sensitivity with considerably lower rates of referral for colposcopy [191,193].

HPV testing has been shown to be of maximal benefit among women older than 30 to 35 years of age [190,192,196,197], in whom the prevalence of latent HPV infections is low. Primary screening via HPV testing in young women would lead to detection of a high number of cases, either without lesions or with LSIL, which have a high probability of spontaneous regression. The most attractive feature of the use of HPV testing in primary screening is the gain in negative predictive value contributed by the joint use of Pap cytology and HPV. This gain approaches 100% for HSIL [192,193,196]. This should permit longer intervals between successive screens since interval lesions are less likely to occur in the absence of high-risk HPV types [198]. Long-term follow-up studies of women screened with HPV and Pap cytology are needed to provide an empirical basis for the duration afforded by the dual negative result on primary screen. The increased screening intervals resulting in fewer repeat tests should reduce costs and allow greater coverage of screening programs. In addition, recent studies have shown the suitability of HPV DNA testing using self-obtained cervicovaginal samples in screening for CIN and cervical carcinoma, a feature which may improve compliance over current screening programmes [195,199]. Yet, the social and medical costs of identifying HPV-positive, cytology-negative women must be considered, for this may result in anxiety and clinical management problems. Indeed, it becomes problematic to identify cytologically negative, HPV-DNA–positive women if timing of HPV testing and consideration of the clinical significance of the HPV latency period issue are not handled appropriately. Consensus guidelines are yet to be developed for the management of women aged 30 to 35 years and older with a positive test for high-risk HPV types but negative cytology.

Management and Treatment

Because cytology is a screening test, not a diagnostic test, cytologically-detected ASCUS and LSIL cases may in fact be HSIL by histology. This occurs in about 30% to 40% of LSIL and 5% to 10% of ASCUS [157,186]. Accordingly, international consensus guidelines [157,160]

recommend that women with these cytological abnormalities be closely followed by Pap cytology every six months to discover those with HSIL. Persistence of ASCUS or LSIL results constitutes grounds for referral for colposcopy and biopsy. All HSIL cases must be immediately referred for colposcopy, either on primary screen or follow-up. More conservative variations of the latter guidelines are used in North America, where ASCUS and LSIL patients are frequently referred to colposcopy and biopsy when first encountered without initial cytological follow-up. As discussed above, guidelines may likely change as HPV testing has become more widely used in different settings.

Management options for LSIL (CIN 1) on histology vary widely across North America, ranging from simple observation to ablative and excisional therapies. Patients with persistent LSIL should be treated chiefly using office-based ablative therapies, because of their increased risk of progression to HSIL [170]. Management guidelines for HSIL (CIN 2 or 3) are well established and recommend colposcopically-directed biopsy with or without endocervical curettage. Ablative therapy such as electrofulguration or cryotherapy for relatively small size (<2.5 cm) exocervical HSILs may be appropriate in patients who can be reliably followed-up, since such therapy results in a 90% cure rate after one treatment and 95% after repeat therapy [200–202]. Large HSILs respond poorly to ablative therapies with cure rates no higher than 50% after repeat therapies [200]. Carbon dioxide laser vaporization results in excellent cure rates (>90%) regardless of lesion size; however, the equipment is expensive, thus precluding its universal availability. Excisional techniques using cold knife, laser, or loop electrodes for any size and distribution of HSIL result in a cure rate of over 90% after a single treatment session. Complications associated with excisional techniques are higher (about 20%) than with ablative methods (about 2%). Among excisional techniques used, the loop electrosurgical excision procedure (LEEP) [or large loop excision of the transformation zone (LLETZ)] provides the most cost-effective means to treat HSILs [201,202].

In conclusion, ablative therapy is appropriate for histologically-proven, small exocervical HSIL provided that invasive cancer has been ruled out and the patient can be reliably followed-up at regular intervals. Of all excisional techniques, the LEEP or LLETZ procedures are preferred to treat large HSILs. Only patients with cytologically and colposcopically unequivocal HSIL should be managed with the "see and treat" electroexcisional approach. Those with borderline lesions should be histologically documented by endocervical curettage and punch biopsies prior to initiating definitive treatment.

Prevention

Recognition that HPV infection is the central cause of cervical cancer and its precursor CIN has created new research fronts in primary and secondary prevention of this disease.

Primary Prevention by Education

Primary prevention of cervical cancer can be achieved through prevention and control of genital HPV infection. Health promotion strategies geared at a change in sexual behavior, targeting all sexually transmitted infections of public health significance, can be effective in preventing genital HPV infection [203,204]. Although there is consensus that symptomatic HPV infection (genital warts) should be managed via treatment, counseling, and partner notification, active case-finding of asymptomatic HPV infection is currently not recommended as a control measure. Further research is needed to determine the effectiveness of such a strategy.

Primary Prevention by HPV Vaccination

Two main types of HPV vaccines are currently being developed: prophylactic vaccines, to prevent HPV infection and associated diseases, and therapeutic vaccines, to induce regression of precancerous lesions or remission of advanced cervical cancer. DNA-free virus-like particles (VLP) synthesized by self-assembly of fusion proteins of the major capsid antigen L1 induce a strong humoral response with neutralizing antibodies. VLPs are thus the best candidate immunogen for HPV vaccine trials. Since protection seems to be type specific production of VLPs for a variety of oncogenic types will be required. Such vaccines are already under evaluation in phase I and II trials in different populations sponsored by pharmaceutical companies and by the NIH [205,206]. Immunization against HPV may have its greatest value in developing countries, where 80% of the global burden of cervical cancer occurs each year, and where Pap screening programs have been largely ineffective.

Secondary Prevention

Organized cytology screening programs have been successful in industrialized countries, but in the third world, these programs lack coverage, accessibility, effectiveness, and acceptability; these conditions are not likely to change soon because of competing public health priorities and cultural factors. General improvement in the socioeconomic status and educational level of the population tends to have a positive impact on the risk of cervical cancer by altering some of the known risk factors such as age at marriage, parity, and healthcare-seeking behavior. Other strategies such as low-intensity cytology screening (e.g., one Pap smear every 10 years after age 35), DVI, and other low-cost technologies need to be further evaluated in randomized controlled trials to determine their cost-effectiveness [157,181].

Although there is enthusiasm concerning the potential utility of HPV testing, either alone or as an adjunct to Pap cytology, for screening CIN, there are pending issues (e.g., test delivery and performance in remote areas, detailed assessment of cost effectiveness in different settings, and evaluation of the duration of the protection conferred by negative results) that need to be solved before existing Pap-based secondary prevention programs can be augmented with HPV testing. Ongoing research on the epidemiology of viral persistence will help to determine the utility of HPV testing as a screening tool for cervical cancer.

Glandular Precursor Lesions

Introduction

Descriptive Epidemiology of Adenocarcinoma of the Uterine Cervix

Compared to squamous cell carcinoma (SCC), adenocarcinoma is a much rarer occurrence in most statistical compilations of cervical cancer incidence or histopathology series. Adenocarcinomas accounted for 13.4% of all invasive cervical cancers registered in the SEER program from 1973 to 1987, including adenosquamous morphology and other glandular types [207]. Unlike cervical SCC, however, the incidence of invasive adenocarcinoma has slowly but steadily increased over the years of the SEER program [208] as well as in many western populations [209]. Age-standardized incidence rates (per 100,000 women, 1970 US population as standard) of adenocarcinoma in the SEER areas by period were: 1973 to 1977, 1.34; 1978 to 1982, 1.28; 1983 to 1987, 1.39; 1988 to 1992, 1.70; 1993 to 1996, 1.73. Analysis by stage of disease yielded similar trends, albeit the increase in incidence seems to have been somewhat more pronounced in locally detected tumors, as opposed to tumors showing regional and distant spread. Given that the incidence of cervical SCC has decreased during the same period, the proportion of adenocarcinomas among all cervical cancers has nearly doubled, from 12.4% in 1973 to 1977 to 24.2% in 1993 to 1996 [208]. The increase in incidence seems to be mostly confined to younger women in many of the populations for which time trends have been analyzed [209,210]. Likely explanations include more active case-finding by Pap cytology screening and a possible cohort effect due to increased prevalence of HPV infection. It cannot be discounted, however, that the increase in incidence may have resulted, to some extent, from changes in morphologic classification during the past three decades [211].

Adenocarcinoma tends to be diagnosed at a younger age than SCC [212] and with extent of disease at diagnosis comparable to SCC [208]. In the SEER program, relative survival rates were slightly lower for adenocarcinoma compared with SCC [208].

Cervical Adenocarcinoma Precursors

The Bethesda classification includes a category of glandular cytological abnormalities indicative of endocervical or endometrial malignancy or its precursors [12–14]. If endocervical, these abnormalities could be indicative of cervical adenocarcinoma or its pre-invasive lesion counterpart, adenocarcinoma-in-situ (AIS). An "equivocal" atypia category of "atypical glandular cells of undetermined significance", or AGCUS (also known as AGUS), has also been proposed by the Bethesda system to indicate glandular cells with changes that may be either due to benign reactive processes or glandular neoplasms [213].

Morphology of Cervical Adenocarcinoma Precursors

Cytology

AGCUS abnormalities originating from the endocervix can generally be recognized based on a larger nuclear size and more abundant cytoplasm compared with those abnormalities originating in endometrial cells. AGCUS findings should be qualified to indicate when a benign reactive process is favored or malignancy is to be ruled out. Lesions considered as indicative of AIS are designated as "atypical endocervical cells, probably neoplastic" in the Bethesda system [12–14]. AIS appears cytomorphologically as sheets of packed glandular cells with clear pseudostratification, high nuclear:cytoplasm ratio, nuclear hyperchromasia, feathering, and palisading borders [15,213]. A lesion severity continuum equivalent to CIN/SIL has not been widely used, although the term "endocervical glandular intraepithelial lesions" has been proposed by some [15]. Endocervical cytology is difficult; false-negative rates in large series ranging from 14% to nearly 100% [211,214,215]. Many cases are missed because their relative rarity precludes developing expertise in their recognition, and many AIS cases are in fact discovered on histology because of coexistent SIL, which is easy to recognize on cytology.

Histology

Histologically, both AIS and invasive forms may be classified as endocervical type, endometrioid type, intestinal type, mixtures of the above, mucoepidermoid, clear cell type, adenoid basal cell carcinoma, adenoid cystic carcinoma, adenoma malignum carcinoma, and glassy cell carcinoma. There is no compelling evidence that the histologic classification can be reproduced in cytology or that it helps cytologic detection. In fact, most cytopathologists simply divide endocervical gland cell neoplasms into well-differentiated and poorly differentiated AIS and invasive cancer [215]. The so-called "endocervical dysplasia" is a highly controversial morphologic entity, and for all purposes, its natural history is poorly documented and understood.

Colposcopy

The majority of AIS cases are not grossly visible and only a few are suspected by colposcopy. They produce no appreciable clinical symptoms or signs such as vaginal bleeding. AIS involves the transformation zone in over two-thirds of cases and is multifocal only occasionally [211,216].

AIS as a Precursor Lesion to Adenocarcinoma

AIS is considered a precursor lesion that may progress to invasive adenocarcinoma. The evidence for this contention includes: (i) there are similar cytologic features in both conditions; (ii) AIS is often contiguous to invasive cancer; (iii) the peak incidence of AIS occurs about 10 years earlier than that of invasive carcinoma [217]; and (iv) the high rate of HPV-DNA detection in both AIS and adenocarcinoma (discussed later) often with the same HPV type distribution including a predominance of HPV type 18 [57,218,219]. It is noteworthy that the glandular epithelium does not accept productive type HPV infections, thus the morphologic alteration commonly found in early LSIL (namely,

koilocytotic atypia) is lacking in endocervical gland cells.

In most series, AIS is associated with HSIL in over 60% of the cases and HPV DNA is found in up to 90% of coexistent lesions [219]. It may be that both the squamous and glandular lesions develop through a process of bidirectional differentiation from subcolumnar reserve cells initially infected with HPV 18 or 16 [211].

Descriptive Epidemiology

AIS is an extremely rare condition. Of the 64,628 incident cases of *in-situ* cervical cancers registered in the SEER program between 1973 and 1987, only 0.7% were of adenocarcinoma (0.6%) or adenosquamous (0.1%) histology [207], for an average of about 30 new cases per year for the SEER areas, or approximately 300 new cases per year if extrapolated to the entire US population. AGCUS diagnoses typically constitute less than 1% of a cytopathology laboratory workload [213]. A large cytopathology series of 177,715 specimens analyzed from 1993 to 1995 revealed AGCUS in 0.66% of the slides, and only 5% of these favored premalignant and malignant lesions. There was a significant increase in the detection rate of AGCUS findings within the same period, from 0.55% to 0.73%, but this was accompanied by a marked decrease in the proportion of such specimens that were subclassified as favoring malignancy or premalignancy [220].

While accurate estimates of progression from AIS to adenocarcinoma are not known, it is estimated that 13 years may elapse in that transition, judging from the mean ages of patients with AIS and adenocarcinoma registered in the SEER program. This is somewhat shorter than the equivalent figure for the transition between CIN and cervical squamous carcinoma, 18 years [217].

Etiology

Risk Factors

There are no published epidemiologic studies of risk factors that have focused exclusively on

AIS. There are only a few studies on the etiology of cervical adenocarcinomas [221–228]. In general, these studies have shown that risk factors are similar to those for cervical SCC including parity, early age at first intercourse, multiple sexual partners, and a history of sexually transmitted diseases, although the associations for adenocarcinomas seem to be weaker than those for SCC concerning sexual behavior, reproductive, or socioeconomic factors [210,225,229].

There is increasing evidence supporting the hypothesis of a hormone–adenocarcinoma relationship. The evidence comes from the following findings: (i) AIS and adenocarcinomas are commonly encountered in pregnant women [211]; (ii) adenocarcinoma or hyperplasia seem to be associated with OC use [226,227,230–233] or with estrogen replacement therapy [228]; and (iii) adenocarcinomas often contain estrogen and progesterone receptors [234].

While earlier studies failed to show a link between OC use and cervical adenocarcinoma, more recent well-conducted case-control studies found an increased risk, including increased risk of adenosquamous carcinomas [221,224,226,227]. RR estimates for women who have ever used OCs are in the range of 2 to 3, and there is a significant trend upward with greater duration of OC use. These associations seem to be independent from those of potential confounders [221,224,226]. However, a more recent study, using more accurate determination of HPV in cervical specimens, found that adjustment for HPV and other potential confounders made the association between OC use and adenocarcinoma disappear, although it persisted significantly elevated for AIS [227]. There seems to be no indication that the effect of OC use in adenocarcinoma is secondary due to a detection bias effect among pill users, since the association persists after adjustment for lifetime number of cervical smears [221,226].

The association between adenocarcinoma risk and hormone replacement therapy seems to be stronger than that for cervical SCCs with a doubling in RRs among women who have ever used hormone replacement therapy. Unopposed estrogens seem to convey much of the risk elevation [228]. The association with OC use and other exogenous estrogens is plausible since progestational agents have been shown to be tumorigenic in nude mice inoculated with baby rat kidney cells infected with HPV 16 and with cellular oncogenes activated [235].

Cigarette smoking and dietary factors such as β-carotene, vitamin C, and folate have not been linked with cervical adenocarcinoma risk [236]. Associations with obesity, hypertension, and diabetes remain to be confirmed [210]. Overall, adenocarcinoma of the cervix has an intermediate risk factor profile between those for cervical SCC and endometrial cancer (see Chapter 17).

Role of HPV Infection

Several studies using *in-situ* hybridization, Southern blot, and PCR methods have demonstrated HPV DNA in AIS and cervical adenocarcinomas [reviewed in 57,211]. The prevalence of HPV DNA in these lesions range from 0% to 69%, using *in-situ* hybridization, and from 15% to 90%, using Southern blot hybridization or PCR. HPV 18 is the predominant type in most studies, in contrast with cervical SCCs, which contain HPV 16 as the prevailing type [57,211,237]. Although the evidence implicating HPV in the genesis of adenocarcinomas is not as abundant as it is for SCC because of the scarcity of large scale molecular epidemiology studies, the association is considered causal for this histological type as well. The IARC evaluation of carcinogenicity for HPV did not specifically qualify the strength of the evidence for adenocarcinomas, but concluded that both HPVs 16 and 18 were human carcinogens for the uterine cervix [57].

Detection and Management

In general, Pap smear screening has not been highly effective in detecting AIS and cervical adenocarcinomas [238]. However, epidemiologic studies have suggested protective effects for shorter smear intervals and for ever being screened [166,225,229]. Pap cytology has higher false-negative rates with adenocarcinomas than with SCCs [211]. This issue is particularly important because a high proportion of rapidly progressing tumors are likely to be adenocarcinomas [217,239].

AGCUS findings should be closely followed-up by repeat cytology if reported as "favors benign atypia". However, patients with persistent AGCUS smears (two) should be referred for colposcopy and biopsy. The same is true for those in whom neoplasia is favored [240,241]. More recently, HPV testing in AGCUS patients has been suggested to be an option as a way to decide who should be sent for colposcopy given the very high prevalence of HPV in AIS [242]. AIS patients should undergo conization with careful consideration given to the extent of the upper excisional margin in the endocervix. At least 12 to 15 mm of internal endocervical tissue should be excised [157]. If fertility preservation is not required, hysterectomy will provide a safer alternative, but conservative treatment by conization offers a viable approach provided that close follow-up monitoring can be guaranteed [241,243].

Conclusions

Of all anatomical sites of cancer, the cervix has been the one most extensively studied with respect to the natural history of precancerous lesions. This is because of the importance of cervical cancer and the accessibility of the cervix for direct visual examination and tissue sampling for microscopy. Pap smear screening offered an earlier solution to the critical problem of the cervical cancer burden throughout the world 40 to 50 years ago. The widespread availability of Pap screening to detect preinvasive cervical lesions has helped decrease the incidence and mortality from cervical cancer from about 40 to 50 women per 100,000, in the early 60s, to around 10 cases per 100,000, in the late 90s in Western developed nations. Substantial progress has also been made in the last 25 years in the identification of the etiological factors of cervical neoplasia, resulting in the acceptance that the disease has a central cause, HPV infection, which may ultimately be proven to be a *sine qua non* condition for neoplastic

development. This has led to promising new avenues in prevention, both primary and secondary. In addition, the enormous progress in molecular biology and epidemiology in the last couple of decades has greatly helped our understanding of the natural history of HPV infection and precancerous lesions of the cervix as well as our understanding of the host and viral characteristics that mediate risk of disease.

The next few years will indicate whether or not the potential exists for preventing persistent HPV infection by immunization, a key first step in moving towards preventing cervical cancer by vaccination of at-risk women throughout the world. Secondary prevention fronts have continued to advance at a fast pace, however, since the vaccine-based approach will take at least a decade to be properly evaluated in controlled trials. The difficulty in properly implementing Pap screening programs in resource-poor countries has spawned new research endeavors into the development and assessment of new and more practical technologies for detection of cervical neoplastic precursors. Informed witnesses of the progress that has characterized the fields of cervical carcinogenesis and the prevention of cervical cancer will be tempted to conclude that possibly no other areas in cancer research have had as coherent a progress in the same time span, and certainly none have as optimistic a prospect.

References

1. Ries LAG, Eisner MP, Kosary CL, et al. (eds) *SEER Cancer Statistics Review, 1973–1997*, Bethesda, MD: National Cancer Institute, 2000.
2. Parkin DM, Pisani P, Ferlay J. Estimates of the worldwide incidence of 25 major cancers in 1990. *Int J Cancer* 1999; 80:827–41.
3. Parkin DM, Pisani P, Ferlay J. Estimates of the worldwide incidence of 18 major cancers in 1985. *Int J Cancer* 1993; 54:594–606.
4. Ferlay J, Parkin DM, Pisani P. *GLOBOCAN: cancer incidence and mortality worldwide. International Agency for Research on Cancer (IARC) Cancer Base 3.* Lyon, International Agency for Research on Cancer, 1998.
5. Muir C, Waterhouse J, Mack T, et al. *Cancer incidence in five continents, Vol. V. IARC Scien-*

tific Publications No. 88, International Agency for Research on Cancer: Lyon, 1987.

6. Pisani P, Parkin DM, Bray F, et al. Estimates of the worldwide mortality from 25 cancers in 1990. *Int J Cancer* 1999; 83:18–29.

7. CDC. Results from the National Breast and Cervical Cancer Early Detection Program, October 31, 1991–September 30, 1993. *MMWR* 1994; 43:530–4.

8. Papanicolaou GN. *Atlas of exfoliative cytology*. Cambridge, MA: Harvard University Press, 1954.

9. Reagan JW, Seidemann IL, Saracusa Y. The cellular morphology of carcinoma in situ and dysplasia or atypical hyperplasia of the uterine cervix. *Cancer* 1953; 6:224–35.

10. Richart RM. Natural history of cervical intra-epithelial neoplasia. *Clin Obstet Gynecol* 1968; 5:748–84.

11. Richart RM. A modified terminology for cervical intraepithelial neoplasia. *Obstet Gynecol* 1990; 75:131–3.

12. Solomon D. The 1988 Bethesda system for reporting cervical/vaginal cytologic diagnoses. Developed and approved at the National Cancer Institute Workshop, Bethesda, Maryland, USA, December, 12–13, 1988. *Acta Cytol* 1989; 33:567–74.

13. Kurman RJ, Malkasian GD Jr, Sedlis A, et al. From Papanicolaou to Bethesda: the rationale for a new cervical cytologic classification. *Obstet Gynecol* 1991; 77:779–82.

14. National Cancer Institute Workshop. The Bethesda System for reporting cervical/vaginal cytologic diagnoses: revised after the second National Cancer Institute Workshop, April 29–30, 1991. *Acta Cytol* 1993; 37:115–24.

15. Meisels A, Morin C. *Cytopathology of the uterus*, 2nd ed. Chicago: ASCP Press, 1997.

16. Lawson HW, Lee NC, Thames SF, et al. Cervical cancer screening among low-income women: results of a national screening program, 1991–1995. *Obstet Gynecol* 1998; 92:745–52.

17. Bjorge T, Gunbjorud AB, Langmark F, et al. Cervical mass screening in Norway—510,000 smears a year. *Cancer Detect Prev* 1994; 18: 463–70.

18. Dietl J, Semm K, Hedderich J, et al. CIN and preclinical cervical carcinoma. A study of morbidity trends over a 10-year period. *Int J Gynaecol Obstet* 1983; 21:283–9.

19. Learmonth GM, Durcan CM, Beck JD. The changing incidence of cervical intra-epithelial neoplasia. *S Afr Med J* 1990; 77:637–9.

20. Utagawa ML, Pereira SM, Cavaliere MJ, et al. Cervical intraepithelial neoplasia in adolescents: study of cytological findings between 1987 and 1995 in Sao Paulo State-Brazil. *Arch Gynecol Obstet* 1998; 262:59–64.

21. Sigurdsson K. Trends in cervical intra-epithelial neoplasia in Iceland through 1995: evaluation of targeted age groups and screening intervals. *Acta Obstet Gynecol Scand* 1999; 78: 486–92.

22. Stern E, Neely PM. Dysplasia of the uterine cervix: incidence of regression, recurrence, and cancer. *Cancer* 1964; 17:508–12.

23. Peritz E, Ramcharan S, Frank J, et al. The incidence of cervical cancer and duration of oral contraceptive use. *Am J Epidemiol* 1977; 106:462–9.

24. Parkin DM, Hodgson P, Clayden AD. Incidence and prevalence of preclinical carcinoma of cervix in a British population. *Br J Obstet Gynaecol* 1982; 89:564–70.

25. Chow WH, Greenberg RS, Liff JM. Decline in the incidence of carcinoma in situ of the cervix. *Am J Public Health* 1986; 76:1322–4.

26. Anderson GH, Boyes DA, Benedet JL, et al. Organisation and results of the cervical cytology screening programme in British Columbia, 1955–85. *Br Med J* 1988; 296:975–8.

27. Miller AB, Knight J, Narod S. The natural history of cancer of the cervix, and the implications for screening policy. In: Miller AB, Chamberlain J, Day NE, Hakama M, Prorok PC (eds) *Cancer screening*. Cambridge (UK): Cambridge Press, 1991, pp. 141–52.

28. Friedell GH, Tucker TC, McManmon E, et al. Incidence of dysplasia and carcinoma of the uterine cervix in an Appalachian population. *J Natl Cancer Inst* 1992; 84:1030–2.

29. Gram IT, Macaluso M, Churchill J, et al. Trichomonas vaginalis (TV) and human papillomavirus (HPV) infection and the incidence of cervical intraepithelial neoplasia (CIN) grade III. *Cancer Causes Control* 1992; 3:231–6.

30. Kainz C, Gitsch G, Heinzl H, et al. Incidence of cervical smears indicating dysplasia among Austrian women during the 1980s. *Br J Obstet Gynaecol* 1995; 102:541–4.

31. New Zealand Contraception and Health Study Group. An attempt to estimate the incidence of cervical dysplasia in a group of New Zealand women using contraception. *Epidemiology* 1995; 6:121–6.

32. Morrison BJ, Coldman AJ, Boyes DA, et al. Forty years of repeated screening: the signifi-

cance of carcinoma in situ. *Br J Cancer* 1996; 74:814–19.

33. Bos AB, van Ballegooijen M, van Oortmarssen GJ, et al. Nonprogression of cervical intraepithelial neoplasia estimated from population-screening data. *Br J Cancer* 1997; 75:124–30.

34. Forsmo S, Buhaug H, Skjeldestad FE, et al. Treatment of pre-invasive conditions during opportunistic screening and its effectiveness on cervical cancer incidence in one Norwegian county. *Int J Cancer* 1997; 71:4–8.

35. Bergstrom R, Sparen P, Adami HO. Trends in cancer of the cervix uteri in Sweden following cytological screening. *Br J Cancer* 1999; 81: 159–66.

36. Blohmer JU, Schmalisch G, Klette I, et al. Increased incidence of cervical intraepithelial neoplasia in young women in the Mitte district, Berlin, Germany. *Acta Cytol* 1999; 43:195–200.

37. Quinn M, Babb P, Jones J, et al. Effect of screening on incidence of and mortality from cancer of cervix in England: evaluation based on routinely collected statistics. *Brit Med J* 1999; 318:904–8.

38. Kibur M, af Geijerstamm V, Pukkala E, et al. Attack rates of human papillomavirus type 16 and cervical neoplasia in primiparous women and field trial designs for HPV16 vaccination. *Sex Transm Infect* 2000; 76:13–17.

39. Sawaya GF, Kerlikowske K, Lee NC, et al. Frequency of cervical smear abnormalities within 3 years of normal cytology. *Obstet Gynecol* 2000; 96:219–23.

40. Sawaya GF, Grady D, Kerlikowske K, et al. The positive predictive value of cervical smears in previously screened postmenopausal women: The Heart and Estrogen/progestin Replacement Study (HERS). *Ann Intern Med* 2000; 133:942–50.

41. National Cancer Institute. Surveillance, Epidemiology, and End Results (SEER) program. Available from: URL: *http://www-seer.ims.nci.nih.gov/*

42. Östor AG. Natural history of cervical intraepithelial neoplasia: a critical review. *Int J Gynecol Pathol* 1993; 12:186–92.

43. Mitchell MF, Hittelman WN, Hong WK, et al. The natural history of cervical intraepithelial neoplasia: an argument for intermediate endpoint biomarkers. *Cancer Epidemiol Biomarkers Prev* 1994; 3:619–26.

44. McIndoe WA, McLean MR, Jones RW, et al. The invasive potential of carcinoma in situ of the cervix. *Obstet Gynecol* 1984; 64:451–8.

45. Melnikow J, Nuovo J, Willan AR, et al. Natural history of cervical squamous intraepithelial lesions: a meta-analysis. *Obstet Gynecol* 1998; 92(4 Pt 2):727–35.

46. Holowaty P, Miller AB, Rohan T, et al. Natural history of dysplasia of the uterine cervix. *J Natl Cancer Inst* 1999; 91:252–8.

47. Harris RW, Brinton LA, Cowdell RH, et al. Characteristics of women with dysplasia or carcinoma in situ of the cervix uteri. *Br J Cancer* 1980; 42:359–69.

48. Brock KE, MacLennan R, Brinton LA, et al. Smoking and infectious agents and risk of in situ cervical cancer in Sydney, Australia. *Cancer Res* 1989; 49:4925–8.

49. Cuzick J, Singer A, De Stavola BL, et al. Case-control study of risk factors for cervical intraepithelial neoplasia in young women. *Eur J Cancer* 1990; 26:684–90.

50. Parazzini F, La Vecchia C, Negri E, et al. Risk factors for cervical intraepithelial neoplasia. *Cancer* 1992; 69:2276–82.

51. Munoz N, Bosch FX, de Sanjose S, et al. Risk factors for cervical intraepithelial neoplasia grade III/carcinoma in situ in Spain and Colombia. *Cancer Epidemiol Biomarkers Prev* 1993; 2:423–31.

52. de Vet HC, Sturmans F. Risk factors for cervical dysplasia: implications for prevention. *Public Health* 1994; 108:241–9.

53. Kjellberg L, Wang Z, Wiklund F, et al. Sexual behaviour and papillomavirus exposure in cervical intraepithelial neoplasia: a population-based case-control study. *J Gen Virol* 1999; 80: 391–8.

54. Franco EL. Viral etiology of cervical cancer: a critique of the evidence. *Rev Infect Dis* 1991; 13:1195–206.

55. zur Hausen H. Papillomaviruses causing cancer: evasion from host-cell control in early events in carcinogenesis. *J Natl Cancer Inst* 2000; 92:690–8.

56. Cox JT. Epidemiology of cervical intraepithelial neoplasia: the role of human papillomavirus. *Baillieres Clin Obstet Gynaecol* 1995; 9:1–37.

57. IARC Working Group. *Human papillomaviruses. IARC Monographs on the evaluation of carcinogenic risks to humans*, Vol. 64. Lyon: International Agency for Research on Cancer, 1995.

58. Hildesheim A, Schiffman MH, Gravitt PE, et al. Persistence of type-specific human papillomavirus infection among cytologically normal women. *J Infect Dis* 1994; 169:235–40.

59. Ho GY, Bierman R, Beardsley L, et al. Natural history of cervicovaginal papillomavirus infection in young women. *N Engl J Med* 1998; 338:423–8.

60. Franco EL, Villa LL, Sobrinho JP, et al. Epidemiology of acquisition and clearance of cervical human papillomavirus infection in women from a high-risk area for cervical cancer. *J Infect Dis* 1999; 180:1415–23.

61. Thomas KK, Hughes JP, Kuypers JM, et al. Concurrent and sequential acquisition of different genital human papillomavirus types. *J Infect Dis* 2000; 182:1097–102.

62. Liaw KL, Hildesheim A, Burk RD, et al. A prospective study of human papillomavirus (HPV) type 16 DNA detection by polymerase chain reaction and its association with acquisition and persistence of other HPV types. *J Infect Dis* 2001; 183:8–15.

63. Schiffman MH, Brinton LA. The epidemiology of cervical carcinogenesis. *Cancer* 1995; 76 (10 Suppl):1888–901.

64. Morrison EA, Ho GY, Vermund SH, et al. Human papillomavirus infection and other risk factors for cervical neoplasia: a case-control study. *Int J Cancer* 1991; 49:6–13.

65. Van Den Brule AJ, Walboomers JM, Du Maine M, et al. Difference in prevalence of human papillomavirus genotypes in cytomorphologically normal cervical smears is associated with a history of cervical intraepithelial neoplasia. *Int J Cancer* 1991; 48:404–8.

66. Kadish AS, Hagan RJ, Ritter DB, et al. Biologic characteristics of specific human papillomavirus types predicted from morphology of cervical lesions. *Hum Pathol* 1992; 23:1262–9.

67. Koutsky LA, Holmes KK, Critchlow CW, et al. A cohort study of the risk of cervical intraepithelial neoplasia grade 2 or 3 in relation to papillomavirus infection. *N Engl J Med* 1992; 327:1272–8.

68. Levine AJ, Harper J, Hilborne L, et al. HPV DNA and the risk of squamous intraepithelial lesions of the uterine cervix in young women. *Am J Clin Pathol* 1993; 100:6–11.

69. Schiffman MH, Bauer HM, Hoover RN, et al. Epidemiologic evidence showing that human papillomavirus infection causes most cervical intraepithelial neoplasia. *J Natl Cancer Inst* 1993; 85:958–64.

70. Bosch FX, Munoz N, de Sanjose S, et al. Human papillomavirus and cervical intraepithelial neoplasia grade III/carcinoma in situ: a case-control study in Spain and Colombia. *Cancer Epidemiol Biomarkers Prev* 1993; 2:415–22.

71. Becker TM, Wheeler CM, McPherson RS, et al. Risk factors for cervical dysplasia in southwestern American Indian women: a pilot study. *Alaska Med* 1993; 35:255–63.

72. Coker AL, Jenkins GR, Busnardo MS, et al. Human papillomaviruses and cervical neoplasia in South Carolina. *Cancer Epidemiol Biomarkers Prev* 1993; 2:207–12.

73. Becker TM, Wheeler CM, McGough NS, et al. Sexually transmitted diseases and other risk factors for cervical dysplasia among southwestern Hispanic and non-Hispanic white women. *JAMA* 1994; 271:1181–8.

74. Brisson J, Morin C, Fortier M, et al. Risk factors for cervical intraepithelial neoplasia: differences between low- and high-grade lesions. *Am J Epidemiol* 1994; 140:700–10.

75. Liaw KL, Hsing AW, Chen CJ, et al. Human papillomavirus and cervical neoplasia: a case-control study in Taiwan. *Int J Cancer* 1995; 62:565–71.

76. Olsen AO, Gjoen K, Sauer T, et al. Human papillomavirus and cervical intraepithelial neoplasia grade II-III: a population-based case-control study. *Int J Cancer* 1995; 61:312–15.

77. Sasagawa T, Dong Y, Saijoh K, et al. Human papillomavirus infection and risk determinants for squamous intraepithelial lesion and cervical cancer in Japan. *Jpn J Cancer Res* 1997; 88:376–84.

78. Liaw KL, Glass AG, Manos MM, et al. Detection of human papillomavirus DNA in cytologically normal women and subsequent cervical squamous intraepithelial lesions. *J Natl Cancer Inst* 1999; 91:954–60.

79. MacLehose RF, Harpster A, Lanier AP, et al. Risk factors for cervical intraepithelial neoplasm in Alaska Native women: a pilot study. *Alaska Med* 1999; 41:76–85.

80. Herrero R, Hildesheim A, Bratti C, et al. Population-based study of human papillomavirus infection and cervical neoplasia in rural Costa Rica. *J Natl Cancer Inst* 2000; 92:464–74.

81. Schiff M, Becker TM, Masuk M, et al. Risk factors for cervical intraepithelial neoplasia in southwestern American Indian women. *Am J Epidemiol* 2000; 152:716–26.

82. Bosch FX, Manos MM, Munoz N, et al. Prevalence of human papillomavirus in cervical cancer: a worldwide perspective. International Biological Study on Cervical Cancer (IBSCC)

Study Group. *J Natl Cancer Inst* 1995; 87: 796–802.

83. Franco EL. Cancer causes revisited: human papillomavirus and cervical neoplasia. *J Natl Cancer Inst* 1995; 87:779–80.

84. Lorincz AT, Reid R, Jenson AB, et al. Human papillomavirus infection of the cervix: relative risk associations of 15 common anogenital types. *Obstet Gynecol* 1992; 79:328–37.

85. Bauer HM, Hildesheim A, Schiffman MH, et al. Determinants of genital human papillomavirus infection in low-risk women in Portland, Oregon. *Sex Transm Dis* 1993; 20:274–8.

86. Herrero R. Epidemiology of cervical cancer. *J Natl Cancer Inst Monogr* 1996; 21:1–6.

87. Holly EA. Cervical intraepithelial neoplasia, cervical cancer, and HPV. *Annu Rev Public Health* 1996; 17:69–84.

88. Walboomers JM, Meijer CJ. Do HPV-negative cervical carcinomas exist? *J Pathol* 1997; 181:253–4.

89. Walboomers JM, Jacobs MV, Manos MM, et al. Human papillomavirus is a necessary cause of invasive cervical cancer worldwide. *J Pathol* 1999; 189:12–19.

90. Franco EL, Rohan TE, Villa LL. Epidemiologic evidence and human papillomavirus infection as a necessary cause of cervical cancer. *J Natl Cancer Inst* 1999; 91:506–11.

91. Franco EL, Villa LL, Rahal P, et al. Molecular variant analysis as an epidemiological tool to study persistence of cervical human papillomavirus infection. *J Natl Cancer Inst* 1994; 86:1558–9.

92. Moscicki AB, Shiboski S, Broering J, et al. The natural history of human papillomavirus infection as measured by repeated DNA testing in adolescent and young women. *J Pediatr* 1998; 132:277–84.

93. Ho GY, Burk RD, Klein S, et al. Persistent genital human papillomavirus infection as a risk factor for persistent cervical dysplasia. *J Natl Cancer Inst* 1995; 87:1365–71.

94. Remmink AJ, Walboomers JM, Helmerhorst TJ, et al. The presence of persistent high-risk HPV genotypes in dysplastic cervical lesions is associated with progressive disease: natural history up to 36 months. *Int J Cancer* 1995; 61:306–11.

95. Londesborough P, Ho L, Terry G, et al. Human papillomavirus genotype as a predictor of persistence and development of high-grade lesions in women with minor cervical abnormalities. *Int J Cancer* 1996; 69:364–8.

96. Nobbenhuis MA, Walboomers JM, Helmerhorst TJ, et al. Relation of human papillomavirus status to cervical lesions and consequences for cervical-cancer screening: a prospective study. *Lancet* 1999; 354:20–5.

97. Ylitalo N, Josefsson A, Melbye M, et al. A prospective study showing long-term infection with human papillomavirus 16 before the development of cervical carcinoma in situ. *Cancer Res* 2000; 60:6027–32.

98. Winkelstein W Jr. Smoking and cervical cancer—current status: a review. *Am J Epidemiol* 1990; 131:945–57.

99. Schiffman MH, Haley NJ, Felton JS, et al. Biochemical epidemiology of cervical neoplasia: measuring cigarette smoke constituents in the cervix. *Cancer Res* 1987; 47:3886–8.

100. Palefsky JM, Holly EA. Molecular virology and epidemiology of human papillomavirus and cervical cancer. *Cancer Epidemiol Biomarkers Prev* 1995; 4:415–28.

101. Lyon JL, Gardner JW, West DW, et al. Smoking and carcinoma in situ of the uterine cervix. *Am J Public Health* 1983; 73:558–62.

102. La Vecchia C, Franceschi S, Decarli A, et al. Cigarette smoking and the risk of cervical neoplasia. *Am J Epidemiol* 1986; 123:22–9.

103. Gram IT, Austin H, Stalsberg H. Cigarette smoking and the incidence of cervical intraepithelial neoplasia, grade III, and cancer of the cervix uteri. *Am J Epidemiol* 1992; 135:341–6.

104. Becker TM, Wheeler CM, McGough NS, et al. Cigarette smoking and other risk factors for cervical dysplasia in southwestern Hispanic and non-Hispanic white women. *Cancer Epidemiol Biomarkers Prev* 1994; 3:113–19.

105. de Vet HC, Sturmans F, Knipschild PG. The role of cigarette smoking in the etiology of cervical dysplasia. *Epidemiology* 1994; 5:631–3.

106. Ho GY, Kadish AS, Burk RD, et al. HPV 16 and cigarette smoking as risk factors for high-grade cervical intra-epithelial neoplasia. *Int J Cancer* 1998; 78:281–5.

107. Phillips AN, Smith GD. Cigarette smoking as a potential cause of cervical cancer: has confounding been controlled? *Int J Epidemiol* 1994; 23:42–9.

108. Brinton LA, Hamman RF, Huggins GR, et al. Sexual and reproductive risk factors for invasive squamous cell cervical cancer. *J Natl Cancer Inst* 1987; 79:23–30.

109. Brinton LA, Reeves WC, Brenes MM, et al. Parity as a risk factor for cervical cancer. *Am J Epidemiol* 1989; 130:486–96.

110. Schneider A, Hotz M, Gissmann L. Increased prevalence of human papillomaviruses in the lower genital tract of pregnant women. *Int J Cancer* 1987; 40:198–201.

111. Pater MM, Mittal R, Pater A. Role of steroid hormones in potentiating transformation of cervical cells by human papillomaviruses. *Trends Microbiol* 1994; 2:229–34.

112. Becker TM, Wheeler CM, McGough NS, et al. Contraceptive and reproductive risks for cervical dysplasia in southwestern Hispanic and non-Hispanic white women. *Int J Epidemiol* 1994; 23:913–22.

113. Molina R, Thomas DB, Dabancens A, et al. Oral contraceptives and cervical carcinoma in situ in Chile. *Cancer Res* 1988; 48:1011–15.

114. Jones CJ, Brinton LA, Hamman RF, et al. Risk factors for in situ cervical cancer: results from a case-control study. *Cancer Res* 1990; 50: 3657–62.

115. Brinton LA. Epidemiology of cervical cancer— overview. *IARC Sci Publ* 1992; 119:3–23.

116. Schiffman MH, Brinton LA, Devesa SS, et al. Cervical Cancer. In: Schottenfeld D, Fraumeni JF, Jr. (eds) *Cancer epidemiology and prevention.* New York: Oxford University Press, 1996, pp. 1090–116.

117. Irwin KL, Rosero-Bixby L, Oberle MW, et al. Oral contraceptives and cervical cancer risk in Costa Rica. Detection bias or causal association? *JAMA* 1988; 259:59–64.

118. Beral V, Hannaford P, Kay C. Oral contraceptive use and malignancies of the genital tract. Results from the Royal College of General Practitioners' Oral Contraception Study. *Lancet* 1988; 2:1331–5.

119. Negrini BP, Schiffman MH, Kurman RJ, et al. Oral contraceptive use, human papillomavirus infection, and risk of early cytological abnormalities of the cervix. *Cancer Res* 1990; 50:4670–5.

120. Gram IT, Macaluso M, Stalsberg H. Oral contraceptive use and the incidence of cervical intraepithelial neoplasia. *Am J Obstet Gynecol* 1992; 167:40–4.

121. Coker AL, McCann MF, Hulka BS, et al. Oral contraceptive use and cervical intraepithelial neoplasia. *J Clin Epidemiol* 1992; 45:1111–18.

122. Potischman N, Brinton LA. Nutrition and cervical neoplasia. *Cancer Causes Control* 1996; 7:113–26.

123. Palan PR, Mikhail MS, Goldberg GL, et al. Plasma levels of β-carotene, lycopene, canthaxanthin, retinol, and α- and τ-tocopherol in cervical intraepithelial neoplasia and cancer. *Clin Cancer Res* 1996; 2:181–5.

124. Giuliano AR. The role of nutrients in the prevention of cervical dysplasia and cancer. *Nutrition* 2000; 16:570–3.

125. Brock KE, Berry G, Mock PA, et al. Nutrients in diet and plasma and risk of in situ cervical cancer. *J Natl Cancer Inst* 1988; 80:580–5.

126. VanEenwyk J, Davis FG, Bowen PE. Dietary and serum carotenoids and cervical intraepithelial neoplasia. *Int J Cancer* 1991; 48:34–8.

127. VanEenwyk J, Davis FG, Colman N. Folate, vitamin C, and cervical intraepithelial neoplasia. *Cancer Epidemiol Biomarkers Prev* 1992; 1:119–24.

128. Liu T, Soong SJ, Wilson NP, et al. A case control study of nutritional factors and cervical dysplasia. *Cancer Epidemiol Biomarkers Prev* 1993; 2:525–30.

129. Kwasniewska A, Charzewska J, Tukendorf A, et al. Dietary factors in women with dysplasia colli uteri associated with human papillomavirus infection. *Nutr Cancer* 1998; 30:39–45.

130. Ziegler RG, Jones CJ, Brinton LA, et al. Diet and the risk of in situ cervical cancer among white women in the United States. *Cancer Causes Control* 1991; 2:17–29.

131. de Vet HC, Knipschild PG, Grol ME, et al. The role of β-carotene and other dietary factors in the aetiology of cervical dysplasia: results of a case-control study. *Int J Epidemiol* 1991; 20: 603–10.

132. Palan PR, Mikhail MS, Basu J, et al. Plasma levels of antioxidant beta-carotene and alpha-tocopherol in uterine cervix dysplasias and cancer. *Nutr Cancer* 1991; 15:13–20.

133. Cuzick J, De Stavola BL, Russell MJ, et al. Vitamin A, vitamin E and the risk of cervical intraepithelial neoplasia. *Br J Cancer* 1990; 62: 651–2.

134. Kwasniewska A, Tukendorf A, Semczuk M. Content of α-tocopherol in blood serum of human Papillomavirus-infected women with cervical dysplasias. *Nutr Cancer* 1997; 28:248– 51.

135. Kwasniewska A, Tukendorf A, Semczuk M. Folate deficiency and cervical intraepithelial neoplasia. *Eur J Gynaecol Oncol* 1997; 18: 526–30.

136. Liu T, Soong SJ, Alvarez RD, et al. A longitudinal analysis of human papillomavirus 16 infection, nutritional status, and cervical dysplasia progression. *Cancer Epidemiol Biomarkers Prev* 1995; 4:373–80.

137. Breitburd F, Ramoz N, Salmon J, et al. HLA control in the progression of human papillomavirus infections. *Semin Cancer Biol* 1996; 7:359–71.

138. Odunsi KO, Ganesan TS. The roles of the human major histocompatibility complex and human papillomavirus infection in cervical intraepithelial neoplasia and cervical cancer. *Clin Oncol (R Coll Radiol)* 1997; 9:4–13.

139. Odunsi K, Terry G, Ho L, et al. Association between *HLA DQB1 * 03* and cervical intraepithelial neoplasia. *Mol Med* 1995; 1:161–71.

140. Odunsi K, Terry G, Ho L, et al. Susceptibility to human papillomavirus-associated cervical intra-epithelial neoplasia is determined by specific *HLA DR-DQ* alleles. *Int J Cancer* 1996; 67:595–602.

141. Hildesheim A, Schiffman M, Scott DR, et al. Human leukocyte antigen class I/II alleles and development of human papillomavirus-related cervical neoplasia: results from a case-control study conducted in the United States. *Cancer Epidemiol Biomarkers Prev* 1998; 7: 1035–41.

142. Maciag PC, Schlecht NF, Souza PS, et al. Major histocompatibility complex class II polymorphisms and risk of cervical cancer and human papillomavirus infection in Brazilian women. *Cancer Epidemiol Biomarkers Prev* 2000; 9: 1183–91.

143. Apple RJ, Erlich HA, Klitz W, et al. HLA DR-DQ associations with cervical carcinoma show papillomavirus-type specificity. *Nature Genet* 1994; 6:157–62.

144. Apple RJ, Becker TM, Wheeler CM, et al. Comparison of human leukocyte antigen DR-DQ disease associations found with cervical dysplasia and invasive cervical carcinoma. *J Natl Cancer Inst* 1995; 87:427–36.

145. Sanjeevi CB, Hjelmstrom P, Hallmans G, et al. Different HLA-DR-DQ haplotypes are associated with cervical intraepithelial neoplasia among human papillomavirus type-16 seropositive and seronegative Swedish women. *Int J Cancer* 1996; 68:409–14.

146. Helland A, Olsen AO, Gjoen K, et al. An increased risk of cervical intra-epithelial neoplasia grade II-III among human papillomavirus positive patients with the HLA-DQA1*0102-DQB1*0602 haplotype: a population-based case-control study of Norwegian women. *Int J Cancer* 1998; 76:19–24.

147. CDC. 1993 Revised classification system for HIV infection and expanded surveillance case definition for AIDS among adolescents and adults. *MMWR* 1992; 41(RR–17):1–19.

148. Wright TC, Jr. Papillomavirus infection and neoplasia in women infected with human immunodeficiency virus. In: Franco EL, Monsonego J (eds) *New developments in cervical cancer screening and prevention*. Oxford: Blackwell Science, 1997, pp. 131–43.

149. Jay N, Moscicki AB. Human papillomavirus infections in women with HIV disease: prevalence, risk, and management. *AIDS Reader* 2000; 10:659–68.

150. Langley CL, Benga-De E, Critchlow CW, et al. HIV-1, HIV-2, human papillomavirus infection and cervical neoplasia in high-risk African women. *AIDS* 1996; 10:413–17.

151. Rezza G, Giuliani M, Branca M, et al. Determinants of squamous intraepithelial lesions (SIL) on Pap smear: the role of HPV infection and of HIV-1-induced immunosuppression. DIANAIDS Collaborative Study Group. *Eur J Epidemiol* 1997; 13:937–43.

152. Maiman M, Fruchter RG, Sedlis A, et al. Prevalence, risk factors, and accuracy of cytologic screening for cervical intraepithelial neoplasia in women with the human immunodeficiency virus. *Gynecol Oncol* 1998; 68:233–9.

153. Massad LS, Riester KA, Anastos KM, et al. Prevalence and predictors of squamous cell abnormalities in Papanicolaou smears from women infected with HIV-1. Women's Interagency HIV Study Group. *J Acquir Immune Defic Syndr* 1999; 21:33–41.

154. Moscicki AB, Ellenberg JH, Vermund SH, et al. Prevalence of and risks for cervical human papillomavirus infection and squamous intraepithelial lesions in adolescent girls: impact of infection with human immunodeficiency virus. *Arch Pediatr Adolesc Med* 2000; 154:127–34.

155. Ellerbrock TV, Chiasson MA, Bush TJ, et al. Incidence of cervical squamous intraepithelial lesions in HIV-infected women. *JAMA* 2000; 283:1031–7.

156. Mandelblatt JS, Kanetsky P, Eggert L, et al. Is HIV infection a cofactor for cervical squamous cell neoplasia? *Cancer Epidemiol Biomarkers Prev* 1999; 8:97–106.

157. Miller AB, Nazeer S, Fonn S, et al. Report on consensus conference on cervical cancer screening and management. *Int J Cancer* 2000; 86:440–7.

158. Gustafsson L, Sparen P, Gustafsson M, et al. Efficiency of organised and opportunistic cyto-

logical screening for cancer in situ of the cervix. *Br J Cancer* 1995; 72:498–505.

159. World Health Organization. *National cancer control programmes: policies and managerial guidelines*. Geneva: World Health Organization, 1995.

160. Miller AB, Chamberlain J, Day NE, et al. Report on a Workshop of the UICC Project on Evaluation of Screening for Cancer. *Int J Cancer* 1990; 46:761–9.

161. U.S. Preventive Services Task Force. *Guide to clinical preventive services*, 2nd ed. Washington, DC: U.S. Department of Health and Human Services, 1996.

162. Smith RA, Mettlin CJ, Davis KJ, et al. American cancer society guidelines for the early detection of cancer. *CA cancer J Clin* 2000; 50: 34–49.

163. Canadian Task Force on the Periodic Health Examination. *The Canadian guide to clinical preventive health care*. Ottawa: Health Canada, 1994.

164. Miller AB, Anderson G, Brisson J, et al. Report of a National Workshop on Screening for Cancer of the Cervix. *Can Med Assoc J* 1991; 145:1301–25.

165. La Vecchia C, Franceschi S, Decarli A, et al. "Pap" smear and the risk of cervical neoplasia: quantitative estimates from a case-control study. *Lancet* 1984; 2:779–82.

166. Herrero R, Brinton LA, Reeves WC, et al. Screening for cervical cancer in Latin America: a case-control study. *Int J Epidemiol* 1992; 21:1050–6.

167. Laara E, Day NE, Hakama M. Trends in mortality from cervical cancer in the Nordic countries: association with organised screening programmes. *Lancet* 1987; 1:1247–9.

168. Benedet JL, Anderson MB, Matisic JP. A comprehensive program for cervical cancer detection and management. *Amer J Obstet Gynecol* 1992; 166:1254–9.

169. McCrory DC, Matchar DB, Bastian L, et al. *Evaluation of cervical cytology. Evidence report/technology assessment No. 5. AHCPR Publication No. 99-E010*. Rockville, MD: Agency for Health Care Policy and Research, U.S. Department of Health and Human Services, February 1999.

170. Franco EL, Duarte-Franco E, Ferenczy A. Cervical cancer: epidemiology, prevention, and role of human papillomavirus infection. *Can Med Assoc J* 2001; 164:1017–25.

171. Koss LG. The papanicolaou test for cervical cancer detection. A triumph and a tragedy. JAMA 1989; 261:737–43.

172. McGoogan E. Advantages and limitations of automated screening systems in developing and developed countries. In: Franco EL, Monsonego J (eds) *New developments in cervical cancer screening and prevention*. London: Blackwell, 1997; pp. 317–22.

173. Wilbur DC, Prey MU, Miller WM, et al. The AutoPap system for primary screening in cervical cytology. Comparing the results of a prospective, intended-use study with routine manual practice. *Acta Cytol* 1998; 42:214–20.

174. Hutchinson ML, Zahniser DJ, Sherman ME, et al. Utility of liquid-based cytology for cervical carcinoma screening: results of a population-based study conducted in a region of Costa Rica with a high incidence of cervical carcinoma. *Cancer* 1999; 87:48–55.

175. Ferenczy A, Robitaille J, Franco E, et al. Conventional cervical cytologic smears vs. ThinPrep smears. A paired comparison study on cervical cytology. *Acta Cytol* 1996; 40:1136–42.

176. Austin RM, Ramzy I. Increased detection of epithelial cell abnormalities by liquid-based gynecologic cytology preparations. A review of accumulated data. *Acta Cytol* 1998; 42:178–84.

177. Stafl A. Cervicography: a new method for cervical cancer detection. *Am J Obstet Gynecol* 1981; 139:815–25.

178. Mould TA, Singer A. Adjuvant tests to cytology: cervicography and the polarprobe. In: Franco EL, Monsonego J (eds) *New developments in cervical cancer screening and prevention*. London: Blackwell, 1997; pp. 406–10.

179. Nuovo J, Melnikow J, Hutchison B, et al. Is cervicography a useful diagnostic test? A systematic overview of the literature. *J Am Board Fam Pract* 1997; 10:390–7.

180. Schneider DL, Herrero R, Bratti C, et al. Cervicography screening for cervical cancer among 8460 women in a high-risk population. *Am J Obstet Gynecol* 1999; 180(2 Pt 1):290–8.

181. Sankaranarayanan R, Wesley R, Somanathan T, et al. Visual inspection of the uterine cervix after the application of acetic acid in the detection of cervical carcinoma and its precursors. *Cancer* 1998; 83:2150–6.

182. Anonymous. Visual inspection with acetic acid for cervical-cancer screening: test qualities in a primary-care setting. University of Zimbabwe/ JHPIEGO Cervical Cancer Project. *Lancet* 1999; 353:869–73.

183. Denny L, Kuhn L, Pollack A, et al. Evaluation of alternative methods of cervical cancer screening for resource-poor settings. *Cancer* 2000; 89:826–33.

184. Manos MM, Ting Y, Wright DK, et al. Use of polymerase chain reaction amplification for the detection of genital human papillomaviruses. *Cancer Cells* 1989; 7:209–14.

185. VanDenBrule AJC, Snijders PJF, Gordijn RLJ, et al. General primer-mediated polymerase chain reaction permits the detection of sequenced and still unsequenced human papillomavirus genotypes in cervical scrapes and carcinomas. *Int J Cancer* 1990; 45:644–9.

186. Manos MM, Kinney WK, Hurley LB, et al. Identifying women with cervical neoplasia: using human papillomavirus DNA testing for equivocal Papanicolaou results. *JAMA* 1999; 281:1605–10.

187. Franco EL, Ferenczy A. Assessing gains in diagnostic utility when human papillomavirus testing is used as an adjunct to papanicolaou smear in the triage of women with cervical cytologic abnormalities. *Am J Obstet Gynecol* 1999; 181:382–6.

188. Anonymous. Human papillomavirus testing for triage of women with cytologic evidence of low-grade squamous intraepithelial lesions: baseline data from a randomized trial. The Atypical Squamous Cells of Undetermined Significance/Low-Grade Squamous Intraepithelial Lesions Triage Study (ALTS) Group. *J Natl Cancer Inst* 2000; 92:397–402.

189. Clavel C, Masure M, Bory JP, et al. Hybrid Capture II-based human papillomavirus detection, a sensitive test to detect in routine high-grade cervical lesions: a preliminary study on 1518 women. *Br J Cancer* 1999; 80:1306–1.

190. Cuzick J, Beverley E, Ho L, et al. HPV testing in primary screening of older women. *Br J Cancer* 1999; 81:554–8.

191. Kuhn L, Denny L, Pollack A, et al. Human papillomavirus DNA testing for cervical cancer screening in low-resource settings. *J Natl Cancer Inst* 2000; 92:818–25.

192. Ratnam S, Franco EL, Ferenczy A. Human papillomavirus testing for primary screening of cervical cancer precursors. *Cancer Epidemiol Biomarkers Prev* 2000; 9:945–51.

193. Schiffman M, Herrero R, Hildesheim A, et al. HPV DNA testing in cervical cancer screening: results from women in a high-risk province of Costa Rica. *JAMA* 2000; 283:87–93.

194. Schneider A, Hoyer H, Lotz B, et al. Screening for high-grade cervical intra-epithelial neoplasia and cancer by testing for high-risk HPV, routine cytology or colposcopy. *Int J Cancer* 2000; 89:529–34.

195. Wright TC Jr, Denny L, Kuhn L, et al. HPV DNA testing of self-collected vaginal samples compared with cytologic screening to detect cervical cancer. *JAMA* 2000; 283:81–6.

196. Cuzick J, Sasieni P, Davies P, et al. A systematic review of the role of human papilloma virus (HPV) testing within a cervical screening programme: summary and conclusions. *Br J Cancer* 2000; 83:561–5.

197. Cuzick J. Human papillomavirus testing for primary cervical cancer screening. *JAMA* 2000; 283:108–9.

198. Rozendaal L, Walboomers JM, van der Linden JC, et al. PCR-based high-risk HPV test in cervical cancer screening gives objective risk assessment of women with cytomorphologically normal cervical smears. *Int J Cancer* 1996; 68:766–9.

199. Sellors JW, Lorincz AT, Mahony JB, et al. Comparison of self-collected vaginal, vulvar and urine samples with physician-collected cervical samples for human papillomavirus testing to detect high-grade squamous intraepithelial lesions. *Can Med Assoc J* 2000; 163:513–18.

200. Ferenczy A. Management of patients with high grade squamous intraepithelial lesions. *Cancer* 1995; 76 (10 Suppl):1928–33.

201. Ferenczy A. Optimal management of cervical cancer precursors: high grade lesion. In: Franco EL, Monsonego J (eds) New developments in cervical cancer screening and prevention. London: Blackwell, 1997, pp. 116–21.

202. Cirisano FD. Management of pre-invasive disease of the cervix. *Semin Surg Oncol* 1999; 16:222–7.

203. Meheus A. Prevention of sexually transmitted infections through health education and counselling: a general framework. In: Franco EL, Monsonego J (eds) *New developments in cervical cancer screening and prevention.* London: Blackwell, 1997; pp. 84–90.

204. Rock CL, Michael CW, Reynolds RK, et al. Prevention of cervix cancer. *Crit Rev Oncol Hematol* 2000; 33:169–85.

205. Breitburd F, Coursaget P. Human papillomavirus vaccines. *Semin Cancer Biol* 1999; 9:431–44.

206. Schiller JT. Papillomavirus-like particle vaccines for cervical cancer. *Mol Med Today* 1999; 5:209–15.

207. Platz CE, Benda JA. Female genital tract cancer. *Cancer* 1995; 75 (1 Suppl):270–94.

208. Smith HO, Tiffany MF, Qualls CR, et al. The rising incidence of adenocarcinoma relative to squamous cell carcinoma of the uterine cervix in the United States—a 24-year population-based study. *Gynecol Oncol* 2000; 78:97–105.

209. Vizcaino AP, Moreno V, Bosch FX, et al. International trends in the incidence of cervical cancer: I. Adenocarcinoma and adenosquamous cell carcinomas. *Int J Cancer* 1998; 75: 536–45.

210. Parazzini F, La Vecchia C. Epidemiology of adenocarcinoma of the cervix. *Gynecol Oncol* 1990; 39:40–6.

211. Ferenczy A. Glandular lesions: an increasing problem. In: Franco EL, Monsonego J (eds) *New developments in cervical cancer screening and prevention*. London: Blackwell, 1997; pp. 122–30.

212. Anton-Culver H, Bloss JD, Bringman D, et al. Comparison of adenocarcinoma and squamous cell carcinoma of the uterine cervix: a population-based epidemiologic study. *Am J Obstet Gynecol* 1992; 166:1507–14.

213. Solomon D, Frable WJ, Vooijs GP, et al. ASCUS and AGUS criteria. International Academy of Cytology Task Force summary. Diagnostic cytology towards the 21st century: an international expert conference and tutorial. *Acta Cytol* 1998; 42:16–24.

214. Gallup DG, Abell MR. Invasive adenocarcinoma of the uterine cervix. *Obstet Gynecol* 1977; 49:596–603.

215. Pacey NF. Glandular neoplasms of the uterine cervix. In: Bibbo M (ed) *Comprehensive cytopathology*. Philadelphia: W.B. Saunders, 1991, 231–256.

216. Ostor AG, Pagano R, Davoren RA, et al. Adenocarcinoma in situ of the cervix. *Int J Gynecol Pathol* 1984; 3:179–90.

217. Plaxe SC, Saltzstein SL. Estimation of the duration of the preclinical phase of cervical adenocarcinoma suggests that there is ample opportunity for screening. *Gynecol Oncol* 1999; 75:55–61.

218. Farnsworth A, Laverty C, Stoler MH. Human papillomavirus messenger RNA expression in adenocarcinoma in situ of the uterine cervix. *Int J Gynecol Pathol* 1989; 8:321–30.

219. Tase T, Okagaki T, Clark BA, et al. Human papillomavirus DNA in adenocarcinoma in situ, microinvasive adenocarcinoma of the uterine cervix, and coexisting cervical squamous intraepithelial neoplasia. *Int J Gynecol Pathol* 1989; 8:8–17.

220. Eddy GL, Ural SH, Strumpf KB, et al. Incidence of atypical glandular cells of uncertain significance in cervical cytology following introduction of the Bethesda System. *Gynecol Oncol* 1997; 67:51–5.

221. Brinton LA, Huggins GR, Lehman HF, et al. Long-term use of oral contraceptives and risk of invasive cervical cancer. *Int J Cancer* 1986; 38:399–44.

222. Kvale G, Heuch I, Nilssen S. Reproductive factors and risk of cervical cancer by cell type. A prospective study. *Br J Cancer* 1988; 58: 820–4.

223. Parazzini F, La Vecchia C, Negri E, et al. Risk factors for adenocarcinoma of the cervix: a case-control study. *Br J Cancer* 1988; 57:201–4.

224. Brinton LA, Reeves WC, Brenes MM, et al. Oral contraceptive use and risk of invasive cervical cancer. *Int J Epidemiol* 1990; 19:4–11.

225. Brinton LA, Herrero R, Reeves WC, et al. Risk factors for cervical cancer by histology. *Gynecol Oncol* 1993; 51:301–6.

226. Ursin G, Peters RK, Henderson BE, et al. Oral contraceptive use and adenocarcinoma of cervix. *Lancet* 1994; 344:1390–4.

227. Lacey JV Jr, Brinton LA, Abbas FM, et al. Oral contraceptives as risk factors for cervical adenocarcinomas and squamous cell carcinomas. *Cancer Epidemiol Biomarkers Prev* 1999; 8: 1079–85.

228. Lacey JV Jr, Brinton LA, Barnes WA, et al. Use of hormone replacement therapy and adenocarcinomas and squamous cell carcinomas of the uterine cervix. *Gynecol Oncol* 2000; 77: 149–54.

229. Kjaer SK, Brinton LA. Adenocarcinomas of the uterine cervix: the epidemiology of an increasing problem. *Epidemiol Rev* 1993; 15: 486–98.

230. Taylor HB, Irey NS, Norris HJ. Atypical endocervical hyperplasia in women taking oral contraceptives. *JAMA* 1967; 202:637–9.

231. Czernobilsky B, Kessler I, Lancet M. Cervical adenocarcinoma in a woman on long-term contraceptives. *Obstet Gynecol* 1974; 43:517–21.

232. Dallenbach-Hellweg G. On the origin and histological structure of adenocarcinoma of the

endocervix in women under 50 years of age. *Pathol Res Pract* 1984; 179:38–50.

233. Chumas JC, Nelson B, Mann WJ, et al. Microglandular hyperplasia of the uterine cervix. *Obstet Gynecol* 1985; 66:406–9.

234. Ford LC, Berek JS, Lagasse LD, et al. Estrogen and progesterone receptor sites in malignancies of the uterine cervix, vagina, and vulva. *Gynecol Oncol* 1983; 15:27–31.

235. Pater A, Bayatpour M, Pater MM. Oncogenic transformation by human papillomavirus type 16 deoxyribonucleic acid in the presence of progesterone or progestins from oral contraceptives. *Am J Obstet Gynecol* 1990; 162: 1099–103.

236. Potischman N. Nutritional epidemiology of cervical neoplasia. *J Nutr* 1993; 123:424–9.

237. Duggan MA, Benoit JL, McGregor SE, et al. Adenocarcinoma in situ of the endocervix: human papillomavirus determination by dot blot hybridization and polymerase chain reaction amplification. *Int J Gynecol Pathol* 1994; 13:143–9.

238. Nieminen P, Kallio M, Hakama M. The effect of mass screening on incidence and mortality of squamous and adenocarcinoma of cervix uteri. *Obstet Gynecol* 1995; 85:1017–21.

239. Hildesheim A, Hadjimichael O, Schwartz PE, et al. Risk factors for rapid-onset cervical cancer. *Am J Obstet Gynecol* 1999; 180:571–7.

240. Cheng RF, Hernandez E, Anderson LL, et al. Clinical significance of a cytologic diagnosis of atypical glandular cells of undetermined significance. *J Reprod Med* 1999; 44:922–8.

241. Soofer SB, Sidawy MK. Atypical glandular cells of undetermined significance: clinically significant lesions and means of patient follow-up. *Cancer* 2000; 90:207–14.

242. Ronnett BM, Manos MM, Ransley JE, et al. Atypical glandular cells of undetermined significance (AGUS): cytopathologic features, histopathologic results, and human papillomavirus DNA detection. *Hum Pathol* 1999; 30:816–25.

243. Nicklin JL, Wright RG, Bell JR, et al. A clinicopathological study of adenocarcinoma in situ of the cervix. The influence of cervical HPV infection and other factors, and the role of conservative surgery. *Aust N Z J Obstet Gynaecol* 1991; 31:179–83.

17
Endometrium

Eduardo L. Franco and Alex Ferenczy

Although separated by only a few centimeters, the transformation zone of the uterine cervix and the endometrial glandular epithelium of the uterine corpus are the sites of neoplastic diseases that have considerably different epidemiologic, histopathologic, and etiologic characteristics. In chapter 16 we described the epidemiology, detection methods, and preventive approaches for squamous and glandular precursor lesions of cervical cancer. This chapter presents the same information for endometrial cancer precursors.

Endometrial carcinomas can be divided into two main types: endometrioid and nonendometrioid. Those with a predominantly endometrioid histology are primarily linked etiologically with hormonal stimulation and related risk factors and are typically responsive to the antiproliferative effects of progesterone. Endometroid type adenocarcinomas are also called type 1 endometrial cancers and account for 80% to 90% of all invasive malignancies of the uterine corpus. Some contain areas of squamous differentiation, which may range from benign to frankly malignant; in the latter case, the lesion is classified as adenosquamous carcinoma. Type 2 or nonendometrioid tumors represent a smaller proportion of neoplasms, have histological features of serous, clear cell, or mixed-type carcinomas, and are not linked to estrogenic effects. Type 2 endometrial carcinomas tend to develop in the postmenopausal atrophic endometria of older women. Endometrial hyperplasia (EH), particularly EH with cytological atypia, is believed to represent the precursor lesion for type 1 endometrial carcinoma. Type 2 cancers are not associated with or preceded by EH; rather, they seem to arise from in situ carcinomas of the surface or glandular epithelium, lesions that are called endometrial intraepithelial carcinoma (EIC).

This duality in the natural history of endometrial cancers has only recently been proposed on the basis of the emerging evidence from studies of computerized morphometry, clonal analysis, and mutations in specific tumor suppressor genes [1–3]. Progress in this area has been delayed by the relative lack of information on the comparative epidemiology of these neoplasms, and by the difficulty in histologically identifying lesions with adequate reproducibility. The following sections review the information on the histopathological definitions of endometrial cancer precursors, and on their epidemiology, detection, and prevention.

Histopathology

Precursors of Type 1 (Endometrioid) Carcinomas

Stroma and glands are the two major components of the normal endometrium. Physiologic or abnormal estrogenic stimulation leads to an increase in the size and number of glands and in the volume of stroma. During the menstrual cycle, the production of progesterone by the corpus luteum counters the proliferative influence of estradiol on glandular and stromal cells.

When conception does not occur, the endometrial lining is then shed, and a new cycle begins. Continued estrogenic stimulation unopposed by progesterone often leads to EH, which is characterized by an overgrowth of the glandular component in favor of the supportive stroma.

Table 17.1 shows the approximate correspondence among the various designations of EH with and without cytological atypia. The World Health Organization (WHO) classification of 1994 provides four categories regrouping the various designations for EH with or without cytological atypia that were common in the histopathology literature [4]. The distinctions are made on the basis of the proportion of glands relative to stroma, crowding of glands, and other features. It also established that the architecture of the lesions be described separately from the presence of atypia. The new nomenclature of endometrial intraepithelial neoplasia (EIN) resulted from a proposal by the Endometrial Collaborative Group, an international consortium of gynecologic pathologists led by Mutter [1,5]. The EIN nomenclature makes a clear distinction between EH and EIN, the latter being considered a genuine

precancerous state, whereas the former is not. It removes the emphasis on the distinction between simple and complex glandular architecture and establishes the importance of the relative fraction of the sectioned tissue that is occupied by stroma versus glands, the volume percentage stroma (VPS). The EIN nomenclature proposes the following necessary criteria for EH: irregular cystically dilated glands, VPS greater than 55%, and no cytological atypia. The necessary criteria for EIN are: cytological atypia, VPS greater than 55%, and total size larger than 1mm [5,6]. The correspondence between diagnostic categories for the WHO and EIN classifications is not absolute, because of the revised architectural and cytological criteria proposed by the latter. Therefore, the correspondence between categories shown in Table 17.1 should be viewed as approximate.

The main argument in support of an unified EIN scheme comes from the recognition that, unlike polyclonal normal or hyperplastic endometrium, EIN is a monoclonal proliferation, a feature also found in endometrial carcinomas. This has been demonstrated by analyses of nonrandom X-chromosome inactivation, clonal propagation of altered microsatellites,

TABLE 17.1. Terminology[1] for endometrial cancer precursor lesions of endometrioid type histology.

WHO classification	Other designations	Main histologic features	Endometrial intraepithelial neoplasia (EIN) nomenclature	Implications for management
Simple endometrial hyperplasia without cytologic atypia	Cystic glandular hyperplasia	Increased number of glands relative to stroma, glands cystically dilated, mild to moderate crowding	Endometrial hyperplasia (EH)	Results from estrogen-induced stimulation, can be managed with progesterone therapy
Complex endometrial hyperplasia without cytologic atypia	Adenomatous hyperplasia	Marked crowding with irregular outlines, little or no stroma		
Simple endometrial hyperplasia with cytologic atypia		In addition to the above: nuclear enlargement, rounding anisokaryosis, and loss of polarity	Endometrial intraepithelial neoplasia (EIN)	Considered a cancer precursor, to be managed by progesterone therapy or surgery
Complex endometrial hyperplasia with cytologic atypia	Atypical adenomatous hyperplasia			

[1] *Source* (World Health Organization classification): Scully RE et al., 1994 [4]. *Source* (EIN nomenclature): Mutter GL, 2000 [1] and Ferenczy A et al., 2000 [5].

and the similarity of acquired mutations of tumor suppressor genes between EIN and endometrial carcinomas, such as *K-ras* and *PTEN* [1,3,5]. In addition, loss of *PTEN* function by mutation or other molecular events seem to occur early in the natural history of EIN and endometrioid carcinomas [7].

Classically, the distinction among EH and atypical EH categories has been plagued by poor inter- and intraobserver agreement [8,9], which has made it difficult for clinical and epidemiologic studies to identify correlates of morphologic attributes. In addition, epithelial metaplastic changes in simple or complex EH lesions may be mistaken for EIN [10]. Use of the new EIN nomenclature is expected to minimize problems related to misclassification of lesions in future studies of natural history and epidemiology. Until now, however, the existing information on the descriptive epidemiology and risk factors of endometrial precursors (to be discussed later) has been based on the WHO classification [4] or on some of the older designations that lacked defined histologic criteria. Since epidemiologic studies strictly based on the EIN nomenclature are not yet available, the following sections on epidemiology, etiology, and prevention will refer only to the conventional designation of EH without and with atypia.

As mentioned above, the EIN nomenclature clearly defines EH with atypia (EIN), but not EH alone, as the actual precursor lesion of endometrial carcinoma. The designation of EH as a precursor lesion does appear, however, in earlier epidemiologic studies that found that women with this type of lesion experienced an elevated risk of endometrial carcinoma compared to those who were lesion-free [11]. It is possible that these findings may have been a result of failure to identify atypia in some cases of EH (that is, misclassification of EH with atypia as EH alone), since strict histological criteria have only recently become established [1,2].

Precursors of Type 2 Carcinomas

Despite their rarity, serous (type 2) carcinomas account for at least half of all endometrial cancer recurrences, and they are associated with a substantially lower survival expectation than that from endometrioid-type neoplasms [12,13]. They are rarely observed in association with areas of concomitant EH [14]. Serous carcinomas tend to occur at relatively older ages than endometrioid (type 1) cancers and in patients with no signs of hyperestrogenism [3,15]. Type 2 carcinomas also tend to develop from atrophic rather than from hyperplastic endometrium [13,16,17]. In addition, unlike type 1 tumors, they tend to lack or to have low levels of progesterone receptors [15]. Loss of *p53* function is a common event in the genesis of serous carcinomas, and it seems to be negatively correlated with hormone receptor levels [14]. The latter differences and the fact that risk factors for type 2 carcinomas tend to differ from those for type 1 tumors [18] have led Sherman to propose the existence of a separate natural history model for EIC as a specific precursor lesion for type 2 endometrial carcinomas [3,19–21].

EIC represents malignant transformation of the atrophic endometrium. It is characterized by single or multilayered pleomorphic gland cells with anaplastic nuclei, abnormal mitotic figures, and apoptotic bodies [3]. This serous carcinoma-in-situ state shares with its resultant invasive serous counterpart the following features: strong, diffuse p53 and Ki-67 immunostaining; an absence of microsatellite instability, and an absence of estrogen and progesterone receptors [3]. As of today, there are no published studies on the epidemiology of EIC, either of the serous or clear-cell type. Therefore, the following sections refer primarily to endometrioid-type cancers and their precursor lesions, EH and EH with atypia.

Descriptive Epidemiology

Incidence

Invasive cancer of the uterine corpus (endometrium) represents 3.8% of all female neoplasms, an estimated 142,000 new cases annually, and is the seventh most common malignancy affecting women worldwide, after cancers of the breast, colon/rectum, uterine cervix, stomach, lung, and ovary [22]. In contrast to the situation regarding cervical cancer, endometrial cancer incidence is higher in developed than in developing countries. Incidence rates (per 100,000 women per year, age-standardized to the world population of 1960) are 15.0 in North America and 11.1 in Western Europe. The average rate for developed countries is 10.7, whereas that for developing areas is 3.1 [22]. Endometrial cancer is the most common uterine malignancy and fourth overall (after those of breast, colon/rectum, and lung) among North American women. An estimated 36,100 new cases occurred in 2000 in the United States [23] and 3,500 in Canada [24].

The average incidence rate of endometrial cancer for the years 1993 to 1997 in the US National Cancer Institute's Surveillance, Epidemiology, and End Results (SEER) program was 21.3 per 100,000 per year (age-standardized to the 1970 United States population) [23]. It affects preferentially white women of relatively older ages, in whom it generally follows a more favorable course than that of cervical cancer. It is not uncommon for endometrial cancer to be a silent disease found at autopsy [25]. Although the annual incidence rate in blacks (14.5 per 100,000) is lower than that in whites (22.3 per 100,000) in the SEER program, the 5-year survival rate for endometrial cancer is much lower for black women, at 59%, compared to 86% for white women [23]. This leads to a higher annual mortality rate among black than in white women at 2.8 and 1.6 per 100,000, respectively [23]. Most of the excess mortality among black women can be explained by factors related to stage of disease, histology, treatment, sociodemographics, hormonal and reproductive variables, coexisting health conditions, and health behavior [26].

Unlike the situation for cervical cancer, screening for endometrial cancer and its precursors is not common medical practice. Therefore, detection of preinvasive endometrial lesions results from incidental findings from histopathological examination of specimens from women who are deemed at high clinical risk for the disease. The SEER program, the only source of population-based information on incidence rates of endometrial neoplasia,

classifies registered cases of preinvasive lesions as in situ cancers of the uterine corpus, without specification of the histological lineage as per the classification schemes described earlier. From 1973 to 1987 there had been 43,364 cases of invasive cancers of the uterine corpus in the SEER program with following histological distribution by types: specified adenocarcinomas, 91.6%; unspecified adenocarcinomas, 0.4%; epidermoid and unspecified carcinomas, 2.3%; sarcomas, 2.1%; other types and unspecified, 3.8%. During the same period the program registered 2,650 cases of in situ cancers of the uterine corpus, or less than 6% of all neoplasms of that anatomical site [27]. While the distribution by histological types of the in situ cancers may have been different than that of the invasive cancers, it is plausible to assume that the vast majority of in situ lesions were of glandular origin.

Figure 17.1 shows incidence rates for invasive and in situ endometrial cancers in the SEER program from 1973 to 1995 calculated from source data in the publicly available CD–ROM [28]. The incidence rate of invasive lesions peaked in 1975 and that for in situ lesions in 1974. Incidence rates of invasive cancer decreased gradually from 1975 to 1986 and have remained fairly constant during the subsequent decade. A similar pattern can be seen for in situ rates except that, with estimates in the early 1990s being 80% lower than when incidence peaked in 1974, the decline was more pronounced. Before peaking in the mid 1970s, rates of invasive cancer increased substantially in the late 1960s, most likely in response to the widespread use of estrogen-only replacement therapy in North America for postmenopausal symptoms. As soon as the association was recognized, the practice of prescribing estrogen without progestin declined dramatically (during the late 1970s), and incidence rates began to decrease shortly thereafter [29,30].

As shown in Figure 17.2, the aforementioned impact of the historical changes in the practice of prescribing unopposed estrogens can be seen exclusively among US white women, who were more likely than black women to have had access to the treatment of menopausal symptoms via hormone replacement therapy. While

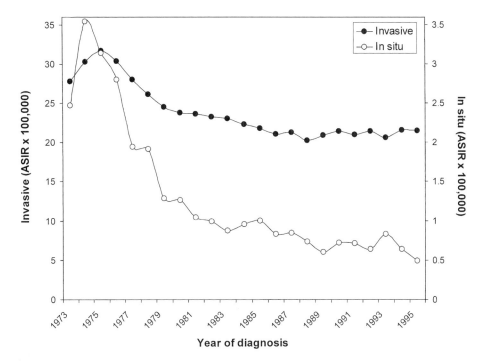

FIGURE 17.1. Age-standardized incidence rates (ASIR) of invasive and in situ endometrial neoplasms in all SEER registration areas from 1973 to 1995. Rates are standardized according to the age structure of the 1970 US population and expressed per 100,000 women.

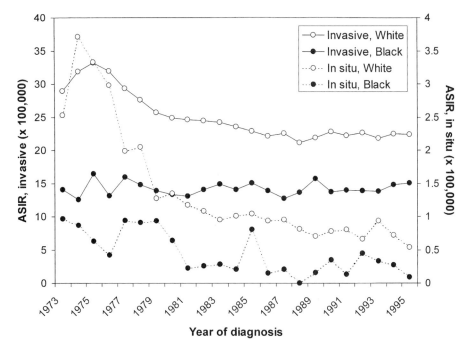

FIGURE 17.2. Race-specific, age-standardized incidence rates (ASIR) of invasive and in situ endometrial neoplasms in the SEER program from 1973 to 1995. Rates are standardized according to the age structure of the 1970 US population and expressed per 100,000 women.

the decline in rates following the peak in the mid-1970s was apparent among white women for both invasive and in situ lesions, there was no similar pattern for black women, whatever the extent of the lesions. For black women, an additional explanation for the lack of correlation between trends in incidence rates and the changes in use of unopposed estrogens may be related to the differences between white and blacks in the histological types of endometrial neoplasms. Compared with white women, blacks tend to have proportionally more type 2, serous endometrial adenocarcinomas [31], which are not etiologically linked to estrogens.

Risk of endometrial neoplasms rises rapidly after the age of 40 and then begins to decline after 70 to 74, in contrast with the risk of cervical cancer, which tends to stabilize after age 40. At approximately age 45, American women begin to have a higher risk of cancer of the endometrium than that of the cervix [29]. The peak age-specific incidence of endometrial neoplasms has changed over time. Figure 17.3

shows age-specific rates for both invasive and in situ lesions in successive periods from 1973 to 1995. During the highest risk period, 1973 to 1975, the incidence rate of invasive endometrial cancer peaked at ages 60 to 64. In subsequent periods, when the overall population incidence was declining, the peak age-specific rate shifted to ages 65 to 69 in 1976 to 1985, and then to 70 to 74 years in 1986 to 1995. To some extent, the shift in peak age-specific incidence can also be observed for in situ lesions. The peak rate in 1973 to 1975 was very pronounced at ages 55 to 59, but in 1986 to 1995, the peak incidence had shifted to later ages, particularly 60 to 64, but with less variation in rates during the postmenopausal years. On average, across all periods of observation, the peak incidence of in situ lesions is about 5 years earlier than that for invasive cancers; this coincides with estimates of mean transit time from atypical hyperplasia to endometrial carcinoma in natural history studies [11,32,33]. It is noteworthy that although rates of both invasive and in situ

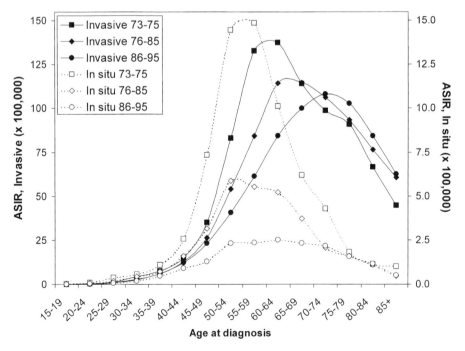

FIGURE 17.3. Age-specific incidence rates (ASIR) of invasive and in situ endometrial neoplasms in the SEER program during successive registration periods from 1973 to 1995. Rates are standardized according to the age structure of the 1970 US population and expressed per 100,000 women.

lesions declined substantially during the 1970s and 1980s the age-specific rates by period are of comparable magnitude after age 70 to 74. This is in line with the expectation that the increase in risk of endometrial neoplasms that followed the widespread use of unopposed estrogens in the late 1960s was predominantly for endometrioid-type tumors, which result from estrogenic stimulation and affect younger women than are affected by type 2, serous or clear cell tumors.

Other Sources of Data

Except for the SEER program's population-based rates of in situ lesions, which likely underestimate the true incidence of these lesions, the other sources of descriptive epidemiologic information on preinvasive endometrial neoplasms are histopathology series, screening studies of peri- and postmenopausal women, and clinical trials of hormonal therapy. These will be briefly reviewed.

EH is a common finding in biopsies or curettage specimens from pre- or postmenopausal women with abnormal uterine bleeding, but not all studies specify the presence of atypia. The prevalence of EH with or without atypia in these patient populations is in the range of 5% to 20%, whereas that of endometrial carcinoma ranges from less than 1% to 18% [34–38]. Expectedly, screening studies of asymptomatic women provide much lower figures. In one US cohort study of 2,586 asymptomatic postmenopausal women who were examined up to 3 times with endometrial sampling followed by cytology and histology, the prevalence rate of endometrial cancers was 7 per 1,000 and the annual incidence was 1.7 per 1,000, with nearly identical rates of EH [39,40]. As a consequence of active screening, this incidence rate is about 50% to 200% higher than the age-specific incidence rates of invasive neoplasms in the SEER program for women at ages 50 to 75. However, the incidence rate of EH in the actively screened cohort was 20- to 50-fold greater than the equivalent age-specific rates of in situ lesions in the SEER program (Figure 17.3). A recent Swedish cohort study found the incidence rate of EH with or without atypia among asymptomatic postmenopausal women to be 44 per 100,000 per year [37], an estimate that is also considerably higher than that of in situ lesions in the SEER program among women of comparable age. One Finnish study of 1,074 postmenopausal women recruited as part of a breast-cancer-screening invitation used Doppler sonography to refer 291 suspicious cases for endometrial biopsy. The latter yielded 16 cases of EH and 2 cases of cancer for presumed prevalences of 1.5% and 0.2%, respectively [41].

Clinical trials of hormone therapy have been able to measure the cumulative incidence of endometrial neoplasms using active follow-up of postmenopausal women. Results differ considerably depending on the type of hormonal treatment. For women on unopposed estrogens the one-year cumulative incidence of EH ranged from 15% to 38% [42–44]. On the other hand, rates for women taking estrogen/progesterone combinations were considerably lower, ranging from less than 0.5% to 5.6% over follow-up periods of up to four years [42–46].

Invasive Cancer Following a Diagnosis of EH

A histopathological diagnosis of EH with atypia (EIN under the new nomenclature discussed previously) in an endometrial biopsy or curettage specimen is frequently equated with an invasive neoplasm upon examination of the hysterectomy specimen. The proportion of "occult cancers" in EH series ranges from 28% to 45%. On the other hand, the risk of endometrial carcinoma is considerably lower for EH without atypia, ranging from 0% to 3% [47–50].

A number of cohort studies have also analyzed the risk of a final diagnosis of endometrial carcinoma during follow-up of women found to have EH on an initial biopsy. Subjects in these studies were followed for periods of 1 to 20 years. Among those with EH without cytological atypia, the cumulative risk of cancer was in the 0% to 8% range. Progression to cancer among those with EH with atypia was much higher, in the range of 25% to 58% [5,32,33,51].

Much of the variation across studies stems from the histological heterogeneity of endometrial cancer precursors. As mentioned previously, defined histological criteria for classifying lesions have become available only very recently [1,3,6]. The relative rarity of EH, with or without atypia, and the historical difficulty in obtaining a set of reproducible histological features that could guide pathologists in their diagnoses of endometrial lesions, has undoubtedly led to substantial misclassification of lesion outcomes in epidemiologic and clinical studies. This state of affairs should be kept in mind when examining the results of the very few studies that have attempted to find etiologic factors for preinvasive endometrial neoplasms. The findings are summarized in the next section.

Etiology

Endometrial cancer risk is most influenced by reproductive and hormonal factors. In many respects, the risk-factor profile for endometrial cancer is opposite to that of cervical cancer. For instance, risk of endometrial cancer and its precursors is positively associated with nulliparity [52,53], high socioeconomic status [54], and, unlike the association with many cancers, there is less risk among women who smoke [55,56]. Estrogenic stimulation and obesity are also important risk factors (to be discussed later). One large case-control study that compared endometrioid-type adenocarcinomas with and without adjacent areas of EH did not find material differences in epidemiologic determinants [57]. This provides indirect evidence that risk-factor profiles for invasive and preinvasive endometrial cancers are similar.

Exogenous Hormones

Exogenous exposure to estrogens, without concomitant intake of progesterone, has the greatest impact on the risk of endometrial cancer and its precursors. Several case-control and cohort studies have demonstrated the effects of estrogen replacement therapy on the risk of endometrial cancer, finding relative risks in the range of 1.5 to 12.0 [reviewed in 30,54,58]. The magnitude of the association with unopposed estrogens is similar for EH for which relative risks were found to be 7 for ever use and 8 to 20 for long-term use [59,60]. Early concerns that the association could be spurious, due to detection bias [61] (increased detection of endometrial cancers among estrogen users because of heightened medical surveillance among these women) have been assuaged by later epidemiologic studies [62].

The aforementioned clinical trials of hormone replacement therapy (see section on Descriptive Epidemiology) have provided unequivocal proof that unopposed estrogen use leads to a 5- to 15-fold higher incidence of EH and EH with atypia than when a progesterone combination is used [42–46,63]. Lesion risk associated with the latter form of replacement therapy is not significantly different from that for women in a placebo control group [63]. In addition, further proof of causality is obtained by studies that show substantial regression of EH or partial regression of EH with atypia following progesterone therapy [33,63,64].

In premenopausal women, sequential-type oral contraceptives (OC), which were largely used in the past, led to substantial increases in risk [65], while modern combination-type OCs generally decrease risk by approximately 50% [30,66,67]. Maximum protection may be conferred on women who receive low-dose estrogen and high-dose progestin [54]. The protective effect of OC use, particularly long term, is also seen for EH [59]. Tamoxifen, a nonsteroidal drug with both estrogen and antiestrogen effects *in vitro* and *in vivo*, has largely been used to treat breast cancer, and as an added benefit, to prevent the occurrence of a second breast cancer during follow-up. Trials of tamoxifen therapy have indicated that, while the beneficial effects of improved survival and reduced risk of second breast cancer primaries are real, a disadvantage is that tamoxifen treatment is associated with an increased risk of endometrial lesions of about 3- to 7-fold [58,68].

Obesity

Obesity is associated with increased endometrial cancer risk (2- to 5-fold), possibly through a combination of mechanisms [30,54,58]. Obese women may be more prone to an increased endogenous production of estradiol. Increased risk may also result from continued anovulation causing progesterone deficiency [30,69]. Obesity, measured as body mass or Quetelet index, has also emerged as a risk factor for EH in a few case-control or case-comparison studies [37,53,59,70], but the association seems to be more evident for postmenopausal women [59].

Other Determinants

Diet has been a notoriously difficulty class of risk factors to assess in epidemiologic studies. Nevertheless, there seems to be a trend for increased endometrial cancer risk associated with high animal fat intake, and dietary differences could help explain the international variation in rates [71]. It is difficult, however, to disentangle the confounding effects of obesity, fat intake, and endogenous estrogens on the risk of the disease. The effect of diet has not been assessed in epidemiologic studies of EH.

The presence of cytological or histopathological abnormalities has also been studied with respect to the risk of endometrial malignancy. A history of endometrial polyps in previous curettage samples is equated with a 3-fold greater risk of cancer [11] or of EH with or without atypia [72]. The presence of atypical endometrial cells on a Pap smear is equated with an elevated risk of endometrial cancer or EH [73]. In addition, the Bethesda system for reporting cervicovaginal cytologic diagnoses (see Chapter 16) states that "normal" endometrial cells on the Pap smear could also be indicative of EH and endometrial cancer [74]. Although this contention has been challenged [75], the empirical evidence for the association between normal endometrial cells on the smear and EH or endometrial cancer emerged as strong in a study that controlled for other cytological features in a multivariate analysis [76].

Detection

High-clinical-risk women are candidates for assessment of endometrial pathology including cancer and its precursors. These women are defined as those with the following conditions: (i) 60 years of age or older; (ii) obesity (with upper body fat pattern) with or without diabetes or hypertension; (iii) use of estrogen-only replacement therapy; (iv) previous breast cancer; (v) tamoxifen therapy for breast cancer; (vi) chronic liver disease; (vii) infertility: low parity, chronic anovulation (polycystic ovarian disease, estrogen-secreting ovarian stroma or tumors). Women receiving unopposed estrogens should undergo endometrial sampling once biennially (risk increases only after 2 years of estrogen use), particularly if endometrial hyperstimulation has previously been documented and has not been treated by short-term administration of progestins. Also, if the informed high-risk woman requests an endometrial evaluation prior to the initiation of or during hormone replacement therapy, or at any time during her periodic health examinations, she should not be deprived of an office-based investigative procedure to rule out endometrial pathology [5]. Endometrial evaluations should also be performed in women with a history of Lynch II syndrome, a condition associated with very high risk for endometrial carcinoma [77].

Patients with perimenopausal or postmenopausal uterine bleeding are high-priority candidates for office-based endometrial examination. Breakdown of endometrial neoplastic tissue results in metrorrhagia, which is viewed by both the patient and her physician as an ominous sign of serious underlying disease. In consequence, diagnostic delays are uncommon in Western populations [67].

A number of methods are presently available for detecting endometrial neoplasms and its precursors in high risk women: (i) cervicovaginal cytology, (ii) endometrial cytology, (iii) endometrial biopsy, (iv) dilatation and curettage (D&C), (v) transvaginal ultrasonography (TVUS), (vi) saline infusion sonography (SIS), (vii) magnetic resonance imaging (MRI) or computerized tomography (CT), and (viii) hysteroscopy.

Cytologic Methods

Presence of endometrial cells on cervical smears is equated with a substantially elevated risk of endometrial hyperplasia [76,78]. However, the main drawbacks of Pap cytology are that it detects mainly advanced endometrial carcinoma and has a high false-negative rate in postmenopausal, asymptomatic endometrial carcinoma patients [6,67].

Cytological assessment is best accomplished with direct sampling of the endometrial lining either by brushing or by aspirating the superficial endometrial mucosa [79]. Numerous endometrial cell samplers are available commercially. Methods based on brushing of the endometrium include: Endo-Pap (Sherwood Medical, Inc., St. Louis, MD), Gynecyte, and Endocyte (Organon Inc., West Orange, NJ). Those based on aspiration of endometrial contents include the Isaacs cell sampler and the Gravlee-jet washer. Rates of diagnostic accuracy with respect to histologically verified carcinoma and atypical EH are in the range of 91% to 100% for brushing methods, and 96% to 100% for those based on aspiration. These estimates have been obtained under controlled clinical conditions and in selected patient populations, and therefore they may not be generalizable to practice conditions [5,80]. The presence of normal endometrial cells on the smear indicates that the patient may either have a normal or a hyperplastic uterine lining. Frequently, EH without cytologic atypia is indistinguishable from normal proliferative endometrium. Unfortunately, most cytology laboratories lack expertise for distinguishing cytologic atypia related to EH from that associated with degeneration or repair. As a result, false-positive rates may be too high to justify the routine use of cytology for detection of endometrial malignancies or EH with atypia. Also, the screening of an endometrial smear is very time-consuming and interpretation is difficult because of the complexity of endometrial gland cell morphology.

Histologic Methods

Histologic sampling is the gold standard for diagnosing either asymptomatic or symptomatic (abnormal uterine bleeding) endometrial neoplasia. Available methods use plastic disposable or metal reusable devices for brushing, aspiration biopsy (Pipelle [Unimar, Inc., Wiltin, CT], Endocell (Wallach Medical Devices, Inc., Milford, CT), Vabra (Cooper Labs., Cedar Knolls, NY), Isaacs cell sampler, Pistolette (Unimed, Lausanne, Switzerland) or suction curettage or stroke biopsy (Kevorkian Device). These are more or less comparable in attaining high diagnostic accuracy [5,79]. The pitfalls of histologic methods are their relatively high cost and discomfort to the patient. The latter leads to low compliance for repeat testing. Conventional curettage is much too costly, and its diagnostic accuracy may not be as high as originally anticipated [81]. Use of endometrial aspirators seems to be the most cost-effective approach and causes the least amount of discomfort for patients [79]; however, the choice of method should be dictated by specific conditions. For instance, severe stenosis of the external/internal os (or internal os spasm) may require prior sequential cyclic treatment with Premarin (Wyeth-Ayerst, St Davids, PA) or Provera (Pharmacia Co., Peapack, NJ) to allow dilatation of the os, and proper assessment of the atrophic endometrium of elderly postmenopausal women may require the use of powerful vacuum aspirators, e.g., Vabra [5]. In general, endometrial biopsies are more difficult to perform in women who are older, nulliparous, or who have undergone radiation treatment [67].

Nowadays, D&C has essentially been replaced by office-based endometrial biopsy using the aforementioned flexible aspiration devices. The latter are more cost-effective than D&C, and the diagnostic yield in both symptomatic and asymptomatic women is similar to D&C; the sensitivity and specificity are on the order of 90% and 95%, respectively [79]. Cervical stenosis prevents successful endometrial sampling in about 10% of the cases [5].

Other Methods

A noninvasive and painless method for assessing the endometrial cavity is TVUS. It is extensively used for screening of asymptomatic women and for increasing follow-up compliance of high-risk patients. TVUS visualizes both the anterior and posterior endometrial linings on a monitor when a 5 MHz probe is placed against the vaginal fornix. The double thickness of the endometrium is measured with accuracy because the endometrio-myometrial junction has a distinct halo-like appearance. TVUS is highly sensitive at a cut-off value of 4 mm for endometrial double thickness in women with postmenopausal bleeding [82] but has low specificity for identifying endometrial carcinoma and its precursors [5]. Recent studies have suggested that specificity may be improved without substantially affecting sensitivity by judiciously defining the cut-off value that is equated with a positive result based on length of time since menopause [80]. The high cost of TVUS is presently the most important barrier to its use as a screening method. SIS measures single endometrial thickness; a 3 mm cut-off value corresponding to endometrial atrophy. SIS is used when TVUS or biopsy are equivocal in relation to symptoms of bleeding [83].

MRI and CT have been of clinical value to obtain preoperative data on the extent and depth of myometrial invasion by endometrial carcinoma rather than for the primary diagnosis of endometrial carcinoma or its precursors [84]. Their role in the diagnosis of endometrial cancer and EH with atypia remains to be determined.

Hysteroscopy is an endoscopic procedure that allows direct inspection of the endometrial cavity by the use of CO_2 gas to expand the uterine cavity. It is of value for obtaining directed biopsies of endometrial lesions and polyps in women with postmenopausal bleeding or in those who undergo tamoxifen treatment [5,67]. Its high cost and the possibility of procedure-associated risks preclude its widespread use as a screening or diagnostic procedure.

Prevention

Screening

Routine screening of asymptomatic women using any of the above techniques for endometrial cancer or its precursors has not been proven to be of benefit [85]. No screening test has been assessed with respect to its impact on mortality from endometrial cancer (see Chapters 22 and 24 on screening). The US National Cancer Institute's Physician's Data Query (PDQ) Program has concluded that there is insufficient evidence to establish whether a decrease in mortality from endometrial cancer occurs with screening by endometrial sampling or TVUS. The level of evidence for this statement comes from studies of multiple-time series with or without intervention and the published opinions of respected authorities based on clinical experience, descriptive studies, or reports of expert committees [86]. An explanation of the PDQ's levels of evidence will be provided in Chapter 24. The existing recommendations for screening certain high risk groups for endometrial neoplasia are based on judgments of presumptive benefit rather than on proof of mortality reduction in these patient groups [86].

Though it is successfully used for screening of cervical cancer, the Pap test lacks sufficient sensitivity to reliably detect endometrial cancer and EH with or without atypia. As mentioned above, however, Pap cytology may help to identify endometrial malignancy, particularly if it reveals the presence of endometrial cells on a smear of a postmenopausal woman not taking exogenous hormones [76,78]. Endometrial aspiration techniques have been proposed as potential screening tools, but studies suffer from verification (diagnostic work-up) bias, which prevents reliable estimation of true sensitivity and specificity values among asymptomatic women. Among women with abnormal uterine bleeding, endometrial sampling has the advantage of being a less invasive alternative to D&C, but issues related to access to the lesions in the endometrial cavity and to sampling error limit the significance of a negative result [86].

Screening for endometrial neoplasms with TVUS has been proposed as beneficial for women receiving long-term tamoxifen therapy [87,88] because of the risks of endometrial diseases associated with this form of treatment. However, TVUS may yield many false-positive results because tamoxifen exerts an echogenic and sonolucent effect in the endometrial stroma and myometrium that may give the appearance of EH or carcinoma [89]. This could result in a large number of unnecessary endometrial biopsies. This problem may be circumvented by using a higher threshold of endometrial thickness than in conventional for TVUS to triage women for biopsy [90]. SIS has not been used for routine screening of endometrial lesions.

In addition to the above pitfalls, it can also be argued that although endometrial carcinoma is common, its attendant morbidity is relatively low as compared with that of other female neoplasms such as breast and cervix cancers. The high cost and discomfort to the patient of most procedures make them unattractive as large-scale, cost-effective screening tools. Moreover, the majority of patients with disease eventually become symptomatic, presenting with abnormal uterine bleeding, which prompts the detection of early clinical stage disease at the time of diagnosis and results in surgical treatment. This contention is supported by the excellent 5-year survival rate (95%) of patients with localized endometrial carcinoma (75% of those in the SEER program) [23]. Unlike cervical cancer, which affects women at relatively earlier ages, the incidence of endometrial carcinoma and its precursors is very low in women younger than 50 years and in those receiving combination-type hormone replacement therapy. Elderly people are difficult to enroll into screening programs, and the drop-out rate is relatively high, particularly given the discomfort caused by the available screening procedures.

Primary Prevention

Considering the similarity of risk factors for both precursor and invasive endometrial lesions, it is plausible to assume that primary prevention strategies aiming at reducing the risk of endometrial cancers will exert an effect at the level of precursors initially. Preventing endometrial cancer via public and professional education seems to be a sensible approach, although evidence of benefit via reductions in incidence and/or mortality is not yet available. Physician education should include increasing awareness of the following tenets:

1. Endometrial cancer is the most common gynecologic malignancy, but one with a low mortality rate.
2. Common risk factors are advanced age, obesity, use of unopposed estrogen therapy, use of tamoxifen, nulliparity, and a family history of breast or colon cancer.
3. Risk can be reduced by early intervention via endometrial biopsy and treatment in the setting of abnormal uterine bleeding,
4. by administering progestational therapy for postmenopausal patients on estrogen-only regimens, and
5. by referring patients who have endometrial or atypical glandular cells on Pap smear to endometrial biopsy.

Public education concerning the risks of endometrial cancer should include: (i) encouraging proper weight maintenance; (ii) increasing awareness of the risks associated with unopposed estrogen therapy, (iii) making known the value of OC use in reducing risk, and (iv) increasing awareness of the most common signs and symptoms of the disease.

A chemopreventive approach based on the administration of gonadotropin-releasing hormone (GnRH) agonists plus low-dose add-back steroid hormones has been proposed to minimize lifetime risks of breast, ovarian, and endometrial cancers [91]. This has been shown to be a promising strategy in reversing endometrial proliferation (to be discussed later), particularly in women at high risk of developing endometrial malignancy (for instance, those on tamoxifen therapy). However, large scale trials are still needed for formal proof of long-term benefit.

Treatment

Consensus treatment guidelines for EH are not available, but medical or surgical treatment have become practice standards. The choice depends on the histopathologic form of hyperplasia, the woman's reproductive status, whether the patient is on estrogen-only replacement therapy, and her general health. For women who desire to conceive, the initial treatment should include progestational suppression, regardless of whether the lesion is classified as EH without or with atypia. Although many lesions respond to exogenous progestogens and/or ovulation inducers, in most cases they tend to recur within a few months to a few years after delivery of the newborn. Medical hormone therapy is also given to women whose general health is unsuitable to withstand surgery.

EH tends to respond well to relatively low-dose progestational therapy [33]. Women who develop EH without or with atypia during estrogen-alone replacement therapy may benefit from the addition of progestins to their replacement regimen. The rare patient (1%) who develops endometrial hyperplasia while on combined cyclic or continuous replacement therapy [63] may benefit from higher doses of combined hormones or from a progestin-only replacement therapy for 3 months as an attempt to revert the hyperplastic endometrium to normal.

Surgery, specifically transabdominal hysterectomy with or without bilateral salpingo-oophorectomy, is recommended for those women who have persistent EH without atypia but are symptomatic (abnormal uterine bleeding) and for postmenopausal women with atypical EH. Surgery is justified in this group in the face of 25 to 35% progression rates to invasion and an 80% rate of failure to respond to progestational therapy [33].

More recently, GnRH agonists, such as leuprolide acetate or triptorelin, have been tried to treat EH with or without atypia [92]. The rationale for this form of treatment is that the endometrium both in health and disease, like the breast and ovary, contains GnRH receptors, and that GnRH agonists may down-regulate GnRH receptors, resulting in a direct antiproliferative effect on endometrial growth [91,93]. However, GnRH therapy is still in its experimental stages, and issues related to short-term recurrence of EH need to be properly addressed.

Conclusions

The vast majority of invasive carcinomas of the endometrium are of endometrioid-type histology. The remote precursor lesion for these neoplasms is EH, which in association with cytological atypia and/or reduction of the volume occupied by stroma versus endometrial glands, becomes an EIN lesion, a condition now accepted as the immediate endometrial cancer precursor. Type 2, nonendometrioid endometrial cancers are rare and seem to originate from EIC as a distinct intragladular or surface epithelium precursor lesion. The evidence from the few epidemiologic and genetic marker studies available indicate that EH with atypia and EIC are true endometrial cancer precursors.

At present there are no screening methods for EH with or without atypia that have been proven to reduce the incidence of or mortality from endometrial cancer, a neoplasm that is associated with remarkably favorable prognosis. Certain high-risk groups (women on unopposed estrogen or tamoxifen therapy) may benefit from close follow-up using endometrial sampling or TVUS, but evidence of benefit that exceeds the costs and discomfort inherent to these procedures is yet to become available. Treatment methods should be tailored to individual cases, and the woman's desire to preserve fertility and other factors should be considered. Progestational therapy can reverse hyperplasia and some cancer precursors, but close follow-up monitoring is needed. Surgery is the definitive treatment strategy for reducing clinical risks of cancer precursor recurrence.

Unlike the precursors of neoplasms of the uterine cervix, which have histological attributes that are easily recognizable and reproducible, EH and EIN have only recently become well defined as endometrial cancer precursors with established histological criteria. Future natural history and epidemiologic investigations, aided by judicious testing for genetic markers of disease progression, should not suffer from the misclassification problems that affected past etiologic studies. Such new studies will be instrumental in testing novel chemotherapeutic approaches and the value of noninvasive screening modalities for endometrial neoplasms.

References

1. Mutter GL. Endometrial intraepithelial neoplasia (EIN): will it bring order to chaos? The Endometrial Collaborative Group. *Gynecol Oncol* 2000; 76:287–90.
2. Mutter GL, Baak JP, Crum CP, et al. Endometrial precancer diagnosis by histopathology, clonal analysis, and computerized morphometry. *J Pathol* 2000; 190:462–9.
3. Sherman ME. Theories of endometrial carcinogenesis: a multidisciplinary approach. *Mod Pathol* 2000; 13:295–308.
4. Scully RE, Bonfiglio TA, Kurman RJ, et al. *Histological typing of female genital tract tumours. World Health Organization International Histological Classification of Tumours*, 2nd ed. Berlin: Springer-Verlag, 1994, pp. 13–28.
5. Ferenczy A, Mutter G. Endometrial hyperplasia and neoplasia: Definition, diagnosis and management Principles. In: Sciarra J (ed) *Gynecology and obstetrics looseleaf CD-ROM*, Lippincott, Williams & Wilkins, 2000. Philadelphia.
6. Mutter GL. Premalignant Lesions of the Endometrium. A project from the Endometrial Collaborative Group. Available at URL: *http://www.endometrium.org/*.
7. Mutter GL, Lin MC, Fitzgerald JT, et al. Altered PTEN expression as a diagnostic marker for the earliest endometrial precancers. *J Natl Cancer Inst* 2000; 92:924–30.
8. Kendall BS, Ronnett BM, Isacson C, et al. Reproducibility of the diagnosis of endometrial hyperplasia, atypical hyperplasia, and well-differentiated carcinoma. *Am J Surg Pathol* 1998; 22:1012–19.
9. Bergeron C, Nogales FF, Masseroli M, et al. A multicentric European study testing the reproducibility of the WHO classification of endometrial hyperplasia with a proposal of a simplified working classification for biopsy and curettage specimens. *Am J Surg Pathol* 1999; 23:1102–8.
10. Silverberg SG. Problems in the differential diagnosis of endometrial hyperplasia and carcinoma. *Mod Pathol* 2000; 13:309–27.
11. Pettersson B, Adami HO, Lindgren A, et al. Endometrial polyps and hyperplasia as risk factors for endometrial carcinoma. A case-control study of curettage specimens. *Acta Obstet Gynecol Scand* 1985; 64:653–9.
12. Hendrickson M, Ross J, Eifel P, et al. Uterine papillary serous carcinoma: a highly malignant form of endometrial adenocarcinoma. *Am J Surg Pathol* 1982; 6:93–108.
13. Sherman ME, Bitterman P, Rosenshein NB, et al. Uterine serous carcinoma. A morphologically diverse neoplasm with unifying clinicopathologic features. *Am J Surg Pathol* 1992; 16:600–10.
14. Moll UM, Chalas E, Auguste M, et al. Uterine papillary serous carcinoma evolves via a p53-driven pathway. *Hum Pathol* 1996; 27:1295–300.
15. Deligdisch L, Holinka CF. Endometrial carcinoma: two diseases? *Cancer Detect Prev* 1987; 10:237–46.
16. Hoffman K, Nekhlyudov L, Deligdisch L. Endometrial carcinoma in elderly women. *Gynecol Oncol* 1995; 58:198–201.
17. Sherman ME, Silverberg SG. Advances in endometrial pathology. *Clin Lab Med* 1995; 15:517–43.
18. Sherman ME, Sturgeon S, Brinton LA, et al. Risk factors and hormone levels in patients with serous and endometrioid uterine carcinomas. *Mod Pathol* 1997; 10:963–8.
19. Ambros RA, Sherman ME, Zahn CM, et al. Endometrial intraepithelial carcinoma: a distinctive lesion specifically associated with tumors displaying serous differentiation. *Hum Pathol* 1995; 26:1260–7.
20. Sherman ME, Bur ME, Kurman RJ. p53 in endometrial cancer and its putative precursors: evidence for diverse pathways of tumorigenesis. *Hum Pathol* 1995; 26:1268–74.
21. Sherman ME, Sturgeon S, Brinton L, et al. Endometrial cancer chemoprevention: implications of diverse pathways of carcinogenesis. *J Cell Biochem Suppl* 1995; 23:160–4.
22. Parkin DM, Pisani P, Ferlay J. Estimates of the worldwide incidence of 25 major cancers in 1990. *Int J Cancer* 1999; 80:827–41.
23. Ries LAG, Eisner MP, Kosary CL, et al. (eds) *SEER Cancer Statistics Review, 1973–1997*. Bethesda, MD: National Cancer Institute, 2000.
24. National Cancer Institute of Canada. *Canadian Cancer Statistics 2000*. Toronto, Canada: National Cancer Institute of Canada, 2000.
25. Dhom G. Epidemiology of hormone-depending tumors. In: Voigt KD, Knabbe C (eds) *Endocrine dependent tumors*. New York: Raven Press, 1991, pp. 26–35.

26. Hill HA, Eley JW, Harlan LC, et al. Racial differences in endometrial cancer survival: the black/white cancer survival study. *Obstet Gynecol* 1996; 88:919–26.

27. Platz CE, Benda JA. Female genital tract cancer. *Cancer* 1995; 75(1 Suppl):270–94.

28. SEER Cancer Incidence Public-Use Database, 1973–1995. August, 1997, submission. US Department of Health and Human Services, April, 1998.

29. Franco EL. Epidemiology of uterine cancers. In: Meisels A, Morin C (eds) *Cytopathology of the uterus*, 2nd Ed. Chicago: American Society of Clinical Pathologists, 1997 (pp. 301–24).

30. Schottenfeld D. Epidemiology of endometrial neoplasia. *J Cell Biochem* 1995; 23(Suppl.): 151–9.

31. Barrett RJ 2nd, Harlan LC, Wesley MN, et al. Endometrial cancer: stage at diagnosis and associated factors in black and white patients. *Am J Obstet Gynecol* 1995; 173:414–22; discussion 422–3.

32. Kurman RJ, Kaminski PF, Norris HJ. The behavior of endometrial hyperplasia. A long-term study of "untreated" hyperplasia in 170 patients. *Cancer* 1985; 56:403–12.

33. Ferenczy A, Gelfand M. The biologic significance of cytologic atypia in progestogen-treated endometrial hyperplasia. *Am J Obstet Gynecol* 1989; 160:126–31.

34. Feldman S, Cook EF, Harlow BL, et al. Predicting endometrial cancer among older women who present with abnormal vaginal bleeding. *Gynecol Oncol* 1995; 56:376–81.

35. Ben-Yehuda OM, Kim YB, Leuchter RS. Does hysteroscopy improve upon the sensitivity of dilatation and curettage in the diagnosis of endometrial hyperplasia or carcinoma? *Gynecol Oncol* 1998; 68:4–7.

36. Farquhar CM, Lethaby A, Sowter M, et al. An evaluation of risk factors for endometrial hyperplasia in premenopausal women with abnormal menstrual bleeding. *Am J Obstet Gynecol* 1999; 181:525–9.

37. Gredmark T, Kvint S, Havel G, et al. Adipose tissue distribution in postmenopausal women with adenomatous hyperplasia of the endometrium. *Gynecol Oncol* 1999; 72:138–42.

38. Anastasiadis PG, Skaphida PG, Koutlaki NG, et al. Descriptive epidemiology of endometrial hyperplasia in patients with abnormal uterine bleeding. *Eur J Gynaecol Oncol* 2000; 21:131–4.

39. Koss LG, Schreiber K, Oberlander SG, et al. Detection of endometrial carcinoma and hyperplasia in asymptomatic women. *Obstet Gynecol* 1984; 64:1–11.

40. Koss LG. Detection of occult endometrial carcinoma. *J Cell Biochem Suppl* 1995; 23:165–73.

41. Vuento MH, Pirhonen JP, Makinen JI, et al. Screening for endometrial cancer in asymptomatic postmenopausal women with conventional and colour Doppler sonography. *Br J Obstet Gynaecol* 1999; 106:14–20.

42. Woodruff JD, Pickar JH. Incidence of endometrial hyperplasia in postmenopausal women taking conjugated estrogens (Premarin) with medroxyprogesterone acetate or conjugated estrogens alone. The Menopause Study Group. *Am J Obstet Gynecol* 1994; 170:1213–23.

43. Archer DF, Furst K, Tipping D, et al. A randomized comparison of continuous combined transdermal delivery of estradiol-norethindrone acetate and estradiol alone for menopause. CombiPatch Study Group. *Obstet Gynecol* 1999; 94:498–503.

44. Kurman RJ, Felix JC, Archer DF, et al. Norethindrone acetate and estradiol-induced endometrial hyperplasia. *Obstet Gynecol* 2000; 96:373–9.

45. Bjarnason K, Cerin A, Lindgren R, et al. Adverse endometrial effects during long cycle hormone replacement therapy. Scandinavian Long Cycle Study Group. *Maturitas* 1999; 32:161–70.

46. Bergeron C, Fox H. Low incidence of endometrial hyperplasia with acceptable bleeding patterns in women taking sequential hormone replacement therapy with dydrogesterone. *Gynecol Endocrinol* 2000; 14:275–81.

47. Baak JP, Wisse-Brekelmans EC, Fleege JC, et al. Assessment of the risk on endometrial cancer in hyperplasia, by means of morphological and morphometrical features. *Pathol Res Pract* 1992; 188:856–9.

48. Hunter JE, Tritz DE, Howell MG, et al. The prognostic and therapeutic implications of cytologic atypia in patients with endometrial hyperplasia. *Gynecol Oncol* 1994; 55:66–71.

49. Janicek MF, Rosenshein NB. Invasive endometrial cancer in uteri resected for atypical endometrial hyperplasia. *Gynecol Oncol* 1994; 52:373–8.

50. Ho SP, Tan KT, Pang MW, et al. Endometrial hyperplasia and the risk of endometrial carcinoma. *Singapore Med J* 1997; 38:11–15.

51. Lindahl B, Willen R. Endometrial hyperplasia following estrogen treatment without the addition of gestagen. A follow-up study after withdrawal of estrogens. *Anticancer Res* 1991; 11: 2071–3.

52. Parazzini F, La Vecchia C, Bocciolone L, et al. The epidemiology of endometrial cancer. *Gynecol Oncol* 1991; 41:1–16.

53. Weber AM, Belinson JL, Piedmonte MR. Risk factors for endometrial hyperplasia and cancer among women with abnormal bleeding. *Obstet Gynecol* 1999; 93:594–8.

54. Daly MB, Bookman MA, Lerman CE. Female reproductive tract: cervix, endometrium, ovary. In: Greenwald P, Kramer BS, Weed DL (eds) *Cancer Prev Control*. New York: Marcel Dekker, 1995, pp. 585–610.

55. Brinton LA, Barrett RJ, Berman ML, et al. Cigarette smoking and the risk of endometrial cancer. *Am J Epidemiol* 1993; 137:281–91.

56. Weir HK, Sloan M, Kreiger N. The relationship between cigarette smoking and the risk of endometrial neoplasms. *Int J Epidemiol* 1994; 23:261–6.

57. Sturgeon SR, Sherman ME, Kurman RJ, et al. Analysis of histopathological features of endometrioid uterine carcinomas and epidemiologic risk factors. *Cancer Epidemiol Biomarkers Prev* 1998; 7:231–5.

58. Grady D, Ernster VL. Endometrial cancer. In: Schottenfeld D, Fraumeni JF Jr (eds) *Cancer epidemiology and prevention*. New York: Oxford University Press, 1996, pp. 1058–89.

59. Kreiger N, Marrett LD, Clarke EA, et al. Risk factors for adenomatous endometrial hyperplasia: a case-control study. *Am J Epidemiol* 1986; 123:291–301.

60. Weiderpass E, Baron JA, Adami HO, et al. Low-potency oestrogen and risk of endometrial cancer: a case-control study. *Lancet* 1999; 353: 1824–8.

61. Horwitz RI, Feinstein AR. Alternative analytic methods for case-control studies of estrogens and endometrial cancer. *N Engl J Med* 1978; 299:1089–94.

62. Rothman KJ, Greenland S. *Modern Epidemiology*, 2nd ed. Philadelphia: Lipincott-Raven, 1998, pp. 139–40.

63. The Writing Group for the PEPI Trial. Effects of hormone replacement therapy on endometrial histology in postmenopausal women. The Postmenopausal Estrogen/Progestin Interventions (PEPI) Trial. *JAMA* 1996; 275:370–5.

64. Grimbizis G, Tsalikis T, Tzioufa V, et al. Regression of endometrial hyperplasia after treatment with the gonadotrophin-releasing hormone analogue triptorelin: a prospective study. *Hum Reprod* 1999; 14:479–84.

65. Beral V. Exogenous sex hormones and cancer. In: Lilienfeld AM (ed) *Reviews in cancer epidemiology*. New York: Elsevier, 1980, pp. 126–30.

66. Kendrick JS, Wingo P, Rubin GL, et al. Combination oral contraceptive use and the risk of endometrial cancer. *JAMA* 1987; 257:796–800.

67. Burke TW, Tortolero-Luna G, Malpica A, et al. Endometrial hyperplasia and endometrial cancer. *Obstet Gynecol Clin North Am* 1996; 23:411–56.

68. Fisher B, Costantino JP, Redmond CK. Endometrial cancer in tamoxifen-treated breast cancer patients: findings from the National Surgical Adjuvant Breast and Bowel Project (NSABP) B-14. *J Natl Cancer Inst* 1994; 86:527–37.

69. Henderson BE, Ross R, Bernstein L. Estrogens as a cause of human cancer. *Cancer Res* 1988; 48:246–53.

70. Baanders-van Halewyn EA, Blankenstein MA, Thijssen JH, et al. A comparative study of risk factors for hyperplasia and cancer of the endometrium. *Eur J Cancer Prev* 1996; 5:105–12.

71. La Vecchia C, Decarli A, Fasoli M, et al. Nutrition and diet in the etiology of endometrial cancer. *Cancer* 1986; 57:1248–53.

72. Bakour SH, Khan KS, Gupta JK. The risk of premalignant and malignant pathology in endometrial polyps. *Acta Obstet Gynecol Scand* 2000; 79:317–20.

73. Cherkis RC, Patten SF Jr, Dickinson JC, et al. Significance of atypical endometrial cells detected by cervical cytology. *Obstet Gynecol* 1987; 69:786–9.

74. Kurman RJ, Solomon D. The Bethesda System for Reporting Cervical/Vaginal Cytologic Diagnoses: Definitions, criteria, and explanatory notes for terminology and specimen adequacy. New York: Springer, 1994.

75. Gomez-Fernandez CR, Ganjei-Azar P, Behshid K, et al. Normal endometrial cells in Papanicolaou smears: prevalence in women with and without endometrial disease. *Obstet Gynecol* 2000; 96:874–8.

76. Nguyen TN, Bourdeau JL, Ferenczy A, et al. Clinical significance of histiocytes in the detection of endometrial adenocarcinoma and hyperplasia. *Diagn Cytopathol* 1998; 19:89–93.

77. Hakala T, Mecklin JP, Forss M, et al. Endometrial carcinoma in the cancer family syndrome. *Cancer* 1991; 68:1656–9.

78. Yancey M, Magelssen D, Demaurez A, et al. Classification of endometrial cells on cervical cytology. *Obstet Gynecol* 1990; 76:1000–5.

79. Ferenczy A. Methods for detecting endometrial carcinoma and its precursors. In: Buchsbaum HJ, Sciarra JJ (eds) *Gynecology and obstetrics,* Vol. 4. New York: Harper & Row, 1982, pp. 1–8.

80. Tsuda H, Kawabata M, Yamamoto K, et al. Prospective study to compare endometrial cytology and transvaginal ultrasonography for identification of endometrial malignancies. *Gynecol Oncol* 1997; 65:383–6.

81. Grimes DA. Diagnostic dilation and curettage: a reappraisal. *Am J Obstet Gynecol* 1982; 142:1–6.

82. Karlsson B, Granberg S, Wikland M, et al. Transvaginal ultrasonography of the endometrium in women with postmenopausal bleeding—a Nordic multicenter study. *Am J Obstet Gynecol* 1995; 172:1488–94.

83. Goldstein SR. Saline infusion sonohysterography. *Clin Obstet Gynecol* 1996; 39:248–58.

84. Takahashi S, Murakami T, Narumi Y, et al. Preoperative staging of endometrial carcinoma: diagnostic effect of T2-weighted fast spin-echo MR imaging. *Radiology* 1998; 206:539–47.

85. Pritchard KI. Screening for endometrial cancer: is it effective? *Ann Intern Med* 1989; 110:177–9.

86. Screening for Endometrial Cancer (PDQ). Screening/Detection—Health Professionals. US National Cancer Institute. Updated: August, 2000. Available at URL: *http://cancernet.nci.nih. gov/pdq/pdq_screening.shtml.*

87. Jordan VC, Morrow M. Should clinicians be concerned about the carcinogenic potential of tamoxifen? *Eur J Cancer* 1994; 30A:1714–21.

88. Suh-Burgmann EJ, Goodman A. Surveillance for endometrial cancer in women receiving tamoxifen. *Ann Intern Med* 1999; 131:127–35.

89. Goldstein SR. Unusual ultrasonographic appearance of the uterus in patients receiving tamoxifen. *Am J Obstet Gynecol* 1994; 170:447–51.

90. Barakat RR. Benign and hyperplastic endometrial changes associated with tamoxifen use. *Oncology* 1997; 11 (2 Suppl 1):35–7.

91. Pike MC, Spicer DV. Hormonal contraception and chemoprevention of female cancers. *Endocr Relat Cancer* 2000; 7:73–83.

92. Agorastos T, Bontis J, Vakiani A, et al. Treatment of endometrial hyperplasias with gonadotropin-releasing hormone agonists: pathological, clinical, morphometric, and DNA-cytometric data. *Gynecol Oncol* 1997; 65:102–14.

93. Spitz IM, Chwalisz K. Progesterone receptor modulators and progesterone antagonists in women's health. *Steroids* 2000; 65:807–15.

18
Ovary

Joellen M. Schildkraut

Ovarian cancer has a prevalence of about 50 per 100,000 and an annual incidence of 14 per 100,000 in the United States [1,2]. The median age at diagnosis of the epithelial form of ovarian cancer, the most common histologic type, is approximately 59 years [3]. In the absence of a family history of ovarian cancer, the lifetime risk of developing this disease is one in 70, compared to breast cancer for which the lifetime risk is one in 8 [4]. With 25,200 new cases per year and about 14,500 deaths, ovarian cancer is the fifth leading cause of cancer death among women and has the highest death rate of the gynecologic cancers [4]. Because ovarian cancer is usually not detected prior to extensive intraperitoneal spread of disease, survival is poor, despite treatment with cytoreductive surgery and combination chemotherapy [5].

The stage at diagnosis is the most important factor in predicting a patient's prognosis for survival from ovarian cancer [6–8]. More than half of patients with ovarian cancer are stage III or IV at the time of diagnosis. The 5-year survival rate for all stages of ovarian cancer is less that 40%, but women diagnosed with stage I disease may have an 80% to 90% survival rate [9–11]. Also, women diagnosed with ovarian cancer confined to the ovaries are approximately four times more likely to survive 5 years than women diagnosed with distant metastatic disease.

Early diagnosis is the key to improving the survival rates of ovarian cancer patients. However, a definable preinvasive lesion in the ovary has not been identified thus far. Since ovarian cancer usually presents in an advanced stage, identification of putative precursors is difficult. Unfortunately there are no recognized symptoms in early stages. Abdominal pain or fullness, early satiety, dyspepsia, frequent urination, or constipation are signals that the disease has spread throughout the pelvic and abdominal cavities. Identification of a sufficiently specific and sensitive screening test for ovarian cancer would have the potential to improve the treatment and survival of ovarian cancer, but none yet exists. Therefore preventive strategies are worthy of consideration.

The Etiology of Ovarian Cancer

Although there are some established risk factors for ovarian cancer, the etiology of this disease is not well understood, and clearly, given the absence of definable precursor lesions, there have been no studies that addressed the epidemiology of precursors to ovarian cancer. However, there are several theories concerning the pathogenesis of ovarian cancer, and there is compelling evidence suggesting that there may be several pathways leading to this disease.

Histopathological Characteristics

The histologic characteristics of ovarian cancers are found in Table 18.1. Ovarian cancer is a collection of diverse pathologic entities that can broadly be characterized as epithelial, germ

TABLE 18.1. Histologic features of ovarian tumors.

	Overall frequency	Proportion malignant	Types
Non epithelial tumors	20%–30%	5%–8%	
Germ cell	15%–20%	3%–5%	Teratoma
			Dysgerminoma
			Endodermal sinus tumor
			Choriocarcinoma
Sex cord-stromal	5%–10%	2%–3%	Fibroma
			Granulosa-theca cell tumor
			Sertoli-Leydig cell tumor
Epithelial tumors	65%–70%	90%	
	60%	25%	Serous
			Mucinous
			Endometrioid
			Clear cell
			Brenner tumor
			Cystadenofibroma

Source: Kumar et al., 1997 [144], with permission.

cell, or sex cord-stromal in origin. The incidence of germ cell tumors peaks in young adulthood, whereas that of sex cord-stromal tumors peaks in middle age [5]. In contrast, patients with epithelial tumors have an older age at onset [5]. Epithelial ovarian cancer constitutes approximately 90% of all ovarian cancer diagnoses and is the focus of this discussion [12]. The most common epithelial histologic subtype of epithelial ovarian cancer is serous carcinoma (~53%) [13]. Other histologic subtypes of epithelial ovarian cancer include mucinous (~16%), endometrioid (~16%), clear cell (~7%), and other (~8%). Most patients with epithelial ovarian cancer remain asymptomatic until they reach an advanced stage that coincides with the time of initial presentation. Approximately 70% of patients present initially with Internal Federation of Gynecology and Obstetrics (FIGO) stage III or IV disease [14]. The incidence of epithelial ovarian cancer is lower in blacks than in whites [15].

Epithelial ovarian cancers are classified either as low malignant potential (LMP; borderline tumors) or invasive malignant lesions. By definition, an LMP tumor has some but not all of the morphologic features of malignancy, and obvious invasion of adjacent stroma is lacking [9]. LMP tumors form 10% to 20% of all ovarian epithelial neoplasms, are mostly seen at younger ages, and exhibit a low level of malignant behavior, although they are considered to be a malignant tumor. LMP tumors are more likely to present as stage I and stage II disease (80%) in contrast to approximately 30% of invasive tumors. At all stages, survival is better among patients with borderline tumors [6,14].

The leading theory for ovarian tumorigenesis is that epithelial ovarian tumors arise from the single cell layer lining the ovarian surface or the ovarian surface epithelium [12]. It has been proposed that the ovarian epithelium is predisposed to undergo a malignant transformation because it is disrupted during every ovulatory event and needs to be repaired (see "incessant ovulation hypothesis" below), or perhaps because it is exposed to high levels of estrogen and other substances in cyst fluid (see "gonadotropin hypothesis", later). Recently, an alternative hypothesis was proposed by Dubeau [16] who, based on evidence observed during embryogenesis, suggested that components of the secondary müllerian system should be considered as having a possible role in ovarian tumorigenesis.

Risk Factors

The variation of epithelial ovarian cancer, with respect to menopausal status, age at onset, stage, histological type, tumor behavior (invasive versus LMP tumors), and survival, likely reflects differences in underlying causes of this disease. Family history, reproductive experiences (including difficulties encountered in infertility treatment), oral contraceptive (OC) use and other factors related to altered hormonal profiles (e.g., menstrual cycle characteristics and tubal ligation) remain the most promising leads to understanding the development of epithelial ovarian cancer. However, ovarian cancer risk factors unrelated to reproductive history and hormone exposures have been reported. Relative risk (RR) estimates for the relationship between some of the most established epidemiologic risk factors are found in Table 18.2.

It has long been established that ovarian cancer risk decreases with high parity [17–19] and OC use [20–22]. Studies have shown that OC use decreases the risk of ovarian cancer overall by approximately 30% to 40%, and that there is a dose-response relationship [22,23]. The protective effect of a single term pregnancy is estimated to be 40% while each subsequent pregnancy decreases risk by an additional 14% [22]. Failed pregnancies confer lesser degrees of protection. Women with low parity or who are nulliparous are at increased risk for developing ovarian cancer. Low parity may be voluntary or involuntary. Conditions associated with low parity including contraception, infertility, and hysterectomy, have been shown to alter ovarian cancer risk [24].

Although infertility and inability to conceive have been reported to be associated with an increased risk of epithelial ovarian cancer, it has also been reported that a life-long irregular menstrual pattern is negatively associated with the risk of ovarian cancer, supporting the idea that anovulation may be protective [25]. Whittemore et al. [22] and Rossing et al. [26] reported data which suggest there is an association between the use of fertility drugs and ovarian cancer, which might explain the association with infertility. These studies suggest that ovulation induction and the hyperstimulatory effects of fertility medications on the ovary increase the risks of ovarian cancer. Some investigators have suggested an alternative explanation for these findings, proposing that

the abnormal hormonal environment experienced by infertile women, rather than exposure to the drug, would explain this apparent association [24,27,28].

TABLE 18.2. Epidemiologic risk factors for epithelial ovarian cancer.

Risk factors[1]	Relative risk/ range of relative risks
Number of full term pregnancies [22]	
0	1.0 (referent)[2]
1	0.60
2	0.53
3	0.48
4	0.36
5	0.33
6+	0.29
Nulliparity [22]	
No	1.0 (referent)[2]
Yes	2.13
Duration of oral contraceptive use (years) [22]	
0	1.0 (referent)[2]
<1	0.93
2–3	0.87
4–5	0.58
6+	0.30
Lactation duration (months) [22]	
0	1.0 (referent)[2]
1–5	0.87
6–11	0.74
12–23	0.69
23+	0.74
History of infertility due to an ovulatory abnormality [22]	
No	1.0 (referent)
Yes	2.1
Tubal ligation [22]	
No	1.0 (referent)
Yes	0.87
Family history of ovarian cancer in a 1° relative [32,34,145]	
No	1.0 (referent)[2]
Yes	2.0–4.0
Talc (application of dusting) powder/talc to peritoneal area [5]	
No	1.0 (referent)
Yes	1.1–3.9

[1] Numbers in brackets are references.
[2] Statistically significant p < 0.05.

Data from case-control studies support that having had a tubal ligation or hysterectomy is associated with a small decrease in the risk of developing ovarian cancer [29,30]. An earlier menopause [29] or hormonal changes, such as lower estradiol and progesterone levels, resulting from tubal ligation or hysterectomy may explain these associations [24,29,30].

One of the most consistent risk factors for ovarian cancer is having had a first degree relative who was diagnosed with the disease [31–33]. RR estimates are in the range of 2.0 to 4.0 [31,32,34]. Family history of breast and colon cancer has also been associated with an increased risk of ovarian cancer [32,35–37]. More recently, a gene causing high breast and ovarian cancer risk, *BRCA1*, was identified [38], and subsequently, a second gene involved in breast-ovarian cancers, *BRCA2* on chromosome 13q, was cloned. It appears that the risk for ovarian cancer associated with *BRCA2* mutations may not be quite as elevated as the risk associated with the *BRCA1* gene [39,40]. Together, it appears that mutations in *BRCA1* and *BRCA2* account for approximately 10% of all cases of ovarian cancer [41]. For ovarian cancer, estimates of lifetime risk for women with a family history of such cancers range from 16% to 80% compared to one in 70 for women without such a family history [42–44]. Risk estimates, derived from family studies for research purposes are likely to be overestimates of the cancer risk associated with *BRCA1* and *BRCA2* mutations and should be interpreted with caution, because these families represent the high penetrant families and are highly selected [45]. The second most common form of hereditary ovarian cancer is associated with hereditary nonpolyposis colorectal cancer syndrome (HNPCC), which involves mutations in mismatch repair genes (i.e., *hMSH2, hMLH1, hPMS1,* and *hPMS2*) [46]. Froggatt et al. [47] recently reported a 20% risk of developing ovarian cancer by age 50 in HNPCC families with a mutation in the *MSH2* gene. Additionally, familial ovarian cancer is likely to be a complex disease resulting from several different susceptibility genes as well as genetic and environmental modifiers. Genetic susceptibility can influence the risk of disease by itself, or it may exacerbate the effect of an environmental risk factor, or the risk factor may exacerbate the genetic effect [48].

Dietary factors (e.g., fat intake and low intake of fruits and vegetables) have received less attention, but the available data provide conflicting evidence of an effect [30,49–51]. The use of talc as an hygienic agent on contraceptive devices and sanitary products has also been associated with an increased risk of ovarian cancer in some studies [52,53]. Obesity, and alcohol, tobacco and caffeine use have occasionally been linked to increased ovarian cancer risk [54].

Some studies have suggested that there may be etiologic differences between the histologic subtypes of epithelial ovarian cancer. A recent study confirmed previous reports indicating a lack of association between parity and OC use, family history of breast cancer, and the risk of mucinous tumors [55]. Researchers found that mucinous cases had not used noncontraceptive estrogens more frequently than controls; in this respect, mucinous cases differed from invasive serous cases and endometrioid cases. The association of epithelial ovarian cancer with dietary intake of saturated fat was stronger for mucinous than for non mucinous cases, and in addition, current cigarette smokers experience close to a 3-fold increased risk for developing ovarian cancer of the mucinous histologic subtype [56].

The extent to which these epidemiologic risk factors represent multiple, distinct causal pathways has not been determined. Furthermore, little is known with regard to the relationship between epidemiologic factors and biological events underlying carcinogenesis.

Pathogenic Models of Ovarian Cancer

Most theories of ovarian carcinogenesis focus on the roles of ovulation and gonadotropins. It has been postulated that epithelial proliferation required to repair ovulatory defects may lead to accumulation of genetic damage. The two major theories that have been associated with the pathogenesis of ovarian cancer are the "incessant ovulation hypothesis" (or "uninterrupted ovulation hypothesis") [57,58] and the "gonadotropin hypothesis" [17,58].

Under the incessant ovulation hypothesis, ovulation leads to entrapment of epithelial cells in the underlying stroma with subsequent formation of inclusion cysts. These cysts could represent precursor lesions in which transformation is facilitated. Proliferation of epithelial cells required to repair the disrupted ovarian surface after ovulation could contribute to carcinogenesis by increasing the likelihood of mutations due to spontaneous errors in DNA synthesis [59,60]. If mutations involve critical growth regulatory genes, this could facilitate clonal expansion of premalignant cells with an increased susceptibility to becoming fully transformed subsequently. Several observations support the premise that ovulation is causally related to the development of ovarian cancer. First, epithelial ovarian cancer is exceedingly rare in women with Turner's syndrome, who are anovulatory. In addition, epithelial ovarian cancer is rare in other animal species, such as rats and mice, which ovulate infrequently, whereas it is common in hens, which like humans, are frequent ovulators [61]. However, women with polycystic ovarian syndrome (PCOS), a disorder characterized by anovulation, were found to have surface epithelial inclusion cysts approximately five times more often than women without PCOS. There is also some indication that women with PCOS are at increased risk for developing ovarian cancer [28]. Both these findings weigh against this hypothesis [62].

The gonadotropin hypothesis is based on the assumption that repetitive exposure to high levels of follicle stimulating hormone (FSH) and luteinizing hormone (LH) during ovulation also could contribute to ovarian carcinogenesis. This model incorporates the "incessant ovulation hypothesis" and a pathogenic model linking ovarian failure, gonadotropins, and ovarian cancer [32,63]. Ovarian damage, manifested by primary and secondary amenorrhea, infertility, premature menopause, and subsequent ovarian cancer is consistent with this model.

A third theory, suggesting that there is pregnancy-dependent clearance of cells that have undergone malignant transformation (apoptosis or programmed cell death) from the ovaries, has been recently proposed [64]. Apoptosis is an important means through which cells that have sustained DNA damage can be eliminated. Progestin (e.g., progesterone and 17-hydroxyprogestereone) levels increase early in pregnancy and are sustained at high levels through gestation [65]. A recent study in primates demonstrated that the progestin component in OC pills induces apoptosis in the ovarian epithelium [66]. Data on the protective effect of a shorter time since last birth and later age at last birth also support this theory. A later pregnancy may be more likely to eliminate a larger accumulation of damaged cells than an earlier pregnancy [67,68].

Finally, Ness and Cottreau [69] recently proposed that an inflammatory reaction induced by ovulatory events, asbestos and talc exposure, endometriosis, or pelvic inflammatory disease might be a pathophysiologic contributor to the development of ovarian cancer. In contrast, tubal ligation and hysterectomy, which are protective factors, may diminish the likelihood that the ovarian epithelium is exposed to environmental initiators of inflammation by severing the pathway from the lower to the upper genital tract and preventing inflammatory substances from ascending through the lower genital tract to the upper genital tract and ultimately to the ovarian epithelium [70]. Inflammation, which entails cell damage, oxidative stress, and elevations of cytokines and prostaglandins, all of which may be mutagenic, is a possible mechanism for DNA damage in the inflammation-induced inclusion cysts. Support for this hypothesis was obtained in a recent case-control study which demonstrated an increased risk of ovarian cancer associated with environmental factors associated with inflammatory responses [69].

Data from epidemiologic studies are not entirely consistent with what the various hypotheses would predict. The incessant ovulation hypothesis assumes an equal protective effect of anovulation due to OC use, pregnancy, earlier menopause, and breast-feeding. Yet, analyses of data from case-control studies indicate that the protective effect of pregnancy and

OC use may not be entirely due to suppression of ovulation [22,71]. For example, in an analysis of 12 case-control studies of epithelial ovarian cancer, a single term pregnancy was estimated to decrease risk by 40%, and each subsequent pregnancy decreased risk by an additional 14%; failed pregnancies conferred lesser degrees of protection [22]. Five years of OC use decreased the risk of ovarian cancer by 50% while decreasing total years of ovulation by only 10% to 20% [22]. It is possible that prolonged interruption of ovarian epithelial proliferation might increase the likelihood of apoptosis of cells that have acquired genetic damage. If this is the case, 5 years of interruption of ovulation could negate the effect of a greater number of years of accumulated genetic damage [68]. Alternatively, it is possible that a greater protective effect due to pregnancy than what would be expected due to anovulation alone may be explained through the modulation of gonadotropin levels [23].

In addition, under the gonadotropin hypothesis, exogenous estrogen exposure would be expected to have a protective effect against developing ovarian cancer, since exogenous estrogen is known to decrease gonadotropin stimulation. However, an association between estrogen replacement therapy and the risk of developing ovarian cancer has not been demonstrated [22]. Gonadotropin levels in postmenopausal women receiving hormone replacement remain higher than those of premenopausal women. Therefore, it is not clear whether the lack of a protective effect of hormone replacement is because levels remain above a critical threshold, or because gonadotropins do not influence the carcinogenic process. Although lactation tends to suppress ovulation, it increases release of FSH; therefore it might not be expected to decrease the risk of developing ovarian cancer. Yet, breast feeding has been shown to be protective in most studies [22]. An association between premature or early menopause, due to high gonadotropin production, and increased risk of ovarian cancer is also consistent with the gonadotropin hypothesis for ovarian cancer risk [32]. However, investigation of the relationship between age at menopause and

ovarian cancer has produced inconsistent results. Some studies have reported increased risks with early menopause [32,72], others with late menopause [18,33], and still others have reported no effects [73,74].

Recent studies suggest that ovulation induction and the hyperstimulatory effects of fertility medications on the ovary increase the risk of ovarian cancer [26,75]. However, it is also possible that elevated gonadotropin or androstenedione levels, which are associated with some conditions of infertility such as PCOS, may be responsible for the increase in risk [28]. As women move into menopause, their hormonal environment changes and becomes more similar to that of women with PCOS, suggesting that hormonal factors may play even a more important role in later onset ovarian cancer.

A strong protective effect related to recent pregnancy or OC use might suggest the importance of apoptosis/cell clearing in the etiology of ovarian cancer. However, an interesting interaction between age at diagnosis and OC use and parity was reported [22]. The protective effect of parity was much stronger in women under age 55 at diagnosis, while the protective effect of OC use was stronger in women diagnosed over age 55. This interaction may reflect a cohort effect due to secular trends in OC formulation or OC use and in family planning practices; however, it also may provide tentative evidence of etiologic heterogeneity with respect to pre- and postmenopausal ovarian cancer. It is possible that later onset ovarian cancer may be etiologically distinct from ovarian cancer with an earlier onset. Ovulation may be more important in the etiology of premenopausal ovarian cancer and different etiologic pathways may be involved in the development of postmenopausal ovarian cancer in women for whom exposure to ovulation occurred in the remote past.

Ovarian cancer is most likely a heterogeneous disease with various underlying causes. It is plausible that there may be coexisting causal pathways, possibly interconnected, in the pathogenesis of ovarian cancer (see Figure 18.1).

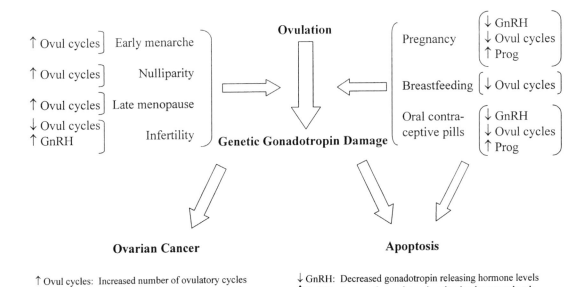

FIGURE 18.1. Integrated pathogenic model for ovarian cancer.

Evidence for the Existence of Precursor Lesions

Proposed precursors of some ovarian cancers include serous inclusion cysts, "dysplasia" of the ovarian surface epithelium or the lining of cysts, borderline tumors (atypical proliferative tumors or LMP tumors), and endometriosis [76]. However, if a histologically definable preinvasive lesion exists in the ovary, it has not been convincingly defined thus far. Since ovarian cancer usually presents at an advanced stage, identification of putative precursors is difficult. It has been suggested that since neither premalignant lesions nor transition from a premalignant to a malignant phase have been described, the premalignant phase is probably of short duration and therefore difficult to observe [62].

Pathologic and Epidemiologic Evidence

Whether ovarian carcinomas develop from malignant transformation of precursor lesions, such as benign cystadenocarcinomas or LMP tumors, from the ovarian surface epithelium or from inclusion cysts, or whether they arise *de novo*, has been the subject of debate [77,78]. However, a high prevalence of hyperplasia and müllerian metaplasia on the surface epithelium or in the inclusion cysts has been reported in patients with epithelial ovarian tumors, suggesting a potential role for these lesions as morphologic precursors of this disease [12, 62]. Additionally, histologic characteristics of ovarian dysplasia adjacent to carcinoma have been found to be the same as those seen in ovaries removed for reasons other than malignancy, suggesting a single underlying pathologic process [79]. Also, ovaries removed by prophylactic oophorectomy reveal ovarian dysplasia and occasionally ovarian carcinoma [80]. Sherman et al. [76] compared histologic findings in benign ovaries among those who were at increased risk of developing ovarian cancer compared to those at normal risk. Although inclusion cysts were identified more frequently among older women, no difference in cyst formation was found in the high-risk group compared to the normal-risk group after age adjustment. There was also an increased frequency of atypia detected among women at high risk compared to those at normal risk, although this was not statistically significant. These results were in contrast to two other studies that reported an increased frequency of inclusion cysts among high-risk subjects, that is, among those who had a family history of breast and ovarian cancer [81,82]. Additionally, inclusion cysts have been found to occur more frequently in ovaries of nulliparous women and women with PCOS, individuals at increased risk of developing ovarian cancer [12,62]; however, these comparisons were not age-adjusted, and it is possible that age differences may explain these findings [76].

Support for the theory that ovarian carcinomas arise *de novo* is seen in the observation that early ovarian carcinomas of high histological grades are observed in the absence of adjacent lower-grade or benign tumors, and low grade or benign tumors appear phenotypically stable over long periods of time, showing no evidence of gradual progression [77]. However, sometimes histologically benign tumors are observed adjacent to ovarian carcinomas, and ovarian tumors are often classified as mixed histological grades, suggesting that the higher-grade lesions arise from low-grade carcinomas by clonal expansion [77].

Zheng et al. [77] did not find the allelic losses in low-grade or benign neoplasms that were found in low-grade or benign areas adjacent to invasive tumors. If benign or low-grade tumors preceded the high-grade tumors, then allelic loss may have predisposed these lesions to progress toward more aggressive lesions. Thus, the possibility of a single lesion with different degrees of maturation in different areas could not be ruled out. Wolf et al. [78] observed that heterogeneous histologic appearance was related to aneuploidy in the tumor components, supporting the possibility that benign and LMP tumors may have genetic aberrations that predispose them to malignant transformation. However, a report of a series of 14 cases of microscopic *de novo* ovarian cancer in otherwise normal-sized ovaries challenges this view for at least a subset of ovarian cancer [2]. Importantly, no temporal relationship between the appearance of the various proposed stages of progression has yet been established.

There have been only a few epidemiologic studies of ovarian cysts, benign ovarian neoplasms, and LMP ovarian tumors. It has been suggested that LMP tumors may be an intermediate form of ovarian cancer, between benign and malignant tumors. Yet LMP tumors are different with respect to biologic and clinical behavior. Although the age at diagnosis of ovarian tumors of LMP is earlier than that of invasive ovarian tumors, the epidemiologic risk factors appear similar, but not identical, to those of invasive ovarian tumors [55,83,84]. A stronger protective effect for OC use among women with LMP tumors compared to invasive tumors has been described [85]. Exposure to fertility drugs was reported to be more strongly associated with increased risk of borderline tumors than with increased risk of invasive tumors [83]. A relationship between an older age at menopause was reported for LMP tumors but not for invasive tumors [85]. In one study, none of the women diagnosed with LMP ovarian tumors reported a family history of ovarian cancer, but three percent of the women with invasive tumors reported such a history [31].

Data from several case-control studies of ovarian cysts and benign ovarian neoplasms suggest some similarities and some differences in risk factors for these versus invasive ovarian cancers [25,85,86]. In one study, comparing women who had given birth with nulliparous women, the risk of ovarian cysts decreased with increasing number of births [25]. A small case-control study of women with benign epithelial ovarian neoplasms, functional ovarian cysts, and dermoid cysts revealed that the etiology of ovary cysts and benign ovarian neoplasms may differ [86]. Recent OC use was associated with reduced risk of all three tumor types. Among benign neoplasms only, an increased risk was associated with nulliparity and infertility, and a decreased risk was associated with multiparity. However, these differences may be explained by the small sample sizes for the different tumor types. The results of a more recent and larger case-control study of benign ovarian tumors, including serous adenomas, teratomas, endometriomas, and mucinous adenomas, were consistent with the finding that oral contraceptives are associated with a reduced risk of benign ovarian tumors [87].

Molecular Markers

The delineation of the molecular biology of ovarian cancer appears to hold some promise for the identification of early lesions of this disease and, more importantly, some such findings may be useful for screening detection of ovarian cancer. It will be critical to identify early molecular alterations that increase risk of ovarian cancer. However, a thorough understanding of the molecular pathogenesis for the particular disease is required to characterize genetic lesions in such a way as to lead to the development of a screening strategy targeting a particular gene or gene product. This is a very complex problem.

Some of the genetic mechanisms that have been studied in relation to the molecular carcinogenesis of ovarian cancer include genes involved in the regulation of cell proliferation, for example, tumor suppressor genes such as *BRCA1* and *BRCA2* and growth factors such as epidermal growth factor (EGF) and transforming growth factor (TGF). Of the molecular genetic lesions currently known to be present in ovarian cancer, mutations or deletions of the *p53* tumor suppressor gene are the most common. These have been found in 40% to 70% of stage III and IV ovarian cancers [88–93] and in 16% to 50% of stage I and II cancers [88–90]. Overexpression of *p53*, which is highly correlated with mutation of the *p53* gene, is much less common in LMP ovarian cancer than in invasive tumors and has been reported to occur within a range of 4% to 24% of LMP [6,94–96]. In addition, well-differentiated tumors are less likely to overexpress *p53* compared to moderately/poorly differentiated tumors [97].

As discussed earlier, in the section entitled "Pathologic and Epidemiologic Evidence", there have been reports of cases in which a transition from normal to neoplastic surface epithelium and focal carcinoma appears on a background of surface epithelium inclusion cysts with varying degrees of cytologic atypia. Such reports support the notion that the origin of these ovarian cancers is from the surface epithelium and its inclusion cysts [2]. However, mutations in the *p53* gene have also been a rare finding in possible precursor lesions such as cystic adenomas. Together, these findings have been interpreted to mean that alterations in the *p53* gene are indicative of a more aggressive disease and tumor progression. However, data from other published reports contradict this interpretation and suggest that *p53* alterations may be an early event in ovarian carcinogenesis. Huston et al. [98] found atypia in the inclusion cysts in eight of thirteen stage III serous ovarian carcinomas. Of these, five exhibited *p53* overexpression. No atypia was observed in the cysts of LMP tumors or normal ovaries. In addition, *p53* expression was also seen more frequently in surface epithelium associated with ovarian serous adenocarcinoma than in normal ovaries. These findings are consistent with the premise that atypia in epithelial inclusion cysts is a precursor of ovarian malignancy, and suggest that *p53* overexpression may precede the onset of cytological abnormalities of invasive but not LMP ovarian tumors. Additionally, investigators recently described the molecular characteristics of an *in situ* ovarian tumor found in a women who underwent prophylactic oophorectomy. The patient had a personal history of a previous primary breast cancer, a family history of both breast and ovarian cancer, and had tested positive for a *BRCA1* mutation. The ovarian tumor exhibited loss of heterozygosity and overexpression of *p53* indicating that *p53* mutation is an early change in ovarian carcinogenesis [99].

The epidemiologic literature assessing the molecular epidemiology of ovarian cancer is sparse. Results of a case-series and case-control analysis also provide evidence for an association of ovarian tumors overexpressing *p53* with lifetime ovulatory cycle exposure, supporting the incessant ovulation hypothesis for ovarian cancer. This suggests that *p53* mutations may be an early event in ovarian cancer pathogenesis [97], and these results are consistent with more than one possible causal pathway in the pathogenesis of ovarian cancer. Since these results were not subsequently confirmed [100], more research into this relationship is required.

Finally, findings from a case report of the same mutation of the p53 gene in both a primary ovarian mucinous adenocarcinoma and a synchronous contralateral ovarian mucinous tumor offer a somewhat different interpretation concerning p53 alterations in LMP tumors and the relationship between tumors of LMP and invasive ovarian tumors. It has been suggested that the presence of a heterogeneous degree of differentiation is indicative of a progressive loss of differentiation, with the metastatic site representing reversibility in morphological differentiation, rather than differentiation among mucinous tumors [101].

In addition to *p53*, overexpression of several other proto-oncogenes, including *MYC* (30%), *EGFR* (35%), and *HER-2/neu* (24%), have been described [14]. As with *p53*, overexpression of these genes has been linked to poor prognosis and advanced disease [102,103]. With the exception of mucinous ovarian tumors, mutation and/or overexpression of the *RAS* oncogenes is uncommon in ovarian cancer. This is consistent with epidemiologic findings and suggests that there may be a difference between the pathogenesis of mucinous ovarian cancer and that of other forms of this disease [14,55,56].

Additional clues to the molecular carcinogenesis of ovarian cancer come from observations of genetic losses on multiple chromosomes. Several chromosomes, including chromosomes 3, 6, 11, and 17, have been identified as having nonrandom deletions in ovarian tumors, suggesting genomic regions where tumor suppressor genes associated with ovarian cancer may be found [104–111]. One example is that of the genetic susceptibility gene for breast and ovarian cancer, *BRCA1*, on chromosome 17q [38,112].

Prevention Strategies

Screening and early detection represent one strategy for decreasing cancer mortality. However, in most cancers in which screening has an impact (such as cervical and colorectal cancer), there is a well-defined preinvasive lesion, and screening efforts focus on detection

and eradication of these precursors. In contrast, the preinvasive lesion that precedes the development of ovarian cancer remains unknown. Easy accessibility of the target organ is another characteristic of cancers in which screening programs have been successful, as this facilitates detection of preinvasive and early invasive changes (for example, as with the breast). Unfortunately, the ovaries are small, relatively inaccessible organs that lie in the peritoneal cavity, and most masses that arise in the ovaries are not malignant or even premalignant.

Screening: Biochemical Markers

Since a premalignant state for ovarian cancer has not yet been identified, the focus of screening strategies has been on the detection of ovarian cancer in an earlier state. One strategy is to identify a highly specific biomarker (or a combination of several biomarkers) that could be applied for early detection.

A number of cell-surface antigens and serum proteins are produced by ovarian tumors and can be assayed using monoclonal antibodies. Some of these assays have been applied clinically as markers of disease status and are useful in the detection of subclinical disease and in the diagnosis of recurrent ovarian cancer. Most known markers are not unique to ovarian cancer. The challenge of finding a highly specific biomarker remains.

Of the biomarkers described for ovarian cancer, CA125 has been the most extensively studied. CA125 is a cell-surface glycoprotein that is detectable in 80% of epithelial ovarian cancer cases [113,114]. CA125 has been shown to be elevated prior to clinical development of primary and recurrent ovarian cancer. However, CA125 is elevated in less than half of the cases of early ovarian cancer, and in premenopausal patients, several benign conditions, including endometriosis, pelvic inflammatory disease, pregnancy, and leiomyoma uteri, are also associated with mild elevations of CA125. Malignancies of the lung, breast, colon, cervix, endometrium, and pancreas have also been associated with elevated CA125 [115]. Interestingly, mucinous neoplasms of the ovary generally are not associated with elevated CA125. A randomized trial of screening with CA125 in normal risk postmenopausal women demonstrated an increased survival duration for ovarian cancer patients, even among women in stages III and IV [116]. However, sensitivity is a concern in premenopausal patients, patients with stage I disease, and for those patients with mucinous tumors [117].

Additional markers that can be assayed using monoclonal antibodies exist, including TAG 72, CA 15-3, CA 54/61, CA 19-9, NB/70K, and OVX1 [14,118]. In addition, lipophosphatidic acid (LPA), measured via mass spectrometry, has shown promise as a biomarker for detection of early stage ovarian cancer [118]. Thus far, it appears that only combinations of these markers are promising although such testing involves considerable laboratory effort.

The possibility of combining methods, specifically CA125 detection and transvaginal ultrasound, to improve specificity and sensitivity of screening, is being investigated in the NCI PLCO (prostate, lung, colorectal, and ovarian) screening trial [119]. Even if a significant reduction in mortality could be demonstrated with a screening program that employed ultrasound and serum markers, this approach has not been shown to be practical because of the high cost associated with screening for low incidence disease.

Chemoprevention

Despite the formidable obstacles to treatment and screening, epidemiologic studies suggest that prevention of ovarian cancer is a realistic goal. In fact, new data reveal a decrease in the incidence rates of ovarian cancer in the United States in women of ages 35 to 59 [120]. The strong protective effect of OC pills against ovarian cancer provides dramatic evidence of the potential efficacy of chemopreventive strategies. Observations concerning the protective effect of a recent last pregnancy, which may be due to apoptosis, also support this concept.

If the mechanism underlying the protective effect of OC pills can be elucidated, then it may be possible to devise a pharmacologic chemopreventive strategy that is more effective than OC pills, while eliminating side effects and not interfering with ovulation. The apoptosis pathway may be a virtually universal safeguard to prevent the persistence and proliferation of damaged cells that can be detrimental to the organism. There is mounting evidence that activation of the apoptosis pathway is the critical mechanism underlying chemopreventive effects of a number of agents including the retinoids [121–129], dietary flavanoids [130], anti-inflammatory drugs [131], monoterpenes [132,133], S-adenosyl-L-methionine [134], and selenium [135,136]. The possibility that oral contraceptive progestin activates the apoptosis pathway in the ovarian epithelium raises the possibility that this class of hormones can be used for chemoprevention of ovarian cancer and provides new hope for reducing the risk of this highly fatal disease.

Prophylactic Surgery

In addition to chemoprevention, prophylactic oophorectomy and interruption of fallopian tubes have been suggested as possible means for reducing a high-risk individual's risk of developing ovarian cancer [34,137,138]. The only published study concerning prophylactic oophorectomy suggests the protective effect may only decrease the risk by two fold [139]. Although prophylactic oophorectomy has a potential benefit, it has also been shown that it may not address the potential future risk of papillary serous carcinoma of the peritoneum, which is a particular issue among women from high-risk families and women with *BRCA1* mutations [140,141].

Conclusions

Thus far, pathologic examination of the ovary has not provided consistent evidence for defining early morphologic changes related to ovarian carcinogenesis [11,12,62,76–78,81,82]. It remains unproven that available ovarian cancer screening technologies can decrease mortality from this disease. The inability to detect a premalignant phase makes early detection of ovarian cancer difficult. However, many forms of cancer are thought to develop through a multistep process of progression from benign to malignant as a series of genetic changes [142]. Although it is not known to what extent this progression theory can explain the natural history of ovarian cancer, the advent of new surgical laparoscopic techniques making the ovaries more accessible can provide laparoscopic biopsy material that may reveal early preinvasive or precancerous lesions. Since there is some indication that molecular markers associated with the early phase of ovarian cancer pathogenesis can be identified, a direct assessment of genetic markers may be necessary for implementing a useful approach for screening [14]. Even if a significant reduction in mortality could be demonstrated, this approach might not be practical because of the low cost-effectiveness associated with screening for a relatively uncommon disease [143]. Therefore, it is important to be able to further delineate high-risk populations to enhance chemopreventive, prophylactic surgery, and screening strategies. Clearly, further studies are required incorporating the epidemiology, pathology, and molecular biology of potential precursors and early lesions of ovarian cancer.

References

1. Wingo PA, Tong T, Bolden S. Cancer statistics, 1995. *CA Cancer J Clin* 1995; 45:8–30.
2. Bell DA, Scully RE. Early de novo ovarian carcinoma. A study of fourteen cases. *Cancer* 1994; 73:1859–64.
3. Amos CI, Shaw GL, Tucker MA, et al. Age at onset for familial epithelial ovarian cancer. *JAMA* 1992; 268:1896–9.
4. American Cancer Society. *Cancer Facts & Figures—1999*. Atlanta: American Cancer Society, 1999, p. 36.
5. Weiss NS. Ovary. In: Schottenfeld D, Fraumeni J (eds) *Cancer epidemiology and prevention*. Philadelphia: WB Saunders Company, 1982, pp. 871–80.
6. Schildkraut JM, Halabi S, Bastos E, et al. Prognostic factors in early-onset epithelial ovarian cancer: a population-based study. *Obstet Gynecol* 2000; 95:119–27.
7. Parker SL, Tong T, Bolden S, et al. Cancer statistics, 1997. *CA Cancer J Clin* 1997; 47:5–27.

8. de Souza PL, Friedlander ML. Prognostic factors in ovarian cancer. *Hematol Oncol Clin North Am* 1992; 6:761–82.
9. Ozols RF, Rubin SC, Dembo AJ, et al. Epithelial ovarian cancer. In: Hoskins WJ, Perez CA, Young RC (eds) *Principles and practice of gynecologic oncology*. Philadelphia: JB Lippincott, 1992, pp. 731–81.
10. Morrow CP. Malignant and borderline epithelial tumors of the ovary: Clinical features, staging, diagnosis, intraoperative assessment and review of management. In: Coppleson M (ed) *Gynecologic oncology: fundamental principles and clinical practice*. Edinburgh: Churchill Livingston, 1992, pp. 889–915.
11. Westhoff C, Randall MC. Ovarian cancer screening: potential effect on mortality. *Am J Obstet Gynecol* 1991; 165:502–5.
12. Scully RE. Pathology of ovarian cancer precursors. *J Cell Biochem Suppl* 1995; 23 (Suppl): 208–18.
13. Russell P, Farnsworth A. *Surgical pathology of the ovaries*. New York: Churchill Livingstone, 1997, p. 231.
14. Teneriello MG, Park RC. Early detection of ovarian cancer. *Cancer J Clin* 1995; 45:71–87.
15. Miller BA, Kolonel LN, Bernstein L, et al. *Racial/ethnic patterns of cancer in the United States*. Bethesda: National Cancer Institute, 1996, p. 101.
16. Dubeau L. The cell of origin of ovarian epithelial tumors and the ovarian surface epithelium dogma: does the emperor have no clothes? *Gynecol Oncol* 1999; 72:437–42.
17. Cramer DW, Hutchinson GB, Welch WR. Determinants of ovarian cancer risk. II. Inferences regarding pathogenesis. *J Natl Cancer Inst* 1983; 71:717–21.
18. Franceschi S, LaVecchia C, Helmrick SP, et al. Risk factors for epithelial ovarian cancer in Italy. *Am J Epidemiol* 1982; 115:714–19.
19. Joly DJ, Lilienfeld AM, Diamond EL, et al. An epidemiologic study of the relationship of reproductive experience to cancer of the ovary. *Am J Epidemiol* 1974; 99:190–209.
20. Rosenberg L, Shapiro S, Stone D. Epithelial ovarian cancer and combination oral contraceptives. *JAMA* 1982; 247:3210–2.
21. Weiss NS, Lyon JL, Liff JM, et al. Incidence of ovarian cancer in relation to the use of oral contraceptives. *Int J Cancer* 1981; 28:669–71.
22. Whittemore AS, Harris R, Itnyre J, et al. Characteristics relating to ovarian cancer risk: collaborative analysis of twelve U.S. case-control

studies. IV. The pathogenesis of epithelial ovarian cancer. *Am J Epidemiol* 1992; 136:1212–20.

23. Risch HA, Weiss NS, Lyon JL, et al. Events of reproductive life and the incidence of epithelial ovarian cancer. *Am J Epidemiol* 1983; 117:128–39.

24. Risch HA, Howe GR. Pelvic inflammatory disease and the risk of epithelial ovarian cancer. *Cancer Epidemiol Biomarkers Prev* 1995; 4:447–51.

25. Parazzini F, La Vecchia C, Negri E, et al. Menstrual factors and the risk of epithelial ovarian cancer. *J Clin Epidemiol* 1989; 42:443–8.

26. Rossing MA, Daling JR, Weiss NS, et al. Ovarian tumors in a cohort of infertile women. *N Engl J Med* 1994; 331:771–6.

27. Bristow RE, Karlan BY. Ovulation induction, infertility, and ovarian cancer risk. *Fertil Steril* 1996; 66:499–507.

28. Schildkraut JM, Schwingl P, Bastos E, et al. Epithelial ovarian cancer risk among women with polycystic ovarian disease. *Obstet Gynecol* 1996; 88:554–9.

29. Cramer DW, Xu H. Epidemiologic evidence for uterine growth factors in the pathogenesis of ovarian cancer. *Ann Epidemiol* 1995; 5:310–4.

30. Risch HA, Jain M, Marrett LD, et al. Dietary fat intake and risk of epithelial ovarian cancer. *J Natl Cancer Inst* 1994; 86:1409–15.

31. Schildkraut JM, Thompson WD. Familial ovarian cancer: a population-based case-control study. *Am J Epidemiol* 1988; 128:456–66.

32. Cramer DW, Hutchinson GB, Welch WR, et al. Determinants of ovarian cancer risk. I. Reproductive experiences and family history. *J Natl Cancer Inst* 1983; 71:711–6.

33. Hildreth NG, Kelsey JL, Livolsi VA. An epidemiologic study of epithelial carcinoma of the ovary. *Am J Epidemiol* 1981; 114:398–405.

34. Kerlikowske K, Brown JS, Grady DG. Should women with familial ovarian cancer undergo prophylactic oophorectomy? *Obstet Gynecol* 1992; 80:700–7.

35. Schildkraut JM, Thompson WD. Relationship of epithelial ovarian cancer to other malignancies within families. *Genet Epidemiol* 1988; 5:355–67.

36. Schildkraut JM, Risch N, Thompson WD. Evaluating genetic associations among ovarian, breast and endometrial cancer: evidence for a breast/ovarian cancer relationship. *Am J Hum Genet* 1989; 86:7204–7.

37. Thompson WD, Schildkraut JM. Family history of gynecologic cancers: Relationships to the incidence of breast cancer prior to age 55. *Int J Epidemiol* 1991; 20:595–602.

38. Miki Y, Swenson J, Shattuck-Eidens D, et al. A strong candidate for the breast and ovarian cancer susceptibility gene *BRCA1*. *Science* 1994; 266:66–71.

39. Wooster R, Neuhausen SL, Mangion J, et al. Localization of a breast cancer susceptibility gene, *BRCA2*, to chromosome 13q12-13. *Science* 1994; 265:2088–91.

40. Wooster R, Bignell G, Lancaster J, et al. Identification of the breast cancer susceptibility gene *BRACA2*. *Nature* 1995; 378:789–92.

41. Claus EB, Schildkraut JM, Thompson WD, et al. The genetic attributable risk of breast and ovarian cancer. *Cancer* 1996; 77:2318–24.

42. Streuwing JP, Hartge P, Wacholder S, et al. The risk of cancer associated with specific mutations of *BRCA1* and *BRCA2* among Ashkenazi Jews. *N Engl J Med* 1997; 336:1401–8.

43. Easton DF, Ford D, Bishop DT. Breast and ovarian cancer incidence in *BRCA1*-mutation carriers. *Am J Hum Genet* 1995; 56:265–71.

44. Ford D, Easton DF, Bishop DT, et al. Risks of cancers in *BRCA1* mutation carriers. *Lancet* 1994; 343:692–5.

45. Burke W, Daly M, Garber J, et al. Recommendations for follow-up care of individuals with cancer susceptibility mutations: *BRCA1* and *BRCA2* associated mutations. *JAMA* 1997; 277:997–1003.

46. Angioli R, Estape R, Mason M, et al. Hereditary and sporadic ovarian cancer: genetic testing and clinical implications. *Int J Oncol* 1998; 12:1029–34.

47. Froggatt NJ, Green J, Brassett C, et al. A common MSH2 mutation in English and North American HNPCC families: origin, phenotypic expression, and sex specific differences in colorectal cancer. *J Med Genet* 1999; 36:97–102.

48. Ottman R. An epidemiologic approach to gene-environment interaction. *Genet Epidemiol* 1990; 7:177–85.

49. Byers T, Marshall J, Graham S, et al. A case-control study of dietary and nondietary factors in ovarian cancer. *J Natl Cancer Inst* 1983; 71:681–6.

50. Cramer DW, Welch WR, Hutchinson GB, et al. Dietary animal fat in relation to ovarian cancer risk. *Obstet Gynecol* 1984; 63:833–8.

51. Slattery ML, Schuman KL, West DW, et al. Nutrient intake and ovarian cancer. *Am J Epidemiol* 1989; 130:497–502.

52. Cramer DW, Welch WR, Scully RE, et al. Ovarian cancer and talc: a case-control study. *Cancer* 1982; 50:372–6.

53. Harlow BL, Cramer DW, Bell DA, et al. Perineal exposure to talc and ovarian cancer risk. *Obstet Gynecol* 1992; 80:19–26.

54. Hartge P, Schiffman MH, Hoover R, et al. A case-control study of epithelial ovarian cancer. *Am J Obstet Gynecol* 1989; 161:10–6.

55. Risch HA, Marrett L, Jain M, et al. Difference in risk factors for epithelial ovarian cancer by histologic type. *Am J Epidemiol* 1996; 144: 363–72.

56. Marchbanks PA, Wilson H, Bastos E, et al. Cigarette smoking and epithelial ovarian cancer by histologic type. *Obstet Gynecol* 2000; 95:255–60.

57. Fathalla MF. Incessant ovulation: a factor in ovarian neoplasia? *Lancet* 1971; 2:163.

58. Pike MC. Age-related factors in cancers of the breast, ovary, and endometrial. *J Chronic Dis* 1987; 40 (Suppl):59–69.

59. Ames BN, Gold LS. Too many rodent carcinogens: mitogenesis increases mutagenesis. *Science* 1990; 249:970–97.

60. Preston-Martin S, Pike ML, Ross RK, et al. Increased cell division as a cause of human cancer. *Cancer Res* 1990; 50:7415–21.

61. Fredrickson TN. Ovarian tumors of the hen. *Env Health Perspect* 1987; 73:35–51.

62. Resta L, Russo S, Colucci GA, et al. Morphologic precursors of ovarian epithelial tumors. *Obstet Gynecol* 1993; 82:181–6.

63. Cramer DW. Epidemiologic aspects of early menopause and ovarian cancer. *Ann NY Acad Sci* 1990; 592:363–75, 390–4.

64. Adami HO, Hsieh CC, Lambe M, et al. Parity, age at first birth, and risk of ovarian cancer. *Lancet* 1995; 344:1250–4.

65. O'Leary P, Boyne P, Flett P, et al. Longitudinal assessment of changes in reproductive hormones during normal pregnancy. *Clin Chem* 1991; 37:667–72.

66. Rodriguez GC, Walmer DK, Cline M, et al. Effect of progestin on the ovarian epithelium of macaques: cancer prevention through apoptosis? *J Soc Gynecol Invest* 1998; 5:271–6.

67. Albrektsen G, Heuch I, Kvale G. Reproductive factors and incidence of epithelial ovarian cancer: A Norwegian prospective study. *Cancer Causes Control* 1996; 7:421–7.

68. Cooper GS, Schildkraut JM, Whittemore AS, et al. Pregnancy recency and risk of ovarian cancer. *Cancer Causes Control* 1999; 10:397–402.

69. Ness RB, Grisso JA, Cottreau C, et al. Factors related to inflammation of the ovarian epithelium and risk of ovarian cancer. *Epidemiology* 2000; 11:111–7.

70. Green A, Purdie D, Green L, et al. Validity of self-reported hysterectomy and tubal sterilisation. The Survey of Women's Health Study Group. *Aust NZ J Public Health* 1997; 21:337–40.

71. Siskind V, Green A, Bain C, et al. Beyond ovulation: oral contraceptives and epithelial ovarian cancer. *Epidemiology* 2000; 11:106–10.

72. Wynder EL, Dodo H, Barber HRK. Epidemiology of cancer of the ovary. *Cancer* 1969; 23: 352–70.

73. Annegers JF, Strom H, Decker DG, et al. Ovarian Cancer: incidence and case-control study. *Cancer* 1979; 43:723–9.

74. Hartge P, Hoover R, McGowan L, et al. Menopause and ovarian cancer. *Am J Epidemiol* 1988; 127:990–8.

75. Whittemore AS, Harris R, Itnyre J, et al. Characteristics relating to ovarian cancer risk: collaborative analysis of twelve U.S. case-control studies. II. Invasive epithelial ovarian cancers in white women. *Am J Epidemiol* 1992; 136: 1184–203.

76. Sherman ME, Lee JS, Burks RT, et al. Histopathologic features of ovaries at increased risk for carcinoma. A case-control analysis. *Int J Gynecol Pathol* 1999; 18:151–7.

77. Zheng J, Wan M, Zweizig S, et al. Histologically benign or low-grade malignant tumors adjacent to high-grade ovarian carcinomas contain molecular characteristics of high-grade carcinomas. *Cancer Res* 1993; 53:4138–42.

78. Wolf NG, Abdul-Karim FW, Schork NJ, et al. Origins of heterogeneous ovarian carcinomas. A molecular cytogenetic analysis of histologically low malignant potential, and fully malignant components. *Am J Pathol* 1996; 149: 511–20.

79. Deligdisch L, Einstein AJ, Guera D, et al. Ovarian dysplasia in epithelial inclusion cysts. A morphometric approach using neural networks. *Cancer* 1995; 76:1027–34.

80. Deligdisch L, Gil J, Kerner H, et al. Ovarian dysplasia in prophylactic oophorectomy specimens: cytogenetic and morphometric correlations. *Cancer* 1999; 86:1544–50.

81. Afify AM, Bielat KL, Eltabbakh GH, et al. Characteristics of ovaries prophylactically removed from women with a family history of ovarian cancer (Abstr). *Mod Pathol* 1998; 11:100A.

82. Salazar H, Godwin AK, Daly MB, et al. Microscopic benign and invasive malignant neoplasms and a cancer-prone phenotype in prophylactic oophorectomies [comments]. *J Natl Cancer Inst* 1996; 88:1810–20.

83. Harris R, Whittemore AS, Itnyre J. Characteristics relating to ovarian cancer risk: collaborative analysis of 12 US case-control studies. III. Epithelial tumors of low malignant potential in white women. Collaborative Ovarian Cancer Group. *Am J Epidemiol* 1992; 136:1204–11.

84. Harlow BL, Weiss NS, Lofton S. Epidemiology of borderline ovarian tumors. *J Natl Cancer Inst* 1987; 78:71–4.

85. Parazzini F, Moroni S, Negri E, et al. Risk factors for seromucinous benign ovarian cysts in northern Italy. *J Epidemiol Community Health* 1997; 51:449–52.

86. Booth M, Beral V, Maconochie N, et al. A case-control study of benign ovarian tumours. *J Epidemiol Community Health* 1992; 46:528–31.

87. Westoff C, Britton JA, Gammon MD, et al. Oral contraceptives and benign ovarian tumors. *Am J Epidemiol* 2000; 152:242–6.

88. Allan LA, Campbell MK, Milner BJ, et al. The significance of *p53* mutations and overexpression in ovarian cancer prognosis. *Int J Gynecol Cancer* 1996; 6:483–90.

89. van der Zee AGJ, Hollema H, Suurmeijer AJH, et al. Value of p-glycoprotein, glutathione s-transferase pi, c-*erb*B-2, and p53 as prognostic factors in ovarian carcinomas. *J Clin Oncol* 1995; 13:70–8.

90. Hartman LC, Posratz KC, Kenney GL, et al. Prognostic significance of p53 immunostaining in epithelial ovarian cancer. *J Clin Oncol* 1994; 12:64–9.

91. Hollstein M, Sidransky D, Vogelstein B, et al. *p53* mutations in human cancers. *Science* 1991; 253:49–53.

92. Marks JR, Davidoff AM, Kerns B, et al. Overexpression and mutation of *p53* in epithelial ovarian cancer. *Cancer Res* 1991; 51:2979–84.

93. Nigro JM, Baker SJ, Preisinger AC, et al. Mutations in the *p53* gene occur in diverse human tumor types. *Nature* 1989; 342:705–8.

94. Berchuck A, Kohler MF, Hopkins MP, et al. Overexpression of *p53* is not a feature of benign and early stage borderline epithelial ovarian tumors. *Gynecol Oncol* 1994; 52: 232–6.

95. Wertheim I, Muto MG, Welch WR, et al. *p53* gene mutation in human borderline epithelial ovarian tumors. *J Natl Cancer Inst* 1994; 86: 1549–51.

96. Eltabbakh GH, Belinson JL, Kennedy AW, et al. *p53* and *HER2/neu* overexpression in ovarian borderline tumors. *Gynecol Oncol* 1997; 65:218–24.

97. Schildkraut JM, Bastos E, Berchuck A. Relationship between lifetime ovulatory cycles of mutant *p53* in epithelial ovarian cancer. *J Natl Cancer Inst* 1997; 89:932–8.

98. Hutson R, Ramsdale J, Wells M. *p53* protein expression in putative precursor lesions of epithelial ovarian cancer. *Histopathology* 1995; 27:367–71.

99. Werness BA, Parvatiyar P, Ramus SJ, et al. Ovarian carcinoma *in situ* with germline *BRCA1* mutation and loss of heterozygosity at *BRCA1* and *TP53*. *J Natl Cancer Inst* 2000; 92:1088–91.

100. Webb PM, Green A, Cummings MC, et al. Relationship between number of ovulatory cycles and accumulation of mutant *p53* in epithelial ovarian cancer. *J Natl Cancer Inst* 1998; 90: 1729–34.

101. Werness BA, DiCioccio RA, Piver MS. Identical, unique *p53* mutations in a primary ovarian mucinous adenocarcinoma and a synchronous contralateral ovarian mucinous tumor of low malignant potential suggest a common clonal origin. *Hum Pathol* 1997; 28:626–30.

102. Berchuck A, Kamel A, Whitaker R, et al. Overexpression of *HER-2/neu* is associated with poor survival in advanced epithelial ovarian cancer. *Cancer Res* 1990; 50:4087–91.

103. Haldane JS, Hird V, Hughes CM, et al. c-*erb*B-2 oncogene expression in ovarian cancer. *J Pathol* 1990; 162:231–7.

104. Jones MH, Nakamura Y. Deletion mapping of chromosome 3p in female genital tract malignancies using microsatellite polymorphisms. *Oncogene* 1992; 7:1631–4.

105. Eccles DM, Brett L, Lessells A, et al. Overexpression of the p53 protein and allele loss at 17p13 in ovarian carcinoma. *Br J Cancer* 1992; 65:40–4.

106. Tsao SW, Mok CH, Oike K, et al. Involvement of *p53* gene in the allelic deletion of chromosome 17p in human ovarian tumors. *Anticancer Res* 1991; 11:1975–82.

107. Eccles DM, Cranston G, Steel CM, et al. Allele losses on chromosome 17 in human epithelial ovarian carcinoma. *Oncogene* 1990; 5:1599–601.

108. Narod SA, Feunteun J, Lynch HT, et al. Familial breast-ovarian cancer locus on chromosome 17q12-q23 [comments]. *Lancet* 1991; 338:82–3.

109. Ehlen T, Dubeau L. Loss of heterozygosity on chromosomal segments 3p, 6q and 11p in human ovarian carcinomas. *Oncogene* 1990; 5:219–23.

110. Lee JH, Kavanagh JJ, Wildrick DM, et al. Frequent loss of heterozygosity on chromosomes 6q, 11, and 17 in human ovarian carcinomas. *Cancer Res* 1990; 50:2724–8.

111. Gallion HH, Powell DE, Morrow JK, et al. Molecular genetic changes in human epithelial ovarian malignancies. *Gynecol Oncol* 1992; 47:137–42.

112. Futreal PA, Liu Q, Shattuck-Eidens D, et al. *BRCA1* mutations in primary breast and ovarian carcinomas. *Science* 1994; 266:120–2.

113. Jacobs I, Bast RC Jr. The CA 125 tumour-associated antigen: a review of the literature. *Hum Reprod* 1989; 4:1–12.

114. Bast RC Jr, Klug TL, St John E, et al. A radioimmunoassay using a monoclonal antibody to monitor the course of epithelial ovarian cancer. *N Engl J Med* 1983; 309:883–7.

115. Niloff JM. Tumor Markers. In: Hoskins WJ, Perez CA, Young RC (eds) *Principles and practice of gynecologic oncology*. Philadelphia: JB Lippincott, 1992, pp. 137–50.

116. Jacobs IJ, Skates SJ, MacDonald N, et al. Screening for ovarian cancer: a pilot randomised controlled trial [comments]. *Lancet* 1999; 353:1207–10.

117. Thompson SD. Ovarian cancer screening: a primary care guide. *Lippincotts Prim Care Pract* 1998; 2:244–50.

118. Xu Y, Shen Z, Wiper DW, et al. Lysophosphatidic acid as a potential biomarker for ovarian and other gynecologic cancers [comments]. *JAMA* 1998; 280:719–23.

119. Schapira MM, Matchar DB, Young MJ. The effectiveness of ovarian cancer screening. A decision analysis model [comments]. *Ann Intern Med* 1993; 118:838–43.

120. Gnagy S, Ming EE, Devesa SS, et al. Declining ovarian cancer rates in U.S. women in relation to parity and oral contraceptive use. *Epidemiol* 2000; 11:102–5.

121. Chan LN, Zhang S, Cloyd M, et al. N-(4-hydroxyphenyl)retinamide prevents development of T-lymphomas in AKR/J mice. *Anticancer Res* 1997; 17:499–503.

122. Ponzoni M, Bocca P, Chiesa V, et al. Differential effects of N-(4-hydroxyphenyl)retinamide and retinoic acid on neuroblastoma cells: apoptosis versus differentiation. *Cancer Res* 1995; 55:853–61.

123. Delia D, Aiello A, Lombardi L, et al. N-(4-hydroxyphenyl)retinamide induces apoptosis of malignant hemopoietic cell lines including those unresponsive to retinoic acid. *Cancer Res* 1993; 53:6036–41.

124. Seewaldt VL, Kim JH, Caldwell LE, et al. All-trans-retinoic acid mediates G1 arrest but not apoptosis of normal human mammary epithelial cells. *Cell Growth Differ* 1997; 8:631–41.

125. Lotan R. Retinoids in cancer chemoprevention. *FASEB J* 1996; 10:1031–9.

126. Sankaranarayanan R, Mathew B. *Retinoids as cancer-preventive agents*. Lyon: IARC Scientific Publications, 1996, pp. 47–59.

127. Toma S, Isnardi L, Raffo P, et al. Effects of all-trans-retinoic acid and 13-cis-retinoic acid on breast-cancer cell lines: growth inhibition and apoptosis induction. *Int J Cancer* 1997; 70: 619–27.

128. Oridate N, Lotan D, Mitchell MF, et al. Inhibition of proliferation and induction of apoptosis in cervical carcinoma cells by retinoids: implications for chemoprevention. *J Cell Biochem* 1995; 23(Suppl):80–6.

129. Dolivet G, Ton Van J, Sarini J, et al. [Current knowledge on the action of retinoids in carcinoma of the head and neck]. *Rev Laryngol Otol Rhinol* 1996; 117:19–26.

130. Kuo SM. Antiproliferative potency of structurally distinct dietary flavonoids on human colon cancer cells. *Cancer Lett* 1996; 110:41–8.

131. Thompson HJ, Jiang C, Lu J, et al. Sulfone metabolite of sulindac inhibits mammary carcinogenesis. *Cancer Res* 1997; 57:267–71.

132. Reddy BS, Wang CX, Samaha H, et al. Chemoprevention of colon carcinogenesis by dietary perillyl alcohol. *Cancer Res* 1997; 57:420–5.

133. Gould MN. Cancer chemoprevention and therapy by monoterpenes. *Environ Health Perspect* 1997; 105:977–9.

134. Pascale RM, Simile MM, De Miglio MR, et al. Chemoprevention by S-adenosyl-L-methionine of rat liver carcinogenesis initiated by 1,2-dimethylhydrazine and promoted by orotic acid. *Carcinogenesis* 1995; 16:427–30.

135. Thompson HJ, Wilson A, Lu J, et al. Comparison of the effects of an organic and an inorganic

form of selenium on a mammary carcinoma cell line. *Carcinogenesis* 1994; 15:183–6.

136. el-Bayoumy K, Upadhyaya P, Chae YH, et al. Chemoprevention of cancer by organoselenium compounds. *J Cell Biochem* 1995; 22(Suppl): 92–100.

137. Grimes DA. The safety of oral contraceptives: epidemiologic insights from the first 30 years. *Am J Obstet Gynecol* 1992; 166:1950–4.

138. Hankinson SE, Hunter DJ, Colditz GA, et al. Tubal ligation, hysterectomy, and risk of ovarian cancer. A prospective study. *JAMA* 1993; 270:2813–8.

139. Struewing JP, Watson P, Easton DF, et al. Prophylactic oophorectomy in inherited breast/ovarian cancer families. *J Natl Cancer Inst Monogr* 1995, 33–5.

140. Tobacman JK, Greene MH, Tucker MA, et al. Intra-abdominal carcinomatosis after prophylactic oophorectomy in ovarian-cancer-prone families. *Lancet* 1982; 2:795–7.

141. Karlan BY, Baldwin RL, Lopez-Luevanos E, et al. Peritoneal serous papillary carcinoma, a phenotypic variant of ovarian cancer: implications for ovarian cancer screening. *Am J Obstet Gynecol* 1999; 180:917–28.

142. Fearon ER, Vogelstein B. A genetic model for colorectal tumorigenesis. *Cell* 1990; 61:759–67.

143. Brucks JA. Ovarian cancer. The most lethal gynecologic malignancy. *Nurs Clin North Am* 1992; 27:835–45.

144. Kumar V, Cotran RS, Robbins SL. *Basic pathology*. Philadelphia: WB Saunders Company, 1997, 614–7.

145. Schildkraut, JM, Thompson, WD. Familial ovarian cancer: a population-based case-control study. *Am J Epidemiol* 1988; 128: 456–66.

19
Vulva and Vagina

Margaret M. Madeleine, Janet R. Daling, and Hisham K. Tamimi

Vulvar and vaginal precursor lesions can either regress spontaneously or lead to in situ or invasive cancer. The anogenital precursor lesions are often multifocal within a site and can occur at multiple sites. Although both vulvar and vaginal neoplasias have risk factors that are similar to cervical neoplasia risk factors, there are important differences between cancers at these sites. The most striking difference between these anogenital lesions is that though possibly all cervical cancer is caused by human papillomaviruses (HPV), there are likely to be non-HPV pathways to vulvar and vaginal cancer. In this chapter, we present the literature on vulvar and vaginal precursor lesions separately to highlight the differences in risk factors between these sites.

Vulvar Precursor Lesions

As with cervical intraepithelial neoplasia (CIN) (see Chapter 16), most vulvar neoplasia is associated with HPV [1]. However, HPV is found less often in invasive vulvar cancer than in invasive cervical cancer, which is almost always related to HPV. Even though in situ vulvar cancer has a low rate of progression [2], the treatment of vulvar intraepithelial neoplasm (VIN) can involve long-term follow-up and the cancer has a high rate of recurrence [3]. VIN is also associated with an increased risk of another genital primary malignancy [4] and with cancers at other sites [5]. Considering that the psychosexual implications for women are

potentially severe [6] and the incidence rate of in situ vulvar cancer is increasing steadily, it is important to study preinvasive vulvar cancer.

Histological Definition

VIN consists of mild, moderate, and severe dysplasia/carcinoma-in-situ, also known as VIN 1 to 3. The degree of dysplasia, from one-third to the full thickness of the epithelium, dictates the grading of the intraepithelial neoplasia. Most reports of vulvar cancer precursors in the literature are confined to discussions of squamous cell VIN 3/in situ disease. Squamous cell in situ vulvar cancer is characterized as having three distinct patterns: warty, basaloid, or keratinizing. Warty and basaloid patterns can appear together and are classified according to the predominant pattern or as mixed. This classic form of in situ vulvar cancer is the most prevalent preinvasive disease of the vulva, is mostly HPV-related, is more often multifocal, and is found in women with a younger mean age. The histology of these lesions may resemble the histology of a spectrum of pathologies ranging from condyloma to cervical intraepithelial neoplasia grades 2 to 3 [7]. One study showed that multifocal in situ vulvar cancer might represent different clones [8].

In contrast, the keratinized or differentiated (simplex) form of in situ carcinoma, which more often progresses to malignant disease, is less frequently associated with HPV and is more often unifocal [9,10]. A recent report by

Pinto et al. [11] found 16.4% (20/122) of kera-tinizing squamous cell cancers to be HPV-positive compared with 50% (18/36) of basaloid and warty invasive tumors. Haefner et al. [7] consider the keratinizing pattern to be a com-ponent of invasive disease and do not classify it as VIN. HPV-negative vulvar cancers with a keratinizing morphology occur in older women and sometimes appear with lichen sclerosis or epithelial hyperplasia. One study reported more loss of heterozygosity among HPV-negative VIN compared with HPV-positive VIN, suggesting that more genetic changes are necessary for oncogenesis in HPV-negative VIN [12].

Other, more-rare histologic types of vulvar precursor lesions include Paget's disease, melanoma-in-situ, basal cell carcinoma, verru-cous carcinoma, and sarcoma [13]. The distrib-ution of the in situ vulvar histologic types in the United States Statistics, Epidemiology, End Results (SEER) cancer registry for 1973 to 1996 is: 77.7% squamous cell carcinoma-in-situ, 20.7% carcinoma-in-situ not otherwise speci-fied, 1.0% Paget's disease, 0.5% nevi and melanomas, and 0.2% other [14].

The distribution of VIN is approximately 7% on the clitoris and introitus, 22% on the per-ineum, and 23% on the labium minorum and majorum, with 42% in two or more areas [15]. The perineal area is reported to be a high-risk area for multifocal VIN and foci of invasion [16].

The natural history of VIN is clearly affected by treatment. In a clinic-based sample of 78 VIN 1 and 2 lesions, 53.0% regressed or remained stable, 20.8% recurred, and 26.4% progressed to a higher stage over 5 to 15 years of evaluation at 6-month intervals [17]. The recurrence rate for in situ lesions ranges from 21% [17] to 36% [18] in case series. The natural history of VIN was observed in one study that reported seven out of eight untreated women progressed to invasive carcinoma within 8 years, including three women in their forties [19]. The prevalence of another primary anogenital lesion preceding VIN, especially CIN, is reported to be about 20% [20]. Two registry-based studies, one in Switzerland [21] and one in the United States [5] reported

significant excess risks of lung, oropharyngeal, skin, and invasive vulvar cancer following VIN.

Descriptive Epidemiology

The highest incidence rates of invasive vulvar cancer are reported in developing countries, with a rate of 4.2 per 100,000 in Sao Paulo, Brazil [22]. The international rates of in situ disease are not reported by the International Agency for Research on Cancer (IARC), so US SEER rates are reported here. According to Woodruff [16], only 44 cases of in situ vulvar carcinoma had been reported in the United States up to 1953; by 1996, 558 cases had been reported in one year in the United States [14]. Sturgeon et al. [23] reported in 1992 that the incidence rate of squamous cell in situ vulvar cancer was increasing, while the rate of invasive cancer was constant. The incidence rate of in situ disease went from 1.3 per 100,000 women between 1973 and 1978 to 3.3 per 100,000 women between 1991 and 1996. In those same time periods, the rate of invasive vulvar cancer changed little, from 1.6 to 1.7 per 100,000 women per year (Table 19.1).

The rate of vulvar cancer is slightly higher for white women than for black women: 3.3 compared to 2.9 per 100,000 women–years for in situ vulvar cancer and 1.8 compared to 1.5/100,000 for the years of 1991 to 1996 (Figures 19.1 and 19.2). The epidemiology of in situ vulvar cancer has changed over time, a larger proportion of in situ disease occurr-ing in younger women in recent years (Table 19.2). The incidence rate of in situ disease among women in the youngest age category in 1991–1996 was triple that in 1973–1978.

The difference between in situ and invasive incidence rates may be due to treatment of in situ disease that prevents progression to inva-sive cancer, or it could be that most in situ vulvar cancer does not precede most invasive cancer, and that the two cancers are largely un-related [24]. Progression from preinvasive to invasive disease has been estimated to be as low as about 3 to 4% [18,25]. Part of the increase in the incidence rate of in situ vulvar cancer may

TABLE 19.1. Incidence rates of vaginal and vulvar cancer, 1973–1996.*

Diagnosis years	Vulva			Vagina		
	In situ	Invasive	Total	In situ	Invasive	Total
1973–78	1.28	1.63	2.91	0.37	0.70	1.06
1979–84	1.83	1.58	3.41	0.37	0.66	1.03
1985–90	2.37	1.73	4.10	0.45	0.64	1.09
1991–96	3.29	1.68	4.97	0.69	0.58	1.27
1973–96	2.27	1.66	3.93	0.48	0.64	1.12

* Incidence rates include all races, ages, and histologies and are from SEER [14]. The rates are per 100,000 women and age-adjusted to the 1970 United States standard.

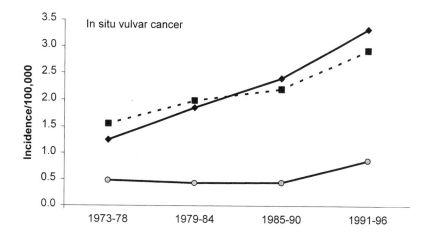

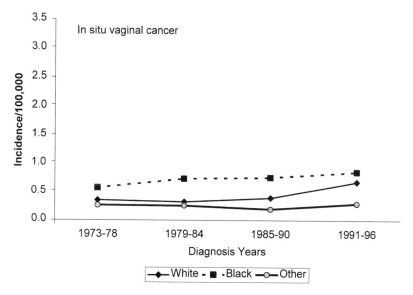

FIGURE 19.1. Incidence rates of in situ vulvar and vaginal cancer, 1973–1996, by race. Rates include women of all ages and histologic types and are from April, 1999 Surveillance, Epidemiology, and End Result (SEER) data. The incidence rates are calculated per 100,000 women and age-adjusted to the 1970 United States standard.

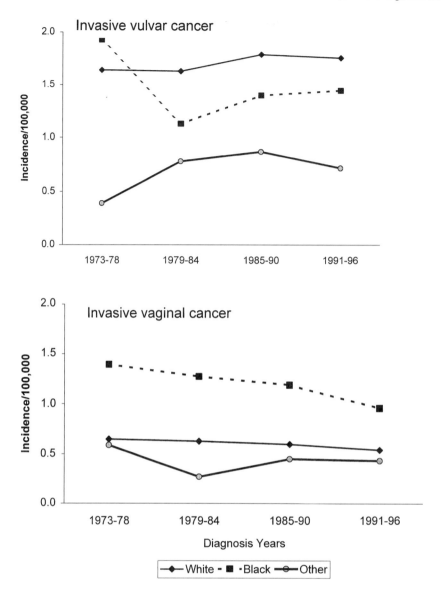

FIGURE 19.2. Incidence rates of invasive vulvar and vaginal cancer, 1973–1996, by race. Rates include women of all ages and histologic types and are from April, 1999 Surveillance, Epidemiology, and End Result (SEER) data [14]. The incidence rates are calculated per 100,000 women and age-adjusted to the 1970 United States standard.

be attributable to greater detection due to increased attention to the vulva by physicians during routine pelvic exams and increased self-detection by patients. If the increased incidence rate reflects a true increase in squamous cell in situ vulvar disease, perhaps there has been increased exposure to HPV through an increase in the number of women who have had multiple sexual partners. There may also be an increased exposure to cofactors such as smoking that may predispose persistently HPV-infected women to vulvar neoplasia [26].

TABLE 19.2. Incidence rates of vaginal and vulvar cancer, 1973–1996, by age at diagnosis.[1]

Diagnosis years	In situ vulva, Age at diagnosis			In situ vagina, Age at diagnosis		
	15–44	45–64	65–79	15–44	45–64	65–79
1973–78	1.20	2.63	2.68	0.21	0.96	0.91
1979–84	2.01	3.37	3.43	0.20	0.82	1.28
1985–90	2.64	4.27	4.43	0.30	1.01	1.17
1991–96	3.59	6.42	5.40	0.51	1.38	2.23
1973–96	2.47	4.29	4.12	0.31	1.06	1.45
Diagnosis years	Invasive vulva, Age at Diagnosis			Invasive vagina, Age at diagnosis		
	15–44	45–64	65–79	15–44	45–64	65–79
1973–78	0.42	2.74	8.06	0.17	1.19	3.46
1979–84	0.42	2.47	7.29	0.21	1.18	2.69
1985–90	0.46	2.84	8.12	0.14	1.14	3.15
1991–96	0.48	2.66	7.62	0.15	1.04	2.66
1973–96	0.45	2.67	7.76	0.17	1.14	2.96

[1] Incidence rates include all races, ages, and histologies and are from SEER [14]. The rates are per 100,000 women and age-adjusted to the 1970 United States standard.

Etiology

In situ vulvar carcinoma is predominantly a neoplasm that affects sexually active women. Case-control studies by Brinton et al. [27] and Sherman et al. [28] reported increased risk of in situ vulvar carcinoma associated with sexual transmission of disease, and/or a history of multiple sexual partners, genital warts, or genital herpes. In recent studies of in situ vulvar cancer, the prevalence of HPV DNA after amplification by polymerase chain reaction ranged from 59% (13/22) [29] to 91.9% (147/160) [30]. The risk of VIN associated with HPV 16 antibody seroprevalence has been measured using virus-like particle assays in two population-based studies (OR = 13.4, 95% CI: 3.9–46.5 [31] and OR = 3.6, 95% CI: 2.6–4.8 [26]). One study found that the seroprevalence of HPV 16 was 18.2% in controls, 22.2% in women with invasive keratinizing vulvar cancer, 50.0% in women with invasive basaloid or warty vulvar cancer, and 59.1% in women with VIN [32].

A history of anogenital cancer at another site, particularly a prior history of cervical cancer, has been reported among women with in situ vulvar cancer. A population-based case-control study by Sherman et al. [20] reported that 23.0% of women with in situ cancer but only 0.9% of controls reported a prior anogenital cancer. In a case series, Buscema et al. [33] reported that 27% of women with VIN had an associated cervical neoplasm.

Cigarette smoking was reported as a potential risk factor for in situ vulvar cancer in some early case reports. Observational studies were able to specify this risk in defined populations that represent the population at risk. In an early case-control study, Brinton et al. [27] found an elevated risk of VIN associated with current smoking (OR = 4.7, 95% CI: 2.2–10.0) but this relationship was not seen with invasive disease (OR = 1.2, 95% CI: 0.6–2.2). In a large case-control study, the relative risk of in situ vulvar cancer associated with current smoking was 6.4 (95% CI: 4.4–9.3) [26], but was lower for women with invasive disease (OR = 3.0, 95% CI: 1.7–5.3). The risks of in situ and invasive disease associated with current smoking were significantly different from each other in the latter study, and the prevalence of current smoking was 63.5%, 42.7%, and 25.4% for women with in situ disease, invasive disease, and controls, respectively. Former smokers in both studies had only modest relative risks associated with VIN (OR = 1.8, 95% CI: 0.7–4.4 [27] and OR = 2.1, 95% CI: 1.4–3.3) [26].

In both of the above case-control studies, the adjusted relative risk of in situ vulvar cancer associated with a history of genital warts was strongly elevated (OR = 18.5, 95% CI: 5.5–62.5 [27] and OR = 5.8, 95% CI: 8.4–29.8 [28]). Since the HPV types most often associated with genital warts are not oncogenic, genital warts may be a marker of exposure to other HPV types and may indicate a lack of ability to mount a sufficient immune response.

Impaired cell-mediated immunity is also associated with VIN, as reported in studies of immunosupressed patients. One study compared 20 women with multiple anogenital neoplasia to 20 control women and found evidence of significantly suppressed T cell ratios and response to mitogens [34]. In another study, the excess of anogenital neoplasia in renal transplant patients was estimated to be 20-fold [35]. In a clinic-based cross-sectional study, 6.1% of 396 HIV-positive women compared with 0.8% of 375 HIV-negative women had VIN [36]. There will soon be a report from linked AIDS and cancer registries of an excess risk of VIN after AIDS diagnosis in the United States [37]. The overall relative risk for vulvar and vaginal in situ cancers in the registry study was 3.9 (95% CI: 2.0–7.0). As the lifespan of women with AIDS and HIV is increased by the use of highly active antiretroviral therapy, increased screening for VIN and other HPV-related anogenital lesions may be indicated. Studies of renal transplant patients, who also suffer from cell-mediated immune suppression, have also noted an increase in HPV-related precursor lesions [38].

Detection

About 45% of women with VIN present with a 6-month history of itching and irritation [33],

symptoms which are also indicative of nonneoplastic infections and dystrophies [39]. Screening by visual inspection of the vulva during routine gynecologic exams may be followed by colposcopy with acetic acid application, cytology, pathology, and HPV testing when indicated. As with cervical neoplasia, the prevention of early vulvar cancer precursor lesions lies in identifying persistent infection with oncogenic HPV types [40].

Prevention

The goal of prevention activities, such as visual examination of the vulva, is to prevent cancer. Since in situ vulvar cancer is often multifocal, the entire anogenital region of women with VIN and other HPV-related lesions should be monitored closely in order to detect new or subsequent lesions at an early stage. The rate of recurrences is high with in situ vulvar cancer, so clinical follow-up of women treated for in situ vulvar cancer usually involves gynecologic visits every 3 to 6 months after initial treatment for many years. Women with a history of anogenital neoplasia, genital warts, impaired immunity, and women who are current cigarette smokers and HPV-positive should be considered to be at higher risk of multifocal or recurrent in situ vulvar cancer. Patients with vulvar condylomata should be examined periodically to detect early neoplasia. Women who are at high risk of vulvar cancer could be taught to practice self-examination [41].

Vaginal Precursor Lesions

Vaginal cancer is one of the rarest of the gynecologic malignancies. Vaginal intraepithelial neoplasia (VAIN) is the precursor lesion for squamous cell invasive vaginal cancer. The natural history of VAIN is thought to be the same as that of cervical intraepithelial neoplasia [42,43]. Progression of VAIN to invasive disease has been described in a number of studies [44–47]. The incidence of VAIN has been increasing as a result of changes in sexual practices starting in the mid-1960s. Improved cytological and colposcopic screening techniques may account in part for the increasing incidence of VAIN [48].

Histologic Definition

VAIN is defined as "the spectrum of intra-epithelial changes beginning with generally well-differentiated neoplasm, traditionally classified as mild dysplasia, and ending with invasive carcinoma" [49]. The changes in the squamous epithelium above the basement membrane include abnormal mitoses, nuclear pleomorphism, loss of polarity, and loss of cell differentiation. VAIN lesions are classified from grades 1 to 3, based on the percentage of cells that are neoplastic [50], that is, grade 1: one-third of the cells from the basement membrane to the surface are undifferentiated; grade 2: more than one-third to up to and including two-thirds of the cells are undifferentiated; grade 3, more than two-thirds of the cells are undifferentiated. When a lesion breaks through the basement membrane into the vaginal mucosa, submucosa, or connective tissue of the vagina, the lesion is diagnosed as "invasive vaginal cancer". The majority (75%) of invasive vaginal cancer is squamous histology, followed by adenocarcinoma (10%), melanoma (5%), and other rare histologies [14]. Subtypes of squamous cell carcinoma include keratinizing, nonkeratinizing, verrucous, and warty. Subtypes of adenocarcinoma include clear cell, endometroid, mucinous, and mesonephic. Not much is known about the precursors for the nonsquamous cell histologies; therefore, this review focuses on the squamous cell cancer precursor, in situ vaginal cancer (VAIN 3).

Descriptive Epidemiology

The incidence rate of vaginal carcinoma-in-situ is 0.7/100,000 and for invasive vaginal cancer is 0.6/100,000, age-adjusted to the 1970 United States standard (Table 19.1). Time trends show an increase in the incidence rate for the most current time period for in situ disease and a decrease in the rate of invasive disease (Table 19.1). In Table 19.2, the incidence rate of in situ vaginal cancer is shown to increase with

increasing age from 0.5/100,000 for women less than 45 years of age, to 1.4/100,000 for women aged 45 to 64, to 2.2/100,000 for women 65 years or older. A similar pattern is seen in the incidence rates for invasive disease: 0.2, 1.0, and 2.7/100,000, respectively. The incidence rates for in situ and invasive vaginal cancer are highest in blacks, followed by whites, and lowest in the "other" racial group category (Figures 19.1 and 19.2). The incidence rate of in situ vaginal cancer has been increasing since 1979 in whites in contrast to women in other racial groups.

Etiology

No epidemiologic studies have been published that have separated the etiologic factors of "in situ" carcinoma of the vagina from invasive carcinoma of the vagina. This is likely due to the very low incidence rate of both these diseases. Brinton et al. [51] reported that risk factors for these diseases were similar, with the exception that vaginal warts were only related to VAIN. In that study, 19 of the cases had a diagnosis of VAIN, whereas 22 had invasive disease. This small number of cases was a limiting factor in determining statistically significant associations; however, in general, many of the risk factors were similar to cervical cancer risk factors. Women with vaginal cancer were more likely to have had two or more abnormal Pap smears, and 6 of the 41 women had a previous diagnosis of cervical cancer. Eighteen of the 41 women with vaginal cancer had a prior hysterectomy, as compared to 17 of 97 controls.

The few case-control studies that have been conducted have suggested a role for hysterectomy in the etiology of in situ and invasive vaginal cancer. The explanations for an association could be: (i) residual cervical disease following hysterectomy for cervical cancer; (ii) multifocal disease due to a common infectious agent (i.e., human papillomavirus); (iii) secondary lesions occuring as a result of radiation therapy for cervical disease; (iv) a new primary tumor from an entirely independent origin; and (v) apical lesions in the 4 to 5% of women who have the transformation zone outside the confines of the cervix [52–54]. Tamimi et al. [55], in an analysis of 118 squamous cell in situ cancers, 36 invasive squamous cell cancers, and 1,958 population-based controls, found that the increased risk of vaginal neoplasia associated with prior hysterectomy was highest among women who had a prior anogenital neoplasia. However, a significant elevation in risk of vaginal neoplasia was found among women with hysterectomy who did not have this history. Herman et al. [56] did not find a relationship between prior hysterectomy and vaginal cancer (16 in situ and 33 invasive case subjects) in a controlled study where they adjusted for age and prior disease of the cervix. As these authors pointed out, since 35% of adult women have had a hysterectomy, one would expect that close to 35% of women with vaginal cancer would have had a prior hysterectomy for benign conditions.

Squamous cell carcinomas of the vagina have been consistently associated with HPV infection. Condylomata occur in the vagina and have been found adjacent to carcinoma in situ of the vagina [57]. Brinton et al. [51], in their case-control study, found that 26% of women with in situ carcinoma of the vagina reported genital warts, compared to 4% of controls. This was similar to the findings of Daling et al. [58], who found that women with in situ and invasive vaginal cancer reported a history of genital warts more often than controls (20.2% for cases versus 4.7% for controls). Tamimi et al. [55] recently updated this study to include 154 cases. The relative risk of vaginal cancer associated with genital warts was 5.3 (95% CI: 3.4–8.3). Tamimi reported that HPV DNA was detected in 47 of 60 (78.3%) of the tumors found in the women with vaginal carcinoma in situ and 12 of 24 (50.0%) of the tumors from women with invasive vaginal cancer. In this study, HPV 16 L1 antibodies were present in 47.9% of the patients and 26.6% of the controls (age-adjusted OR = 2.6, 95% CI: 1.8–3.8). Ostrow et al. [59], Kiyahu et al. [60], Ikenberg et al. [61], and Okagaki et al. [62] have also reported finding HPV DNA in the tumors of women with vaginal cancer. Sugase and Matsukura [63] reported that 59 of 71 VAIN cases were positive for the HPV capsid antigen by immuno-histochemistry, but when an HPV 58 probe and blot hybridization were used, all 71 VAIN cases harbored a single HPV type at more 1,000 viral copies. They identified 15 different HPV types. The finding of numerous HPV types among women with in situ or invasive vaginal cancer is consistent with that of Daling et al. [64], who found that 15 of 43 HPV DNA positive tumors harbored HPV types other than type 16, 18, 31, 33, or 35, the types most often detected in vulvar and cervical tumors. The consistent finding of HPV DNA in the tumors, and the strong association of VAIN and invasive vaginal cancer with multiple lifetime sexual partners, clearly indicate that squamous cell in situ and invasive vaginal cancers are primarily sexually transmitted diseases [55].

Current cigarette smoking has been found to be a strong risk factor for cervical cancer [18,65,66], and it is also related to risk of in situ and invasive vaginal cancer [51,55,64]. Tamimi et al. [55] found that 40.2% of women with in situ carcinoma of the vagina and 50.0% of women with invasive carcinoma of the vagina were current smokers at diagnosis, compared to 23.6% of controls. After adjusting for age and number of lifetime sexual partners, the relative risk for in situ and invasive vaginal cancer (combined case group) was 1.7 (95% CI: 1.2–2.6). The mechanism by which current cigarette smoking increases the risk of squamous cell anogenital tumors is not clear; however, it may be due to systemic immunosuppression [67–69]. Another mechanism by which tobacco smoking may be a causative factor in anogenital cancer is the potential for nicotine to block apoptosis, an important mechanism in the regulation of cancer cell growth [70–72].

Predisposing factors for vaginal cancer also include a history of pelvic radiation for other anogenital cancers. Patients treated for cervical cancer by radiation have a 3-fold increased risk of a second malignancy in the vulva or vagina [73]. Clear cell adenocarcinoma of the vagina has been associated with in utero exposure to diethylstilbestrol (DES), a synthetic estrogen used between 1940 and 1970 to prevent spontaneous abortion [74–77]. The precursor lesion for this disease is thought to be vaginal adenosis. Herbst [78] showed that the frequency of the development of glandular tissue in the vagina was related to the gestational age at the initiation of DES and was correlated to the total dose of the drug ingested. Reports of squamous cell carcinoma of the vagina in DES-exposed women have also been published [79,80].

Detection

Most VAIN lesions are asymptomatic and are found by routine cytopathologic follow up of patients with previous anogenital disease [81,82]. Occasionally, vaginal discharge or bleeding may lead to the diagnosis. Abnormal vaginal cytology should be evaluated by a colposcopy-directed biopsy. In general, VAIN presents as acetowhite lesions that do not stain well [83].

Prevention

VAIN that follows cervical disease should be preventable or at least detected at an early stage. Careful inspection of the upper vagina for VAIN prior to hysterectomy for cervical neoplasia is important. One study recommended that the vaginal cuff should not be closed in patients undergoing hysterectomy for cervical disease, since occult foci of neoplastic epithelium might be present [84]. Women with a history of anogenital cancer or HPV infection should be screened routinely due to the multicentric character of this disease. Although cytologic screening among women with hysterectomy for benign disease has been stated to not be warranted, this group merits continued surveillance [85]. Since current smoking is a strong risk factor for squamous cell anogenital carcinoma, women who develop one of these tumors or their precursor lesions should be counseled about smoking cessation.

Conclusions

Vulvar and vaginal cancer precursor lesions are predominantly squamous cell neoplasias that contain HPV DNA. Other risk factors that are similar to CIN include current smoking, a history of prior genital warts or anogenital neoplasia, and multiple sexual partners. Unlike cervical cancer, vulvar and vaginal neoplasias are rare, and prevention beyond visual examination is not a part of routine gynecologic care. Women with impaired immunity (e.g., organ transplant recipients, acquired immunodeficiency syndrome patients, and patients who are treated with corticosteroids) should be screened periodically. A history of previous HPV-related diseases should be obtained in these women before determining the frequency of cytologic screening.

The overall patterns of incidence seem to be similar between vulvar and vaginal cancers in the United States. The incidence of VIN3 is increasing more sharply than that of VAIN3, but the incidence of invasive vaginal and vulvar cancer remains steady or has started to decline. Outstanding questions concerning the etiology and prevention of in situ vulvar cancer are becoming more important as the incidence rate has increased. There are few studies of these rare lesions, but future studies will give us a more thorough understanding of their natural history and etiology.

References

1. IARC Monographs on the Evaluation of carcinogenic risks to humans. Human Papillomaviruses. Lyon, France. 1995; 64:106–7.
2. Iversen T, Tretli S. Intraepithelial and invasive squamous cell neoplasia of the vulva: trends in incidence, recurrence, and survival rate in Norway. *Obstet Gynecol* 1998; 91:969–72.
3. Kuppers V, Stiller M, Somville T, et al. Risk factors for recurrent VIN: role of multifocality and grade of disease. *J Reprod Med* 1997; 42: 140–2.
4. Hording U, Daugaard S, Junge J, et al. Human papillomaviruses and multifocal genital neoplasia. *Int J Gynecol Pathol* 1996; 15:230–4.
5. Sturgeon SR, Curtis RE, Johnson K, et al. Second primary cancers after vulvar and vaginal cancers. *Am J Obstet Gynecol* 1996; 174:929–33.
6. Thuesen B, Angeasson B, Bock JE. Sexual function and somatopsychic reactions after local excision of vulvar intra-epithelial neoplasia. *Acta Obstet Gynecol Scand* 1992; 71:126–8.

7. Haefner HK, Tate JE, McLachlin CM, et al. Vulvar intraepithelial neoplasia: age, morphological phenotype, papillomavirus DNA, and coexisting invasive carcinoma. *Hum Pathol* 1995; 26:147–54.

8. Lin MC, Mutter GL, Trivijisilp P, et al. Patterns of allelic loss (LOH) in vulvar squmous carcinomas and adjacent noninvasive epithelia. *Am J Pathol* 1998; 152:1313–8.

9. Crum CP. Pathobiology of vulvar squamous neoplasia. *Curr Opin Obstet Gynecol* 1997; 9:63–9.

10. Park JS, Jones RW, McLean MR, et al. Possible etiologic heterogeneity of vulvar intraepithelial neoplasia. *Cancer* 1991; 67:1599–607.

11. Pinto AP, Signorello LB, Crum CP, et al. Squamous cell carcinoma of the vulva in Brazil: prognostic importance of host and viral variables. *Gynecol Oncol* 1999; 74:61–7.

12. Flowers LC, Wistuba II, Scurry J, et al. Genetic changes during the multistage pathogenesis of human papillomavirus positive and negative vulvar carcinomas. *J Soc Gynecol Invest* 1999; 6:213–21.

13. Morely GW. Cancer of the vulva: a Review. *Cancer* 1981; 48:597–601.

14. Surveillance, Epidemiology, and End Results (SEER) Program Public-Use CD-ROM (1973–1996), National Cancer Institute, DCPC, Surveillance Program, Cancer Statistics Branch, Version 2.0, 1999.

15. Ragnarsson B, Raabe N, Williems J, et al. Carcinoma in situ of the vulva: long term prognosis. *Acta Oncol* 1987; 26:277–80.

16. Woodruff JD. Carcinoma in situ of the vulva. *Clin Obstet Gynecol* 1985; 28:230–9.

17. Basta A, Adamek K, Piynski K. Intraepithelial neoplasia and early stage vulvar cancer. Epidemiological clinical and virological observations. *Eur J Gynaec Oncol* 1999; 20:111–4.

18. Hording U, Junge J, Poulsen H, et al. Vulvar intrepithelial neoplasia III: a viral disease of undetermined progressive potential. *Gynecol Oncol* 1995; 56:276–9.

19. Jones RW, Rowan DM. Vulvar intraepithelial neoplasia III: a clinical study of the outcome in 113 cases with relation to later development of invasive vulvar carcinoma. *Obstet Gynecol* 1994; 84:741–5.

20. Sherman KJ, Daling JR, Chu J, et al. Multiple primary tumors in women with vulvar neoplasms: a case-control study. *Br J Cancer* 1988; 57:423–7.

21. Levi F, Randimbison L, La Vecchia C. Descriptive epidemiology of vulvar and vaginal cancers in Vaud, Switzerland, 1974–1994. *Ann Oncol* 1998; 9:1229–32.

22. IARC: Cancer Incidence in Five Continents. Lyon: IARC Scientific Publications, 1996; 6.

23. Sturgeon SR, Brinton LA, Devesa SS, et al. In situ and invasive vulvar cancer incidence trends (1973–1987). *Am J Obstet Gynecol* 1992; 166:1482–5.

24. Kurman RJ, Trimble CL, Shah KV. Human papillomavirus and the pathogenesis of vulvar carcinoma. *Curr Opin Obstet Gynecol* 1992; 4:582–5.

25. Iversen T, Tretli S. Intraepithelial and invasive squamousa cell neoplasia of the vulva: trends in incidence, recurrence and survival rate in Norway. *Obstet Gynecol* 1998; 91:969–72.

26. Madeleine MM, Daling JR, Carter JJ, et al. Cofactors with human papillomavirus in a population-based study of vulvar cancer. *J Natl Cancer Inst* 1997; 89:1516–23.

27. Brinton LA, Nasca PC, Mallin K, et al. Case-control study of cancer of the vulva. *Obstet Gynecol* 1990; 75:859–66.

28. Sherman KJ, Daling JR, Chu J, et al. Genital warts, other sexually transmitted diseases, and vulvar cancer. *Epidemiology* 1991; 2:247–62.

29. Nuovo GJ, Delvenne P, MacConnell P, et al. Correlation of histology and detection of human papillomavirus DNA in vulvar cancers. *Gynecolog Oncol* 1991; 43:275–80.

30. Shera K. Personal communication, 2000.

31. Hildesheim A, Han C-L, Brinton LA, et al. Human papillomavirus type 15 and risk of preinvasive and invasive vulvar cancer: results from a seroepidemiological case-control study. *Obstet Gynecol* 1997; 90:748–54.

32. Sun Y, Hildesheim A, Brinton LA, et al. Human papillomavirus-specific serologic response in vulvar neoplasia. *Gynecol Oncol* 1996; 63:200–3.

33. Buscema J, Woodruff JD, Parmley TH, et al. Carcinoma in situ of the vulva. *Obstet Gynecol* 1980; 55:225–30.

34. Carson LF, Twiggs LB, Fukushima M, et al. Human genital papilloma infections: an evaluation of immunologic competence in the genital neoplasia-papilloma syndrome. *Am J Obstet Gynecol* 1986; 155:784–9.

35. Sillman FH, Sentovich S, Shaffer D. Anogenital neoplasia in renal tansplant patients. *Ann Transplan* 1997; 2:59–66.

36. Chiasson MA, Ellerbrock TV, Bush TJ, et al. Increased prevalence of vulvovaginal condyloma and vulvar intraepithelial neoplasia in women infected with the human immunodeficiency virus. *Obstet Gynecol* 1997; 89:690–4.

37. Frisch M. Personal Communication, 2000.
38. Bouwes Bavinck JN, Berkhout RJ. HPV infections and immunosuppression. *Clinics Dermatol* 1997; 15:427–37.
39. Edwards CL, Tortolero-Luna G, Linares AC, et al. Vulvar intraepithelial neoplasia and vulvar cancer. *Gynecol Cancer Prev* 1996; 23:295–324.
40. Burk RD. Pernicious papillomavirus infection. [editorial]. *N Engl J Med* 1999; 341:1687–8.
41. Lawhead RA, Majmudar B. Early diagnosis of vulvar neoplasia as a result of vulvar self examination. *J Reprod Med* 1990; 35:1134–7.
42. Gallup DG, Morley G. Carcinoma in situ of the vagina. *Obstet Gynecol* 1975; 46:334–40.
43. Geelhoed GW, Henson DE, Taylor PT, et al. Carcinoma in situ of the vagina following treatment for carcinoma of the cervix. *Am J Obstet Gynecol* 1976; 124:510–6.
44. Lee RA, Symmonds RE. Recurrent carcinoma in situ of the vagina in patients previously treated for in situ carcinoma of the cervix. *Obstet Gynecol* 1976; 48:61.
45. Petrelli ES, Townsend DE, Morrow CP. Vaginal intraepithelial neoplasia. Biologic aspects and treatment with topical 5-flourouracil and the carbon dioxide laser. *Am J Obstet Gynecol* 1980; 138:321.
46. Aho M, Vesterinen E, Meyer B, et al. Natural history of vaginal intraepithelial neoplasia. *Cancer* 1991; 66:195–7.
47. Lenehan PM, Meffe F, Lickrish GM. Vaginal intraepithelial neoplasia: biologic aspects and management. *Obstet Gynecol* 1986; 68:333–7.
48. Minucci D, Cinel A, Insacco E, et al. Epidemiological aspects of vaginal intraepithelial neoplasia (VAIN). *Clin Exp Obstet Gynecol* 1995; 1:36–42.
49. Ferenczy A, Wright TC. Anatomy and histology of the cervix. In: Kurman RJ (ed) *Blaustein's Pathology of the Female Genital Tract*, 4th ed. New York: Springer-Verlag, 1994, p. 185.
50. Wharton JT, Guillermo T-L, Linares AC, et al. Vaginal intraepithelial neoplasia and vaginal cancer. *Gynecol Cancer Prev* 1996; 23:325–45.
51. Brinton LA, Nasca PC, Mallin K, et al. Case-control study of in situ and invasive carcinoma of the vagina. *Gynecol Oncol* 1990; 38:49–54.
52. Kalogirou D, Antoniou G, Karakitsos P, et al. Vaginal intraepithelial neoplasia (VAIN) following hysterectomy in patients treated for carcinoma in situ of the cervix. *Eur J Gynecol Oncol* 1997; 3:188–91.
53. Chen N-J, Okuda H, Sekiba K. Recurrent carcinoma of the vagina following Okabayashi's radical hysterectomy for cervical carcinoma. *Gynecol Oncol* 1985; 20:10–6.
54. Ireland D, Monaghan JM. The management of the patient with abnormal vaginal cytology following hysterectomy. *Br J Obstet Gynecol* 1988; 95:973–5.
55. Tamimi H. Paper presented at 18th International Conference of Human Papillomavirus; 2000 July 23–8; Barcelona, Spain.
56. Herman JM, Homesley HD, Dignan MB. Is hysterectomy a risk factor for vaginal cancer? *JAMA* 1986; 256:601–3.
57. Campion MJ. Clinical manifestations and natural history of genital human papillomavirus infection. *Obstet Gynecol Clin North Am* 1987; 73:40–6.
58. Daling JR, Sherman KJ, Hislop TG, et al. Cigarette smoking and the risk of anogenital cancer. *Am J Epidemiol* 1992; 135:180–9.
59. Ostrow RS, Manias DA, Clark BA, et al. The analysis of carcinomas of the vagina for human papillomavirus DNA. *Int J Gynecol Pathol* 1988; 7:308–14.
60. Kiyabu MT, Shibata D, Arnheim N, et al. Detection of human papillomavirus in formalin-fixed, invasive squamous carcinomas using the polymerase chain reaction. *Am J Surg Pathol* 1989; 13:221–4.
61. Ikenberg H, Runge M, Goppinger A, et al. Human papillomavirus DNA in invasive carcinoma of the vagina. *Obstet Gynecol* 1990; 76:432–8.
62. Okagaki T, Twiggs LB, Zachow KR, et al. Identification of human papillomavirus DNA in cervical and vaginal intraepithelial neoplasia with molecularly cloned virus-specific DNA probes. *Int J Gynecol Pathol* 1983; 2:153–9.
63. Sugase M, Matsukura T. Distinct manifestations of human papillomaviruses in the vagina. *Int J Cancer* 1997; 72:412–5.
64. Daling JR, Madeleine MM, Sherman KJ, et al. Anogenital tumors associated with human papillomavirus. In: Fortner JG, Rhoads JE (eds) *Accomplishments in cancer research*. Philadelphia: Lippincott, 1992, pp. 280–6.
65. Daling JR, Madeleine MM, McKnight B, et al. The relationship of human papillomavirus-related cervical tumors to cigarette smoking, oral contraceptive use, and prior herpes simplex virus type 2 infection. *Cancer Epidemiol Biomarkers Prev* 1996; 5:541–8.

66. Winkelstein W. Smoking and cervical cancer—current status. A review. *Am J Epidemiol* 1990; 131:945–57.
67. Poppe WAJ, Ide PS, Drijkoningen M, et al. Tobacco smoking impairs the local immunosurveillance in the uterine cervix. *Gynecol Obstet Invest* 1995; 39:34–8.
68. Poppe WAJ, Peeters R, Drijkoningen M, et al. Cervical cotinine and macrophage-Langerhans cell density in the normal human uterine cervix. *J Gynecol Obstet Invest* 1996; 41:253–9.
69. Hughes DA, Haslam PL, Townsend PJ. Numerical and functional alternations in circulatory lymphocytes in cigarette smokers. *Clin Exp Immunol* 1985; 61:459–66.
70. Heusch WL, Maneckjee R. Signalling pathways involved in nicotine regulation of apoptosis of human lung cancer cells. *Carcinogenesis* 1998; 19:551–6.
71. Wright SC, Zhong J, Zheng H, et al. Nicotine inhibition of apoptosis suggests a role in tumor progression. *FASEB J* 1993; 7:1045–51.
72. Wright SC, Zhong J, Larrick JW. Inhibition of apoptosis as mechanism of tumor promotion. *FASEB J* 1994; 8:654–60.
73. Boice JD Jr, Day NE, Anderson A, et al. Second cancers following radiation treatment for cervical cancer. An international collaboration among cancer registries. *J Natl Cancer Inst* 1985; 74:955–75.
74. Herbst AL, Ulfelder H, Poskanzer DC. Adenocarcinoma of the vagina: association of maternal stilbestrol therapy with tumor appearance in young women. *N Engl J Med* 1971; 284:878–81.
75. Melauck S, Cole P, Anderson D, et al. Rates and risks of diethylstilbestrol related to clear cell adenocarcinoma of vagina and cervix. *N Engl J Med* 1987; 316:514–6.
76. Greenwald P, Barlow JJ, Nasca et al. Vaginal cancer after maternal treatment with synthetic estrogens. *N Engl J Med* 1971; 284:390–2.
77. Robboy SJ, Noller KL, O'Brien P, et al. Increased incidence of cervical and vaginal dysplasia in 3,980 diethylstilbestrol-exposed young women. *JAMA* 1984; 252:2979–83.
78. Herbst AL, Poskanzer DC, Robboy SJ, et al. Prenatal exposure to stilbestrol: a prospective comparison of exposed female offspring with unexposed controls. *N Engl J Med* 1975; 292: 334–9.
79. Bornstein J, Kaufman RH, Adam E, et al. Human papillomavirus associated with vaginal intraepithelial neoplasia in women exposed to diethylstilbestrol in utero. *Obstet Gynecol* 1987; 70:75–80.
80. Faber K, Jones M, Tarraza HM. Case Report. Invasive squamous cell carcinoma of the vagina in a diethylstilbestrol-exposed woman. *Gynecol Oncol* 1990; 37:125–8.
81. Woodruff JD. Carcinoma in situ of the vagina. *Clin Obstet Gynecol* 1981; 24:485–501.
82. MacLeod C, Fowler A, Dalrymple C, et al. High-dose-rate brachytherapy in the management of high-grade intraepithelial neoplasia of the vagina. *Gynecol Oncol* 1997; 65:74–7.
83. Davis GD. Colposcopic examination of the vagina. *Contemp Colposcopy* 1993; 20:217–28.
84. Sillman FH, Fruchter RG, Chen Y-S, et al. Vaginal intraepithelial neoplasia: risk factors for persistence, recurrence, and invasion and its management. *Am J Obstet Gynecol* 1997; 176: 93–9.
85. Benedict JL, Sanders BH. Carcinoma in situ of the vagina. *Am J Obstet Gynecol* 1984; 148:695–700.

20
Prostate

James R. Marshall and David P. Wood, Jr.

High-grade prostatic intraepithelial neoplasia (HGPIN) has received increasing attention in the past decade as a precursor for prostate cancer (PC). Study of this condition holds the potential for describing the etiology and course of PC, and for evaluating chemotherapeutic alternatives and options. In this chapter, the significance of PC is discussed, as are the nature of HGPIN, the evidence linking HGPIN to cancer of the prostate, and the implications of HGPIN for prostate cancer prevention, especially for chemoprevention.

Significance of PC

It has been estimated that in the United States in 1999 there were 179,000 new cases of prostate cancer and 37,000 deaths from prostate cancer [1]. This makes prostate cancer the highest incidence, single-site cancer among men and the second highest single-site cancer cause of death among men in the United States.

The Clinical Course of PC

The major means of therapy for prostate cancer, even when it is confined to the prostate, are surgery and irradiation. Surgery, generally regarded as the only definitively curative approach, results in substantial side effects, including a high probability of incontinence and of impotence [2–8].

There is a need for additional information on the clinical course of prostate cancer. Even more acutely needed are means by which prostate cancer can be prevented. Identification of a precursor lesion, so that those at elevated risk can be identified and treated, is an important priority.

Occult and Clinical PC

Internationally, there is substantial variation in the incidence rates of prostate cancer. The prostate cancer rate in the United States, for example, is several times that of Japan, and this difference is probably not due to diagnostic differences [9]. However, autopsy series in which latent or undiagnosed cancer of the prostate has been identified show much less marked variations. In these series, United States blacks have the highest percentage of latent cancer of the prostate, at approximately 37%. United States whites have an only slightly lower percentage of 35%. The percentages for Japanese in Hawaii and in Japan, respectively, are 26% and 21% [10]. Mortality rates do not show international differences as great as those for PC incidence. African Americans have an annual age-adjusted mortality rate of approximately 44 per 100,000 person–years, and United States non-Hispanic whites have a rate approximately half that: 21.1 per 100,000 person–years. Japanese and Chinese, on the other hand, have mortality rates of 8.4 and 7.4 per 100,000 person-years, respectively. The proportion of men who are diagnosed with PC is many times the proportion who actually die from it [9]. Thus, a 50-year-old man with a 25-year life expectancy has a probability of 42% of developing microscopic prostate cancer, a 9% probability of developing clinically identified prostate cancer, and a 3% probability of developing fatal prostate cancer [9]. These data suggest that many men have PC, but are unaware of it. It is tempting to conclude that some asymptomatic men whose disease is uncovered by screening would not ever have experienced symptoms or disability due to PC. However, some are cured by treatment. We do not at present possess the means to accurately identify those men who will profit most from treatment. Clearly, identification of those at increased risk of aggressive disease would be an advance.

The Nature of HGPIN

HGPIN can be described as a disturbance of tissue formation around the ducts of the prostate. Brawer has specified that this disturbance involves both dysplasia and proliferation of the lumenal prostate cells [11]. HGPIN tissue is recognizable as prostate, largely divisible into ducts and stroma, with the alteration of structure generally slight. Normal prostate ducts are lined with basal cells, and the basal cells are covered by a lumenal layer of secretory cells. In HGPIN the secretory cells become irregular and enlarged. They are characterized by irregular and clumped chromatin within the nuclei. The individual cells begin to closely resemble cancer cells [11]. The cells also crowd one another and pile up. The layer of basal cells becomes degraded, and gaps develop between the cells and in the basal membrane [12]. Although four distinct patterns of HGPIN have been identified—the tufting, micropapillary, flat, and cribriform patterns—the significance of these patterns is not well understood [13].

The cells of HGPIN are characterized by genetic instability and allelic loss [14]. Chromosomal abnormalities and anomalies are elevated, as in early cancer. It is possible to describe a continuum ranging from healthy tissue to HGPIN to cancer; along that continuum, a progression of molecular and cellular disturbances reflects increasing genetic damage. Thus, for examples, *p53* mutations appear to be as elevated in HGPIN as in PC in comparison with normal tissue [15]. As HGPIN advances, microvessel density appears to rise above the level usually seen in normal tissue. This microvessel density begins to approximate that found in PC [12,16].

In general, morphometric, differentiation and stromal markers, growth factors and receptors, oncogenes, and tumor suppressor genes all seem to be present in HGPIN at levels intermediate between those of the normal prostate and PC [16].

The Epidemiology of HGPIN

Although premalignant change in prostatic tissue was first reported in the 1920s, consensus about the most common form of premalignant change was reached only recently [17]. The term, *prostatic intraepithelial neoplasia* was adopted. Initially categorized in terms of three stages or grades, the highest two grades have since been collapsed to form the category "high-grade prostatic intraepithelial neoplasia." HGPIN is of interest since it appears to be linked to PC. It is not symptomatic, and there is no recognized and acceptable treatment for it; the interventions which appear to affect it are administered to treat PC. Since it does not produce symptoms, and since it is not readily treatable, it is usually only discovered clinically as a by-product of the search for PC. It is identified by biopsy, prostatectomy, or post mortem. The seminal work of Sakr et al. [18,19] shows that the prevalence of HGPIN rises two to three decades before the incidence of PC begins to rise. Sakr's research also shows that African Americans have a higher prevalence of HGPIN at a younger age than whites. Little else is known about the epidemiology of HGPIN. Similarities and contrasts between the etiology and epidemiology of HGPIN and those of PC have not been documented. Whether the factors that increase the presence of HGPIN or that lead HGPIN to progress to PC are the same as those that give rise to HGPIN is not known. Clearly, if HGPIN is to fulfill its promise as a surrogate marker for

PC risk, there will need to be study of the epidemiology of its development and course.

The Link of HGPIN to PC

Several lines of evidence tend to implicate HGPIN as premalignant with a high likelihood of proceeding to PC. The fact that the prevalence of HGPIN begins to rise steeply two to three decades before the incidence and prevalence of PC peak suggests that HGPIN could well be present for two to three decades before it proceeds to PC [17]. The greater prevalence of HGPIN among African Americans than among European Americans is consistent with African Americans' substantially higher PC incidence and mortality rates as compared to those of Caucasian Americans [18].

Co-occurrence of HGPIN and PC

The regional distribution of HGPIN within the prostate parallels the regional distribution of prostate cancer. Both of these conditions are most frequently found in the peripheral, rather than in either the transitional or central zones of the prostate [11]. Brawer has pointed out that HGPIN is seen without cancer present, but that cancer is rarely seen without HGPIN present [11]. This suggests that HGPIN develops, and that cancer develops from it. When HGPIN is multifocal, as it often is, PC tends to be also [11]. It has already been noted in the previous section that the characteristics of HGPIN with respect to morphometry, differentiation, growth factors, oncogenes, and tumor suppressor genes are intermediate between those for normal tissue and those for prostate cancer. Several genetic changes, including changes in genes located on chromosomes 7q, 8p, 8q, 10q, 16q, and 18q, are found both in HGPIN and PC [16,20]. These and other changes are found more commonly in HGPIN than in normal tissue, more commonly in PC than in HGPIN. The pattern of these changes argues that HGPIN is an intermediate stage in the causal process transforming normal tissue to cancer [17].

Some of the strongest evidence linking HGPIN to PC is the observation that HGPIN lesions can be seen occasionally to contain foci of microinvasion in which the secretory cells appear to be growing through gaps in the basal membrane of prostatic ducts into the stromal tissue and into adjacent ducts [21]. Da Silva et al. [21] evaluated nuclear chromatin patterns using quantitative morphometry and observed similarities between HGPIN and prostate cancer. They also observed, however, that the cells most directly involved in microinvasion appeared more normal than HGPIN or cancer cells. The sources of this discontinuity between HGPIN and early transition to cancer and invasion are not well understood. It is possible that a vigorous clone of HGPIN cells is responsible for invasion through the basal cell layer, but that obvious abnormality returns after invasion [22]. In any case, there is evidence indicating that HGPIN disrupts the basal cell layer and membrane, and that this disruption is associated with early invasion in prostate cancer [22].

HGPIN and Risk of PC

Additional evidence that HGPIN is a premalignant lesion for prostate cancer is that its presence marks substantially increased risk of both synchronous and metachronous prostate cancer. Davidson et al. [23] compared two groups of men who had been biopsied: men with HGPIN and men in a control group. Men whose initial biopsies revealed HGPIN were rebiopsied within a period ranging from two to 1,200 days; the median interval was 221 days, or about seven months. Controls—men whose initial biopsies revealed neither HGPIN nor adenocarcinoma—were reevaluated by biopsy within a period ranging from six to 1,400 days; the median interval was 440 days, or about 14 months. The subjects in the two groups were matched for age and reason for biopsy (induration, elevated PSA, a nodule, or abnormal transrectal ultrasound). Davidson et al. [23] evaluated subsequent biopsy findings for men in both groups, observing that, among men with no HGPIN found, the subsequent probability of diagnosed prostate cancer was about 13%.

Among men with HGPIN, that probability was near 35%. It is pertinent that the mean follow-up period for men with HGPIN was only about half as long as that for controls: thus, the predictive value of HGPIN for subsequent PC was probably underestimated in this study. Prostate-specific antigen (PSA) predicted the presence and subsequent risk of prostate cancer [24], and did also in the study of Davidson et al. [23]. However, HGPIN alone does not appear to substantially increase the level of PSA; apparently, increased PSA occurs relatively late in the carcinogenic process. Thus, the links of PSA and HGPIN to prostate cancer can be readily separated for evaluation of their predictive abilities regarding prostate cancer; HGPIN predicts subsequent PC, with PSA held constant.

A somewhat different perspective on the link of HGPIN to prostate cancer is provided by the work of O'Dowd et al. [25], who reported on the discovery of PC among 81,000 patients in the year following their biopsy-based diagnosis of: (1) no evidence of malignancy, (2) HGPIN, or (3) glands suspicious for cancer in the presence of HGPIN. Of the 81,000 noncancer patients, O'Dowd et al. identified 6,000 who returned for a follow-up biopsy within one year. O'Dowd et al. discovered that, among those with HGPIN, the probability of a subsequent cancer diagnosis was about 23%. On the other hand, if a man had a lesion identified as suspicious for malignancy, or a lesion that was suspicious for malignancy in the presence of HGPIN, that man's probability of subsequent cancer was between 40 and 53%. At the other end of the spectrum, a man with no evidence of malignancy in his initial biopsy had a probability of subsequent prostate cancer detection of about 20%, which is very nearly that of a man with HGPIN. The source of the difference in the findings of O'Dowd et al., as opposed to those of Davidson et al. [23], is not clear. It is possible that some of those lesions identified in Davidson et al. as HGPIN would, in O'Dowd et al., have been characterized as suspicious, or as suspicious and HGPIN. Both studies were based on widely recognized pathology criteria. Nonetheless, subtle diagnostic differences, which could have noteworthy effects, are

possible. It is also important that, among the men studied by O'Dowd et al., only about 5% of those with no evidence of malignancy on the first examination returned for a subsequent examination and biopsy. It was among these very select men that the cancer detection rate on return biopsy was 20% [24], a proportion 50% higher than that observed in Davidson et al. How those men differed from the other 95% who were not biopsied again is not clear. On the other hand, of the men with HGPIN on the initial diagnosis, nearly 27% appeared for rebiopsy. About a third of those initially identified with a suspicious lesion or with a suspicious lesion and HGPIN returned within a year for follow-up. Even these follow-up examination rates are low and not in keeping with what is regarded as standard clinical care for a man with a very high-risk preneoplastic condition [11–14,16,17,22,23]. These low rates suggest that substantial follow-up bias could have confounded the results of O'Dowd et al. In addition, the follow-up time in the study of O'Dowd et al. was one year. In the study of Davidson et al., it was up to three years; however, O'Dowd et al. stated that within the first year, there was no association between the time of repeat biopsy and the probability that cancer was identified. For men with an HGPIN lesion, a suspicious lesion and HGPIN, or no evidence of malignancy, the probability of PC being subsequently diagnosed, from the first to the last quarter of the following year, remained about the same. Thus, for example, for men with a suspicious HGPIN lesion and acinar glands suspicious for cancer, the probability of subsequent diagnosis of cancer remained at about 50%, whenever the subsequent biopsy was performed. For men with a suspicious lesion, the probability of subsequent diagnosis hovered around 40%. For men with HGPIN or with no evidence of malignancy, the probability of subsequent prostate cancer identification remained around 20% to 25%. There is substantial need for studies evaluating the longer-term course of HGPIN. The maximum follow-up time in the study of O'Dowd et al. was one year; the maximum follow-up in the study of Davidson et al. was three years; however, the median follow-up time in both studies was less than one year. If the link of HGPIN to PC is as strong as it is believed to be, longer-term follow up of HGPIN patients should show substantially increased probability of subsequent PC.

HGPIN and PC: Implications for Prevention

Bacus et al. [26] have suggested that a promising strategy for cancer chemoprevention in general would be to focus on specific categories of precursor lesions, especially on intraepithelial neoplasia, using quantitative morphometry to assess response to a chemopreventive agent. Bartels et al. have developed such morphometry and applied it to HGPIN [27,28], using such quantitative markers as degradation of the basal cell layer in ducts and glands affected by HGPIN, size of nuclei and nucleoli, and characteristics of the nuclear chromatin within HGPIN lesions, including the intensity of staining of nuclei and the spatial distribution and clumping of nuclear chromatin within the nucleus.

It is readily possible to identify HGPIN as present or not present in a gland or in a series of glands within a given prostate [29]. Because of the heterogeneity of the prostate, the degree to which the presence or the extent of HGPIN in a single gland or duct characterizes the extent of HGPIN in an entire prostate, however, is not as clear. The signicance of percentage of the area within a biopsy occupied by an HGPIN lesion, the extent to which HGPIN lesions are dysplastic, the percentage of non-stromal tissue taken up by HGPIN, and the percentage of ductal tissue taken by HGPIN [30] need to be explored. Clearly, if progression or reversion of HGPIN within a gland is to be made useful as a quantitative indicator, it will be necessary to develop guidelines on the extent to which a tissue can be seen as progressing in terms of HGPIN. To the degree that there may be several dimensions to the progression of HGPIN, it may be necessary to use multidimensional scaling to describe such change.

HGPIN as a Premalignant Lesion

HGPIN is the most promising intermediate endpoint that can be identified and used as a basis for PC prevention to date. In contrast, it is important to recognize that PSA is of use for prevention in only a very limited sense. PSA has not yet been successfully used as a marker of preneoplasia; it has been used only as a marker of the presence of malignancy. Thus, monitoring of PSA levels does not prevent cancer; rather, it leads to earlier diagnosis of cancer. It may lessen the sequelae of diagnosis and treatment. Whether it does, however, has not been firmly established [3–8].

HGPIN is also a useful surrogate marker because neither surgery nor irradiation is typically used to treat it. Certain men may be seen to have HGPIN for years without cancer ever being discovered. The progression to cancer of even an active, advanced PIN lesion has been estimated to take at least two to three years [31]. Inasmuch as HGPIN has been seen in men in their thirties and forties, among whom the diagnosis of invasive PC is rare, HGPIN may even be present for several years before malignancy develops to a detectable, much less clinical point. This extremely long preclinical diagnostic phase of the course of HGPIN, providing abundant opportunity for observation of the waxing and waning of dysplasia, makes HGPIN a useful target of chemoprevention [32].

Most evidence suggests that HGPIN is the lesion most proximal to PC [33,19,34]. Given the high probability that HGPIN will progress to PC [23], the study of HGPIN's progression to prostate cancer will afford tremendously increased power for statistical evaluation of any given effect of a chemopreventive agent [35]. It may also mean that chemopreventive agents of value for PC should be those that are relatively late acting. It is possible to follow the progression of HGPIN to PC under the influence of a chemopreventive agent with a study utilizing several hundred HGPIN patients and three to five years of observation. Thousands of subjects and five to ten years of observation would be required if such a study were to be undertaken among men at average risk.

If HGPIN is to be a useful marker of cancer risk, it is important that it be reversible [35]. It appears to be. Bostwick has reported that androgen deprivation and irradiation lead to decreases in the extent of PIN lesions [36]. Bostwick is testing Flutamide, an androgen inhibitor, in a randomized-controlled trial as a means of decreasing the extent of HGPIN.

HGPIN as a Surrogate Endpoint Biomarker

Kelloff et al. [35] have suggested HGPIN as a likely target of chemopreventive studies. They have proposed, however, the HGPIN will need to be validated as a marker of PC. The usefulness of HGPIN as a marker and target for chemopreventive trials of any given drug will probably depend on two factors. The first of these will be the correlation between the effect of the drug on the extent of HGPIN and the effect of that drug or agent on cancer risk. The second is the magnitude of the change in the extent of HGPIN relative to the change in cancer risk. Evaluating these criteria will require that studies be instituted in which it is possible to estimate the impact of the chemopreventive agent on the risk of PC, with consideration of changes in the extent of HGPIN. If HGPIN changes predict changes in risk as well as the agent does, they can be said to "explain" the effect of the agent on risk. Evaluating the association of the agent with risk, within categories of HGPIN, would vitiate that association. Such a study would, of course, be a substantial undertaking.

Chemopreventive Options

A number of chemopreventive options appear to present testing opportunities. Androgen is widely believed to increase PC risk [37,38]. The most important chemopreventive strategies are directed toward androgen suppression, which is already widely used as a means to retard the growth of prostate cancer. The data describing the association of androgen and PC risk factor are myriad. However, studies by Vatten et al. [39] and by Nomura et al. [40] suggest that androgen has no bearing on the risk of prostate cancer. On the basis of the fact that prostate cancer risk appears to increase at the same time as androgen in the male is declining, Prehn has suggested that it may be the decline in androgen, rather than the level of it, that increases PC risk [41]. As noted, however, there is a great deal of interest in androgen metabolism and its alteration. Cote et al. [42] reported on the use of the 5-alpha reductase inhibitor Finasteride, which inhibits the conversion of testosterone to its more biologically active form, dihydrotestosterone [42]. Contrary to expectation, Finasteride was associated with a slight increase in the risk of PC development among men who had HGPIN and elevated PSA levels, and who had undergone prostatic biopsy [42]. On the other hand, androgen deprivation appears to decrease the prevalence and extent of HGPIN among men with PC scheduled for prostatectomy [43].

A number of retinoid compounds have been used for chemoprevention at a number of sites. Giovannucci observed no association of retinol with prostate cancer risk or with the risk of advanced prostate cancer [44]. However, two carotenoids—β-carotene, which is readily metabolized to retinol, and lycopene, which is structurally quite similar to β-carotene—have been associated with some protection against PC [45,46].

The most promising agent linked to a decrease in PC risk appears to be the antioxidant metal selenium. One of the key protective characteristics of selenium appears to be its antioxidative activity. Clark et al. [47] observed a decrease in PC risk of approximately 60% in a randomized, double-blind controlled clinical trial of selenium, among men who had been diagnosed for nonmelanoma skin cancer [47]. This observation from an experimental trial follows a number of other nonexperimental studies [48,49].

We are presently engaged in an efficient approach to testing selenium as a means of protecting against PC, evaluating selenium in a chemoprevention trial focused on men with HGPIN. In light of evidence that the short-term incidence of PC among with men with HGPIN could be as high as 50%, men with HGPIN are appropriate subjects for a chemoprevention trial. After initial biopsy identifying HGPIN, all participants will be rebiopsied before randomization to lessen the probability that they have PC missed by the first biopsy [34,50,51]. The primary study outcome will be progression of HGPIN to PC, with secondary endpoints including proliferation, apoptosis, and changes in ductal, glandular, cellular, and nuclear morphometry. This study will be carried out in collaboration between the University of Arizona and the Southwest Oncology Group. The agent will be 200 μg selenium as L-selenomethionine compared to placebo. Each patient will be treated for up to three years when a final end-of-study prostate biopsy is scheduled. This study can be carried out with 470 randomized patients, 235 per arm. This will require initially enrolling over 1,000 patients, given that as many as 50% may be excluded from the trial on the basis of cancer being detected in their rebiopsy, but a study with 470 randomized patients will provide 90% power with a two-sided alpha level of .05 to detect a one-third reduction in the three-year incidence rate of PC [20]. This study will also generate substantial power to identify any sizeable increase in the probability of side effects resulting from increased selenomethionine intake of 15% or more. The contrast between the necessary size of this HGPIN trial and the upcoming SELECT trial, which will test 200 μg per day of selenomethionine in combination with vitamin E administration (Scott Lippman, personal communication), is instructive; the SELECT trial will require randomization to a two-by-two factorial study of 32,800 men at average risk of prostate cancer, and these men will have to be followed for seven or more years.

The α-Tocopherol β-Carotene Study (ATBC) was intended to test the use of α-tocopherol as an agent to protect against heart disease; the same study also evaluated β-carotene as protective against lung cancer [52]. Apparently, neither agent provided the expected protection: α-tocopherol did not lessen heart disease, and β-carotene actually increased lung cancer [52]. However, α-tocopherol did induce a 30% decrease in PC. Issuing as it did from a large clinical trial, this finding has generated tremendous optimism about the chemopreventive potential of vitamin E. Thus, in the 32,800-man SELECT trial, 400 μg of α-tocopherol will be administered in a two-by-two factorial design with 200 μg of selenium. In assembling the Southwest Oncology Group trial of selenium among HGPIN patients, the investigators considered a two-by-two factorial study design with vitamin E as the second agent. It was estimated that this study would require randomizing only about 1,000 subjects in total. The focus on a high-risk population of men at increased PC risk does enable a significantly smaller study to be conducted.

Vitamin D has been proposed as an agent that might decrease PC risk, so several vitamin D analogs are being considered and tested [35,53,54]. Inasmuch as the body tightly regulates tissue levels of vitamin D, it will be interesting to assess the impact of this in upcoming studies.

Nonsteroidal, anti-inflammatory drugs (NSAIDs) have been the subject of a great deal of investigation as protective against cancer in general [55]. As understanding of NSAIDS has advanced, it has become clear that they affect two cyclooxygenase systems. The first of these, cyclooxygenase-1, is linked to processes of cellular maintenance and repair. NSAIDs which have appreciable cyclooxygenase-1 activity often induce bleeding disorders. On the other hand, agents which focus on cyclooxygenase-2 appear to have no such bleeding-induction limitations. Thus, cyclooxygenase-2 inhibitors have been proposed as a promising option for prostate cancer prevention [56]; they have not been widely studied over extended time spans, so it is not completely established that they are safe enough for testing against PC.

A great deal of interest has been expressed in the possible effects of phytoestrogens and phytochemicals as protective against cancer in general. The evidence that lipids have been seen to be a risk factor for prostate cancer [57,58], could be reflective of low fruit and vegetable intake, and of elevated intake of animal products or lipids. Several phytoestrogenic or phytochemical product sources, such as soy, green tea, and fructose, are under investigation [59–61]. Among the effects of fruit and vegetable intakes could be antioxidant protection. Indeed, inasmuch as oxidative damage linked to smoking appears to increase prostate cancer risk [44], the protective effects of fruits and vegetables could be linked to their antioxidant capacity. Giovannucci et al. [44], in reporting on the impact of lycopene in decreasing the risk of prostate cancer, referred to its powerful role as an antioxidant [44]. The Physician's Health Study, a randomized prevention trial of β-carotene to protect against cancer, documented that either lycopene or β-carotene decreases risk in isolation [45]. The combination of the two, however, adds very little to the protection afforded by either alone. In addition in the Physician's Health Study, it was seen that β-carotene administration in the presence of low baseline plasma β-carotene was associated with decreased prostate cancer risk [46]. If the subject's baseline β-carotene blood level was high, however, the administration of β-carotene in the experimental study made little difference [46].

Questions about HGPIN and PC Prevention

It is worth recognizing the limitations of our present knowledge. First, it will be necessary to better understand the sensitivity and specificity of HGPIN as a predictor or as a marker of PC risk. Those with HGPIN appear to be at substantially increased risk. Whether PC ever develops in the absence of HGPIN is not well understood. Brawer's claim [11] that PC is almost never seen without HGPIN present suggests that HGPIN is a necessary predecessor of PC. Whether substantial numbers of people who develop HGPIN never develop prostate cancer has not yet been well documented. We do not at present have adequate information on the typical time lag between the identification of HGPIN and the appearance of PC. It has been suggested that this time lag is at least two to three years, and demographic data suggest that it could be two to three decades. There have been relatively few studies of the actual process of transformation of HGPIN to PC,

however. Our studies of tissue in which HGPIN is present show relatively small numbers of foci in which HGPIN, even if severe, is in the process of transformation into PC [21,27,28]. Studies focused on the transition of HGPIN to an invasive state are badly needed; these may describe the actual point where the benign lesion, HGPIN, becomes malignant.

It may be instructive to compare the link of HGPIN and PC to the link between the adenomatous polyp and the risk of colon cancer. It has been known for several decades that a relatively small percentage of adenomatous polyps progress to become cancerous [62]. Colon cancer rarely or never occurs except by progression of an adenomatous polyp that was already present. There is a good deal less information on the course of HGPIN. This is partly because of the considerable inaccessibility of the prostate to visual inspection. In similar fashion, the degree to which HGPIN actually is transformed—the percentage of HGPIN lesions that actually become cancerous—is in need of additional study. The discovery of HGPIN on a biopsy predicts a high risk of subsequent cancer. The probability that HGPIN will eventuate in cancer, if there have been two or more prostatic biopsies with none positive for cancer, is not well known. Davidson et al. [23] did not identify samples of subjects with two negative biopsies. The imminence of PC risk for such subjects needs further study.

Conclusions

The purpose of this chapter has been to focus on the promise of HGPIN as a precancerous condition that could be well studied as a subject of PC chemoprevention clinical trials. PC is a condition for which chemoprevention and other preventive activity are warranted: it causes substantial morbidity and mortality. Although PC treatment may be increasing in efficacy, it exacts severe costs. Prevention is desirable, chemoprevention especially so. A rational approach to PC prevention would be to focus on HGPIN. The nature of HGPIN has been described, and the link of HGPIN to PC has been discussed. HGPIN appears to hold more promise as a focus of chemoprevention than any other PC endpoint. It increases risk, and it appears to be treatable by chemoprevention. A number of promising chemopreventive agents have been identified and are ready for experimental study, including androgen suppressors, retinoids, selenium, vitamin E, vitamin D, and several nonsteroidal anti-inflammatory drugs.

The limitations of HGPIN as a precancerous condition and as a subject of chemopreventive studies must be recognized. Most significantly, the sensitivity and specificity of HGPIN as a marker of metachronous prostate cancer risk has not been well described. The time required for the transition from HGPIN to PC is deserving of substantially greater study. Knowledge of the epidemiology of HGPIN is almost nonexistent. Unfortunately, the dependence of HGPIN identification on highly invasive diagnostic techniques presents a severe challenge to conventional epidemiologic approaches. Nonetheless, better understanding of this almost certainly premalignant lesion holds great promise for prevention and especially for chemoprevention of PC.

References

1. *Cancer Facts & Figures—1999*. Atlanta: American Cancer Society; 1999.
2. Chodak GW, Thisted RA, Gerber GS, et al. Results of conservative management of clinically localized prostate cancer [comments]. *N Engl J Med* 1994; 330:242–8.
3. Fleming C, Wasson JH, Albertsen PC, et al. A decision analysis of alternative treatment strategies for clinically localized prostate cancer. Prostate Patient Outcomes Research Team [comments]. *JAMA* 1993; 269:2650–8.
4. Johansson JE, Holmberg L, Johansson S, et al. Fifteen-year survival in prostate cancer. A prospective, population-based study in Sweden [comments] [published erratum appears in *JAMA* 1997; 278:206]. *JAMA* 1997; 277:467–71.
5. Gerber GS, Thisted RA, Scardino PT, et al. Results of radical prostatectomy in men with clinically localized prostate cancer [comments]. *JAMA* 1996; 276:615–9.
6. Catalona WJ, Smith DS. 5-year tumor recurrence rates after anatomical radical retropubic prosta-

tectomy for prostate cancer [comments]. *J Urol* 1994; 152:1837–42.
7. Walsh PC, Partin AW, Epstein JI. Cancer control and quality of life following anatomical radical retropubic prostatectomy: results at 10 years [comments]. *J Urol* 1994; 152:1831–6.
8. Walsh PC. Re: Quality of life: radical prostatectomy versus radiation therapy for prostate cancer. *J Urol* 1996; 155:2038–9.
9. Ross R, Schottenfeld D. Prostate cancer. In: Schottenfeld D, Fraumeni J Jr (eds) *Cancer epidemiology and prevention*, 2nd ed. New York: Oxford University Press, 1996, pp. 1180–206.
10. Yatani R, Chigusa I, Akazaki K, et al. Geographic pathology of latent prostatic carcinoma. *Int J Cancer* 1982; 29:611–6.
11. Brawer MK. Prostatic intraepithelial neoplasia: a premalignant lesion. *J Cell Biochem* 1992; 16G (Suppl):171–4.
12. Bostwick DG. Prospective origins of prostate carcinoma. Prostatic intraepithelial neoplasia and atypical adenomatous hyperplasia. *Cancer* 1996; 78:330–6.
13. Bostwick DG, Amin MB, Dundore P, et al. Architectural patterns of high–grade prostatic intraepithelial neoplasia. *Hum Pathol* 1993; 24:298–310.
14. Bostwick DG. Clinical utility of prostatic intraepithelial neoplasia. *Mayo Clin Proc* 1995; 70:395–6.
15. Yasunaga Y, Shin M, Fujita MQ, et al. Different patterns of p53 mutations in prostatic intraepithelial neoplasia and concurrent carcinoma: analysis of microdissected specimens. *Lab Invest* 1998; 78:1275–9.
16. Bostwick DG, Pacelli A, Lopez-Beltran A. Molecular biology of prostatic intraepithelial neoplasia. *Prostate* 1996; 29:117–34.
17. Bostwick DG. Progression of prostatic intraepithelial neoplasia to early invasive adenocarcinoma. *Eur Urol* 1996; 30:145–52.
18. Sakr WA, Grignon DJ, Crissman JD, et al. High grade prostatic intraepithelial neoplasia (HGPIN) and prostatic adenocarcinoma between the ages of 20–69: an autopsy study of 249 cases. *In Vivo* 1994; 8:439–43.
19. Sakr WA. Prostatic intraepithelial neoplasia: A marker for high-risk groups and a potential target for chemoprevention. *Eur Urol* 1999; 35:474–8.
20. Montironi R, Mazzucchelli R, Marshall JR, et al. Prostate cancer prevention: review of target populations, pathological biomarkers, and chemopreventive agents. *J Clin Pathol* 1999; 52:793–803.

21. da Silva VD, Montironi R, Thompson D, et al. Chromatin texture in high grade prostatic intraepithelial neoplasia and early invasive carcinoma. *Anal Quant Cytol Histol* 1999; 21: 113–20.

22. Bostwick DG, Brawer MK. Prostatic intraepithelial neoplasia and early invasion in prostate cancer. *Cancer* 1987; 59:788–94.

23. Davidson D, Bostwick DG, Qian J, et al. Prostatic intraepithelial neoplasia is a risk factor for adenocarcinoma: predictive accuracy in needle biopsies. *J Urol* 1995; 154:1295–9.

24. Gann PH, Hennekens CH, Stampfer MJ. A prospective evaluation of plasma prostate-specific antigen for detection of prostatic cancer [comments]. *JAMA* 1995; 273:289–94.

25. O'Dowd GJ, Miller MC, Orozco R, et al. Analysis of repeated biopsy results within 1 year after a noncancer diagnosis. *Urology* 2000; 55: 553–9.

26. Bacus JW, Boone CW, Bacus JV, et al. Image morphometric nuclear grading of intraepithelial neoplastic lesions with applications to cancer chemoprevention trials. *Cancer Epidemiol Biomarkers Prev* 1999; 8:1087–94.

27. Bartels PH, Montironi R, Hamilton PW, et al. Nuclear chromatin texture in prostatic lesions. I. PIN and adenocarcinoma. *Anal Quant Cytol Histol* 1998; 20:389–96.

28. Bartels PH, Montironi R, Thompson D, et al. Statistical histometry of the basal cell/secretory cell bilayer in prostatic intraepithelial neoplasia. *Anal Quant Cytol Histol* 1998; 20:381–8.

29. Epstein JI, Grignon DJ, Humphrey PA, et al. Interobserver reproducibility in the diagnosis of prostatic intraepithelial neoplasia. *Am J Surg Pathol* 1995; 19:873–86.

30. Montironi R, Bartels PH, Thompson D, et al. Prostatic intraepithelial neoplasia. Quantitation of the basal cell layer with machine vision system. *Pathol Res Pract* 1995; 191:917–23.

31. Newling D. PIN I-III: when should we interfere? *Eur Urol* 1999; 35:504–7.

32. Zlotta AR, Schulman CC. Clinical evolution of prostatic intraepithelial neoplasia. *Eur Urol* 1999; 35:498–503.

33. Karp JE, Chiarodo A, Brawley O, et al. Prostate cancer prevention: investigational approaches and opportunities. *Cancer Res* 1996; 56:5547–56.

34. Bostwick DG, Burke HB, Wheeler TM, et al. The most promising surrogate endpoint biomarkers for screening candidate chemopreventive compounds for prostatic adenocarcinoma in short-term phase II clinical trials. *J Cell Biochem* 1994; 19(Suppl):283–9.

35. Kelloff G, Lieberman R, Brawer M, et al. Strategies for chemoprevention of prostate cancer. *Prostate Cancer Prostat Dis* 1998; 5:1–7.

36. Bostwick DG, Neumann R, Qian J, et al. Reversibility of prostatic intraepithelial neoplasia: implications for chemoprevention. *Eur Urol* 1999; 35:492–5.

37. Ross RK, Pike MC, Coetzee GA, et al. Androgen metabolism and prostate cancer: establishing a model of genetic susceptibility. *Cancer Res* 1998; 58:4497–504.

38. Gann PH, Hennekens CH, Ma J, et al. Prospective study of sex hormone levels and risk of prostate cancer [comments]. *J Natl Cancer Inst* 1996; 88:1118–26.

39. Vatten LJ, Ursin G, Ross RK, et al. Androgens in serum and the risk of prostate cancer: a nested case-control study from the Janus serum bank in Norway. *Cancer Epidemiol Biomarkers Prev* 1997; 6:967–9.

40. Nomura AM, Stemmermann GN, Chyou PH, et al. Serum androgens and prostate cancer. *Cancer Epidemiol Biomarkers Prev* 1996; 5:621–5.

41. Prehn RT. On the prevention and therapy of prostate cancer by androgen administration. *Cancer Res* 1999; 59:4161–4.

42. Cote RJ, Skinner EC, Salem CE, et al. The effect of finasteride on the prostate gland in men with elevated serum prostate-specific antigen levels [comments]. *Br J Cancer* 1998; 78:413–8.

43. Ferguson J, Zincke H, Ellison E, et al. Decrease of prostatic intraepithelial neoplasia following androgen deprivation therapy in patients with stage T3 carcinoma treated by radical prostatectomy. *Urology* 1994; 44:91–5.

44. Giovannucci E, Ascherio A, Rimm EB, et al. Intake of carotenoids and retinol in relation to risk of prostate cancer. *J Natl Cancer Inst* 1995; 87:1767–76.

45. Gann PH, Ma J, Giovannucci E, et al. Lower prostate cancer risk in men with elevated plasma lycopene levels: results of a prospective analysis. *Cancer Res* 1999; 59:1225–30.

46. Cook NR, Stampfer MJ, Ma J, et al. Beta-carotene supplementation for patients with low baseline levels and decreased risks of total and prostate carcinoma [see comments]. *Cancer* 1999; 86:1783–92.

47. Clark LC, Dalkin B, Krongrad A, et al. Decreased incidence of prostate cancer with selenium supplementation: results of a double-

blind cancer prevention trial. *Br J Urol* 1998; 81:730–4.

48. Yoshizawa K, Willett WC, Morris SJ, et al. Study of prediagnostic selenium level in toenails and the risk of advanced prostate cancer [comments]. *J Natl Cancer Inst* 1998; 90:1219–24.

49. Comstock GW, Bush TL, Helzlsouer K. Serum retinol, beta-carotene, vitamin E, and selenium as related to subsequent cancer of specific sites. *Am J Epidemiol* 1992; 135:115–21.

50. Nelson PS, Gleason TP, Brawer MK. Chemoprevention for prostatic intraepithelial neoplasia. *Eur Urol* 1996; 30:269–78.

51. Weinstein MH, Epstein JI. Significance of high-grade prostatic intraepithelial neoplasia on needle biopsy. *Hum Pathol* 1993; 24:624–9.

52. Beta Carotene Cancer Prevention Study Group: The Alpha-Tocopherol. The effect of vitamin E and beta-carotene on the incidence of lung cancer and other cancers in male smokers. *N Engl J Med* 1994; 330:1029–35.

53. Feldman D. Androgen and vitamin D receptor gene polymorphisms: the long and short of prostate cancer risk [editorial; comment]. *J Natl Cancer Inst* 1997; 89:109–11.

54. Habuchi T, Suzuki T, Sasaki R, et al. Association of vitamin D receptor gene polymorphism with prostate cancer and benign prostatic hyperplasia in a Japanese population. *Cancer Res* 2000; 60: 305–8.

55. Lim JT, Piazza GA, Han EK, et al. Sulindac derivatives inhibit growth and induce apoptosis in human prostate cancer cell lines. *Biochem Pharmacol* 1999; 58:1097–107.

56. Masferrer JL, Leahy KM, Koki AT, et al. Antiangiogenic and antitumor activities of cyclooxygenase-2 inhibitors. *Cancer Res* 2000; 60:1306–11.

57. Bosland MC, Oakley-Girvan I, Whittemore AS. Dietary fat, calories, and prostate cancer risk [editorial; comment]. *J Natl Cancer Inst* 1999; 91:489–91.

58. Giovannucci E, Rimm EB, Colditz GA, et al. A prospective study of dietary fat and risk of prostate cancer [comments]. *J Natl Cancer Inst* 1993; 85:1571–9.

59. Gupta S, Ahmad N, Mohan RR, et al. Prostate cancer chemoprevention by green tea: in vitro and in vivo inhibition of testosterone-mediated induction of ornithine decarboxylase. *Cancer Res* 1999; 59:2115–20.

60. Zhou JR, Gugger ET, Tanaka T, et al. Soybean phytochemicals inhibit the growth of transplantable human prostate carcinoma and tumor angiogenesis in mice. *J Nutr* 1999; 129:1628–35.

61. Giovannucci E, Rimm EB, Wolk A, et al. Calcium and fructose intake in relation to risk of prostate cancer. *Cancer Res* 1998; 58:442–7.

62. Lev R. *Adenomatous polyps of the colon: pathobiological and clinical features*. New York: Springer-Verlag; 1990.

21
Bladder

Kamal S. Pohar and Carlos Cordon-Cardo

Despite the rising incidence of and significant mortality rates attributed to bladder cancer, our understanding of the biology of the disease has improved considerably over the past decade. Translating these novel biological discoveries into therapies or strategies to manage patients who are suspected to have or who have been diagnosed with bladder cancer is the ultimate goal. This chapter begins with a description of the epidemiology and natural history of bladder cancer. A summary of the nonrandom chromosomal alterations as determined by conventional cytogenetics, interphase cytogenetics, and comparative genomic hybridization follows. The reported alterations of both oncogenes and tumor suppressor genes in bladder cancer will be outlined and described in the context of possible novel therapies targeting these alterations. Given that several investigators have hypothesized that certain specific chromosomal abnormalities and mutations play definite roles in bladder tumor development, while other alterations correlate with tumor progression, a model will be described for the molecular basis of certain known malignant phenotypes. The model will be extended to help understand the biological and clinical significance of various preneoplastic lesions. Finally, the reported literature in the areas of chemoprevention and screening of bladder cancer will be summarized. Emphasis will be placed on how biological findings have impacted the development of tests for screening for bladder cancer.

Epidemiology and Natural History of Bladder Cancer

Bladder cancer is one of the most commonly diagnosed malignancies worldwide. The incidence is highest in developed countries, ranking as the sixth most frequent neoplasm [1]. It occurs more commonly in males, with a sex ratio of greater than 3:1, possibly suggesting sex-linked etiologic factors. In the United States, bladder cancer is ranked as the fourth most common malignancy among men and is the sixth most common malignancy among women. Approximately 90% of the malignant tumors of the bladder are of epithelial origin, the vast majority being transitional cell carcinomas (TCC) [2,3]. Bilharzial-related bladder cancer (BBC), resulting from colonization of the bladder by *Schistosoma hematobium*, is the most common malignant neoplasm in Egypt and also occurs with a high frequency in other regions of the Middle East and East Africa [4]. The pathologic features of BBC are different from those described for conventional TCC of the bladder. Specifically, these is a much higher incidence of squamous metaplasia and squamous cell carcinoma (SSC) reported for patients with BBC [5].

The association between exposure to specific environmental factors and the risk of developing a urothelial tumor has been revealed by a series of epidemiologic studies [4]. Cigarette smoke is considered to be the most important risk factor for the development of bladder cancer [6]. Two agents present in cigarette smoke, 2-aminonaphthalene (2-AN) and 4-aminobiphenyl (4-ABP), have been causally linked to the development of bladder cancer. Another proven bladder carcinogen is the aromatic amine, benzidine. In addition, exposure to potassium arsenite and ingestion of large quantities of phenacetin have been reported to be associated with uroepithelial transformation. Finally, infection of the bladder by human papilloma virus, predominantly type 16, has been associated with the development of bladder cancer in roughly 8% of superficial bladder tumors [7]. Other risk factors found to have inconsistent associations with risk include coffee, alcohol, the use of sweeteners, and fat intake [4].

TCC can been classified into two groups with distinct behavioral and molecular profiles: low-grade tumors (always papillary and usually superficial), and high-grade tumors (either papillary or nonpapillary, and often invasive) [8,9]. Superficial bladder tumors (stages Ta [superficial], Tis [in situ], and T1 [early invasive]) account for 75% to 85% of neoplasms at clinical presentation, while the remaining 15% to 25% are invasive (T2, T3, T4) or metastatic (N+, M+) [6]. Greater than 70% of patients treated for a superficial bladder tumor will subsequently develop one or more recurrent tumors, and about one-third of these patients will progress to muscle invasive disease [1].

Criticism has been directed at the nomenclature used when referring to bladder cancer today. The criteria used to define certain bladder lesions have been confusing, and this has resulted in discrepancies in interpretation of pathologic findings amongst investigators. Additional problems relate to whether preneoplastic lesions should be identified and reported, given that considerable difference of opinion exists among clinical investigators regarding the significance of identifying such morphologic changes. For example, it is difficult to definitively attribute certain hyperplastic changes or everted papillomas as being significant preexisting conditions (i.e., precursors) for the development of overt papillary transitional cell carcinomas of low-grade. Even the term used to describe a benign uroepithelial neoplasm, "papilloma", has not been uniformly agreed upon internationally as a distinct entity [1,10]. The other precursor lesions described within today's nomenclature relate more to the flat carcinoma-in-situ (CIS) pathway of tumorigenesis, including the changes known as intra-urothelial neoplasms (IUNs) [11]. This latter group includes simple hyperplasia (IUN-I), atypical urothelial hyperplasia (IUN-II) and dysplasia or marked atypia (IUN-III). Multiple morphologic criteria have been used in the diagnosis of dysplasia, and all of the criteria do not need to be present to fulfill the diagnosis. Some authors have advocated the use of the terms mild, moderate, and severe dysplasia, analogous to the classification scheme used for the cervix [10]. Others have suggested the term CIS grades 1, 2, and 3 for mild, moderate and severe dysplasia, respectively [5]. Several studies have revealed the importance of diagnosing concomitant dysplasia, as it increases the risk of tumor progression for patients affected with superficial bladder tumors [12,13]. Finally, squamous metaplasia followed by dysplastic changes is accepted as the premalignant lesion associated with squamous cell carcinoma in BBC. Regardless of the terminology, it is becoming increasingly evident that morphological changes and their clinical manifestations are preceded by molecular and biochemical alterations.

Additional concepts should be taken into consideration when determining the appropriate management of patients diagnosed with muscle-invasive bladder cancer. Despite radical surgery and adjuvant radiotherapy and/or chemotherapy, the overall cure rate for such cancer remains in the range of 20% to 50%. Several groups of investigators have reported that mutations and altered patterns of expression of genes involved in the *RB* and *p53* pathways occur in a significant proportion of patients with advanced bladder cancer, ranging from 40% to 70% [14]. Moreover, it has been reported that such alterations may represent a major cause of treatment failure and subsequent death. In addition, distant micrometastatic disease, unrecognized at the time of initial diagnosis and treatment, occurs in a significant proportion of patients and is another leading cause of treatment failure and subsequent death [15]. Since selection criteria to determine treatment for a particular tumor in a particular patient are incompletely defined, new biological determinants are needed for treatment selection and for monitoring of specific therapy.

It is well known that morphologically similar tumors may behave in radically different manners, a fact that seriously hampers the ability to accurately predict clinical outcome and creates uncertainty regarding the therapeutic strategy implemented in any given case. The use of modern molecular and immunochemical techniques has led to remarkable progress in our understanding of cell growth, differentiation, senescence, maintenance of genomic integrity, and programmed cell death. These are key concepts in tumor development and progression. Studies involving biologic markers that correlate with tumor behavior and response to therapy are now underway. Similarly, prospective clinical studies, utilizing well-characterized cohorts of patients and properly selected normal, premalignant, and tumor paired samples, are needed to better delineate the role of mutations or altered patterns of expression occurring amongst specific genes. These, in turn, may impact on the management of patients diagnosed with bladder cancer.

Chromosomal Alterations in Bladder Cancer

Bladder cancer cells can be cultured successfully, thus allowing the performance of cytogenetic studies. However, preneoplastic lesions have not been assessed using this approach due to the difficulty in successfully culturing these lesions, even over the short term. Conventional cytogenetics, interphase cytogenetics, and comparative genomic hybridization (CGH) have revealed that preneoplastic and neoplastic bladder lesions contain nonrandom chromosomal aberrations. The most common and consistent alterations appear to be deletions, in contrast to the alterations found in most other solid neoplasms, namely, translocations.

Initial studies of bladder tumors identified monosomy of chromosome 9 [16,17] and interstitial deletions of chromosome 13 [16] as frequent events. Other common abnormalities included trisomy of chromosome 7 and deletions affecting chromosomes 11p and 3p [18,19]. Karyotype and interphase cytogenetic analyses have confirmed previously reported data in addition to providing evidence for novel alterations. For example, Tyrkus et al. analyzed 17 CIS lesions of the bladder and found no chromosome 9 alterations, but did identify nonrandom chromosomal changes involving chromosomes 1, 5, 8 and 11 [20]. Hopman et al. reported chromosomal alterations at 1q12, as well as numerical abnormalities of chromosomes 7, 9, 11 and 18 [21]. In an independent study, Waldman et al. also reported numerical alterations of chromosomes 7, 9, and 11 [22].

Fluorescence in situ hybridization (FISH) assays have also been utilized to assess gene amplification and copy number gains in bladder cancer. Moreover, the use of gene-specific probes has allowed interphase cytogenetics to evaluate particular molecular alterations in the context of tumor development and progression. For example, Sauter et al. reported amplification of ERBB2 (17q21) in 10 of 141 bladder tumors using a dual-labeling hybridization assay [23]. Gene amplification was associated with protein overexpression and was found only in tumors with aneusomy of chromosome 17, which occurred more frequently in muscle invasive tumors.

A similar approach was used for the analysis of cMYC copy number in 87 bladder tumors [24]. Obvious amplification was found in 3 cases, while 32 of the remaining 84 tumors showed a low level of increase in the cMYC copy number. There was no association between a low level of copy number increase and protein overexpression. However, there were strong associations between cMYC gains and tumor grade, stage and Ki-67 labeling index, which is consistent with a role for chromosome 8 alterations in bladder cancer progression.

FISH assays have also been utilized for analyses of specific gene losses. Physical TP53 gene deletion (at 17p13) was studied in 151 bladder tumors [25]. A strong correlation was found between losses at 17p and tumor grade and stage (p < 0.01). Using centromeric probes, Y chromosome loss was reported as a frequent finding in bladder tumors [26]. Nullisomy and monosomy for chromosome Y was seen in 23 of 68 (34%) and in 28 of 68 (41%) tumors, respectively.

The use of gene-specific probes for *CDKN2/INK4A* and *IFNA*, genes located at 9p21, revealed homozygous deletions of *CDKN2/INK4A* without homozygous deletions of *IFNA* in 5 of 17 (29%) superficial tumors (pTa or pT1) studied [27]. One additional tumor had both genes deleted and one tumor showed deletion of *IFNA* without deletion of *CDKN2/INK4A*. These data confirm the frequent and early nature of 9p21 alterations in bladder cancer (discussed later). FISH has also been utilized to evaluate specimens following bladder irrigation [28]. Labeled probes to centromeric sequences for chromosomes 1, 7, 9, 11, 15 and 17 were used on samples from 76 patients who were being monitored for recurrent bladder tumors. This study revealed that 24% of patients with a history of bladder cancer, but no clinical evidence of bladder tumor recurrence, exhibited monosomy of chromosome 9.

Use of comparative genomic hybridization has allowed for the generation of a map of a DNA sequence copy number as a function of chromosomal location throughout the entire genome [29]. In this technique, differentially labeled test DNA from tumor samples and normal reference DNA are hybridized simultaneously to normal chromosome spreads. Regions of gain or loss of DNA sequences are seen as changes in the ratio of intensities of fluorochromes along target chromosomes. Using this innovative method, loci not previously recognized as altered in bladder tumors have been identified. The analysis of genomic imbalance in 26 bladder tumors revealed losses on 11p, 11q, 8p, 9, 17p, 3p, and 12q in more than 20% of the tumors [30]. Bands involved in gains of over 10% were 8q21, 13q21-q34, 1q21, 3q24-q26, and 1p22 [30]. Additional molecular genetic studies may lead to the characterization of tumor suppressor genes and oncogenes residing in these regions, and these genes may play a crucial role in bladder cancer develop-

ment and progression. More recent publications confirm the nature of these alterations in bladder cancer in addition to identifying novel regions of amplification, which include 5p11-p13, 7q21-q31, and 17q24-q25 [31,32].

Alterations of Oncogenes in Bladder Tumors

The first mutation of the *RAS* family of oncogenes, a point mutation in codon 12 of the H-*RAS* gene (11p15.1), was identified in a bladder cancer cell line, T24 [33]. The frequency of mutations of the *RAS* genes in bladder cancer has been controversial. Before the advent of the polymerase chain reaction (PCR), it was estimated that the prevalence of point mutations in *RAS* oncogenes ranged from 10% to 16% [34,35]. The predominant alteration identified was that of codon 12 of *H-RAS*. In addition, *K-RAS* mutations were reported infrequently and no *N-RAS* mutations were identified. However, more recent reports, utilizing a PCR-based method, have revealed that approximately 40% of bladder tumors harbor *H-RAS* codon 12 mutations [36,37]. Other studies have confirmed the high frequency of *H-RAS* point mutations. Ooi et al. analyzed a cohort of 124 patients with Ta or T1 lesions and found that codon 12, G to T substitution, was associated with both recurrent and nonrecurrent primary bladder tumors [38]. In addition, this substitution was found in tumors of patients who experienced both disease progression and nonprogression. Fitzgerald et al. reported the detection of mutations in exon 1 of the *H-RAS* gene in urine sediments from 44 of 100 prospectively evaluated patients presenting with bladder neoplasms [39]. More recent studies have generated additional controversy as to the frequency of *H-RAS* mutations in primary bladder tumors. In an analysis of 19 bladder tumors, Przybojewska et al. reported that 84% of them had mutations detected on the basis of a PCR-RFLP assay [40]. However, Cattan et al. found only one *H-RAS* mutation in 87 primary bladder tumors analyzed [41]. Saito et al. reported mutations in 12% of 50 bladder cancer patients studied, which may represent a more accurate reflection of the true prevalence of mutation [42].

Overexpression and/or amplification of epidermal growth factor receptor (EGF-R) has been reported in bladder cancer. Neal et al. observed increased expression of EGF-R in invasive bladder tumors compared with superficial bladder tumors, demonstrating that overexpression was associated with higher grades and stages of bladder cancer, in addition to being an independent prognostic factor of survival [43,44]. Messing et al. noticed that EGF-R was expressed at detectable levels only in the basal layer of the normal urothelium, whereas increased expression in both the basal and suprabasal layers was identified in transitional cell carcinomas [45]. Rao et al. also found increased expression of EGF-R in areas of dysplastic urothelium, postulating that overexpression of EGF-R may be an early event in bladder carcinogenesis [46]. In another study, Nguyen et al. reported that overexpression of EGF-R was not an independent prognostic marker of survival for patients with advanced bladder cancer [47]. A recent study provides evidence for the coexpression of EGF-R and transforming growth factor (TGF)-α, its physiological ligand, in bladder tumors. This finding has critical connotations, since it implies the oncogenic activation of the receptor by the ligand, giving growth advantage to the tumor cells expressing such a phenotype. In addition to coexpression, a significant correlation exists between the TGF-α protein level and the EGF-R protein level, and this association becomes more significant with increasing tumor stage [48]. These data would lend support to the theory that the EGF-R signaling pathway is functional in certain bladder tumors and may be a novel therapeutic target for the well-characterized monoclonal antibody, C225, which in turn has been demonstrated to have antitumor activity [49].

Amplification of the c-erbB-2 gene, also known as HER-2/NEU (Her-2), was found in 1 of 14 bladder tumors studied by Wood et al. [50]. Overexpression of Her-2 mRNA and protein was also demonstrated in this tumor. In addition, 5 cases displayed high levels of mRNA with no signs of gene amplification, but only 3 of these 5 cases had protein overexpression. Sato et al. observed Her-2 protein (p185) overexpression in 23 of 88 bladder tumors and found a significant association between Her-2 protein overexpression and poor clinical outcome [51]. In a more recent study, Underwood et al. studied Her-2 status in 236 bladder tumors [52]. Sixteen of 89 patients with recurrent disease had evidence of Her-2 amplification; however, gene amplification was not observed in any patient with nonrecurrent tumor. A strong association between Her-2 amplification and disease progression was found. Nevertheless, protein overexpression could not be linked to disease progression, as was the case in the study by Sato et al. [51]. Her-2 gene amplification was also found to be of prognostic significance in a multivariate analysis for disease-specific survival, however, tumor grade and stage were the most significant independent prognostic factors in this analysis. Additional studies corroborate the finding of gene amplification of Her-2 in a significant proportion of patients with bladder cancer, and again it has been reported that this genetic alteration correlates with tumor grade and stage as well as with survival by multivariate analysis [53,54]. In a combined immunohistochemical and FISH study, alterations in the genotype and phenotype of EGF-R and Her-2 genes and their encoded products were evaluated in premalignant lesions of the urinary bladder [55]. FISH analysis showed Her-2 amplification in selected CIS cases. In addition, EGF-R overexpression and diffuse Her-2 positivity were associated with an increased Ki-67 proliferative index. However, only diffuse Her-2 immunoreactivity demonstrated a significant association with advanced dysplasia. More recently, a humanized anti-Her-2 antibody has been utilized for the treatment of patients with breast cancer. It has been suggested that amplification of Her-2 is a critical event in breast cancer progression and as a result such a strategy blocks tumor growth and induces tumor regression. Give that Her-2 overrepresentation is a relatively common event in bladder tumors, this therapeutic approach may hold future promise in the treatment of patients with bladder cancer.

The analysis of the *p53* regulatory pathway has yielded a novel cellular proto-oncogene product, mdm2 or p90. This protein binds to p53 and acts as a negative regulator, inhibiting its transcriptional activity [56] and targeting its ubiquitin-dependent degradation [57]. The *MDM2* gene is located on the long arm of chromosome 12 (12q13-14) and is transactivated by p53 [58]. Lianes et al. characterized the frequency and clinical relevance of identifying *MDM2* and *TP53* alterations in patients diagnosed with a bladder tumor [59]. This study revealed that 26 of 87 tumors studied had abnormally high levels of mdm2 protein; however, only one case demonstrated *MDM2* gene amplification. There was a striking association between mdm2 overexpression and low-grade/low-stage bladder tumors (p < 0.01). Based on these results, it was concluded that aberrant mdm2 phenotypes are frequent events in bladder cancer and may be involved in tumorigenesis or early tumor progression in urothelial neoplasms. In an independent study that lacked clinicopathological correlations, Barbareschi et al. reported mdm2 nuclear overexpression in 5 of 25 bladder tumors [60]. More recent studies demonstrate an even higher overexpression of mdm2 in superficial bladder tumors. Overexpression of mdm2 occurred in tumors with and without p53 overexpression [61].

Alterations of Tumor Suppressor Genes in Bladder Tumors

The studies of inheritance and cancer predisposition that led to the concept of tumor suppressor genes, conducted by Knudson, were based on the retinoblastoma model. Today, it is widely accepted that germ-line mutations in certain tumor suppressor genes, for example *RB* (retinoblastoma), *TP53* (Li-Fraumeni syndrome), and *APC* (familial adenomatous polyposis of colorectum), predispose an individual to the development of certain tumors. Even though the etiology of bladder cancer is largely unknown, the vast majority of patients do not have a family history of bladder cancer, sug-

gesting that germ-line mutations are not common. Nevertheless, a recent review of the literature suggests the clustering of transitional cell carcinomas within families, arguing in favor of a germ-line mutation in selected cases [62]. It has also been established that the tumor suppressor genes listed above are also common somatic mutational events in a variety of tumors, including bladder cancer (discussed later).

In the remainder of this section of our review, we will concentrate on outlining the molecular genetic studies pertinent to the majority of bladder tumors, namely those diagnosed in a nonfamilial inheritance pattern. Through these molecular studies, abnormalities of certain bona fide or candidate tumor suppressor genes have been identified and postulated to be involved in the development or progression of bladder tumors. In addition, these studies have confirmed previous cytogenetic observations, namely the loss of heterozygosity (LOH) of the short arm of chromosome 11 and 9q as well as LOH of 17p as frequent events in bladder cancer [63–65].

A combined molecular genetics and immunopathology approach was used by Presti et al. [66] to survey five suspected or established tumor suppressor gene regions (3p21-25, 11p15, 13q14, 17p11-13, and 18q21) in 34 unselected patients. An immunohistochemical (IHC) assay was also utilized for the analysis of the retinoblastoma gene product (pRB). This study demonstrated that tumor grade correlated with deletions of 3p and 17p, while tumor stage correlated with deletions of 3p, 17p, and altered pRB expression. This study also revealed that deletions of 17p (the *TP53* locus) and 18q occurred only in muscle-invasive bladder tumors, whereas deletions of 3p and 11p occur in both superficial and invasive bladder tumors. Dalbagni et al. [8] followed this study by the analysis of 60 paired bladder tumors and normal tissues using polymorphic DNA markers on eighteen different chromosomal arms. Distinct genotypic patterns were associated with early and late stages of bladder cancer. Correlation of genetic alterations with clinicopathological data suggested the existence of two different genetic pathways for the evolution of superficial bladder tumors. Briefly, 9q deletions were found in 60% of the informative cases, confirming previous reports. Moreover, 9q deletions were the sole abnormality found in a subset of the bladder tumors studied, suggesting the presence of a candidate tumor suppressor gene on chromosome 9. In addition, no Ta tumor demonstrated 5q alterations, however 3 of 10 T1 and 8 of 26 T2+ tumors demonstrated LOH of 5q, suggesting that 5q deletions may be involved in the transition from superficial (Ta) to early invasive (T1) tumors. Allelic loss of 17p was detected in 21 of 47 informative cases. Deletions were not identified among Ta tumors, however 21 of 38 invasive tumors exhibited 17p LOH. These findings support the involvement of 17p in the progression of bladder cancer. Allelic deletion of 3p was not present in any of the informative Ta tumors, however 18 of 33 invasive tumors had such alterations. A statistically significant association between various pathological parameters of poor outcome and 3p LOH was demonstrated. Other allelic losses (i.e., 11p, 6q and 18q) were frequently detected, but these were not associated with clinicopathologic factors of poor outcome [8].

Habuchi et al. investigated the role of allelic losses of seven chromosomal arms (1p, 3p, 9q, 10q, 11p, 13q, and 17p) in 49 bladder tumors [67]. 9q LOH was found to be a common event. In addition, invasive bladder tumors exhibited higher frequencies of 17p and 13q losses when compared with noninvasive bladder tumors. Deletions of the long arm of chromosome 13, including the RB locus (13q14), were independently reported by two groups [68,69]. In one of these studies, Cairns et al. used intragenic RB probes and found that 28 of 94 informative cases had LOH of the RB locus and 26 of these 28 cases were muscle-invasive tumors [69].

Growth control of mammalian cells is accomplished largely by the action of the pRB protein, which regulates exit from the G1 phase, and the p53 protein, which triggers growth arrest or apoptotic processes in response to cellular stress [14]. In tumorigenesis, RB and p53 serve collaborative roles, as evidenced by their frequent alterations in human tumors, the fact that many different tumor types exhibit mutations of both RB and p53, and the fact that several oncoviruses need to inactivate both proteins in order for cells to be transformed. The mechanistic basis for this dual requirement stems, in part, from the deactivation of a p53-dependent cell suicide program that would normally be brought about as a response to unchecked cellular proliferation resulting from RB-deficiency.

The potential relevance of pRB alterations in bladder cancer was disclosed in two independent studies [70,71]. Using a mouse monoclonal antibody (mAb) and IHC in frozen tissue sections of 48 primary bladder tumors, Cordon-Cardo et al. found detectable levels of pRB expression in 34 cases and loss of pRb expression in the other 14 [70]. Thirteen of the 38 patients diagnosed with muscle-invasive tumors were categorized as pRB negative, while only one of the 10 superficial tumors had the negative pRB phenotype. The survival was significantly decreased in pRB negative patients compared to those with pRB expression (p < 0.001). Similarly, Logothetis et al. found that a significant number of locally advanced tumors had a loss of pRB expression [71]. Specifically, 43 patients were evaluated using the Rb-WL-1 polyclonal antiserum and IHC. Negative pRB expression was reported in 37% of the tumor specimens analyzed. A significant decrease in disease-free survival was found for patients with negative pRB expression. Taken together, these data suggest that loss of pRB expression occurs in all grades and stages of bladder cancer but appears to be more common in muscle-invasive bladder tumors.

As mentioned, inactivation of the RB gene is an important event in bladder cancer [72]. Besides its genetic inactivation, RB has also been reported to be altered by epigenetic phenomena, such as enhanced cyclin D1 activity (discussed later). Cote et al. compared levels of pRB expression in a well-characterized cohort of bladder cancer patients. As expected, patients with undetectable pRB had worse clinical outcomes than those having moderate levels of pRB expression. However, another important finding was that the outcome for patients with tumors showing the highest levels of pRB was virtually identical to those with undetectable pRB [73]. This finding has been explained by the likely inactivation of pRB by hyperphosphorylation, which is probably secondary to posttranscriptional modifications in response to other alterations in the *RB* pathway. Examples may include high levels of cyclin D1 and low levels of p16 cyclin-dependent kinase activity.

The clinical implications of detecting *TP53* mutations and altered patterns of its encoded product (p53) in bladder tumors was the focus of a series of early investigations [8,74,75]. Such studies revealed that *TP53* mutations were common events in bladder cancer and were positively associated with tumor grade and stage. In studies designed to evaluate the sensitivity and specificity of different laboratory assays directed at identifying *TP53* mutations (including IHC with mAB PAb1801, restriction fragment length polymorphisms (RFLP), PCR–single-strand conformation polymorphisms (PCR-SSCP), and sequencing) a strong association was demonstrated between p53 nuclear overexpression and 17p LOH ($p < 0.001$). Similarly, a strong association ($p < 0.001$) between p53 nuclear overexpression and detection of *TP53* mutations by SSCP and sequencing was also demonstrated [76,77]. These studies demonstrated that p53 nuclear accumulation correlated highly with mutations in the gene, although the concordance was not 100%. The aim of a group of analyses that followed was to investigate the hypothesis that altered patterns of p53 expression correlated with tumor progression in patients with bladder tumors [78,79]. These studies proved that altered p53 expression is associated with disease progression and death due to bladder cancer. Moreover, p53 alterations were found to be an independent predictor of tumor recurrence and survival. Importantly, the study of Esrig et al. [79] demonstrated that invasive, organ-confined bladder tumors with p53 alterations were associated with disease progression, and that the widely accepted prognostic factors, grade and stage of the tumor, were not as predictive on a

multivariate analysis [79]. These results support the use of molecular determinants in supplementing and even perhaps replacing standard descriptive parameters of assessing prognosis of bladder cancer (i.e., grade and stage of the tumor). Alterations of *TP53* have been identified in dysplastic lesions of the urinary bladder, implying a potential prerequisite for involvement of p53 in bladder carcinogenesis [9,80,81]. Finally, it is now established that alterations in the p53 pathway are important in bladder cancer. Stein et al. demonstrated that the expression of p21 (Waf1/Cip1) in p53-altered tumors (through p53-independent pathways) could abrogate the deleterious effects of p53 alterations [82]. Therefore, understanding the status of the pathways through which the important tumor suppressor genes act (p53 and Rb) provides more relevant biological information than the status of the gene alone.

The cooperative effects of p53 and pRb alterations in superficial bladder tumors were recently revealed [73,83]. Cancer is a multistep genetic process involving alterations of oncogenes and tumor suppressor genes. Both p53 and Rb play important roles in cell cycle regulation and bladder cancer progression. However, a proportion of tumors display no alteration of p53 but still progress, and the same holds true for Rb alterations. Nevertheless, alterations in either p53 or Rb are necessary components of bladder cancer progression. As mentioned above, both p53 and Rb exert control on the cell cycle at the G1/S phase transition, through independent but interrelated pathways [84]. Alterations in one pathway may lead to dysregulation in the other pathway. For example, p53-mediated loss of p21 expression may result in phosphorylation and inactivation of pRb. Likewise, loss of pRb expression through genetic alterations may result in bypass of p53-mediated G1 arrest. Furthermore, it has recently been shown that germ-line mutations in *p53* and *Rb* may have cooperative tumorigenic effects in mice [85]. Therefore, one can reason that alterations in both p53 and Rb may act in a cooperative or synergistic way to promote bladder tumor progression in humans.

The cooperative nature of alterations affecting p53 and RB is reflected in the fact that patients exhibiting alterations of both proteins have significantly higher rates of tumor recurrence and decreased rates of survival when compared with patients with no alterations of either p53 or Rb. Furthermore, patients with alterations in only one of these proteins have intermediate rates of tumor recurrence and survival [73,83]. These studies demonstrated that concomitant alterations in both p53 and Rb have further negative effects on recurrence and survival compared with alterations in either one alone; the majority of patients with bladder cancer who have alterations in both p53 and Rb will suffer from tumor recurrence and eventually die of their disease, no matter what the stage of disease at presentation. Furthermore, patients with bladder cancers that show no evidence of alterations in either Rb or p53 have very low rates of recurrence, again regardless of disease stage. Thus, knowledge of both the p53 and the Rb status provides more specific information about the most likely outcome for the patient. Because tumorigenesis and progression is a process involving multiple genetic defects, it is likely that alterations in other pathways (e.g., involving oncogenes) will also affect bladder cancer progression. Thus, knowledge of the status of multiple pathways will be important in assessing the prognosis of patients with bladder (and other) cancers, in addition to having important implications for the clinical management of the disease.

Loss of genetic material on chromosome 9 has been shown to be an early abnormality detected in bladder tumors (discussed previously). More recently, the existence of two altered loci, one in each of both chromosome 9 arms, was postulated [86,87]. A detailed analysis conducted by Orlow et al. on 73 bladder tumors showed that two regions, one on 9p at the interferon cluster (9p21), and the other on 9q associated with the q34.1-2 bands, have the highest frequencies of allelic losses [88]. The 9p21 region has been found to be mutated frequently in a wide variety of human tumor cell lines, and the search for a putative tumor suppressor gene in this region led to the characterization of the so-called multiple

tumor suppressor 1 (*MTS1*) gene [89]. It was confirmed that the *MTS1* gene was the previously identified *INK4A/CDKN2* (p16) gene [90]. In addition to p16, the *INK4B/MTS2* (p15) gene is found in tandem at 9p21 [91]. These genes encode members of a new family of negative cell cycle regulators, whose products function as cyclin-dependent kinase inhibitory molecules [14]. Additional complexity at this locus results from the discovery that exon 2 of p16 is utilized, albeit in a different reading frame, by a second *INK4A*-encoded gene product, termed p19ARF (ARF being the acronym of alternative reading frame) [92]. Thus, the *INK4A* gene contains two distinct exon 1's (exon 1A and exon 1B) which assemble at the same acceptor site of exon 2 but produce two different proteins: p16 and p19/ARF, respectively [93]. Overexpression of p19ARF has been shown to induce G1 as well as G2M arrest through mechanisms that do not involve inhibition of known Cdks. Several independent groups of investigators showed that genetic alterations, mainly of p16 with concomitant effects on p19ARF and p15, are common events in bladder cancer. Orlow et al. recently reported an overall frequency of deletions and rearrangements for the p16 and p15 genes of 19% and 18%, respectively [94] in bladder cancer. Moreover, this study revealed that p16 and p15 alterations were associated with low-stage, low-grade bladder tumors. It should be emphasized that only Ta and T1, but not *in situ* lesions, showed deletions of either p16 or p15. Since p16 alterations occur independently of *p53* mutations [95], and *p53* mutations are frequent events in Tis bladder tumors, data from that report further support the hypothesis that bladder carcinogenesis may develop through two distinct molecular pathways [8,9]. Furthermore, evidence has accumulated revealing that the two products encoded by *INK4A* impact on the two prototype tumor suppressors, p16 through RB and p19ARF through p53, positioning the single gene *INK4A* at the nexus of the two most critical tumor suppressor pathways controlling neoplasia [96]. This, in turn, may explain the high frequency of mutations of this gene in human cancer.

Bladder Cancer as a Model for the Study of Preneoplastic Lesions and Tumor Progression

The molecular abnormalities reported to date, as well as the natural history of bladder cancer, have allowed the proposal of a working model for tumor development and progression of this group of neoplastic diseases [8,9,97]. It is the hypothesis of several groups of investigators that some specific chromosomal abnormalities and mutations of certain genes play a definite role in bladder tumor development, while other alterations seem to correlate with tumor progression (Figure 21.1). This model describes the molecular basis for differences in bladder tumor behavior well known to clinicians [3]. It shows that superficial papillary tumors of the bladder have a distinct molecular phenotype compared with the more dangerous flat CIS lesions. In addition, this model demonstrates the important molecular alterations that can be exploited in identifying premalignant lesions and the biological potential of such alterations.

Regarding preneoplastic conditions, the need now is to conduct in-depth molecular analyses utilizing well-characterized lesions, including those described above. This will hopefully provide evidence for the clinical relevance of detecting genetic instability, as well as primary genetic or epigenetic alterations, in otherwise morphologically normal appearing urothelium and preneoplastic lesions. Supporting evidence exists within the literature to indicate that papillary hyperplasia of the bladder, in a significant proportion of patients, is a precancerous lesion that subsequently progresses to a papillary bladder tumor. Chow et al. studied 15 papillary hyperplastic lesions for loss of heterozygosity (LOH) at 17 microsatellite markers on 9 chromosomal arms and demonstrated that chromosomal arm 9q was the most frequently lost [98]. Similarly, Czerniak et al. detected a high proportion of allelic losses in dysplastic lesions of the bladder [99]. As with hyperplastic lesions of the bladder, CIS of the bladder is often associated with LOH of chromosome 9 (24 of 31 patients), equally distributed between the short and long arms of chromosome 9. In addition, the following chromosomal arms de-

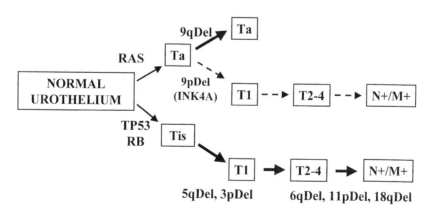

FIGURE 21.1. Working model for bladder cancer progression. Molecular analyses conducted by several independent groups, including our laboratory, have revealed that genetic alterations follow a sequence of events leading to bladder cancer progression. Distinct genotypic patterns have been associated with early versus late stages of bladder cancer. Chromosome 9 deletions are observed in most superficial papillary non-invasive tumors (Ta), but are only detected in a rather limited subset of invasive bladder neoplasms. However, deletions of 3p, 5q, 11p, 13q (*RB* locus), 17p (*TP53* locus), and 18q (*DCC* locus) appear to be absent in Ta tumors, but are identified in invasive bladder carcinomas. Based on these data, a model for bladder tumor progression has been proposed, in which two separate genetic pathways characterize the evolution of superficial bladder neoplasms.

monstrated frequent LOH in CIS lesions: 14q, 8p, 17p, 13q, 11p, and 4q [100]. The above studies provide evidence for LOH in similar chromosomal arms when hyperplasia, dysplasia, and CIS of the bladder are compared to primary bladder tumors. As a result, these lesions should be given strong consideration as being precancerous.

There are other alterations affecting differentiation antigens that have also been implicated in tumorigenesis and tumor progression in bladder cancer [101]. For example, phenotypic biochemical markers such as G-actin and M344 antigen occur as early events in uroepithelial transformation [46,102,103]. Blood group antigen alterations have been identified even in dysplasias of the urothelium [104,105]. Similarly, unscheduled expression of cytokeratin 20 has been reported as a marker of urothelial dysplasia [106]. In addition, it is now understood that the formation of neovasculature (angiogenesis) is an important event in the progression of bladder cancer [107,108], although the role of angiogenesis and cell matrix interactions in the development of early preinvasive lesions is not well understood. It is noted, however, that even CIS is associated with the formation of a neovasculature (an event that has long been used by urologists to identify early lesions cystoscopically), and therefore angiogenic regulation may be important in the maintenance of pre-invasive lesions.

Clinical advances in bladder cancer require the development of novel animal models paralleling the human disease. Several groups have engineered transgenic model systems that specifically target expression to the urothelium. This is achieved in specific models by the use of the uroplakin promoter to drive expression of selected oncogenes implicated in human bladder cancer. An important transgenic model is that of the uroplakin promoter driving the expression of the SV40T transgene, whose product is known to be responsible for inactivation of both p53 and pRB. Zhang et al. demonstrated that transgenic mice bearing a low copy number of the SV40T transgene developed CIS of the bladder, whereas those bearing high copy numbers developed not only CIS of the bladder but also invasive TCC of the bladder [109]. Crossing these transgenic mice with "knockout" models of tumor suppressor genes thought to be involved in bladder cancer is a logical extension of such preliminary studies, and these murine models are currently being engineered. In an alternative model, Wu et al. have engineered a transgenic system in which an *H-Ras* mutant is driven by the same uroplakin promoter. This model resulted in early hyperplastic changes within the bladder, which progress to nodular hyperplasia, and overt superficial papillary bladder tumors (Wu et al., personal communication).

High-throughput assays and bioinformatics, developed and validated by groups networking with one another, will be instrumental in elucidating the components of the regulatory and signaling pathways involved in bladder tumorigenesis and cancer progression. The implementation of hypothesis-generating studies linking clinical protocols with biological markers is a logical extension of the work that is being currently conducted. This undertaking needs to be performed with rigorous statistical methods. The definition and development of a standard method to test marker/disease associations, which will translate into validation studies, is also of importance in the molecular classification of preneoplastic and neoplastic lesions.

Chemoprevention of Bladder Cancer

Bladder cancer is appropriate for chemoprevention trials as the natural history of the disease is characterized by multiple tumor recurrences. While 13-*cis*-retinoic acid has been reported to be effective in preventing superficial bladder tumor recurrences, it is also associated with numerous side effects including conjunctivitis, pruritis, and joint or orbital pain [110]. A study involving 65 patients reported that high-dose multivitamins (40,000 U of vitamin A, 100 mg of vitamin B6, 2,000 mg of vitamin C, 400 U of vitamin E and 90 mg of zinc) decreased the rate of recurrence of superficial bladder tumors in patients receiving these high-dose vitamins compared to patients receiving the minimal daily requirement doses of these vitamins. However, the results of this study should be interpreted with caution due to the small number of patients and the fact that all patients were treated with intravesical bacillus Calmette-Guerin (BCG) with or without percutaneous BCG [111]. In addition to vitamins, polyamine synthesis inhibitors have been studied as chemopreventive agents for bladder cancer. Difluoromethylornithine (DFMO), an inhibitor of ornithine decarboxylase, the rate-limiting enzyme in polyamine synthesis, has also been studied in several animal models with some success in preventing tumor growth [112]. Furthermore, animal models have demonstrated that the agent oltipraz can protect against chemically-induced carcinogenesis in the lung, stomach, colon and bladder. Specifically, oltipraz inhibits carcinogenesis induced by polycyclic aromatic hydrocarbons and N-nitrosamines. Both of these agents are present in tobacco, and therefore oltipraz may be useful in preventing bladder cancer in smokers, as they are known to be at increased risk for this disease [113].

More recent data suggest that cyclooxygenase-2 (COX-2) inhibitors may be the most promising chemopreventive agents for patients at risk for developing bladder cancer. Studies have demonstrated that COX-2 immunoreactivity was absent in normal urothelium and low-grade urothelial tumors. However, the majority of high-grade urothelial tumors (i.e., invasive bladder cancers and carcinoma-in-situ lesions) express COX-2, suggesting a possible role of COX-2 in the progression of bladder cancer and supporting its potential as a therapeutic target in bladder cancer [114,115]. The chemopreventive potential of a selective COX-2 inhibitor, nimesulide, was evaluated in a rat model of bladder cancer. The study demonstrated that nimesulide was capable of preventing bladder tumor recurrences in a dose-dependent manner [116]. Phase II clinical trials, evaluating the efficacy of a COX-2 inhibitor in preventing superficial bladder tumor recurrences in humans have been initiated in different institutions.

Screening for Bladder Cancer

As the natural history of bladder cancer is characterized by multiple tumor recurrences and risk of disease progression, it is imperative that screening tests of high sensitivity and specificity are available for evaluating patients at increased risk of developing bladder cancer or for patients previously treated for superficial bladder cancer. Cystoscopy is the gold standard against which all other tests are compared. However, this test is both invasive and costly. As a result considerable emphasis is being placed on developing noninvasive tests for screening for bladder cancer. Currently, the following noninvasive tests are either being used in clinical practice or undergoing evaluation as screening tests for bladder cancer: urine cytology, bladder tumor antigen (BTA) TRAK assay (Bard Diagnostic Sciences, Redmond, WA), nuclear matrix protein (NMP) 22 test (Matritech, Newton, MA), fibrin degradation product (FDP) assay (PerImmune, Rockville, MD), hyaluronic acid (HA)-hyaluronidase (HAase) urine test, and urine detection of survivin.

As the gold standard for the noninvasive screening tests of bladder cancer, urine cytology is inadequate due to its low sensitivity and subjective diagnostic criteria. This has led to the development of the other screening tests and each of these tests should be compared to the results of urine cytology. The overall sensitivity of urine cytology has been reported to be between 40 and 60%, with higher sensitivities being reported from studies with a higher proportion of patients diagnosed with high-grade tumors [117,118]. Although urine cytology has a low sensitivity, it has consistently demonstrated excellent specificity.

The BTA TRAK assay is based on the detection of the human complement factor H-related protein in the urine. It is a quantitative assay that utilizes a pair of monoclonal antibodies incorporated into a "sandwich" enzyme immunoassay. The BTA TRAK assay, like urine cytology, displays a higher rate of bladder cancer detection with increasing tumor grade and stage. Overall, the sensitivity of the BTA

TRAK assay has been reported as 68%. This test is hampered by false-positive results in 48% of patients with lower urinary tract infections and in 43% of patients with urolithiasis [119]. The NMP 22 test is an immunoassay that measures a nuclear mitotic apparatus protein in the urine. An increase of at least tenfold in this protein has been shown to occur in cancerous tissue when compared with normal tissue, and in transformed cell lines when compared to normal tissue cell lines [120]. It is difficult to interpret the existing literature for the value of this test in the screening of patients for bladder cancer, as no universally accepted cutoff value exists, given that significant variances occur in normal NMP 22 levels.

Bladder cancers produce an angiogenic factor known as vascular endothelial growth factor. This factor is known to increase vessel wall permeability in the tumor which results in leakage of plasma proteins, including plasminogen and fibrinogen, into the extravascular space. The conversion of fibrinogen to fibrin exposes lysine residues to which plasminogen binds. This binding results in the conversion of plasminogen to plasmin, which in turn degrades fibrin and fibrinogen into fibrin degradation products. These products are released into the circulation and, in patients with bladder cancer, are detectable in the urine [121,122]. The FDP assay qualitatively measures intact fibrinogen and fibrin/fibrinogen degradation products in the urine using a hemagglutination immunoinhibition system in which formalin-treated sheep red blood cells are sensitized to human fibrinogen. These cells agglutinate in the presence of antibodies to FDP. The reported sensitivities of urine FDP in detecting bladder cancer vary widely with rates reported between 48% and 80% [118,123]. The utility of urine FDP in the detection of CIS remains controversial, and additional studies in this patient population are necessary.

Hyaluronic acid (HA) is a glycosaminoglycan that is involved in tumor adhesion and migration. The HA levels are three- to five-fold higher in bladder tumor tissue extracts than in normal bladder extracts and are not associated with tumor grade [124]. Many closely related endoglycosidases degrade HA and are collectively referred to as hyaluronidases (HAases). Pham et al. have demonstrated that HAase levels are six- to seven-fold higher in grade 2 and 3 bladder tumor extracts compared with the levels in normal bladder and grade 1 bladder tumor tissue extracts [125]. The HA-HAase test is comprised of two similar ELISA-like assays, the HA test and HAase test. Since the HA test detects bladder cancer regardless of tumor grade and the HAase test preferentially detects higher grade bladder cancers, combining the tests appears to be a rational strategy for not only detecting the presence of bladder cancer but also tumor grade. The overall sensitivity and specificity of the HA-HAase test to detect bladder cancer have been reported to be 92 and 85%, respectively [126].

A novel modulator of the cell death/viability balance in cancer was recently identified as survivin, a member of the inhibitor of apoptosis gene family [127]. Consistent with the hypothesis of deregulated apoptosis leading to or contributing to the development of certain cancers, survivin was present in 78% of bladder cancers but not detected in normal urothelium [128]. Smith et al. recently investigated the potential suitability of survivin detection in urine as a novel marker of the presence of bladder cancer. Survivin was detected in all 46 patients with evidence of bladder cancer and was not detected in the urine of any healthy volunteers or in the urine of patients with prostate, kidney, vaginal, or cervical cancer [129].

Despite its relative inadequacy, urine cytology remains the gold standard against which other noninvasive tests for the screening of bladder cancer must be compared. Many of the novel tests described above offer future promise in the screening of patients for bladder cancer. Whether these tests alone or in combination will outperform current screening protocols remains to be determined.

References

1. Reuter VE, Melamed MR. The lower urinary tract. In: Sternberg SS (ed) *Diagnostic surgical pathology*. New York: Raven Press, 1989, pp. 1355–92.
2. Mostofi FK, Sobin LH, Torloni H. Histologic typing of urinary bladder tumours. In: *Interna-*

tional histological classification of tumors, Vol. 10. Geneva: The World Health Organization, 1973.

3. Koss L. *Atlas of tumor pathology: Tumors of the urinary bladder (Fasicle 11)*, 2nd ed. Washington: Armed Forces Institute of Pathology, 1975.

4. Zhang Z-F, Steineck G. Epidemiology and Etiology of Bladder Cancer. In: Raghavan D, Scher HI, Leibel SA, Lange P (eds) *Principles and practice of genitourinary oncology*. Philadelphia: JB Lippincott Company, 1997, pp. 215–22.

5. Mostofi FK, Sesterhenn IA. Pathology of epithelial tumors and carcinoma in situ of bladder. *Prog Clin Biol Res* 1984; 62:55–74.

6. Prout GR. Bladder carcinoma and a TNM system of classification. *J Urol* 1997; 117:583–8.

7. Simoneau M, LaRue H, Fradet Y. Low frequency of human papillomavirus infection in initial papillary bladder tumors. *Urol Res* 1999; 27:108–14.

8. Dalbagni G, Presti J, Reuter V, et al. Genetic alterations in bladder cancer. *Lancet* 1993; 324:469–71.

9. Spruck CH, Ohneseit PE, Gonzalez-Zulueta M, et al. Two molecular pathways to transitional cell carcinoma of the bladder. *Cancer Res* 1994; 54:784–8.

10. Johansson SL, Cohen SM. Pathology of Bladder Cancer. In: Raghavan D, Scher HI, Leibel SA, Lange P (eds) *Principles and practice of genitourinary oncology*. Philadelphia: JB Lippincott Company, 1997, pp. 207–13.

11. Koss L. *Diagnostic cytology and its histopathologic bases*, 4th ed. Philadelphia: JB Lippincott Company, 1992.

12. Kiemeney LA, Witjes JA, Heijbroek RP, et al. Dysplasia in normal-looking urothelium increases the risk of tumour progression in primary superficial bladder cancer. *Eur J Cancer* 1994; 30:1621–5.

13. Igawa M, Urakami S, Shirakawa H. A mapping of histology and cell proliferation in human bladder cancer: an immunohistochemical study. *Hiroshima J of Med Science* 1995; 44: 93–7.

14. Cordon-Cardo C. Mutation of cell cycle regulators: biological and clinical implications for human neoplasias. *Am J Pathol* 1995; 147: 545–60.

15. Pantel K, Cote RJ, Fodstad O. Detection and clinical importance of micrometastatic disease. *J Natl Cancer Inst* 1999; 91:1113–24.

16. Gibas Z, Prout GR, Connolly JG, et al. Non-random chromosomal changes in transitional cell carcinoma of the bladder. *Cancer Res* 1984; 44:1257–64.

17. Atkin NB, Baker MC. Cytogenetic study of ten carcinomas of the bladder: involvement of chromosomes 1 and 11. *Cancer Genet Cytogenet* 1985; 15:253–68.

18. Babu VR, Lutz MD, Miles BJ, et al. Tumor behavior in transitional cell carcinoma of the bladder in relation to chromosomal markers and histopathology. *Cancer Res* 1987; 47:6800–5.

19. Vanni R, Scarpa RM, Nieddu M, et al. Cytogenetic investigation on 30 bladder carcinomas. *Cancer Genet Cytogenet* 1998; 30:35–42.

20. Tyrkus M, Powell I, Fakr W. Cytogenetic studies of carcinoma in situ of the bladder: prognostic implications. *J Urol* 1992; 148:44–6.

21. Hopman AHN, Moesker O, Smeets W, et al. Numerical chromosome 1, 7, 9, and 11 aberrations in bladder cancer detected by in situ hybridization. *Cancer Res* 1991; 51:644–51.

22. Waldman FM, Carroll PR, Kerschmann R, et al. Centromeric copy number of chromosome 7 is strongly correlated with tumor grade and labeling index in human bladder cancer. *Cancer Res* 1991; 51:3807–13.

23. Sauter G, Moch H, Moore D, et al. Heterogeneity of *erbB-2* gene amplification in bladder cancer. *Cancer Res* 1993; 53:2199–203.

24. Sauter G, Carroll P, Moch H, et al. C-myc copy number gains in bladder cancer detected by fluorescence in situ hybridization. *Am J Pathol* 1995; 146:1131–9.

25. Sauter G, Deng G, Moch H, et al. Physical deletion of the *p53* gene in bladder cancer. *Am J Pathol* 1994; 144:756–66.

26. Sauter G, Moch H, Wagner U, et al. Y chromosome loss detected by FISH in bladder cancer. *Cancer Genet Cytogenet* 1995; 82:163–9.

27. Balazs M, Carroll P, Kerschmann R, et al. Frequent homozygous deletion of cyclin-dependent kinase inhibitor 2 (*MTS1*, p16) in superficial bladder cancer detected by fluorescence in situ hybridization. *Genes Chromosom Cancer* 1997; 19:84–9.

28. Wheeless LL, Reeder JE, Han R, et al. Bladder irrigation specimens assayed by fluorescence in situ hybridization to interphase nuclei. *Cytometry* 1994; 17:319–26.

29. Kallioniemi A, Kallioniemi OP, Sudar D, et al. Comparative genomic hybridization for molecular cytogenetic analysis of solid tumors. *Science* 1992; 258:818–21.

30. Kallioniemi A, Kallioniemi OP, Citro G, et al. Identification of gains and losses of DNA sequences in primary bladder cancer by comparative genomic hybridization. *Genes Chromosom Cancer* 1995; 12:213–19.

31. Simon R, Burger H, Semjonow A, et al. Patterns of chromosomal imbalances in muscle invasive bladder cancer. *Int J Oncol* 2000; 17:1025–9.

32. Koo SH, Kwon KC, Ihm CH, et al. Detection of genetic alterations in bladder tumors by comparative genomic hybridization and cytogenetic analysis. *Cancer Genet Cytogenet* 1999; 110: 87–93.

33. Reddy EP, Reynolds RK, Santos E, et al. A point mutation is responsible for the acquisition of transforming properties by the *T24* bladder carcinoma oncogene. *Nature* 1982; 300:149–52.

34. Fujita J, Srivastava SK, Kraus MH. Frequency of molecular alterations affecting ras protooncogenes in human urinary tract tumors. *Proc Natl Acad Sci* 1985; 82:3849–53.

35. Nagata Y, Abe M, Kobayashi K, et al. Point mutations of *c-ras* genes in human bladder cancer and kidney cancer. *Jap J Cancer Res* 1990; 81:22–7.

36. Czerniak B, Deitch D, Simmons H, et al. *Ha-ras* gene codon 12 mutations and DNA ploidy in urinary bladder carcinomas. *Br J Cancer* 1990; 62:762–3.

37. Czerniak B, Cohen GL, Elkind P, et al. Concurrent mutations of coding and regulatory sequences of the *Ha-ras* gene in urinary bladder carcinomas. *Hum Pathol* 1992; 23:1199–204.

38. Ooi A, Herz F, Setsuko I, et al. *Ha-ras* codon 12 mutation in papillary tumors of the urinary bladder. A retrospective study. *Int J Oncol* 1994; 4:85–9.

39. Fitzgerald JM, Ramchurren N, Rieger K, et al. Identification of H-ras mutations in urine sediments complements cytology in the detection of bladder tumors. *J Natl Cancer Inst* 1995; 87:129–33.

40. Przybojewska B, Jagiello A, Jalmuzna P. *H-RAS*, and *N-RAS* gene activation in human bladder cancers. *Cancer Genet Cytogenet* 2000; 121:73–7.

41. Cattan N, Saison-Behmoaras T, Mari B, et al. Screening of human bladder carcinomas for the presence of *Ha-ras* codon 12 mutation. *Oncol Rep* 2000; 7:497–500.

42. Saito S, Hata M, Fukuyama R, et al. Screening of *H-ras* gene point mutations in 50 cases of bladder carcinoma. *Int J Urol* 1997; 4:178–85.

43. Neal DE, Marsh C, Bennet MK, et al. Epidermal growth-factor receptors in human bladder cancer: comparison of invasive and superficial tumors. *Lancet* 1985; 1:366–8.

44. Neal DE, Sharples L, Smith K, et al. The epidermal growth factor receptor and the prognosis of bladder cancer. *Cancer* 1990; 65:1619–25.

45. Messing EM. Clinical implications of the expression of epidermal growth factor receptors in human transitional cell carcinomas. *Cancer Res* 1990; 50:2530–7.

46. Rao JY, Hemstreet GP, Hurst RE, et al. Alterations in phenotypic biochemical markers in bladder epithelium during tumorigenesis. *Proc Natl Acad Sci* 1993; 90:8287–91.

47. Nguyen PL, Swanson PE, Jaszcz W, et al. Expression of epidermal growth factor receptor in invasive transitional cell carcinoma of the urinary bladder: a multivariate survival analysis. *Am J Clin Pathol* 1994; 101:166–76.

48. Thogersen VB, Jorgensen PE, Sorensen BS, et al. Expression of transforming growth factor alpha and epidermal growth factor receptor in human bladder cancer. *Scand J Clin Lab Invest* 1999; 59:267–77.

49. Perrotte P, Matsumoto T, Inoue K, et al. Antiepidermal growth factor receptor antibody C225 inhibits angiogenesis in human transitional cellcarcinoma growing orthotopically in nude mice. *Clin Cancer Res* 1999; 5:257–65.

50. Wood D, Wartinger DD, Reuter V, et al. DNA, RNA and immunohistochemical characterization of the *HER-2/neu* oncogene in transitional cell carcinoma of the bladder. *J Urol* 1991; 146:1398–401.

51. Sato K, Moriyama M, Mori S, et al. An immunohistologic evaluation of *c-erbB-2* gene product in patients with urinary bladder carcinoma. *Cancer* 1992; 70:2493–8.

52. Underwood M, Barlett J, Reeves J, et al. *C-erbB-2* gene amplification: a molecular marker in recurrent bladder tumors? *Cancer Res* 1995; 55:2422–30.

53. Lonn U, Lonn S, Friberg S, et al. Prognostic value of amplification of c-erb-B2 in bladder carcinoma. *Clin Cancer Res* 1995; 10:1189–94.

54. Miyamoto H, Kubota Y, Noguchi S, et al. *C-ERBB-2* gene amplification as a prognostic marker in human bladder cancer. *Urology* 2000; 55:679–83.

55. Wagner U, Sauter G, Moch H, et al. Patterns of *p53*, *erB-2*, and *EGF-r* expression in premalig-

nant lesions of the urinary bladder. *Hum Pathol* 1995; 26:970–8.

56. Oliner JD, Kinzler KW, Metlzer PS, et al. Amplification of a gene encoding a p53 associated protein in human sarcomas. *Nature* 1992; 358:80–3.

57. Haupt Y, Maya R, Kazaz A, et al. Mdm2 promotes the rapid degradation of p53. *Nature* 1992; 387:296–9.

58. Momand J, Zambetti G, Olson D, et al. The mdm-2 oncogene product forms a complex with the p-53 protein and inhibits *TP53*-mediated transactivation. *Cell* 1992; 69:1237–45.

59. Lianes P, Orlow I, Zhang ZZ, et al. Altered patterns of *MDM2* and *TP53* expression in human bladder cancer. *J Natl Cancer Inst* 1994; 86: 1325–30.

60. Barbareschi M, Girlando S, Fellin G, et al. Expression of mdm2 and p53 proteins in transitional cell carcinoma. *Urology Res* 1995; 22: 349–52.

61. Pfister C, Larue H, Moore L, et al. Tumorigenic pathways in low-stage bladder cancer based on *p53, MDM2* and *p21* phenotypes. *Int J Cancer* 2000; 89:100–4.

62. Kiemeney LA, Schoenberg M. Familial transitional cell carcinoma. *J Urol* 1996; 156:867–72.

63. Fearon ER, Feinberg AP, Hamilton SH, et al. Loss of genes on the short arm of chromosome 11 in bladder cancer. *Nature* 1985; 318:377–80.

64. Tsai YC, Nichols PW, Hiti AL, et al. Allelic losses of chromosomes 9, 11, and 17 in human bladder cancer. *Cancer Res* 1990; 50:44–7.

65. Olumi AF, Tsai YC, Nichols PW, et al. Allelic loss of chromosomes 17p distinguishes high grade from low grade transitional cell carcinoma of the bladder. *Cancer Res* 1990; 50: 7081–3.

66. Presti JC, Reuter VE, Galan T, et al. Molecular genetic alterations in superficial and locally advanced human bladder cancer. *Cancer Res* 1991; 51:5405–9.

67. Habuchi T, Ogawa O, Kakehi Y, et al. Accumulated allelic losses in the development of invasive urothelial cancer. *Int J Cancer* 1993; 53: 579–84.

68. Ishikawa J, Xu H-J, Hu S-X, et al. Inactivation of the retinoblastoma gene in human bladder and renal cell carcinomas. *Cancer Res* 1991; 51: 5736–43.

69. Cairns P, Proctor AJ, Knowles MA. Loss of heterozygosity at the RB locus is frequent and correlates with muscle invasion in bladder carcinoma. *Oncogene* 1991; 6:2305–9.

70. Cordon-Cardo C, Wartinger D, Petrylak D, et al. Altered expression of the retinoblastoma gene product is a prognostic indicator in bladder cancer. *J Natl Cancer Inst* 1992; 84: 1251–6.

71. Logothetis CJ, Xu H-J, Ro JY, et al. Altered retinoblastoma protein expression and known prognostic variables in locally advanced bladder cancer. *J Natl Cancer Inst* 1992; 84:1256–61.

72. Xu HJ, Cairns P, Hu SX, et al. Loss of Rb protein expression in primary bladder cancer correlates with loss of heterozygosity at the Rb locus and tumor progression. *Int J Cancer* 1993; 53:781–4.

73. Cote RJ, Dunn MD, Chatterjee SJ, et al. Elevated and absent of *pRb* expression is associated with bladder cancer progression and has cooperative effects with p53. *Cancer Res* 1998; 58:1090–4.

74. Sidransky D, Von Eschenbach A, Tsai YC, et al. Identification of *p53* gene mutations in bladder cancers and urine samples. *Science* 1991; 252: 706–9.

75. Fujimoto K, Yamada Y, Okajima E, et al. Frequent association of *p53* gene mutation in invasive bladder cancer. *Cancer Res* 1992; 52: 1393–8.

76. Esrig D, Spruck, CH, III, Nichols PW, et al. P53 nuclear protein accumulation correlates with mutations in the *p53* gene, tumor grade, and stage in bladder cancer. *Am J Pathol* 1993; 143:1389–97.

77. Cordon-Cardo C, Dalbagni D, Saez GT, et al. *TP53* mutations in human bladder cancer: Genotypic versus phenotypic patterns. *Int J Cancer* 1994; 56:347–53.

78. Sarkis AS, Dalbagni G, Cordon-Cardo C, et al. Nuclear overexpression of p53 protein in transitional cell bladder carcinoma: a marker for disease progression. *J Natl Cancer Inst* 1993; 85:53–9.

79. Esrig D, Elmajian D, Groshen S, et al. Accumulation of nuclear p53 and tumor progression in bladder cancer. *N Engl J Med* 1994; 331: 1259–64.

80. Soini Y, Turpeenniemi-Hujanan T, Kamel D, et al. p53 immunohistochemistry in transitional cell carcinoma and dysplasia of the urinary bladder correlates with disease. *Br J Cancer* 1993; 68:1029–35.

81. Schmitz-Drager BJ, van Roeyen CR, Grimm MO, et al. p53 accumulation in precursor lesions and early stages of bladder cancer. *World J Urol* 1994; 12:79–83.

82. Stein JP, Ginsberg DA, Grossfeld GD, et al. The effect of *p21WAF1/CIP1* expression on tumor progression in bladder cancer. *J Natl Cancer Inst* 1998; 90:1072–9.

83. Cordon-Cardo C, Zhang ZF, Dalbagni G, et al. Cooperative effects of *p53* and *pRB* alterations in primary superficial bladder tumors. *Cancer Res* 1997; 57:1217–21.

84. Cote RJ, Chatterjee SJ. Molecular determinants of outcome in bladder cancer. *The Cancer J (Scient Am)*, 1999; 5:2–15.

85. Williams BO, Remington L, Albert DM, et al. Cooperative tumorigenic effects of germline mutations in *Rb* and *p53*. *Nat Genet* 1994; 7:480–4.

86. Miyao N, Tsai YC, Lerner SP, et al. Role of chromosome 9 in human bladder cancer. *Cancer Res* 1993; 53:4066–70.

87. Cairns P, Shaw ME, Knowles MA. Preliminary mapping of the deleted region of chromosome 9 in bladder cancer. *Cancer Res* 1993; 53: 1230–2.

88. Orlow I, Lianes P, Lacombe L, et al. Chromosome 9 deletions and microsatellite alterations in human bladder tumors. *Cancer Res* 1994; 54: 2848–51.

89. Kamb A, Gruis NA, Weaver-Feldhaus J, et al. A cell cycle regulator potentially involved in genesis of many tumor types. *Science* 1994; 264: 436–40.

90. Serrano M, Hannon GJ, Beach D. A new regulatory motif in cell-cycle control causing specific inhibition of cyclin D/CDK4. *Nature* 1993; 366:704–7.

91. Hannon GJ, Beach D. p15INK4B is a potential effector of TGF-β-induced cell cycle arrest. *Nature* 1994; 371:257–61.

92. Quelle DE, Zindy F, Ashum RA, et al. Alternative reading frames of the *INK4A* tumor suppressor gene encode two unrelated proteins capable of inducing cell cycle arrest. *Cell* 1995; 83:993–1000.

93. Robertson KD, Jones PA. The human ARF cell cycle regulatory gene promoter is a CpG island which can be silenced by DNA methylation and down-regulated by wild-type p53. *Mol Cell Biol* 1998; 18:6457–73.

94. Orlow I, Lacombe L, Hannon GJ, et al. Deletion of the p16 and p15 genes in human bladder tumors. *J Natl Cancer Inst* 1995; 87: 1524–9.

95. Gruis NA, Weaver-Feldhaus J, Liu Q, et al. Genetic evidence in melanoma and bladder cancers that p16 and p53 function in separate pathways of tumor suppression. *Am J Pathol* 1995; 146:1199–206.

96. Pomerantz J, Schrieber-Agus N, Liegoeis N, et al. The *Ink4a* tumor suppressor gene product, p19/Arf, interacts with MDM2 and neutralizes MDM2's inhibition of p53. *Cell* 1998; 92:713–23.

97. Cordon-Cardo C, Dalbagni D, Sarkis A, et al. Genetic alterations associated with bladder cancer. In: DeVita VT, Hellman S, Rosenberg SA (eds) *Important advances in Oncology*. Philadelphia: JB Lippincott Company, 1994, pp. 71–83.

98. Chow NH, Cairns P, Eisenberger CF, et al. Papillary urothelial hyperplasia is a clonal precursor to papillary transitional cell bladder cancer. *Int J Cancer* 2000; 89:514–18.

99. Czerniak B, Li L, Chaturvedi V, et al. Genetic modeling of human urinary bladder carcinogenesis. *Genes Chromosom Cancer* 2000; 27: 392–402.

100. Rosin MP, Cairns P, Epstein JI, et al. Partial allelotype of carcinoma in situ of the human bladder. *Cancer Res* 1995; 55:5213–6.

101. Fradet Y, Cordon-Cardo C. Tumor markers in the management of bladder cancer. In: Raghavan D, Scher HI, Leibel SA, et al. (eds) *Principles and practice of genitourinary oncology*. Philadelphia: JB Lippincott Company, 1996, pp. 231–238.

102. Bonner RB, Hemstreet GP III, Fradet Y, et al. Bladder cancer risk assessment with quantitative fluorescence image analysis of tumor markers in exfoliated bladder cells. *Cancer* 1993; 72:2461–9.

103. Hemstreet GP III, Hurst RE, Bonner RB, et al. Alterations in phenotypic biochemical markers in bladder epithelium during tumorigenesis. *Proc Natl Acad Sci* 1993; 90:8287–91.

104. Yamada T, Fukui I, Kobayashi T. The relationship of ABH(O) blood group antigen expression in intraepithelial dysplastic lesions to clinicopathologic properties of associated transitional cell carcinoma of the bladder. *Cancer* 1991; 67:1661–6.

105. Orlow I, Lacombe L, Pellicer I, et al. Genotype and phenotype characterization of the histo-blood group ABO(H) in primary bladder tumors. *Int J Cancer* 1998; 75:819–24.

106. Harnden P, Eardley I, Joyce AD, et al. Cytokeratin 20 as an objective marker of urothelial dysplasia. *Br J Urol* 1996; 78:870–5.

107. Bochner BH, Cote RJ, Weidner N, et al. Tumor angiogenesis is an independent prognostic factor in invasive transitional cell carcinoma

of the bladder. *J Natl Cancer Inst* 1995; 87: 1603–12.

108. Grossfeld GD, Ginsberg DA, Stein JP, et al. Thrombospondin-1 expression in transitional cell carcinoma of the bladder: association with p53 alterations, tumor angiogenesis and tumor progression. *J Natl Cancer Inst* 1997; 89: 219–27.

109. Zhang ZT, Pak J, Shapiro E, et al. Urothelium-specific expression of an oncogene in transgenic mice induced the formation of carcinoma in situ and invasive transitional cell carcinoma. *Cancer Res* 1999; 59:3512–17.

110. Prout GR Jr, Barton BA. 13-cis-retinoic acid in chemoprevention of superficial bladder cancer. The National Bladder Cancer Group. *J Cell Biochem* 1992; 161:148–52.

111. Lamm DL, Riggs DR, Shriver JS, et al. Megadose vitamins in bladder cancer: a double-blind clinical trial. *J Urol* 1994; 151:21–6.

112. Moon RC, Detrisac CJ, Thomas CF, et al. Chemoprevention of experimental bladder cancer. *J Cell Biochem* 1992; 161:134–8.

113. Kensler TW, Helzlsouer KJ. Oltipraz: clinical opportunities for cancer chemoprevention. *J Cell Biochem* 1995; 22:101–7.

114. Komhoff M, Guan Y, Shappell HW, et al. Enhanced expression of cyclooxygenase-2 in high grade human transitional cell bladder carcinomas. *Am J Pathol* 2000; 157: 29–35.

115. Mohammed SI, Knapp DW, Bostwick DG, et al. Expression of cyclooxygenase-2 (COX-2) in human invasive transitional cell carcinoma (TCC) of the urinary bladder. *Cancer Res* 2000; 59:5647–50.

116. Okajima E, Denda A, Ozono S, et al. Chemopreventive effects of nimesulide, a selective cyclooxygenase-2 inhibitor, on the development of rat urinary bladder carcinomas initiated by N-butyl-N-(4-hydroxybutyl) nitrosamine. *Cancer Res* 1998; 58:3028–31.

117. Grossman HB. New methods of detection of bladder cancer. *Semin Urol Oncol* 1998; 16: 17–22.

118. Ramakumar S, Bhuiyan J, Besse JA, et al. Comparison of screening methods in the detection of bladder cancer. *J Urol* 1999; 161:388–94.

119. Ellis WJ, Blumenstein BA, Ishak LM. Clinical evaluation of the BTA TRAK assay and comparison to voided urine cytology and the Bard BTA test in patients with recurrent bladder tumors. *Urology* 1997; 50:882–7.

120. Keese SK, Briggman JV, Thill G, et al. Utilization of nuclear matrix proteins for cancer diagnosis. *Crit Rev Eukaryot Gene Expr* 1996; 6:189–214.

121. Ewing R, Tate GM, Hetherington JW. Urinary fibrin/fribrinogen degradation products in transitional cell carcinoma of the bladder. *Br J Urol* 1987; 59:53–9.

122. Jayachandran S, Unni Moopan MM, Wax SH, et al. The value of urinary fibrin/fibrinogen degradation products as tumor markers in urothelial carcinoma. *J Urol* 1984; 132:21–6.

123. Schmetter BS, Habicht KK, Lamm DL, et al. A multicenter trial evaluation of the fibrin/fibrinogen degradation products test for detection and monitoring of bladder cancer. *J Urol* 1997; 158:801–5.

124. Lokeshwar VB, Obek C, Soloway MS, et al. Tumor associated hyaluronic acid: a new sensitive and specific urine marker for bladder cancer. *Cancer Res* 1997; 57:773–9.

125. Pham HT, Block NL, Lokeshaw VB, et al. Tumor-derived hyaluronidase: a diagnostic urine marker for high grade bladder cancer. *Cancer Res* 1997; 57:778–85.

126. Lokeshwar VB, Block NL: HA-Haase urine test: A sensitive and specific method for detecting bladder cancer and evaluating its grade. *Urol Clin NA* 2000; 27:53–61.

127. Ambrosini G, Adida C, Altieri DC. A novel antiapoptosis gene, survivin, expressed in cancer and lymphoma. *Nat Med* 1997; 17: 2941–53.

128. Swana HS, Grossman D, Anthony JN, et al. Tumor content of the antiapoptosis molecule survivin and recurrence of bladder cancer. *N Engl J Med* 1999; 341:452–3.

129. Smith SD, Wheeler MA, Plescia J, et al. Urine detection of survivin and diagnosis of bladder cancer. *JAMA* 2000; 285:324–8.

Part IV
Control of Cancer Precursors

22
Screening

Anthony B. Miller

Screening is based on the expectation that the early detection of cancer, in what has been called the Detectable Preclinical Phase (DPCP) [1], will result in a reduction in mortality from the disease. For most cancers for which screening is currently contemplated, the DPCP comprises an early (asymptomatic) cancer, not a cancer precursor. This is true for screening for cancers of the breast, lung, prostate, skin, and stomach. However, for some of these sites (e.g., breast and prostate), presumed cancer precursors are known. For two other cancers, screening is either primarily (cervix) or partly (colorectum) directed to the detection of precursors.

If screening directed primarily toward the detection of precursors is effective, the development of invasive cancer will be prevented. Therefore, an effective program for screening for cancer precursors will result in a reduction in cancer incidence as well as a reduction in cancer mortality. Reduction in incidence then becomes the primary criterion by which one evaluates whether screening for precursors is effective. This is strikingly different from screening dependent on finding early cancers, in which the initial effect on incidence will be an increase, followed by stabilization with continued screening. This is because the time of diagnosis of the cancer is brought forward (the lead time effect), together in some instances with an increase in the diagnosis of lesions which although labeled as cancer, would never have presented clinically in the person's lifetime in the absence of screening (the overdiag-

nosis effect). Incidence will never fall below the baseline level if screening is continued, but if it ceases, there will be a temporary fall below the baseline followed by a return to the baseline after the lead time (and overdiagnosis) effects dissipate.

The remainder of this chapter focuses primarily on the evidence relating to screening for precursors of cervix and colorectal cancer, but includes a brief review of the possible relevance of screening for precursors of some other cancers.

Cancer of the Uterine Cervix

Cancer of the cervix has a well-defined DPCP lasting many years, if not decades, for the majority of cases [2]. The study of cohorts of screened women over long periods has led to recognition of both the length of time that progression usually takes and the fact that the majority of detectable precursors do not progress, but rather regress to normal epithelium after a variable period [2]. An important implication of this natural history is that management of the majority of these lesions must be conservative. Otherwise, a substantial majority of women detected as having the precursor lesions will receive unnecessary treatment, with risk of complications. Furthermore, such treatment represents unnecessary expenditure for the health care system.

Although the majority of cervical cancer precursors destined to progress do so over a decade or more, there are exceptions. Cases do occur that progress rapidly through the DPCP, and that are not amenable to detection in any program with a reasonable frequency of re-screening. These cases contribute to the irreducible minimum of cervical cancer so that the maximum impact that can be expected of any screening program is to reduce the incidence of invasive cancer of the cervix to about 80% of baseline [3].

A Note on Terminology

In the original World Health Organization (WHO) classification for cervical cytology [4], the appearance of the cells was classified according to whether they were thought to represent the histologic changes in the cervix [5]. In these classifications, the precursors of cancer of the cervix were considered in two groups: carcinoma-in-situ, a full thickness change in the squamous epithelium of the cervix with nuclei that appeared malignant but without invasion of the basement membrane; and various degrees of dysplasia, which involved lesser degrees of involvement of the epithelium without full thickness change. The degrees of dysplasia were identified as mild, moderate and severe. In the hands of experienced observers, the distinction between carcinoma-in-situ and severe dysplasia was usually made consistently. Subsequently, Richart [6] proposed the cervical intraepithelial neoplasia (CIN) terminology, categorizing mild dysplasia as CIN 1, moderate dysplasia as CIN 2, and severe dysplasia and carcinoma-in-situ combined as CIN 3. However in 1989, the "Bethesda" system was promulgated in the United States, in which CIN 1 was combined with cellular evidence of HPV effects as low-grade squamous intraepithelial lesions (LSIL) and CIN 2 and 3 were combined as high-grade squamous intraepithelial lesions (HSIL) [7], so the previous attempt to link cytology to histology was largely abandoned. Although the intent was to simplify reporting and facilitate clinical management, while avoiding some of the observer variation inseparable from a multigrade system, the impact of the spread of this system on understanding of the natural history of the precursors

has been adverse, as will be discussed further.

The Natural History of Carcinoma in Situ of the Cervix

When data began to become available from the early screening programs for cancer of the cervix, it was noticed that the number of cases of carcinoma-in-situ of the cervix was far greater than was "required" to account for the incidence of invasive cancer of the cervix in the absence of screening. The difference between the cumulative incidence of carcinoma-in-situ by age and the sum of the cumulative incidence of invasive cancer and prevalent (non-progressed) cases of carcinoma-in-situ, in the early British Columbia data, was called the "yawning gap" [8]. There seemed to be several potential explanations for this gap. The first was false-negative error. If a case of carcinoma-in-situ was missed at the first or subsequent screens, but was diagnosed subsequently at a later screen, the cumulative incidence of carcinoma-in-situ would be increased artefactually, and the prevalence of carcinoma-in-situ would be reduced, thus contributing to the gap. The second potential explanation was denominator error. If women who returned for re-screening did so after a change of name as a result of marriage, or if the initial records were so deficient that the initial and subsequent screens could not be linked in the laboratory's file, then the prevalence would be reduced artefactually by the inclusion of women screened a second or third time, with lower risk of disease. The effect on the cumulative incidence of carcinoma in situ would be to lower it, and so again the yawning gap would be increased. A third potential explanation was that there was a cohort effect. If more recent birth cohorts had a greater lifetime risk of disease than older cohorts, then a gap would be created, as the younger cohorts in a cross-sectional study would largely comprise those at risk for carcinoma-in-situ, whereas the older cohorts would be at risk for invasive carcinoma. The remaining explanation was regression of carcinoma-in-situ. To be specific, if all the other explanations were discounted, then the apparent excess of carcinoma-in-situ would be explained by the fact that not all cases are destined to progress to invasive cancer; nor are they otherwise destined to remain unchanged in a woman. Rather, some would regress to lesser degrees of abnormality or even to normal epithelium.

The British Columbia cohort study was set up to evaluate these different explanations for the yawning gap. It was found that the gap persisted in spite of corrections for the false-negative error and denominator error, and that the two cohorts 15 years of age apart had almost identical risks of carcinoma-in-situ at comparable ages [8]. Thus the only remaining explanation for the gap was regression, which probably occurred in 40% to 60% of the detectable cases, especially at younger ages. An extension of this study, including a younger cohort, confirmed these conclusions [9].

The Natural History of Dysplasia of the Cervix

In the British Columbia Cohort Study, the inclusion of identified cases of dysplasia contributed nothing to progressive disease. Indeed, the majority of these cases appeared to regress, confirming that only among those cases that progressed to carcinoma-in-situ was there a risk of invasive carcinoma [8]. However, the British Columbia data did not distinguish between separate degrees of dysplasia. Therefore, to address this deficiency, a large cohort of women in Toronto whose records of cytological examinations spanned many years was studied [10]. The pathologists serving this laboratory had made a consistent attempt to identify the different degrees of dysplasia cytologically and only referred women for further assessment if there was cytological evidence of progression. By linking the records extracted from the laboratory with those of the Ontario Cancer Registry, women who were subsequently diagnosed with carcinoma-in-situ or invasive carcinoma of the cervix were identified [10]. Once again there was evidence of regression. The maximum extent of regression occurred in those with cytological evidence of mild dysplasia; but in addition, over 50% of those with cyto-

logical evidence of moderate dysplasia showed regression. Progression to severe dysplasia or worse within 10 years occurred in only 10% of those with mild dysplasia and in 32% of those with moderate dysplasia. Most of these progressions occurred within 5 years. Equally as important, a category identified in the laboratory as minimal dysplasia, a grouping that encompasses those that in the Bethesda system would be labelled as ASCUS, hardly showed any evidence of progression at all. Therefore, the results of the study supported the conclusions of a Canadian workshop [11], which proposed that there is prognostic value in the classification of moderate dysplasia separately from severe dysplasia, and that cytologic surveillance rather than immediate referral to colposcopy should be recommended for those with a cytologic diagnosis of mild dysplasia.

Frequency of Rescreening

A critical study which increased our understanding of the appropriate approach to rescreening was that coordinated by the International Agency for Research on Cancer (IARC) [12]. This study largely provided the basis for international recommendations for three yearly or even less frequent repeat screening and underlined the importance of concentrating screening between the ages of 35 and 64 [13]. However, an underlying difficulty with these recommendations is that probably the most successful screening program in the world is the organized program in Finland which screened only every 5 years and achieved the levels of success that the IARC model suggested would require screening every three years. A reevaluation of the British Columbia data [14] showed that although the median duration of progression from carcinoma-in-situ to invasive cancer in the IARC study was on the order of 5 to 8 years, this was calculated by including cancers detected by screening, for which prognosis is extremely good and for which the disease process is affected by the lead time gained by screening. Correcting for cancers detected by screening resulted in a median duration of progression from carcinoma-in-situ to invasive cancer of 15 years. The implication of this is that screening every 5, not 3 years, will give a 90% reduction in invasive cancer incidence and mortality.

Using these data, it is possible to recompute some of the inferences from the IARC [12] model. In a low-incidence country, nearly maximal benefit is obtained from screening every 5 years with little additional gain from starting screening at age 20 rather than at 25 or 26. Extending this to high-incidence countries, even screening every 10 years between the ages of 35 and 64, which amounts to only three tests in a lifetime, will result in almost a 70% reduction in invasive cancer.

It is important to remember that these effects are achieved only with efficient laboratories and full compliance. However, screening every 10 years with 80% compliance is over twice as efficient and considerably more effective than screening every three years with only 40% compliance. Even 100% compliance of women at an early age, as in maternal and child health programs, is far less efficient and not as effective as screening every ten years with 80% compliance [13].

HPV DNA Testing

Oncogenic types of human papillomaviruses (HPV) can be found in nearly all cancers of the cervix. The evidence that certain types of HPV cause cancer of the cervix has been categorized as *sufficient* by IARC [15]. However, most developed countries that have invested resources in the early detection of precursors of the disease have shown a major impact of such approaches, and it is not yet clear whether HPV testing can improve this situation, though it could enable more efficient and effective concentration on those at greatest risk of the disease, especially if testing was restricted to those of age 35 and greater to allow time for transitory infections in younger women to resolve spontaneously. A study in the UK on older women suggested that a combination of HPV testing and cytology could permit longer screening intervals for those negative on both, which could reduce the overall cost of the program [16].

The potential role of HPV DNA testing in developing countries has been evaluated in studies in South Africa [17] and Costa Rica [18]. Both studies raise questions about what criteria should be used when new tests are developed in order to evaluate whether they should be used in substitution for the older established test. The most rigorous criteria would be for the new test to be required to demonstrate:

- at least as great an efficacy as the old in a randomized screening trial with invasive cancer as the endpoint,
- at least as good cost-effectiveness (when used in the most optimal way), and
- at least as good acceptability to the target population.

However, the studies in South Africa [17] and Costa Rica [18] were not trials, but comparisons of sensitivity and specificity of detection of presumed precursors. The difficulty here is that we need to know which precursors will result in the development of invasive cancer. That is, we need to understand the natural history of the disease. This is recognized by Wilson and Junger [19] as one of the requirements for a screening program.

It is intuitively appealing to test for the presence of the virus believed to cause the disease, especially if the test for the virus is very sensitive, and provided that the test can be performed locally and does not cost too much. If it is known that the test is sufficiently sensitive, it can be assumed that any apparent precursor detected by another means that did not test positive for the oncogenic virus was not a relevant precursor. However, there is a major difficulty if we have evidence that one approach to testing for the virus is less sensitive than another, especially under circumstances when we know that the majority of the precursors will not progress to invasive disease. It could be that the very ones we miss with the less sensitive test are those that will progress. Under such states of uncertainty, we should reject the less sensitive approach to testing, especially if it also has lower specificity. On both counts therefore, the self-collected approach to specimen collection, which was evaluated by Wright et al. [17], fails in comparison to clinician-obtained samples, as its sensitivity was reported to be 64% for HSIL or worse and its specificity was 83%, compared to 84% and 84% for clinician-obtained tests and 61% and 97% for cytology.

Schiffman et al. [18] used two different assays for HPV DNA. The first generation assay had a sensitivity of 75% for HSIL or worse, and a specificity of 93%, compared to a sensitivity of 78% for cytology and a specificity of 94% if ASCUS was used as the cut-point for referral for colposcopy. The second generation assay had lower levels of detection which led to an increase in sensitivity to 88%, but a reduction in specificity to 88%.

Unfortunately, in neither study was sufficient information given to allow assessment of the sensitivity and specificity of HPV testing for detection of CIN 3. Both studies confused the issue by adding cases of invasive cancer to the high-grade lesions. Only "downstaging", an approach now replaced by visual inspection with acetic acid application (VIA), was designed to detect invasive cancers earlier. Since cervical cytology is known to be insensitive for invasive cancer, as the consequent blood and necrotic debris masks cells indicative of cancer, it is the visual component of all the tests evaluated in these studies (with the exception of self-collection) which should be detecting the clinically invasive cancers. However, a greater difficulty is the utilization in these studies of the High-Grade designation, encompassing both cytologically diagnosed CIN 2 as well as CIN 3. In this context, we are not interested in CIN 2, as the majority of such lesions will regress spontaneously, and it is the sensitivity with regard to CIN 3 which is critical. This is an example of the utilization of the Bethesda classification in a circumstance in which it was not meant to apply, namely the classification of the histologic findings after biopsy.

There is at least one other component required if HPV testing is to be used with confidence. It is important to know what causes persistence of infection with oncogenic HPV viruses, and what causes precursors to progress and not regress. Is there a single cocarcinogen or two or more? It is unlikely to be a feature of the virus, given the high prevalence of nonper-sistent infection in young women, so a refined HPV test will not provide the answer. It may be a feature of the host, or it may be something else, as yet unenvisaged.

In the meantime, it is important to remember that the major cost element in screening is the cost of the test itself and the cost of all the staff, equipment, and supplies required to perform the test and provide the report. The next most important cost element is the provision of diagnosis and management for those deemed to test positive. The poorer the specificity, the greater such costs will be.

At present, it seems unlikely that a country that cannot deliver cervical cytology could deliver HPV testing. Under such circumstances, it is VIA which appears to have the greatest promise [20], providing it can be allied to a simplified approach to colposcopy, so that its major disadvantage, poor specificity, does not result in an impossible additional burden.

Implications

In all countries, the incidence of invasive cancer of the cervix peaks at around age 55, and invasive cases are rare before age 30. However, carcinoma-in-situ and the dysplastic lesions that comprise the DPCP are detectable in some women even from the age of 15. This has led many to start screening in women even younger than 20 years of age, in spite of the extensive evidence from many countries that programs that start at age 25 are equally effective, and that programs that do not start until age 35 are even more cost-effective [21]. In reality it is necessary to time smears to detect those precursor lesions that are destined to progress to invasive cancer if left undetected. The large majority of precursor lesions will not have progressed if the first smear is delayed to age 35. Initiating screening at age 35 thus becomes the major priority for countries with restricted resources.

Colon and Rectum Cancer

Adenomatous polyps of the colon and rectum are regarded as the precursors of colon and rectal cancers [22]. Their development and progression mark the early stages of a sequence of genetic changes that eventually result in the development of invasive cancer [23]. However, autopsy studies show that detectable polyps are present in 30% or more of older adults [24], so only a proportion of polyps progress to colon or rectal cancer. Further, it is not clear that cancers only arise from preexisting polyps. Indeed, it is possible that dysplastic change in the colonic epithelium could progress to cancer without passing through a detectable polyp phase [25].

Of the screening tests for colorectal cancer, only the fecal occult blood test (FOBT) has been evaluated by completed randomized screening trials [24]. FOBTs are relatively insensitive for polyp detection, and to date, there have been no reports that the incidence of colorectal cancer has fallen following their use.

Endoscopy has been proposed as the means to remove adenomatous polyps of the colon and rectum and thus reduce colorectal cancer incidence [26]. Several years ago, on the basis of findings in an observational study, it was claimed that the incidence of rectal cancer was reduced following rigid sigmoidoscopy [27]. Yet such a conclusion was almost certainly incorrect [28]. Recently, as a result of the follow-up of the United States National Polyp Study, a similar claim was made for colonoscopy [29]. Yet a similar bias was almost certainly operating. If people who have had a colonoscopy or sigmoidoscopy and have been found to be free of cancer are followed, they represent a group of people who will have a low risk of developing disease for some time. This has been called the healthy screenee effect [30]. The only way to establish whether it is possible to reduce the incidence of colon and rectal cancer by flexible sigmoidoscopy or colonoscopy is through a randomized screening trial in which one group is randomized to receive screening endoscopy, and the other group consists of unscreened controls who receive usual care. The United States Prostate, Lung, Colon and Ovary trial is evaluating flexible sigmoidoscopy at 3 or 5 year intervals [31], a trial in the UK is evaluating one-time flexible sigmoidoscopy [32], and a new trial evaluating colonoscopy will commence shortly in the United States. In the mean time, it can be concluded that, as yet, there is no definitive evidence that removing precursors of colon or rectal cancer reduces the incidence of either cancer.

Breast Cancer

As indicated above, breast screening is designed principally to detect invasive cancers early. However, one effect of mammography screening for breast cancer is to detect in situ cancers of the breast, as the calcification associated with comedo types of ductal carcinoma-in-situ (DCIS) leads to their detection, biopsy, and excision. Many seem to believe that the detection of DCIS is one of the benefits derived from breast screening. Indeed, aggressive screening for what was then called minimal breast cancer used to be advocated strongly, in the belief that only by the detection of such lesions would breast cancer mortality be reduced [33]. Minimal breast cancer, as then defined, consisted of two components, invasive breast cancers of less than 10 mm in size, and DCIS. Data that enable the contribution of the detection of minimal breast cancers to the reduction in breast cancer potentially achieved by screening have recently become available from the 11 to 16-year follow-up of the Canadian National Breast Screening Study among women of ages 50 to 59 on entry (CNBSS 2) [34]. This study was designed to assess whether annual two-view mammography screening, together with annual screening by breast physical examinations and the teaching of breast self-examination (the MP group), resulted in a greater breast cancer mortality reduction than screening by breast physical examinations and the teaching of breast self-examination alone (the PO group). Each group was just under 20,000 women in total, with identical distribution of risk factors for breast cancer (CNBSS was an individually randomized trial, randomization being conducted with 5-year age strata and center). Of the 267 invasive breast cancers detected on screening in the MP group, 48 were less than 10 mm in size, compared to only 6 of 148 in the PO group. Furthermore, in addition,

71 in situ breast cancers were detected in the MP group but only 16 in the PO group. However, no reduction was found in breast cancer mortality over an average of 13 years follow-up on the addition of mammography (a cumulative rate ratio of 1.02, 95% CI: 0.78, 1.33). Thus the greater detection of "minimal" breast cancers in the MP group (an excess of 97) had no impact on breast cancer mortality. Further, there was no evidence that the detection of the in situ cancers resulted in a reduction in breast cancer incidence. The cumulative numbers of invasive breast cancers (including those ascertained after the end of the 4 to 5 year screening period) was 622 in the MP group and 610 in the PO. Thus at present, there is no evidence that the detection of breast cancer precursors is of any value in screening. This conclusion almost certainly applies to atypical hyperplasia of the breast also. These lesions, which are markers of increased risk of breast cancer in either breast [35] (DCIS is a marker of increased risk in the same breast [36]), are also detected and removed in breast screening programs. However, apart from their indication of future risk to the patient, their removal appears to provide no direct benefit.

The DCIS that is detectable clinically or by screening, therefore, is largely either a marker of that precursor elsewhere in the same breast, a marker of slowly growing invasive cancer already present in the same breast, or the end stage of a process well recognized for cancer of the cervix, namely the final stage of the process of regression of the majority of the precursors that are detectable [37]. Fisher and Fisher [38] have reported that, in their experience with about 10,000 cases of DCIS associated with invasive cancer, unequivocal microscopic extension of DCIS through its basement membrane into the surrounding stroma has rarely been observed. They also note that, although about 40% of recurrences of DCIS in the same breast are invasive, the survival of such patients was 98%, again suggesting a qualitatively different natural history from classic invasive ductal carcinoma. This seems to be an example of length bias, and fits strongly with the data from the CNBSS cited above.

Endometrial Cancer

Endometrial hyperplasia is regarded as a precursor of endometrial cancer. However, there have been no reports of screening for this precursor. Endometrial sampling is carried out for the detection of endometrial cancer, as for example, in the later stages of recruitment for the National Surgical Adjuvant Breast and Bowel Project (NSABP) trial of tamoxifen for treatment of breast cancer [39]. However that trial was not designed in a way that enables the efficacy of endometrial sampling to be evaluated, though it is clear that the sampling that was performed did not prevent endometrial cancer occurring in higher incidence in the tamoxifen compared to the control group.

Prostate Cancer

Prostate intraepithelial neoplasia (PIN) is a possible precursor of prostate cancers [40]. It may be detected in those who receive sextant biopsies as part of the diagnostic process following an abnormal prostate cancer screening test, and in some cases, there may be difficulty in distinguishing this condition from invasive cancer of the prostate in such biopsy material. Often such detection is accidental, as PIN is not associated with elevation of prostate-specific antigen (PSA) levels [40]. Furthermore, no evidence has been reported that would suggest its detection in prostate cancer screening is of value in reducing the incidence of the disease.

Conclusions

Theoretically, screening that results in the detection of a cancer precursor is the ideal strategy for reducing cancer incidence, as it prevents the development of invasive cancer. However, as yet, only for cancer of the cervix is such a screening strategy established. There are reasons to hope that such a strategy may also be successful for colon and rectal cancer screening; currently, the evidence in favor of the effectiveness of this approach is not yet sufficiently strong, but randomized screening trials are in progress in an attempt to obtain such evidence. For all other cancers for which screening is currently contemplated, there is no evidence in favor of screening for precursors as a viable strategy. Part of the difficulty may be that some of the presumed precursors are not precursors at all, but simply markers of increased risk, as may be true for DCIS of the breast, for example. It is quite possible that the true invasive cancer precursors are largely not detectable with current screening methods.

It has been well demonstrated for cancer of the cervix that detection of precursors will result in the overtreatment of many individuals not destined to develop invasive cancer, and this also seems likely to be true for cancers of the colon and rectum. For breast cancer, the detection of DCIS in the CNBSS led to an excess of mastectomies in the mammography-containing arms compared to the controls [41]. This makes it essential that management for these conditions should be conservative, with opportunities provided for natural regression, if it is going to occur.

There is some hope that biological markers of progression of neoplasia could facilitate screening. Perhaps only for cancer of the cervix is this likely to become a reality in the short term, if the utility of HPV testing is confirmed [16]. However, even here, there is a danger of over treatment, as the large majority of women who develop HPV infection will have a self-limiting condition that does not become persistent and increase risk of progression to invasive cancer. Therefore, the same caveats as for the recognized precursors apply also to HPV testing. As yet, no other biological markers are used for screening, except for serum PSA for prostate cancer screening, and CA 125 for ovarian cancer screening. However in both instances, what is sought is early invasive cancer, not cancer precursors.

References

1. Cole P, Morrison AS. Basic issues in population screening for cancer. *J Natl Cancer Inst* 1980; 64:1263–72.

2. Miller AB. Cervix cancer. In: Kramer BS, Gohagan JK, Prorok PC (eds) *Cancer screening, theory and practice*. New York: Marcel Dekker, Inc; 1999; pp. 195–217.

3. Miller AB. Editorial: Failures of cervical cancer screening. *Am J Public Health* 1995; 85:761–2.

4. Riotton G, Christopherson WM. *Cytology of the female genital tract. International Histological Classification of Tumours*, No. 8. Geneva: World Health Organization, 1973.

5. Poulsen HE, Taylor CW. *Histological typing of female genital tract tumours. International Histological Classification of Tumours*, No. 13. Geneva: World Health Organization, 1975.

6. Richart RM. The patient with an abnormal Pap smear: screening techniques and management. *N Engl J Med* 1980; 302:332–4.

7. National Cancer Institute Workshop. The 1998 Bethesda System for reporting cervical/vaginal cytological diagnoses. *JAMA* 1989; 262:931–4.

8. Boyes DA, Morrison B, Knox EG, et al. A cohort study of cervical cancer screening in British Columbia. *Clin Invest Med* 1982; 5:1–29.

9. Miller AB, Knight J, Narod S. The natural history of cancer of the cervix, and the implications for screening policy. In: *Cancer screening*, Miller AB, Chamberlin J, Day NE, et al. (eds) Cambridge: Cambridge University Press, 1991, pp. 144–52.

10. Holowaty P, Miller AB, Rohan T, et al. The natural history of dysplasia of the uterine cervix. *J Natl Cancer Inst* 1999; 91:252–8.

11. Miller AB, Anderson G, Brisson J, et al. Report of a National Workshop on Screening for Cancer of the Cervix. *Can Med Assoc J* 1991; 145:1301–25.

12. IARC Working Group on Cervical Cancer Screening. Summary chapter. In: Hakama M, Miller AB, Day NE (eds) *Screening for cancer of the uterine cervix*, IARC Scientific Publications No. 76. Lyon: International Agency for Research on Cancer, 1986, pp. 133–42.

13. Miller AB. *Cervical cancer screening programmes. Managerial guidelines*. Geneva: World Health Organization, 1992.

14. van Oortmarssen GJ, Habbema JDF. Duration of preclinical cervical cancer and reduction in incidence of invasive cancer following negative Pap smears. *Int J Epidemiol* 1995; 24:300–7.

15. *IARC Monographs on the evaluation of carcinogenic risks to humans.* Vol. 64. *Human Papillomaviruses.* Lyon: International Agency for Research on Cancer, 1995.

16. Cuzick J, Beverley E, Ho L, et al. HPV testing in primary screening of older women. *Br J Cancer* 1999; 81:554–8.

17. Wright TC, Denny L, Kuhn L, et al. HPV DNA testing of self-collected vaginal samples compared with cytologic screening to detect cervical cancer. *JAMA* 2000; 283:81–6.

18. Schiffman M, Herrero R, Hildesheim A, et al. HPV DNA testing in cervical cancer screening. Results from women in a high risk province of Costa Rica. *JAMA* 2000; 283:87–93.

19. Wilson JMG, Junger G. *Principles and practice of screening for disease*, Public health paper (No. 34). Geneva: World Health Organization, 1968, p. 26.

20. Miller AB, Nazeer S, Fonn S, et al. Report on consensus conference on cervical cancer screening and management. *Int J Cancer* 2000; 86: 440–7.

21. Miller AB, Chamberlain J, Day NE, et al. Report on a workshop of the UICC Project on evaluation of screening for cancer. *Int J Cancer* 1990; 46:761–9.

22. Muto T, Bussy H, Morson B. The evolution of cancer of the colon and rectum. *Cancer* 1975; 36:2251–70.

23. Fearon E, Vogelstein B. A genetic model for colorectal tumorigenesis. *Cell* 1990; 61:759–67.

24. Mandel JS. Advances in screening for colorectal cancer. In: Miller AB (ed) *Advances in cancer screening*. Boston: Kluwer Academic Publishers, 1996, pp. 51–76.

25. Eide TJ. Natural history of adenomas. *World J Surg* 1990; 15:3–6.

26. Winawer SJ, O'Brien MJ, Waye JD, et al. Risk and surveillance of individuals with colorectal polyps. *Bull World Health Org* 1990; 68:789–95.

27. Gilbertsen VA, Nelms JM. The prevention of invasive cancer of the rectum. *Cancer* 1978; 41:1137–9.

28. Miller AB. Review of sigmoidoscopic screening for colorectal cancer. In: Chamberlain J, Miller AB (eds) *Screening for gastro-intestinal cancer*. Hans Huber: Toronto, 1988, pp. 3–7.

29. Winawer SJ, Zauber AG, Ho MN, et al. Prevention of colorectal cancer by colonoscopic polypectomy. *N Engl J Med* 1993; 329:1977–81.

30. Morrison AS. *Screening in chronic disease*, 2nd ed. New York: Oxford University Press, 1992, p. 112.

31. Gohagan JK, Prorok PC, Kramer BS, et al. The Prostate, Lung, Colorectal, and Ovarian cancer screening trial of the National Cancer Institute. *Cancer* 1995; 75:1869–73.

32. Atkin WS, Cuzick J, Northover JMA, et al. Prevention of colorectal cancer by once-only sigmoidoscopy. *Lancet* 1993; 341:736–40.

33. Moskowitz M, Pemmaraju S, Fidler JA, et al. On the diagnosis of minimal breast cancer in a screenee population. *Cancer* 1976; 37:2543–52.

34. Miller AB, To T, Baines CJ, et al. The Canadian National Breast Screening Study—2: Breast cancer detection and mortality in women age 50–59 on entry, the extended follow-up. *J Natl Cancer Inst* 2000; 92:1490–9.

35. Page DL, Dupont WD, Rogers LW, et al. Atypical hyperplastic lesions of the female breast. A long-term follow-up study. *Cancer* 1985; 55: 2698–708.

36. Page DL, Dupont WD, Rogers LW, et al. Intraductal carcinoma of the breast: follow-up after biopsy only. *Cancer* 1982; 49:751–8.

37. Miller AB, Borges AM. Intermediate histologic effect markers for breast cancer. In: Miller AB, Bartsch H, Boffetta P, et al. (eds) Biomarkers in chemoprevention of cancer. IARC Sci Pub No. 154. Lyon: International Agency for Research on Cancer, 2001, pp. 171–5.

38. Fisher ER, Fisher B. Relation of a recurrent intraductal carcinoma (ductal carcinoma *in situ*) to the primary tumor. *J Natl Cancer Inst* 2000; 92:288–9.

39. Fisher B, Costantino JP, Wickerman DL, et al. Tamoxifen for prevention of breast cancer. Report of the National Surgical Adjuvant Breast and Bowel Project P-1 study. *J Natl Cancer Inst* 1998; 90:1371–88.

40. van der Kwast TH. Intermediate biomarkers for chemoprevention of prostate cancer. In: Miller AB, Bartsch H, Boffetta P, et al. (eds) *Biomarkers in chemoprevention of cancer*. IARC Sci Pub No. 154. Lyon: International Agency for Research on Cancer, 2001, pp. 199–205.

41. Miller AB. May we agree to disagree, or how do we develop guidelines for breast cancer screening in women? *J Natl Cancer Inst* 1994; 86:1729–31.

23
Chemoprevention

Gary J. Kelloff and Caroline C. Sigman

Carcinogenesis Is the Target for Cancer Chemoprevention

Clinical cancer is the end of a chaotic process, termed carcinogenesis, which in humans often requires two to three decades. This process involves progressive disorganization observed at the molecular, cellular and tissue levels. The resulting clinical cancers are characterized by unregulated proliferation and cellular heterogeneity, and consequently very few are amenable to therapeutic intervention. During carcinogenesis, molecular targets become less available, normal cell function and structure are disrupted, and aneusomy increases. Rapid advances in genomics, molecular and cellular biology, and tissue pathology are providing the tools for identifying and evaluating significant events in carcinogenesis. Particularly, these research findings allow characterization of early stages of carcinogenesis when cell function is still sufficiently intact, and cells are sufficiently homogenous that precursor targets are available for preventive interventions.

Seminal work by Wattenberg and Sporn more than two decades ago started a new discipline in oncology, chemoprevention, which is the use of drugs, biologics, or nutrients to inhibit, delay, or reverse carcinogenesis. Chemoprevention can be applied at any time in the process before invasive disease [1–3]. Since that time, remarkable progress has been made in developing chemoprevention strategies, starting with research on mechanisms of chemopreventive drugs and assays for evaluating these drugs in animal models [e.g., 1–3], and spearheaded in the clinic by Hong's early studies on prevention of head and neck carcinogenesis [4,5].

Developing Feasible Chemopreventive Intervention Strategies Involves Cancer Precursors, Particularly Precancer (Intraepithelial Neoplasia)

More than 80% of human cancers are epithelial in origin, and in many target organs, such cancers are almost always preceded by a precursor lesion termed precancer or intraepithelial neoplasia (IEN). Molecular, cellular and tissue changes in precancers, leading to superficial tumors and finally to invasive disease, usually occur over many years. For example, the process may require 30 years or more in the breast [6,7] and 10 to 45 years in the colorectum [8,9] and prostate [10]. The prolonged time course of precancer provides multiple opportunities for chemoprevention—that is, opportunities for interventions when the mutations are fewer, even before tissue-level phenotypic changes are evident. However, the long latency also presents significant challenges for the clinical phase of chemopreventive drug development. Particularly challenging are the large numbers of subjects required for clinical studies, the long study durations, and the associated high costs of demonstrating clinical efficacy. We and others have described these challenges and proposed strategies to address them [e.g., 11–20].

The "gold standard" for chemoprevention trials has been primary prevention—that is, large multiyear randomized controlled cancer incidence and/or mortality reduction studies in subjects at relatively low risk (asymptomatic with normal or with somewhat elevated risk based on family history, the presence of genetic lesions such as polymorphisms in carcinogen activating or deactivating enzymes, or on the basis of lifestyle factors). Recently, the designs for such studies have focused on reducing the number of subjects required and on building in data monitoring to detect significant results at the earliest possible time points. An example is the completed successful trial of tamoxifen (20 mg/day) as a chemopreventive for estrogen receptor (ER)-positive breast cancer [21]. The study size was optimized by defining a minimum risk level (age of 60 years or more, age 35 to 59 years with a five-year predicted risk of 1.66%, or history of lobular carcinoma in situ). Nonetheless, 13,388 women were enrolled and treated for an average of 47.7 months, and the risk of invasive breast cancer was reduced from 4.34% in the placebo control group to 2.2% in the tamoxifen group (p < 0.00001). It is clear, even with efforts to minimize study size and duration, that such primary prevention designs are feasible and practical for only a few agents.

An alternative approach is evaluating agents for reducing cancer incidence in subjects with previous cancers or precancer. Numerous ongoing studies are evaluating the effects of treatment with potential chemopreventive agents on cancer incidence in subjects with previous cancers or IEN such as colorectal adenomas and prostatic intraepithelial neoplasia (PIN) [reviewed in 11,14–16]. These subjects are considered to be at high risk for developing cancers in tissue that is histologically related to tissue from which the original lesion arose. Slaughter et al. [22] coined the term "field cancerization" to describe the early evidence of carcinogenesis found in normal-appearing mucosa of patients with previous head and neck cancers. In fact, the lifetime risk for a second primary tumor of the aerodigestive tract following a squamous cell cancer of the head or neck has been estimated at 20 to 40% [23]. As Hong [16] has noted, chemopreventive treatment regimens can be matched to the subjects' degree of risk, so that patients with previous cancers with high rates of recurrence and/ or new primaries may be treated (in fact, may require treatment) with more aggressive, and potentially more toxic regimens than asymptomatic subjects. For example, Hong's vanguard randomized, placebo-controlled chemoprevention trial in 103 head and neck cancer patients [5] demonstrated a significant decrease in second primary tumors after high-dose adjuvant 13-cis-retinoic acid (ca. 4.1–8.2 μmol/ kg-bw/day) for one year. Second primaries were seen in 24% (12 patients) of the placebo group, but in only 4% of the treatment group. This approach has clear advantages over primary prevention studies in requiring far fewer subjects and shorter time frames for detecting clinically significant outcomes. The promising results of this study benefitted the patients studied and provided a rationale for longer-term administration to less ill cohorts. Often the drug dose will have to be reduced in the less ill cohorts because of toxicity, but this incremental approach provides the opportunity to evaluate chemopreventive activity at early stages of carcinogenesis when efficacy may be seen at the lower drug doses.

Cancer Prevention and Other Clinical Benefit of Treating Precancers

A third model that provides rational and efficient paths for developing chemopreventive agents, and more importantly, potentially huge public health benefits, is treatment directed specifically to preventing or eradicating precancer (Table 23.1). For developing cancer chemopreventive drugs, a primary quality of IEN is their potential as surrogate endpoints for cancer incidence. However, treatment of

TABLE 23.1. Incidence and multiyear time course for progression of precancers in selected cancer targets.[1]

Target organ	Precancer (IEN)	Estimated incidence/prevalence	Years for precancer formation	Years for progression from precancer to cancer
Prostate	PIN	40% to 50% of men ages 40 to 60 years	20	≥10 to latent cancer; 3–15 additional years to cancer
Breast	DCIS	46,000 new cases in US women in 2000	14–18 from atypical hyperplasia	6–10
Colon	Adenoma	30% to 40% of the Western population ages ≥60 years	5–20	5–15
Bladder	Ta, T1, TIS	37,500 cases in US for 1997	20	<5
Esophagus	Barrett's metaplasia	0.4% of the Western population	5–20	5–20 to severe dysplasia; 3–4 additional years to cancer

[1] *Abbreviations*: DCIS, ductal carcinoma *in situ*; IEN, Intraepithelial neoplasia; PIN, prostatic intraepithelial neoplasia; TIS, transitional cell carcinoma-*in-situ*.
Source: Adapted from Kelloff et al. [24].

IEN may also provide direct clinical benefits (in addition to the potential for cancer prevention). These benefits include reduced morbidity, enhanced quality of life, delayed surgery, and increased intervals for surveillance requiring invasive procedures.

Subjects at high cancer risk associated with genetic predisposition form one set of cohorts that may derive direct clinical benefit from prevention of precancers. For example, colorectal adenomas are IEN that are well-documented precursors of colorectal cancer [8,9]. Familial adenomatous polyposis (FAP) is characterized by germline mutations in the adenomatous polyposis coli (APC) tumor suppressor gene. Usually starting when they are teenagers, patients with FAP develop hundreds of colorectal adenomatous polyps. If untreated, FAP subjects will almost certainly develop colorectal cancer by age 50 [25]; they are also at risk for developing other lesions, particularly duodenal polyps and cancers. Once adenomas begin to appear, these patients are monitored by periodic colonoscopy (at approximately six-month intervals), removal of existing polyps, and cancer screening. When the polyp burden becomes unmanageable, most patients have partial or total colectomies. Thereafter, they continue to be monitored. Agents which prevent or slow the progression of the adenomas could benefit these subjects by delaying the need for colectomy and increasing the intervals between surveillance colonoscopies and cancer screenings. In fact, a recent study, conducted

as part of a chemoprevention development program for the selective cyclooxygenase-2 inhibitor, celecoxib [26], led to accelerated Food and Drug Administration (FDA) marketing approval of celecoxib as an adjunct to standard care for the regression and reduction of adenomatous polyps in FAP.

Another example is preventing precancers with high rates of recurrence. New adenomas occur within 1 to 3 years post-resection in approximately 30% of patients with sporadic colorectal adenomas or cancers [27]. These patients are screened routinely at 1 to 5 year intervals, receiving colonoscopies with removal of new lesions. Preventive treatment could potentially provide benefit by reducing the new polyp burden, thereby decreasing surgical intervention with its associated morbidity, increasing the screening interval, and lowering healthcare costs.

Treating IEN for which organ removal or other major surgery with high morbidity is the standard of care is a third example of direct clinical benefit from treating precancer. Current treatment for Barrett's esophagus, a precursor of esophageal cancer, may involve partial or total esophagectomy [28]. Because of the high rate of their recurrence and potential for progression, treatment of superficial bladder cancers includes periodic surveillance (every three months) and removal of new lesions, and may include cystectomy [29]. In both diseases, surgical treatment has profound detrimental effects on quality of life. Both are examples of situations in which preventive agents could provide clinical benefit by reducing the need for these surgeries.

Strategies for Using Precancers in Evaluating Chemopreventive Drugs

The development of chemopreventive drugs using precancers as surrogate endpoints is now quite feasible. This promising and challenging effort requires criteria for defining endpoints and selecting chemopreventive drugs, quantitative methods for measuring effects, criteria for establishing efficacy, and innovative clinical trial designs. We have also discussed these subjects in previous publications that may be of interest to the reader [13–15,18,20,30].

Two factors are especially important in developing these strategies. First, the number of precancers far exceeds the number of cancers that subsequently develop in the target tissue, and behavioral (e.g., smoking history), environmental (e.g., hormonal status), and coexisting disease (e.g., immune system competence) factors may influence progression in individual subjects. Therefore, strategies using precancers as surrogate endpoints should include methods for ensuring that the chemopreventive treatment is effective against those precancers that are likely to progress. Second, chemopreventive agents are required to have minimal toxicity because of their long-term, even lifetime, administration to relatively healthy people. Short-term studies with precancers may not provide sufficient safety data to support such use. Development strategies should include specific plans for long-term postmarketing follow-up of successful agents.

Early Associated Biomarkers Used in Conjunction with Precancers

As stated above, IEN such as colorectal adenomas, PIN, and cervical intraepithelial neoplasia (CIN) embody the abnormal cancer phenotype, and as such, are currently the most promising surrogate endpoints for clinical chemoprevention studies in epithelial tissues [19,30,31]. Although shorter than the period for developing cancer, the latency for IEN progression can also be lengthy compared with the practical time frame for a chemopreventive intervention study. The use of early biomarkers to characterize the stage of IEN progression may allow shorter study durations and also help address the problem of identifying IEN most likely to progress.

Many such carcinogenesis biomarkers of cellular and molecular events are possibilities. For example, cellular biomarkers such as nuclear and nucleolar morphology, mitotic index, and DNA ploidy are being evaluated in ongoing studies [14,20]. Possibly useful genotypic biomarkers include loss of heterozygosity (LOH) and gene amplification, either at specific gene loci (e.g., those for tumor suppressors such as *p53* or tumor growth accelerators such as *c-erbB2*) or at panels of microsatellite loci where mutations indicate increasing genomic instability [20,32]. Both phenotypic and genotypic changes may also be manifested by molecular biomarkers [20,30]. For example, excess proliferation might be associated with increased levels of cellular antigens such as proliferating cell nuclear antigen (PCNA) or Ki-67/MIB-1 or overexpression of growth factors such as epidermal growth factor (EGF), transforming growth factor (TGF)α, and insulin-like growth factor (IGF)-I; reduced propensity to undergo apoptosis may be detected by increased expression of *bcl-2*. Aberrant differentiation may result in changes in G-actin, cytokeratins, and blood-group antigens. Other molecular biomarkers may reflect general changes in cell growth control. These include TGF-β, cyclins, p53 and other tumor suppressors, as well as mutations and overexpression of oncogenes associated with carcinogenesis such as *ras* and the transcription factors *myc*, *fos* and *jun*. Tissue- and drug-related biomarkers may also be useful. Examples of tissue-related biomarkers are the expression of estrogen receptors in breast and prostate specific antigen (PSA) in prostate. Drug-related biomarkers associated with chemopreventive

activity include inhibition of ornithine decarboxylase (ODC) by difluoromethylornithine (DFMO) [30], upregulation of the
retinoid receptor RARβ by 13-*cis*-retinoic
acid [33], and inhibition of prostaglandin bio-
synthesis by nonsteroidal antiinflammatory
drugs [30].

Criteria for Precancers and Early Associated Biomarkers as Surrogate Endpoints in Clinical Chemoprevention Studies

Surrogate endpoints for cancer should be
selected within the context of carcinogenesis at
the target site. The assurance that the chemopreventive agent can modulate the IEN and/or
other biomarker(s) chosen as surrogate endpoints is clearly critical. For example, the
regression of CIN II has been demonstrated
with all-*trans*-retinoic acid [34]. Celecoxib [26]
and sulindac [35] have been shown to regress
colorectal adenomas. Hyperproliferation [25]
and apoptosis [36,37] are examples of the
earlier biomarkers listed that have been modulated in colorectal adenomas. While they will
more often be risk biomarkers, genetic lesions
or their encoded products can be modulated in
certain circumstances. For example, mutations
resulting in *ras* oncogene overexpression could
be overcome by inhibiting farnesyl protein
transferase. Ras farnesylation is required for
activation of the oncogene [38].

As noted above, the surrogate endpoint
should have short latency compared with
cancer incidence—ideally, months or a few
years and not the many years and decades
required for cancers to develop. For early Phase
II exploratory trials, short-latency biomarkers
may provide useful information regardless of
the temporal and pathological closeness to
cancer. For example, 2 to 8 week chemopreventive interventions in patients scheduled for
definitive surgical treatment of IEN or early
cancers in breast and prostate may explore

primarily changes in cell proliferation kinetics
rather than actual progression of ductal
carcinoma-*in-situ* (DCIS) or PIN to cancer,
and may be used to establish dose–response to
the agent [14,19].

Clinical study cohorts should be matched to
the chemopreventive agent being evaluated.
The agent ideally should be investigated first in
subjects whose disease or risk of disease can
be modified by the presumed mechanism of
the agent within relatively short studies (most
Phase II and early Phase III chemoprevention
studies now in progress have durations of one
month to three years). The chemopreventive
agent's effects should also be easily measured
in the subject population. Tissues that are more
accessible and that can be monitored without
biopsy or can be fully visualized (e.g., colon,
skin, cervix) may provide better sites for definitive efficacy trials than less accessible tissues
(e.g., prostate, ovary). This is not to say that
chemopreventive agents will not be effective in
more difficult settings, but that initial demonstration of chemopreventive activity may be
best carried out where fewer obstacles to measurement exist. It is important that chemoprevention trials work within the constraints of
standard treatment, so that subjects' safety is
not compromised. For example, in trials in subjects with small colon adenomas (<1 cm diameter), this may result in frequent monitoring
and removal of any adenomas larger than 1 cm
diameter.

Considerations in validation of IEN and
early associated biomarkers as surrogate endpoints are that the biomarkers are expressed
differentially in normal and high-risk tissue,
and that a temporal progression can be shown
from normal tissue to IEN to cancer. The
sensitivity and specificity of the biomarkers
as measures of cancer are also important.
They should appear with high frequency in
precancers or high-risk tissue. They should
be specific for cancer in that their response
to other diseases or to conditions such
as normal growth or wound healing should
not be as extensive or should follow a
different pattern from that observed during
carcinogenesis.

Correlation of Genotype to Phenotype to Validate Precancers as Surrogates for Cancer

Carcinogenesis progression has been mapped in target tissues by the appearance of specific molecular and more general genotypic damage associated with increasingly severe dysplastic phenotypes [e.g., 32,38–48], the seminal work being that of Fearon and Vogelstein in the colon [38, see also 48]. Examples of genetic progression models that have been developed include those for colon [38,48], brain [39], bladder [40–44], head and neck [32], lung [45,46], and cervix [47]. Measures of these genotypic changes used in conjunction with IEN histopathology currently have the highest potential as surrogate endpoints [19,20,31].

Phenotypic and Genotypic Surrogate Endpoints to Establish Chemopreventive Efficacy

To establish chemopreventive efficacy, we expect that it will be critical to ensure that most of the precancers are prevented, or that the lesions prevented are those with potential to progress. The fraction of IEN that will progress have particular characteristics predisposing them to develop into cancers. These characteristics may be manifested in tissue histopathology. For example, the potential of colorectal adenomas to progress to cancer correlates to histological growth pattern, size, and severity of dysplasia [26,49,50]. However, since the histopathological changes are preceded or accompanied by progressive genetic damage, drug-induced prevention or regression of IEN determined by histopathology may not always be sufficient to determine chemopreventive efficacy. The evaluation should usually also consider the specific and general genotypic effects comprising the progression models for carcinogenesis as well as molecular pathology. Determining that a reduced incidence of new

precancers is due to chemoprevention could require that the genotype of the target tissue in agent-treated subjects, especially in any new precancers, is equivalent to or shows less genetic progression than that of placebo-treated subjects [20]. Similarly, in studies with regression of existing precancers as the endpoint, where regression is incomplete, the remaining lesions in the agent-treated subjects should probably have genotypes equivalent to or showing less progression than placebo control subjects. Otherwise, chemopreventive efficacy established solely on the basis of phenotypic regression would in most cases require near complete regression of existing lesions. Similarly, phenotypic chemoprevention could in most cases only be demonstrated rigorously by near complete inhibition of new lesions. With less than this level of efficacy, it is possible that the remaining lesions are those that will continue to progress to cancer. However, if the posttreatment genotype showed decreased incidence of cancer-related changes (either in specific genes or in more general measures of genomic instability) compared with baseline, significantly less than near complete regression could be considered prevention. Also, less than complete inhibition of phenotypic progression could establish chemopreventive efficacy, if most of the lesions in the active intervention group exhibited a genotype with cancer-related changes that had not progressed beyond those of the baseline lesions or placebo controls. This outcome would be further supported if the genotype of normal-appearing tissue in the target was also stable or showed reduced cancer-related changes compared with baseline or placebo controls.

Cohorts for Clinical Chemoprevention Studies with Precancers

One criterion used for selecting these cohorts is expectation of a high incidence of the precancer, or observable progression of the precancer under study within a reasonable time period. Patients with superficial bladder cancer are appropriate subjects for chemoprevention studies because their high incidence of precancer results in a cancer recurrence rate of approximately 50% within 6 to 12 months [51] and 60% to 75% within 2 to 5 years [52,53]. Similar high rates of recurrence or new lesions apply to colorectal adenomas [54]. Studies in these settings would appear to be particularly promising for the validation of surrogate endpoints, which may then be suitable for application in cohorts without previous precancers.

Germline mutations and other genetic and molecular evidence of susceptibility may also be used to define high-risk cohorts. For example, subjects with FAP [55] and the recent successful study with celecoxib in this cohort [26] were cited earlier. Fabian has described high-risk breast cancer subjects suitable for chemoprevention studies based on the presence of early biomarkers of carcinogenesis, including atypical hyperplasia, aneuploidy, and overexpression of p53 and EGF receptor (EGFR), as well as the potential use of these biomarkers as surrogate endpoints for breast-cancer prevention trials [56].

As described earlier, patients scheduled for surgical treatment of precancer or early cancer provide cohorts for obtaining early evidence of efficacy. Agents are administered to these patients during the several week time period after diagnostic biopsy and before more definitive surgery, so that modulation of biomarkers in the precancer/cancerous, and, if possible, normal-appearing tissue in the target organ can be assessed [14,19].

Methods for Evaluating Precancers

To date, more than 50 clinical chemoprevention studies with IEN and early associated biomarkers as endpoints have been reported to be completed or in progress [11,14,19]. Although many are early developmental and validation studies that have not been undertaken to support chemoprevention indications, most are randomized, double-blinded and placebo-

controlled. Usually, the primary endpoint is histological modulation of the precancer. This modulation may be evaluated by both classical pathological techniques and quantitatively by morphometry and cytophotometry using computer-assisted image analysis (CAIA).

As suggested by the discussion above, high priority is also given to early biomarkers measuring genotypic changes correlating to the carcinogenesis progression model for the targeted cancer. Westra and Sidransky [57] and Mao et al. [58] found that the phenotype of the whole tissue does not always reflect underlying genotypic changes that will contribute to new lesions, thus underscoring the need to evaluate genotypic changes in normal-appearing epithelia surrounding precancers. Progressive genomic instability, as measured by LOH or amplification at specific microsatellite loci, was used by Sidransky and colleagues [32] to characterize head and neck carcinogenesis. These biomarkers are potential surrogate endpoints in the head and neck, and may also prove useful in other tissues where microsatellite instability is a predominant feature of carcinogenesis—for example, in hereditary nonpolyposis colorectal cancer (HNPCC)-associated cancers and some sporadic colorectal cancers. For all the biomarkers, it is highly desirable to measure modulation quantitatively as the difference (Δ) between the biomarker value at the end of treatment and baseline, and so baseline biopsies or other tissue measurements are important. However, biopsies may induce changes in tissue, such as increased rates of proliferation, that are associated with tissue healing and repair. These effects may confound biomarker results, particularly in very short-term studies. Thus, samples from subjects treated with chemopreventive agents should be compared with those from placebo-treated or untreated control subjects for more accurate estimates of chemopreventive activity.

New technology such as computer-assisted pathology, high-volume gene-chip-based assays, and improved diagnostic tools such as the confocal microscope, the lung-imaging fluorescence endoscope for visualizing bronchial tissue, and the magnifying endoscope for colorectal monitoring will be critical to assuring the adequate development of surrogate endpoints for chemoprevention studies.

Quantitative evaluation is important, since it is very likely that qualitative measures will be too crude and lack the reproducibility to detect carcinogenesis-associated changes. Endpoints measured by CAIA, including both nuclear and nucleolar morphometry and cytophotometry, should prove valuable in this regard. Adequate performance ensures that a small trial with limited tissue availability will produce meaningful results. Quantitative nuclear and nucleolar morphometric changes may be used to describe the histopathology that characterizes progression of precancers. Their promise is based on gradient changes associated with increasing IEN severity. Several computer-assisted imaging systems are commercially available. These systems essentially consist of a light microscope, a light sensor, a digitizer to convert the light to computer-readable form, and a computer with appropriate software to analyze the tissue measurements. Examples of these measurements are nuclear size, shape, texture, and pleomorphism, and nucleolar number, size, shape, position, and pleomorphism. CAIA is also useful for cytometry including measurements of cellular proliferation and DNA ploidy that typify IEN histopathology.

The supporting technology as well as the data generated from the Human Genome Project and the Cancer Gene Anatomy Program have provided the means to look quantitatively at general genetic damage as well as specific genetic changes at the molecular level. Much of the work in this area has involved gene sequence comparisons. For example, the measurement of microsatellite instability (MI), using reverse transcription polymerase chain reaction (RT-PCR) at pre-defined markers, has been described above for detection of gene expression changes at loci relevant to carcinogenesis. MI is evidenced by amplification or LOH at these loci. However, although quantitative, this technique looks only at DNA sequences and not at specific gene functions. Comparative gene hybridization (CGH) is being used to approach the evaluation of functional changes. In this technique, gene chips with specific gene sequences (cDNA) and mutations are made (e.g., wild-type and well-characterized mutations in *p53*). Corresponding changes in genes in tissue undergoing carcinogenesis can be evaluated by hybridizing the tissue DNA to the specialized chips. Many different commercial gene chip packages are now made. More importantly, the capability for making individualized gene chips with specific genes is now available. Besides evaluating changes in tissues undergoing carcinogenesis, these chips may be designed to evaluate subjects at risk, for example, those carrying specific germline mutations and genetic polymorphisms.

Fluorescent *in situ* hybridization (FISH) and particularly chromosome *in situ* hybridization (CISH) are also powerful techniques to quantify potential functional changes in carcinogenesis-related genes. Both techniques involve labeling specific gene products related to carcinogenesis. FISH applies a fluorescent label to a gene product of interest. CISH applies different labels (different colors) to wild and mutant gene products, allowing the comparison of different relative amounts at different stages of carcinogenesis and before and after treatment with chemopreventive agents [59].

Brown and Botstein [60] reviewed the potential of functional genomics in biology—the utility ranging from analyzing a mutant phenotype to subcellular localization of gene products (i.e., relative expression in specific tissues), to uncovering patterns of expression along signal transduction pathways. Genomic chip arrays, now being produced for analysis of genetic information on specific target organs, number in some cases in the thousands of genes, and the volume of data being produced will require very sophisticated data analysis to define and quantify contributors to risk. To this end, proven cases from archival specimens from properly designed tissue banks will help provide the endpoints and validation needed. Further, the use of specimens from preclinical and clinical chemoprevention interventions in which known effective drugs are compared to placebo controls, may provide insights as to which single moieties or patterns in this pleiotropic process are the most important.

In this regard the results of quantitative morphometric analysis in the breast, correlating morphometric changes to dysplasia severity, have been presented recently [61,62].

Precancer Sampling Issues

Although rapid advances in genomics and proteomics are leading to improvements in the specificity and sensitivity with which moieties present in the serum from microscopic disease are detected, IEN is currently measured primarily through biopsies, with advances in *in vivo* imaging modalities providing promise for less invasive detection. The challenge for detection by these technologies differs among key human cancer target organs. Access by direct visualization of colon, upper aerodigestive/head and neck/lung, bladder, cervix/endometrium, and skin provides advantage over less accessible targets such as breast, prostate, pancreas, ovary and liver. In some cases in which the tissue can be directly visualized, the amount of abnormal tissue can be quantified; therefore, the extent of modulation by chemopreventive drugs can also be quantified. In tissues that cannot be directly visualized, these measurements are more qualitative since they are limited by the accuracy of the tissue sampling methods used.

Detection of PIN is an example of sampling issues that must be addressed in chemoprevention studies using surrogate endpoints in tissues difficult to visualize [63]. In men of 50 years or older, high-grade PIN (HGPIN) prevalence is 50%. However, of all sextant prostate biopsies taken in this subpopulation for any reason, when no cancer is present, only 5% HGPIN incidence is detected. In the general population, less than 1% HGPIN incidence is detected in sextant prostate biopsies. These discrepancies, most probably due to inability to ensure adequate tissue sampling in the prostate, call for standardized measurement methods. The number and location of samples from invasive cancer, IEN, and adjacent tissue that appears normal, as well as the thickness/number of histologic sections processed and scored, are important parameters that affect variability,

accuracy, and reproducibility in all tissues. In prostate and other tissues, current approaches for refining the measurement of prevalence and extent of IEN involve calculating the area and volume of IEN and digital imaging of the tissue.

Validation of Precancers Using Animal Models

The evaluation of surrogate endpoints benefits from targeted research using animal models which mimic specific characteristics of human carcinogenesis. Particularly, the correlation of surrogate endpoint modulation with effects on cancer incidence and cancer-related mortality in such models can provide strong evidence validating the surrogate endpoint. This correlation can strengthen efficacy claims prior to definitive clinical validation. Transgenic and knock-out mice, which carry well-characterized genetic lesions predisposing to carcinogenesis, are proving to be good models for biomarker evaluation. An example is the inhibition of colorectal adenomas in the *Min* mouse, which carries an APC gene lesion [64,65]. Also, a human papilloma virus (HPV)-infected (K14-HPV16 heterozygote), estradiol-treated mouse develops cervical squamous carcinomas that result from progression of CIN-like lesions [66]. These lesions can be inhibited by the antiproliferative and potential chemopreventive agent, DFMO. A key contribution to future development of such animal models will be identification of specific cancer-related genes (e.g., in the Cancer Genome Anatomy Project) which can be applied to the construction of animal models for evaluating chemopreventive efficacy.

Extensive biomarker research and development is also being carried out in carcinogen-induced animals, as well as in carcinogen-induced transgenic mice. For example, CAIA morphometric measures have been used to follow skin carcinogenesis in benzo(*a*)pyrene (B(*a*)P)-induced SENCAR mice and esophageal cancer in nitrosamine-induced rats; the chemopreventive agents DFMO and phenethylisothiocyanate, respectively, inhibit early lesions as well as cancers in these models [67].

Besides gene chip technologies, new cell and organ culture technologies and newer information on genetic susceptibility to cancer may be used to evaluate chemopreventive agents and targets. The primary objective is to develop models that closely mimic human carcinogenesis. For example, raft cultures, which allow evaluation of stromal–epithelial interactions, cells from transgenic mice, and cells from subjects carrying known cancer-predisposing genes (e.g., Li-Fraumeni syndrome, APC mutations) are being explored. Currently, adequate animal models do not exist for evaluating chemopreventive efficacy in some major cancer sites—for example, lung (squamous cell carcinomas), prostate, ovary, brain, pancreas and ER–breast cancer. An important area of research in the near term will be development of animal models (transgenics or carcinogen-induced) for these cancers.

It may be possible to more closely approximate human carcinogenesis by manipulating two or more carcinogenesis-associated genes, including modifier genes, in a single animal. For example, it might be feasible to knock out *p53* in an animal that already carries another tumor suppressor defect (e.g., *Apc* or *p16*). Studies are now being done on *Min* and *Apc* 1638 mice also carrying genes allowing error-prone DNA repair [68].

The treatment of transgenic and gene knock-out mice with carcinogens may prove to be particularly effective as a strategy for modeling human carcinogenesis at specific cancer targets. For example, the chemopreventive effects of various agents are being evaluated in *p53* mutant and gene knock-out mice also treated with carcinogens (e.g., B(*a*)P or *N*-nitrosonornicotine (NNK) to induce lung tumors, or dimethylhydrazine to induce colon tumors) [69].

Future for Using Precancers in the Development of Chemopreventive Drugs

This chapter has focused on what we believe are critical scientific and practical aspects of using precancers and early associated biomarkers as surrogate endpoints to characterize cancer chemopreventive efficacy (Table 2. Hopefully, this material will serve as a b for designing effective clinical developme strategies for chemopreventive drugs. As we'v discussed here and previously, the multipath multifocal nature of carcinogenesis, as well as the very small percentage of early lesions that progress to cancers and the long time required for cancers to develop, suggest that, initially, the most successful strategies will use well-defined precancers as the surrogate endpoints for cancer incidence. Despite their close temporal and histologic association with cancers, only a relatively small percentage of IEN will progress. Therefore, determination of chemopreventive efficacy will rely on assurance that the lesions most likely to progress are inhibited (e.g., the genotype of any posttreatment lesions should be equivalent to or indicative of less progression than baseline lesions). The phenotypic changes seen in IEN during short-term studies are likely to be subtle; therefore, quantitative measurements such as CAIA are desirable; similarly, the evaluation of genotypic changes requires sensitive, quantitative analysis of gene expression such as that afforded by the various DNA microarray techniques. Standardization is critical, including determination of adequate sampling, handling of nonrelated biopsy effects, and appropriate timing of biomarker assessment relative to normal biological cycles (e.g., timing for measurement of breast cell proliferation during the menstrual cycle). The gold standard for validating surrogate endpoints is comparison with cancer incidence reduction. The resources (e.g., time and number of subjects) required to successfully complete such validation are enormous, and we believe that alternative strategies are needed to ensure that surrogate endpoint-based chemoprevention indications are feasible. One possible strategy is to demonstrate clinical benefit in the prevention or treatment of IEN (as described above for FAP, sporadic colorectal adenomas, superficial bladder cancers, and Barrett's esophagus). A second approach would be to follow the pathway for gaining accelerated marketing approval as defined by the FDA. This mechanism allows early marketing approval based on surrogate endpoints

TABLE 23.2. Potential precancer surrogate endpoints at major cancer target sites.[1]

Target/cohort(s)	IEN endpoint	Histological/ genotypic endpoint(s)	Other potential endpoints
Prostate Patients with PIN Presurgical early prostate cancer patients	PIN regression/ prevention	*Histopathology* Nuclear morphometry (nuclear texture and shape (roundness)), nucleolar morphometry (size and number of nucleoli), DNA ploidy *Genotype* Chromosome 8p LOH and 8q amplification, Fourier transform-infrared spectroscopy of DNA structure	Proliferation (MIB-1 and proliferating cell nuclear antigen (PCNA)) Apoptosis (number of apoptotic bodies, transglutaminase, *bcl*-2) Differentiation (Lewis[Y] antigen, kallikrein hK2 expression, androgen receptor expression) Cell regulatory molecules (c-*erb*B-2, TGF-β, p53) Invasion/metastasis (angiogenesis, PSA)
Breast Atypical hyperplasia, previously treated LCIS, DCIS or minimally invasive breast cancers Atypical hyperplasia/ epithelial hyperplasia and one or more biomarker abnormalities Presurgical mammo-graphically-detected DCIS and minimally invasive cancers	Hyperplasia/DCIS prevention/ regression	*Histopathology* Mammographic density Nuclear morphometry, DNA ploidy	Proliferation (MIB-1, PCNA) Apoptosis (*bcl*-2) Differentiation (sialyl Tn-antigen) Cell regulatory molecules (EGFR/c-*erb*B-2, estrogen receptor, IGF-1, p53)
Colon FAP HNPCC Previous colorectal cancers, previous/ current colorectal adenomas	Colorectal adenomas prevention/ regression	*Histopathology* Nuclear morphometry (nuclear texture and shape), nucleolar morphometry (size and number of nucleoli), DNA ploidy *Genotype* Chromosome 5, 17, 18 LOH and *ras* mutations, microsatellite instability, DNA methylation pattern	Proliferation (expansion of the proliferative compartment in colon crypts measured, for example, by BrdU uptake, S-phase fraction, PCNA, MIB-1, ratio of proliferation to apoptosis) Apoptosis (apoptotic bodies by confocal laser microscopy, TUNEL assay) Differentiation (Lewis[x], Lewis[y], T, Tn, and sialyl Tn antigens, apomucins) Cell regulatory molecules (p53)
Lung Chronic smokers with proven bronchial dysplasia	Bronchial dysplasia regression	*Histopathology* Nuclear morphometry (pleomorphism), DNA ploidy *Genotype* Chromosome LOH at 3p21, 3p24-25, 5q and 9p and in *FRA3B/FHIT* gene, mutagen sensitivity	Proliferation (PCNA) Apoptosis (*bcl*-2) Cell regulatory molecules (telomerase, EGFR, p53)

TABLE 23.2. *Continued*

Target/cohort(s)	IEN endpoint	Histological/ genotypic endpoint(s)	Other potential endpoints
Bladder Ta, T1 superficial bladder cancer Ta, T1 ± TIS superficial bladder cancer treated with BCG	Superficial bladder cancer prevention	*Histopathology* DNA ploidy *Genotype* Chromosome LOH in urine	Proliferation (PCNA, M344) Differentiation (G-actin [92,93]) Cell regulatory molecules (EGFR)
Head and Neck Previous head and neck cancers Dysplastic oral leukoplakia	Dysplasia prevention/ regression	*Histopathology* DNA ploidy *Genotype* Chromosome LOH	Proliferation (PCNA, MIB-1) Cell regulatory molecules (EGFR, c-erbB-2, RARβ, TGF-α, TGF-β)
Cervix CIN II/III	CIN regression	*Histopathology* Nuclear morphometry (pleomorphism, DNA content), DNA ploidy *Genotype* Chromosomal LOH	Proliferation (PCNA [94]) Differentiation (keratins) Cell regulatory molecules (EGFR, Ras expression/mutation)
Esophagus Barrett's esophagus	Barrett's dysplasia prevention/ regression	*Histopathology* Nuclear morphometry (pleomorphism, DNA content), nucleolar morphometry (size and number of nucleoli), DNA ploidy	Proliferation (PCNA, MIB-1) Apoptosis Cell regulatory molecules (EGFR, p53)
Skin Actinic keratosis Previous nonmelanoma skin cancer	Actinic keratosis prevention/ regression	*Genotype* p53	Proliferation (PCNA, ODC activity) Cell regulatory molecules (EGFR, TGFβ, p53)

[1] *Abbreviations*: BCG, *Bacillus Calmette-Guerin*; BrdU, bromodeoxyuridine; CIN, cervical intraepithelial neoplasia; DCIS, ductal carcinoma-*in-situ*; EGFR, epidermal growth factor receptor; FAP, familial adenomatous polyposis; *FHIT*, fragile histidine triad (gene); FISH, fluorescent *in situ* hybridization; *FRA3B*, fragile region A3B (gene); HNPCC, hereditary non-polyposis colorectal cancer; HPV, human papilloma virus; IGF, insulin-like growth factor; LCIS, lobular cell carcinoma-*in-situ*; LOH, loss of heterozygosity; ODC, ornithine decarboxylase; PCNA, proliferating cell nuclear antigen; PIN, prostatic intraepithelial neoplasia; PSA, prostate specific antigen; RAR, retinoic acid receptor; TGF, transforming growth factor; TIS, transitional cell carcinoma *in situ*; TUNEL, terminal deoxynucleotidyl transferase-mediated dUTP-biotin nick end labeling.
Source: Adapted from Kelloff et al. [20].

for disease incidence in the setting of a life-threatening disease such as cancer with strong scientific-support. As has been recently demonstrated by the approval of celecoxib for treatment of colorectal polyps in FAP patients within the context of standard-of-care, successful strategies for cancer prevention will be a combination of the two approaches. Accelerated approval may be obtained on the basis of short clinical studies suggesting clinical benefit in treatment of precancers in high-risk cohorts, with follow-up studies required to confirm this activity for precancer treatment or prevention in larger cohorts in longer-term studies and, ultimately, for prevention or reduction of cancer risk.

References

1. Sporn MB. Approaches to prevention of epithelial cancer during the preneoplastic period. *Cancer Res* 1976; 36:2699–702.

2. Wattenberg LW. Inhibition of chemical carcinogenesis. *J Natl Cancer Inst* 1975; 60:11–18.

3. Wattenberg LW. Chemoprevention of cancer. *Cancer Res* 1985; 45:1–8.

4. Hong WK, Endicott J, Itri LM, et al. 13-*cis*-retinoic acid in the treatment of oral leukoplakia. *N Engl J Med* 1986; 315:1501–5.

5. Hong WK, Lippman SM, Itri LM, et al. Prevention of second primary tumors with isotretinoin in squamous-cell carcinoma of the head and neck. *N Engl J Med* 1990; 323:795–801.

6. Frykberg ER, Bland KI. In situ breast carcinoma. *Adv Surg* 1993; 26:29–72.

7. Page DL, Dupont WD, Rogers LW, et al. Atypical hyperplastic lesions of the female breast. A long-term follow-up study. *Cancer* 1985; 55: 2698–708.

8. Bruzzi P, Bonelli L, Costantini M, et al. A multicenter study of colorectal adenomas—rationale, objectives, methods and characteristics of the study cohort. *Tumori* 1995; 81:157–63.

9. Day DW, Morson BC. The adenoma-carcinoma sequence. In: Bennington JL (ed.) *The pathogenesis of colorectal cancer.* Philadelphia: WB Saunders Co., 1978, pp. 58–71.

10. Bostwick DG. Prostatic intraepithelial neoplasia (PIN): current concepts. *J Cell Biochem* 1992; 16 (Suppl H):10–19.

11. Kelloff GJ, Boone CW, Steele VE, et al. Progress in cancer chemoprevention: perspectives on agent selection and short-term clinical intervention trials. *Cancer Res* 1994; 54 (Suppl):2015–24.

12. Lippman SM, Benner SE, Hong WK. Cancer chemoprevention. *J Clin Oncol* 1994; 12:851–83.

13. Kelloff GJ, Johnson JR, Crowell JA, et al. Approaches to the development and marketing approval of drugs that prevent cancer. *Cancer Epidemiol Biomarkers Prev* 1995; 4:1–10.

14. Kelloff GJ, Hawk ET, Crowell JA, et al. Strategies for identification and clinical evaluation of promising chemopreventive agents. *Oncology* (*Huntington*) 1996; 10:1471–80, 1484.

15. Kelloff GJ, Hawk ET, Karp JE, et al. Progress in clinical chemoprevention. *Semin Oncol* 1997; 24:1–13.

16. Hong WK, Sporn MB. Recent advances in chemoprevention of cancer. *Science* 1997; 278: 1073–7.

17. Lippman SM, Lee JJ, Sabichi AL. Cancer chemoprevention: progress and promise. *J Natl Cancer Inst* 1998; 90:1514–28.

18. Sporn MB, Suh N. Chemoprevention of cancer. *Carcinogenesis* 2000; 21:525–30.

19. Kelloff GJ. Perspectives on cancer chemoprevention research and drug development. *Adv Cancer Res* 2000; 278:199–334.

20. Kelloff GJ, Sigman CC, Johnson KM, et al. Perspectives on surrogate endpoints in the development of drugs that reduce the risk of cancer. *Cancer Epidemiol Biomarkers Prev* 2000; 9:127–34.

21. Fisher B, Costantino JP, Wickerham DL, et al. Tamoxifen for prevention of breast cancer: report of the National Surgical Adjuvant Breast and Bowel Project P-1 Study. *J Natl Cancer Inst* 1998; 90;1371–88.

22. Slaughter DP, Southwick HW, Smejkal W. "Field cancerization" in oral stratified squamous epithelium. Clinical implications of multicentric origin. *Cancer* 1953; 6:963–8.

23. Benner SE, Hong WK, Lippman SM, et al. Intermediate biomarkers in upper aerodigestive tract and lung chemoprevention trials. *J Cell Biochem* 1992; 16G:33–8.

24. Kelloff GJ, Sigman CC, Hawk ET, et al. Surrogate end-point biomarkers in chemopreventive drug development. In: Miller AB, Bartsch H, Boffetta P, et al. (eds) *Biomarkers in cancer prevention,* IARC Scientific Publications No. 154. Lyon: International Agency for Research on Cancer, 2001, pp. 13–26.

25. Lipkin M. Biomarkers of increased susceptibility to gastrointestinal cancer: new application to studies of cancer prevention in human subjects. *Cancer Res* 1988; 48:235–45.

26. Steinbach G, Lynch PM, Phillips RK, et al. The effect of celecoxib, a cyclooxygenase-2 inhibitor, in familial adenomatous polyposis. *N Engl J Med* 2000; 342:1946–52.

27. Hamilton SR. Pathology and biology of colorectal neoplasia. In: Young GP, Levin B, Rozen P (eds) *Prevention and early detection of colorectal cancer: principles and practice,* London: WB Saunders, 1996, pp. 3–21.

28. Roth JA, Putnam JB Jr, Rich TA, et al. Cancers of the gastrointestinal tract: cancer of the esophagus. In: DeVita VT Jr, Hellman S, Rosenberg SA (eds) *Cancer: principles & practice of oncology,* 5th ed. Philadelphia: Lippincott-Raven Publishers, 1997, pp. 970–1251.

29. Linehan WM, Cordon-Cardo C, Isaacs W. Cancers of the genitourinary tract. In: DeVita VT Jr, Hellman S, Rosenberg SA (eds) *Cancer: principles & practice of oncology,* 5th ed. Philadelphia: Lippincott-Raven Publishers, 1997, pp. 1253–395.

30. Kelloff GJ, Boone CW, Crowell JA, et al. Surrogate endpoint biomarkers for Phase II cancer chemoprevention trials. *J Cell Biochem* 1994; 19 (Suppl):1–9.

31. Boone CW, Kelloff GJ, Steele VE. Natural history of intraepithelial neoplasia in humans with implications for cancer chemoprevention strategy. *Cancer Res* 1992; 52:1651–9.

32. Califano J, van der Riet P, Westra W, et al. Genetic progression model for head and neck cancer: implications for field cancerization. *Cancer Res* 1996; 56:2488–92.

33. Lotan R, Xu X-C, Lippman SM, et al. Suppression of retinoic acid receptor-β in premalignant oral lesions and its up-regulation by isotretinoin. *N Engl J Med* 1995; 332:1405–10.

34. Meyskens FL Jr, Surwit E, Moon TE, et al. Enhancement of regression of cervical intraepithelial neoplasia II (moderated dysplasia) with topically applied all-*trans*-retinoic acid: a randomized trial. *J Natl Cancer Inst* 1994; 86: 539–43.

35. Giardiello FM, Hamilton SR, Krush AJ, et al. Treatment of colonic and rectal adenomas with sulindac in familial adenomatous polyposis. *N Engl J Med* 1993; 328:1313–16.

36. Bedi A, Pasricha PJ, Akhtar AJ, et al. Inhibition of apoptosis during development of colorectal cancer. *Cancer Res* 1995; 55:1811–16.

37. Stoner GD, Budd GT, Ganapathi R, et al. Sulindac sulfone induced regression of rectal polyps in patients with familial adenomatous polyposis. *Adv Exp Med Biol* 1999; 470:45–53.

38. Fearon ER, Vogelstein B. A genetic model for colorectal tumorigenesis. *Cell* 1990; 61:759–67.

39. Sidransky D, Mikkelsen T, Schwechheimer K, et al. Clonal expansion of p53 mutant cells is associated with brain tumor progression. *Nature* 1992; 355:846–7.

40. Sidransky D, Messing E. Molecular genetics and biochemical mechanisms in bladder cancer. Oncogenes, tumor suppressor genes, and growth factors. *Urol Clin North Am* 1992; 19:629–39.

41. Sidransky D, Frost P, Von Eschenbach A, et al. Clonal origin bladder cancer. *N Engl J Med* 1992; 326:737–40.

42. Rosin MP, Cairns P, Epstein JI, et al. Partial allelotype of carcinoma *in situ* of the human bladder. *Cancer Res* 1995; 55:5213–16.

43. Mao L, Schoenberg MP, Scicchitano M, et al. Molecular detection of primary bladder cancer by microsatellite analysis. *Science* 1996; 271: 659–62.

44. Simoneau AR, Jones PA. Bladder cancer: the molecular progression to invasive disease. *World J Urol* 1994; 12:89–95.

45. Thiberville L, Payne P, Vielkinds J, et al. Evidence of cumulative gene losses with progression of premalignant epithelial lesions to carcinoma of the bronchus. *Cancer Res* 1995; 55: 5133–9.

46. Kishimoto Y, Sugio K, Hung JY, et al. Allele-specific loss in chromosome 9p loci in preneoplastic lesions accompanying non-small-cell lung cancers. *J Natl Cancer Inst* 1995; 87:1224–9.

47. Larson AA, Liao S-Y, Stanbridge EJ, et al. Genetic alterations accumulate during cervical tumorigenesis and indicate a common origin for multifocal lesions. *Cancer Res* 1997; 57:4171–6.

48. Ilyas M, Straub J, Tomlinson IPM, et al. Genetic pathways in colorectal and other cancers. *Eur J Cancer* 1999; 35:335–51.

49. Muto T, Bussey HJR, Morson BC. The evolution of cancer of the colon and rectum. *Cancer* 1975; 36:2251–70.

50. Hamilton SR. The adenoma-adenocarcinoma sequence in the large bowel: variations on a theme. *J Cell Biochem* 1992; 16 (Suppl G):41–6.

51. Soloway MS, Perito PE. Superficial bladder cancer: diagnosis, surveillance and treatment. *J Cell Biochem* 1992; 16 (Suppl I):120–7.

52. Herr HW, Jakse G, Sheinfeld J. The T1 bladder tumor. *Semin Urol* 1990; 8:254–61.

53. Harris AL, Neal DE. Bladder cancer—field versus clonal origin. *N Engl J Med* 1992; 326:759–61.

54. Winawer SJ, Zauber AG, O'Brien MJ, et al. Randomized comparison of surveillance intervals after colonoscopic removal of newly diagnosed adenomatous polyps. *N Engl J Med* 1993; 328:901–6.

55. Burt RW. Cohorts with familial disposition for colon cancers in chemoprevention trials. *J Cell Biochem* 1996; 25 (Suppl):131–5.

56. Fabian CJ, Kamel S, Zalles C, et al. Identification of a chemoprevention cohort from a population of women at high risk for breast cancer. *J Cell Biochem* 1996; 25 (Suppl):112–22.

57. Westra WH, Sidransky D. Phenotypic and genotypic disparity in premalignant lesions: of calm water and crocodiles. *J Natl Cancer Inst* 1998; 90:1500–1.

58. Mao L, El-Naggar AK, Papadimitrakopoulou V, et al. Phenotype and genotype of advanced premalignant head and neck lesions after chemopreventive therapy. *J Natl Cancer Inst* 1998; 90:1545–51.

59. Hittelman WN, Kim HJ, Lee JS. Detection of chromosome instability of tissue fields at risk: *in situ* hybridization. *J Cell Biochem* 1996; 25 (Suppl):57–62.

60. Brown PO, Botstein D. Exploring the new world of the genome with DNA microarrays. *Nature Gen* 1999; 21 (Suppl):33–7.

61. Sneige N, Lagios MD, Schwarting R, et al. Interobserver reproducibility of the Lagios nuclear grading system for ductal carcinoma *in situ*. *Hum Pathol* 1999; 30:257–62.

62. Bacus JW, Boone CW, Bacus JV, et al. Image morphometric nuclear grading of intraepithelial neoplastic lesions with applications to cancer chemoprevention trials. *Cancer Epidemiol Biomarkers Prev* 1999; 8:1087–94.

63. Kelloff GJ, Lieberman RL, Steele VE, et al. Chemoprevention of prostate cancer: concepts and strategies. *Eur J Urol* 1999; 35:342–50.

64. Su L-K, Kinzler KW, Vogelstein B, et al. Multiple intestinal neoplasia caused by a mutation in the murine homolog of the APC gene. *Science* 1992; 256:668–70.

65. Jacoby RF, Marshall DJ, Newton MA, et al. Chemoprevention of spontaneous intestinal adenomas in the *Apc*Min mouse model by the nonsteroidal anti-inflammatory drug piroxicam. *Cancer Res* 1996; 56:710–14.

66. Arbeit JM, Howley PM, Hanahan D. Chronic estrogen-induced cervical and vaginal squamous carcinogenesis in human papillomavirus type 16 transgenic mice. *Proc Natl Acad Sci USA* 1996; 93:2930–5.

67. Boone CW, Stoner GD, Bacus JV, et al. Quantitative grading of rat esophageal carcinogenesis using computer-assisted image tile analysis. *Cancer Epidemiol Biomarkers Prev* 2000; 9: 495–500.

68. Edelmann W, Yang K, Kuraguchi M, et al. Tumorigenesis in *MLH1* and *MLH1/Apc1638N* mutant mice. *Cancer Res* 1999; 59:1301–7.

69. Zhang Z, Liu Q, Lantry LE, et al. A germ-line *p53* mutation accelerates pulmonary tumorigenesis: *p53*-independent efficacy of chemopreventive agents green tea or dexamethasone/*myo*-inositol and chemotherapeutic agents taxol or adriamycin. *Cancer Res* 2000; 60:901–7.

24
Evidence-Based Policy Recommendations on Screening and Prevention

Eduardo L. Franco and Thomas E. Rohan

This chapter presents an overview of the scientific evidence for existing policies and recommendations concerning screening for and prevention of specific types of cancer. Much of the research on the efficacy of specific screening and preventive interventions has focused on precancerous or early cancerous lesions, such as high grade dysplasias of the uterine cervix, oral leukoplakias, and colonic adenomas. In fact, the most widely studied screening intervention in cancer, the Pap test, is based on the cytological identification of precancerous lesions that can be treated or excised, with consequent arrest of neoplastic development in the cervix. However for many cancer sites, screening interventions have been evaluated with respect to detection of early invasive cancers. The same applies to the evaluation of primary prevention strategies. Though the most convincing evidence of efficacy comes from a reduction in mortality and/or incidence of cancers, many studies have used generally accepted intermediate endpoints, such as large adenomatous polyps for colorectal cancer prevention and high-grade squamous intraepithelial lesions of the cervix.

Ideally, clinical and public health practice guidelines should reflect not only the availability of empirical evidence but also the strength of evidence as judged by expert reviews of published data. The most persuasive arguments for the efficacy of screening come from conclusive randomized controlled trials (RCTs), investigations that typically take many years to complete, particularly if they focus on later endpoints in the natural history of cancer, that

is, the occurrence of invasive cancer or cancer-specific death. Such studies are not always feasible, however, because of ethical reasons—for example, when discovery of the intermediate endpoint is already an accepted basis for treatment, such as in high-grade cervical lesions—or because they would have to be extremely large to the point of being impractical (e.g., rare cancers such as neuroblastoma).

Studies in which baseline screening or primary prevention information on all subjects is subsequently linked with national or regional incidence or mortality databases, without active surveillance of lesions have served a useful purpose in providing evidence of benefit (or lack therof) for interventions. However, the increased concern in Western populations about individual privacy has led to a tendency for funding agencies and ethical review boards to require more stringent justification for record linkage studies. In consequence, trials focusing on intermediate endpoints (precancer lesions or suitable biomarkers) have become more widely accepted, especially because the use of surrogate markers in cancer research has become better understood and such studies can be carried out in a shorter period of time and with greater statistical power (see chapters by Schatzkin and Kelloff and Sigman).

The new era of evidence-based medicine has spawned a number of consortia of biomedical researchers specializing in the practice of reviewing published clinical and epidemiological evidence on a systematic basis and ranking the available evidence in terms of type of study, quality of the information, and generalizability of the results to different health care settings. These consortia are affiliated with government agencies, professional societies, or with private nonprofit organizations dedicated to the improvement of healthcare delivery. This review summarizes the recommendations on screening and prevention from some of the more influential of these organizations in North America and internationally and provides their assessment of the weight and quality of the scientific evidence in support of these interventions.

Evidence for Screening Interventions

National Institutes of Health Physician's Data Query Program

The Physician's Data Query (PDQ) database program maintained by the US National Cancer Institute is a permanent review group that continuously scans the literature to assess the quality of the evidence for oncological practices, including screening interventions and prevention strategies [1]. With respect to screening, the PDQ program produces summary statements of screening efficacy for specific tests or procedures. The assessment of the evidence and the summaries are prepared by the PDQ Screening and Prevention Editorial Board based upon both continuing review of the published scientific evidence and recommendations by professional bodies. Members

of the Editorial Board represent the fields of oncology, cancer prevention, statistics, epidemiology, and economics. This group meets bimonthly to review and update information on cancer screening and early detection. The expertise of the Editorial Board is supplemented by Advisory Boards, which include over 100 specialists who review information regularly and suggest changes or updates to the main Editorial Board.

Table 24.1 summarizes the levels of evidence for statements of screening efficacy by the PDQ. Proof of mortality reduction in RCTs is assigned the highest level of evidence. Lower levels of evidence are obtained from case-control and cohort studies and other information such as the incidence of cancer before and after introduction of a particular screening intervention. Measures of improved outcome for determining screening efficacy are ranked from the most persuasive to the least persuasive as follows: (i) decrease in cause-specific mortality; (ii) reduction in incidence of advanced-stage cancers; (iii) increase in survival; (iv) shift in disease stage [2].

Table 24.2 presents the evidence for efficacy of specific screening tests and cancer sites from the PDQ program (with updated information as of August, 2000, and for some sites, November, 2000). Many of the screening tests described in the table are able to detect cancer precursor lesions in the respective organs or sites (e.g., Pap test, mammography, sigmoidoscopy, oral exfoliative cytology, and skin examination), whereas the remainder are able to detect early invasive cancers. RCTs have

TABLE 24.1. Levels of evidence for statements of screening efficacy from the US National Cancer Institute's Physician's Data Query program.

Level of evidence	Assessment of the evidence by expert review
1	Evidence obtained from at least one well-designed and conducted randomized controlled trial
2	Evidence obtained from well-designed and conducted controlled trials without randomization
3	Evidence obtained from well-designed and conducted cohort or case-control analytic studies, preferably from more than one center or research group
4	Evidence obtained from multiple-time series with or without intervention
5	Opinions of respected authorities based on clinical experience, descriptive studies, or reports of expert committees

Source: Kramer BS, 1995 [1], with permission.

TABLE 24.2. NCI-PDQ program's summaries of evidence for the efficacy of specific screening tests in reducing mortality from cancer.

Cancer site	Screening test	Evidence of benefit	Level of evidence[1]
Uterine cervix	Pap cytology	Yes	3, 4, 5
Breast	Mammography with or without clinical	40–49 years: Yes	1, 2, 3, 5
	breast examination	50–69 years: Yes	1, 2, 3, 5
		70+ years: Uncertain	5
		<40 years: No data	5
Colorectal	Fecal occult blood	Yes	1
	Sigmoidoscopy	Yes	3, 4, 5
	Digital rectal examination	No	3 (limited)
Bladder	Hematuria, cystoscopy, cytology	Insufficient	5
Endometrium	Endometrial sampling or transvaginal	Insufficient	5
	ultrasound		
	Pap cytology	No	5
Liver	α-fetoprotein and/or ultrasound	Insufficient	5
Lung	Chest X-ray and/or sputum cytology	No	1, 3
Neuroblastoma	Vanillylmandelic acid and homovanillic acid	No	3, 4, 5
Mouth	Oral examination or cytology	Insufficient	5
Ovary	CA 125, transvaginal ultrasound, pelvic exam	Insufficient	4, 5
Prostate	Digital rectal examination, transrectal	Insufficient	5
	ultrasound, or prostate-specific antigen		
Skin	Physical examination	Insufficient	5
Stomach	Endoscopy	Insufficient	3 + 4 (limited), 5
Testicular	Physical examination	Insufficient	5

[1] See Table 1 for explanation on levels of evidence.

been conducted for only a few of the more common screening techniques—mammography in breast cancer screening being the one most thoroughly studied in several trials worldwide [3], with unequivocal evidence of benefit among women of ages 50 to 69.

Pap cytology is often considered the most successful cancer screening test. There is widespread acceptance that Pap screening has reduced mortality from cervical cancer in most Western countries, but the evidence comes from observational epidemiologic studies, such as case-control and cohort investigations [4,5] (level 3), time series analysis showing that mortality decreased after the introduction of organized screening [6] (level 4), and geographical comparisons showing that the reduction in mortality was proportional to screening coverage [7] (level 4). In addition, there are numerous consensus statements from expert groups attesting to the effectiveness of the Pap test as an established medical procedure (level 5). The weight of the evidence in favor of Pap cytology obviates the need to have its screening efficacy scrutinized further in an RCT. In fact, such a proposition would be ethically untenable given that the Pap test is a widely accepted medical procedure.

Table 24.2 shows that sufficient evidence for screening effectiveness has been obtained for two screening tests other than Pap cytology and mammography: guaiac-based fecal occult blood (FOB) testing and sigmoidoscopy in colorectal cancer, albeit with quantitatively different levels of evidence. Biennial FOB testing was evaluated in RCTs in Europe [8,9] and in the US [10,11] with a 15% to 21% reduction in mortality, whereas sigmoidoscopy has been assessed in observational studies and by expert review groups [12]. Removal of adenomas found on sigmoidoscopy, particularly the ones with severely dysplastic areas, decreases subsequent colorectal cancer risk [13,14].

As yet there is no evidence of benefit for the remaining screening tests in reducing cancer mortality (Table 24. 2) but many continue to be investigated in a variety of study designs in clinical and population-based settings (e.g., the National Institutes of Health (NIH)-coordinated Prostate, Lung, Colorectal, and

Ovarian (PLCO) Cancer Screening Trial [15]). Conclusive evidence of no benefit has been obtained for Pap cytology in endometrial cancer, for chest X-ray and sputum cytology in lung cancer, and for urinary metabolite tests in neuroblastoma.

A number of novel screening tests not included in Table 24.2 are currently being evaluated in epidemiologic studies and RCTs. Noteworthy among them are automated cytology methods and human papillomavirus (HPV) testing, for detecting preinvasive cervical lesions, and spiral computerized tomography (CT), for detecting incipient, potentially precancerous lung lesions [16]. As yet, there is insufficient evidence to support using automated cytology methods and HPV testing to replace Pap testing in cervical cancer screening, although these new tests seem to have higher sensitivity and at least comparable specificity to the latter when older women are screened [17,18] (see Chapter 16). Spiral CT has been introduced in a clinical research capacity and on a limited basis, in clinical practice in the United States, amidst considerable controversy following the long-term follow-up results of the Mayo Lung Project [19], an RCT that showed no reduction in lung cancer mortality in men receiving frequent chest X-ray examinations (see Chapter 13). Chest X-ray detected many incipient lesions that did not progress to cancer in the latter trial, underscoring the concern that spiral CT, owing to its much greater imaging sensitivity, will unveil many more such lesions. Consequently, a relatively greater proportion of patients will have to undergo unnecessary invasive treatment procedures. A new feasibility trial has been funded recently by NIH (NCI-P00-0171) to examine the acceptability by current and former smokers of participating in a subsequent larger RCT that will compare spiral CT with chest X-rays for lung cancer screening.

United States and Canadian Task Forces

Two other organizations noteworthy for their systematic approach in reviewing the evidence for the effectiveness of cancer screening inter-

ventions are the US Preventive Services Task Force (USPSTF) [20] and the Canadian Task Force on the Periodic Health Examination (CTFPHE) [21]. These two organizations have cooperated in reviewing the appropriateness of a wide range of clinical preventive services in use in North America, including screening tests for early detection of disease, immunizations to prevent infections, and counseling for disease risk reduction. Both task forces rank the quality of the published evidence via the same descriptors adopted by the PDQ program (Table 24.1). However, these organizations do not merely rank the quality of evidence but go one step further by making specific graded recommendations for or against adoption of procedures as part of standard clinical practice. The strength of the recommendations for adoption of a particular screening intervention is graded according to the classification shown in Table 24.3 [20,21]. Assessment of screening test accuracy and the documentation of favorable clinical outcomes, in addition to reduction in mortality from cancer, are important criteria guiding the recommendations by these two task forces. Unfortunately, unlike the PDQ Editorial Board, which meets bimonthly, these two groups do not meet frequently enough to review the published evidence that accumulates continuously in most areas of screening and prevention.

Table 24.4 summarizes both task forces' recommendations concerning the application of cancer screening tests among asymptomatic persons [20,21]. A grade "A" recommendation (good supporting evidence) was given in only two instances by the USPSTF: Pap cytology and mammography among women 50 to 69 years old; and only once by the somewhat more conservative CTFPHE: to mammography in the same age group. The Canadian task force assigned a "B" recommendation (fair supporting evidence) to the Pap test. The degree of evidence is shown in parentheses next to the scores for practice recommendations (Table 24.4). FOB and sigmoidoscopy attained "B" grade recommendations by the USPSTF but failed to be supported by the CTFPHE, which concluded its report with a statement of insufficient evidence concerning efficacy ("C" rec-

TABLE 24.3. Strength of recommendations used by the US Preventive Services Task Force (USPSTF) and by the Canadian Task Force on the Periodic Health Examination (CTFPHE) for assessing clinical preventive services, including screening for cancer.

Strength of recommendations	Description
A	There is good evidence to support the recommendation that the condition[1] be specifically considered in a periodic health examination.
B	There is fair evidence to support the recommendation that the condition be specifically considered in a periodic health examination.
C	There is insufficient evidence to recommend for or against the inclusion of the condition in a periodic health examination, but recommendations may be made on other grounds.
D	There is fair evidence to support the recommendation that the condition be excluded from consideration in a periodic health examination.
E	There is good evidence to support the recommendation that the condition be excluded from consideration in a periodic health examination.

[1] *Condition* in the context of this chapter, implies a particular screening test.
Source: US Preventive Services Task Force, 1996 [20], and Canadian Task Force on the Periodic Health Examination, 1994 [21].

ommendation) for both procedures. Most of the screening tests shown in the table attain at most a "C" recommendation, with several noteworthy negative recommendations, such as urine sediment tests for bladder cancer, and biochemical and clinical tests for ovarian, pancreatic, and prostate cancer, which received "D" scores (fair evidence against). The only frankly negative recommendation ("E" grade: good evidence against) was assigned by the CTFPHE for sputum cytology in lung cancer screening. As mentioned above, an important caveat in interpreting the recommendations by the two task forces is the fact that they do not include the more recent published evidence appearing in the last five (for the American) or six (for the Canadian) years. Therefore, they predate key consensus guidelines that addressed some controversial topics, such as the use of mammography among women 40 to 49 years of age [22], or the more recent evidence in favor of HPV testing in screening for cervical cancer precursors (see Chapter 16).

Other Systematic Reviews

Of paramount importance among the international consortia of clinicians and epidemiologists producing reviews of evidence for health care interventions is the Cochrane Collaboration. This group was inspired by the work of Archie Cochrane, a British epidemiologist who proposed continuous systematic reviews of all relevant RCTs of healthcare interventions. The Cochrane Centre began with seed funds from the United Kingdom's National Health Service and was initially based at Oxford University in 1992. The initiative quickly expanded to include centers around the world, and in 1993, the "Cochrane Collaboration" was founded [23]. Cochrane reviews are the principal output of the Collaboration and are published electronically in successive issues of the Cochrane Database of Systematic Reviews [24]. Preparation and maintenance of Cochrane reviews is the responsibility of international collaborative review groups which cover most of the important areas of healthcare and follow a rigidly defined set of guidelines for reviewing the evidence from RCTs in their specific areas. Whenever appropriate, Cochrane reviews provide a meta-analysis of study results, that is, summary estimates of screening benefit (for instance, the net percent reduction in mortality due to the intervention) averaged across all RCTs with comparable design and outcomes.

Many of the Cochrane reviews cover relevant areas in cancer control and prevention. However, unlike the dedicated function of the PDQ program at NCI and the periodic task force evaluations in North America described above, Cochrane reviews must rely on the ad

TABLE 24.4. Summary of recommendations (with quality of the evidence[1]) by the US Preventive Services Task Force (USPSTF) and by the Canadian Task Force on the Periodic Health Examination (CTFPHE) with respect to the effectiveness of cancer screening tests.

Cancer site	Screening test	USPSTF (1996)	CTFPHE (1994)
Uterine cervix	Pap cytology	A (II-2, II-3)	B (II-2)
	Cervicography or colposcopy	C (III)	not assessed
	HPV testing	C (III)	D (II-2)
Breast	Mammography with or without clinical breast examination	40–49 yrs: C (I)	40–49 yrs: D (I)
		50–69 yrs: A (I, II-2)	50–69 yrs: A (I)
		70+ yrs: C (I, II-3, III)	70+ yrs: not assessed
	Annual clinical breast examination	40–49 yrs: C (III)	not assessed
		50–59 yrs: C (I)	
		60+ yrs: C (III)	
	Routine breast self-examination	C (I, II-2, III)	C (II-2)
Colorectal	Fecal occult blood	B (I, II-1, II-2)	C (I)
	Sigmoidoscopy	B (II-2, II-3)	C (II-2)
	Digital rectal examination	C (III)	not assessed
	Colonoscopy	C (III)	C (III)
Bladder	Dipstick for hematuria	D (II-2, III)	D (II-2)
	Urine cytology	D (III)	D (II-2)
Lung	Chest X-ray	D (I, II-1, II-2)	D (I)
	Sputum cytology	D (I, II-1, II-2)	E (I)
Mouth	Oral examination	C (III)	C (II-2)
Ovary	CA 125, transvaginal ultrasound, pelvic exam	D (II-3, III)	D (II-2)
Pancreas	Abdominal palpation, ultrasound, serum markers	D (III)	D (II-2)
Prostate	Digital rectal examination	D (II-2)	C (II-2)
	Transrectal ultrasound	D (II-2, III)	D (II-3)
	Prostate-specific antigen	D (I, II-2, III)	D (II-3)
Skin	Physical examination	C (II-3, III)	C (II-3)
Testicular	Physical examination	C (III)	C (III)

[1] Quality of evidence indicated in parentheses correspond to scores for the descriptions in Table 1 based on the following equivalency: I = 1, II-1 = 2, II-2 = 3, II-3 = 4, III = 5. The CTFPHE assessment includes only the highest attained score. See also Table 3 for descriptions of recommendations.
Source: US Preventive Services Task Force, 1996 [20], and Canadian Task Force on the Periodic Health Examination, 1994 [21].

hoc assembly of volunteer experts who agree to target a specific maneuver for assessment. For this reason, the number of completed protocols on cancer screening that provide informative conclusions is still relatively small. As of November 2000, of the twelve cancer screening-related procedures that were listed in the Cochrane database of systematic reviews, only three had been completed (Table 24.5). They are included here, however, because of the potential interest in the conclusions to be reached by the pending review protocols and because many of the interventions refer to cancer precursors.

In addition to the above systematic reviews, several others, undertaken by different expert panels assembled by government agencies in North America and in Europe, have focused specifically on certain screening interventions. A few of these reviews are germane to the topic of screening for cancer precursors and are worth mentioning because of their scope. The US Agency for Healthcare Research and Quality (formerly the Agency for Health Care Policy and Research) has produced systematic reviews of the efficacy and costs of Pap cytology in cervical cancer screening [28] and of different screening methods for the detection of colorectal lesions [29]. In Canada, the Canadian Coordinating Office for Health Technology Assessment has produced a comprehensive review of the techniques available for cervical cancer screening, including conventional and automated cytology methods and HPV testing [30]. In the UK, the National Coordinating Centre for Health Technology Assessment has

TABLE 24.5. Screening interventions and related procedures relevant to cancer control that either have been evaluated or are under review by the Cochrane Collaboration as of November, 2000.

Review status	Screening intervention or related procedure [reference]	Conclusion
Completed	Screening for colorectal cancer using the fecal occult blood test [25]	Average reduction in colorectal cancer mortality: 16% (95% CI: 7%–23%) but harmful effects and costs need to be assessed.
	Surgery for cervical intraepithelial neoplasia [26]	No differences among 7 techniques in disease eradication; Large loop excision of the transformation zone yields best specimens for histology.
	Collection devices for obtaining cervical cytology specimens [27]	Extended tip spatulas of various designs are better than Ayre's spatule for sampling endocervical cells specially in combination with a cytobrush.
Under review	Adenoma surveillance on incidence and mortality from colorectal cancer	
	Mammographic screening for breast cancer	
	Strategies for inviting women to participate in breast cancer screening	
	Interventions to encourage the uptake of cervical cancer screening	
	α-fetoprotein and/or liver ultrasound for liver cancer screening among hepatitis B carriers	
	Screening for lung cancer	
	Strategies for detecting colon cancer and/or dysplasia in inflammatory bowel disease patients	
	Therapies for the eradication of *Helicobacter pylori*	
	Interventions for treating oral leukoplakia	

Source: Abstracts of Cochrane Reviews, 2000 [24].

reviewed the evidence for the efficacy of HPV testing [31] and of liquid cytology methods [32] in cervical cancer screening. The latter reviews are more extensive in scope and in their review of study methodology than the PDQ program and North American task forces, and include detailed analyses of costs for the various procedures. On the other hand, the conclusions are more qualitative than quantitative in terms of specific recommendations.

Evidence for Interventions Aiming at Primary Prevention

The same agencies or consortia described above have also produced systematic reviews of evidence for the effectiveness of primary prevention strategies. A compilation of these systematic reviews is presented below.

National Institutes of Health Physician's Data Query Program

The PDQ program defines cancer prevention as the reduction of cancer mortality via reduction in the incidence of cancer. Its panel of experts have assessed a number of plausible interventions, such as avoiding intake of carcinogens or altering their metabolism and modifying lifestyle or dietary practices, that affect cancer risk. These assessments have taken into account not only the potential benefit of the strategy in the general population but also among high-risk individuals who carry genetic predispositions. The summaries are updated bimonthly by the PDQ Editorial Board as new evidence becomes available in the published literature [33].

As with the statements about screening efficacy described above, the PDQ assessments are

TABLE 24.6. Levels of evidence for summary statements on the efficacy of prevention strategies assessed by the US National Cancer Institute's Physician's Data Query program.

Assessment of the evidence by expert review	Type of endpoint	Outcome	Level of evidence
Evidence obtained from at least one well-designed and conducted randomized controlled trial with:	Cancer	Mortality	1ai
		Incidence	1aii
	Intermediate endpoint[1]	Incidence	1b
Evidence obtained from well-designed and conducted nonrandomized controlled trials with:	Cancer	Mortality	2ai
		Incidence	2aii
	Intermediate endpoint	Incidence	2b
Evidence obtained from well-designed and conducted cohort or case-control analytic studies, preferably from more than one center or research group with:	Cancer	Mortality	3ai
		Incidence	3aii
	Intermediate endpoint	Incidence	3b
Ecologic (descriptive) studies (e.g., international patterns studies, migration studies) with:	Cancer	Mortality	4ai
		Incidence	4aii
	Intermediate endpoint	Incidence	4b
Opinions of respected authorities based on clinical experience or reports of expert committees (e.g., any of the above study designs using nonvalidated surrogate endpoints)			5

[1] A generally accepted intermediate endpoint (e.g., large adenomatous polyps for colorectal cancer prevention; high-grade squamous intraepithelial lesions of the cervix).
Source: National Cancer Institute [34].

summarized by varying levels of evidence that support a given statement. Table 24.6 shows the different degrees of quality of evidence assigned to these assessments [34]. The most convincing evidence is that obtained from well-designed and well-conducted RCTs with cancer-specific mortality as the endpoint (level 1ai). Frequently, however, mortality endpoints are not realistic, and other relevant endpoints are utilized, such as cancer occurrence (level 1aii) or an intermediate endpoint defined at a cancer precursor stage in the natural history of the disease (level 1b), for example, a dysplastic preinvasive lesion of the cervix or an adenomatous polyp of the colon. RCTs are also more the exception than the rule among the study designs used to ascertain the role of risk factors or preventive strategies. In general, preventive practice has to rely on evidence obtained by nonrandomized trials with sufficient follow-up (level 2) or on observational epidemiologic studies with individuals as the unit of observation, that is, cohort or case-control investigations (level 3). Less convincing evidence is that obtained in ecologic studies (level 4) that examine variation in cancer morbidity or mortality on entire populations or groups of individuals as a function of the putative average exposure to risk factors. Also included in this category of evidence are studies that establish temporal or geographical relations, or migrant studies. The same suffix assignment based on the type of outcome (ai = mortality, aii = cancer, or b = intermediate endpoint) is made to levels 2, 3 and 4 by PDQ reviewers. Finally, the weakest level of evidence is that concluded by expert panel assessments produced without the availability of the latter study types (level 5).

Table 24.7 summarizes the levels of evidence for specific prevention strategies for individual sites of cancer. For most statements the evidence comes from observational epidemiologic studies and/or opinions of expert panels. Whenever level-1 type evidence (RCTs) is lacking, the rationale for the strategy relies mostly on the facts that increased risk was found for a given exposure in epidemiologic studies, and that decreasing the exposure intensity or eliminating it completely will lead presumably to a reduction in cancer incidence (e.g., dietary modifications leading to a reduction of the constituent associated with risk). Alternatively, it is the exposure itself that seems to lead to a reduction in risk—e.g., exercise in relation to breast cancer—which makes the rationale for a preventive benefit more obvious. Exceptionally, observational epidemiologic studies are able to estimate the actual impact of the elimination of an exposure that leads to increased risk of cancer, for example, smoking cessation in lung and upper aero-digestive tract cancers.

Of particular interest in recent years is research on chemopreventive agents to reduce cancer risk (see chapter on chemoprevention). Table 24.7 lists three such chemopreventive strategies in which favorable RCT-type evidence (level 1) is already available: tamoxifen in breast cancer [35], nonsteroidal anti-inflammatory drugs (NSAIDs) in adenomatous polyps [36], and progestins in endometrial cancer associated with hormone replacement therapy [37]. The original rationale for incorporating the latter preventive maneuvers in RCTs was based on the results from epidemiologic studies and on secondary clinical outcomes in therapeutic trials of cancer treatment.

TABLE 24.7. NCI-PDQ program's summaries of evidence for the efficacy of specific prevention strategies for cancer.

Cancer site	Prevention strategy	Level of evidence[1]
Uterine cervix	Barrier methods of contraception	3ai, 4ai, 5
	Smoking cessation	3ai, 4ai, 5
	Increased intake of micronutrients and carotenoids	3ai
	Health education to lead to behavior modification with diminished exposure	5
Breast	Tamoxifen in women at increased risk for breast cancer	1aii
	Avoidance of unnecessary breast irradiation	3aii
	Controlling exposure to alcohol (conflicting evidence)	3aii
	Exercise at certain ages	3aii
	Reducing dietary fat consumption (conflicting evidence)	4ai, 5
Colorectal	Reducing dietary total fat, protein, calories, alcohol, and meat	3aii, 4aii
	Cereal fiber supplementation and diets low in fat and high in fiber, fruits, and vegetables do not reduce rate of adenoma recurrence	1b
	Nonsteroidal anti-inflammatory drugs (piroxicam, sulindac, aspirin) to prevent adenoma formation or cause adenomatous polyps to regress among familial adenomatous polyposis patients	1b, 3ai, 3aii
	Smoking cessation to prevent adenomas and cancer	3aii
Endometrium	Progestins to prevent cancer associated with estrogen replacement	1aii, 2aii, 3aii, 5
	Use of combination oral contraceptives	3aii, 5
	Avoidance of tamoxifen use	1aii, 3aii, 5
Lung	Smoking cessation	3ai, 4ai, 5
	Avoidance of pharmacological doses of β-carotene among smokers	1a
Oral	Smoking cessation and avoidance of smokeless tobacco	3aii, 5
	Reducing alcohol consumption	3aii, 5
	Increasing dietary intake of fruits and vegetables	3aii, 5
	Avoidance of sunlight exposure (lip cancers)	3aii, 5
Ovary	Sustained use of combination oral contraceptives	3aii
Prostate	Reducing dietary fat consumption	3aii, 4ai, 5
Skin	Reducing ultraviolet radiation exposure (nonmelanoma skin cancer)	1b, 3aii, 5
	Avoidance of sunburns, especially in childhood and adolescence (melanoma)	3aii, 4aii, 5
Stomach	Avoidance of excessive salt intake	3, 5
	Increasing dietary intake of fruits and vegetables, cereals, carotenoids, vitamin C, allium compounds, green tea	3aii, 5

[1] See Table 6 for explanation of levels of evidence.
Source: National Cancer Institute [34].

On the other hand, RCTs of chemoprevention can also lead to results that are dramatically different from what would be expected on the basis of epidemiologic evidence from observational studies. A case in point is the evolution in the understanding of the role of β-carotene as a micronutrient with cancer-preventive potential. During the last quarter century, a substantial body of epidemiologic evidence from case-control and cohort studies has implicated a high dietary intake of fruits and vegetables, a high estimated β-carotene index diet, and high serum levels of β-carotene with a lower risk of many malignant epithelial tumors, particularly lung cancer. This provided the rationale for chemopreventive RCTs of β-carotene to prevent mortality from lung cancer among high risk persons. As shown in Table 24.7, the unequivocal conclusions from two well conducted RCTs, the NCI α-Tocopherol β-carotene (ATBC) trial [38] and the β-Carotene and Retinol Efficacy Trial (CARET) [39] have led the PDQ program to assert with a "1a" level of evidence that intake of β-carotene supplementation at pharmacological doses is to be avoided because it could lead to an increased risk of lung cancer among smokers. The ATBC trial enrolled male smokers and the CARET trial enrolled both male and female smokers and exsmokers and asbestos-exposed persons and the two trials differed in the doses of β-carotene that were administered, namely 20 mg/day and 30 mg/day, respectively. The conclusions from both studies were consistent with a deleterious effect of β-carotene as investigated. The RRs of lung cancer and overall mortality in the ATBC trial were 1.18 (95%CI: 1.03–1.36) and 1.08 (95%CI: 1.01–1.16), respectively [38]. The same RRs in the CARET trial were 1.28 (95%CI: 1.04–1.57) and 1.17 (95% CI: 1.03–1.33), respectively [39]. Interestingly, both studies found negative associations between plasma β-carotene levels and lung cancer rates, which is consistent with the epidemiologic evidence that formed the basis for these trials. This indicates that high levels of β-carotene in plasma may be a marker of increased dietary intake of fruits and vegetables, which in itself may confer the health benefit. These results have led to a rethinking of the rationale for chemopreventive trials of lung cancer.

US and Canadian Task Forces

The two North American task forces tend to view preventive strategies differently in terms of how globally the evidence is assessed. While the CTFPHE examined each maneuver in the context of specific cancers [21], the USPSTF examined the overall potential benefits for many different clinical outcomes simultaneously (i.e., cancer, cardiovascular, etc.) [20]. The USPSTF also tends to provide separate assessments for the effects of the risk determinant itself and of counseling to modify exposure to it.

The USPSTF assigns an "A" grade recommendation with level of evidence II-2 (refer to Tables 24.3 and 24.4 for an explanation of the score system) to the efficacy of a multiple-outcome risk reduction secondary to cessation of tobacco use. On the other hand, this agency provides different recommendations concerning counseling strategies to curb tobacco use: A, level I, for clinician counseling of all smoking patients and the use of nicotine patches or gum as adjuncts to counseling; C, level I, for clonidine as an adjunct to counseling; and C, level III, for clinician counseling of children and adolescents [20]. The Canadian task force assigns an "A" grade recommendation of level I for smoking reduction for preventing oral and lung cancers (B for pancreatic cancer) and "A" and "B" grades for counseling and referral strategies to prevent or reduce smoking [21].

Regarding interventions for gynecologic cancers, the USPSTF assigns an "A" grade recommendation with level II-2 for avoidance of high-risk sexual activity and use of barrier methods of contraception to prevent cervical cancer. A "B" recommendation (level II-2) is assigned to the use of oral contraceptives to prevent ovarian and endometrial cancers. On the other hand, the agency views counseling measures to reduce risk of these diseases somewhat less confidently by assigning them a "C" recommendation with level III evidence [20].

Other Systematic Reviews

Most Cochrane reviews that are applicable to cancer prevention have focused on tobacco cessation strategies. As of November, 2000, the Cochrane database contained 21 completed reviews dealing with tobacco addiction that ranged from counseling interventions to techniques involving specific aids, both conventional and unconventional (acupuncture, antidepressants, aversive smoking, nicotine-replacement therapies, and various forms of counseling). A number of these interventions were deemed efficacious by the review groups, such as prescription of the antidepressants bupropion and nortriptyline; of drugs that aid withdrawal from nicotine, for example, clonidine, mecamylamine, nicotine replacement therapy; individual counseling by health care providers; group therapy; and self-help interventions [40]. An additional completed review on interventions for encouraging sexual behavior modification intended to prevent cervical cancer concluded that sexual education interventions involving women of low socioeconomic status are effective in leading to short-term reduction of sexual risk behaviors and thus have the potential to reduce transmission of HPV infection [41]. The Cochrane database also contained several ongoing review protocols covering the following interventions that are germane to cancer prevention: therapy for the eradication of *Helicobacter pylori* infection, prophylactic mastectomy for the prevention of breast cancer, and drugs for preventing lung cancer.

Quantifying the Importance of the Risk Factor That Is Amenable to an Intervention Strategy

An important aspect in the assessment of the evidence and public health impact of a particular prevention strategy is the population attributable risk proportion (PARP) associated with a particular risk factor that is amenable to intervention. The PARP estimate represents the proportion of all cancer cases that are attributable to the exposure to a given risk factor (under the assumption that the risk factor is causally related to the disease), and is thus, a useful measure for agencies establishing policy targets in cancer prevention. Its calculation is dependent on two other quantities: the relative risk (RR), which is measured in case-control or cohort studies; and the exposure prevalence in the population, which is obtained in health surveys or estimated in the same studies that generated the RR estimates [42]. A highly prevalent risk factor whose strength of association with cancer is high will be equated to a high PARP. For instance, the RR for the association between tobacco smoking and lung cancer risk is relatively high (average RR = 10), and smoking prevalence can be 40% to 50% in some Western populations, which yields a PARP of approximately 80%. That is, four-fifths of all lung cancers are attributable to smoking. In theory at least, one can expect that elimination of smoking will lead to this much of a reduction in lung cancer incidence over time. Occasionally, important risk factors turn out to be less important in terms of overall risk attribution in the population. For instance, the association between a history of ulcerative colitis and colorectal cancer risk is of high magnitude (RR = 20). However, ulcerative colitis is a rare clinical condition in the population with a prevalence of less than 0.1%, which indicates that at most 2% of all colorectal cancers occurring in the population would be due to this condition as a primary cause. The same analogy applies to hepatitis B carrier status and liver cancer risk in North America. While the RR for the relation is high (RRs = 10–20) the prevalence of the exposure is relatively low (<1%). On the other hand, hepatitis B carrier status is very frequent in East Asia and Africa, and thus the potential for a substantial impact of a mass immunization program against hepatitis B virus would be very high. It is easy to see also how an association of presumably low magnitude, such as that between hot *maté* (a type of tea widely consumed in Southern South America) drinking and oral cancer (RR = 1.5) can have a great regional impact on disease occurrence. *Maté* is consumed by approximately 80% of all adults in parts of Southern Brazil, Uruguay, and

Argentina. At this level of exposure, about 30% of all oral cancers can be attributed to *maté* drinking, which translates to a sizable expectation for incidence reduction subsequent to a hypothetically successful public education campaign about the effects of hot *maté* consumption as a putative preventive strategy [42]. Similar considerations apply to the role of environmental tobacco smoke, a recognized risk factor with a relatively weak association with cancer risk the abolition or amelioration of which would potentially have a substantial impact on cancer prevention because of the high prevalence of the exposure.

Practice Recommendations

Numerous government and nongovernmental agencies, medical professional societies, and healthcare organizations have established specific practice recommendations concerning screening and prevention. While some of these groups adopt policy guidelines based solely on scientific evidence that has been carefully reviewed as per the mechanisms described in this chapter, others have a more liberal interpretation of the published data or consider additional circumstances such as delivery costs and prevailing practices. Even when agencies adopt practice guidelines based on careful review of the evidence, pressure from the public and professionals may eventually contribute to the reversal or retraction of such recommendations. In cancer screening, the best example was the retraction by NIH of the conclusions from its consensus conference on mammography among women of ages 40 to 49 [22]. The original main conclusions (*"... data currently available do not warrant a universal recommendation for mammography for all women in their forties ... each woman should decide for herself whether to undergo mammography"*) created substantial controversy and political pressure from the United States Congress [43].

A key factor in the implementation of policy guidelines based on best available evidence is the general structure of the healthcare delivery system. Many countries with an universal payor system of socialized medicine tend to examine overall benefits of screening and prevention strategies in relation to delivery costs and are generally more restrictive in their acceptance of novel technologies. Health technology assessments by Canadian and Western European agencies tend to give far more weight to evidence of effectiveness from RCTs that show reductions in mortality from cancer as the endpoint. On the other hand, in the United States, with its decentralized healthcare system that is free of direct governmental control, policy agencies tend to accept evidence from a broader spectrum of sources and tend to view more favorably RCTs with cancer precursor or cancer occurrence endpoints. A case in point is the traditionally liberal (in the sense of adopting recommendations more broadly) stance taken by the American Cancer Society, arguably the most influential private organization in the United States in setting standards of oncological practice. This agency advocates yearly mammography among women 40 to 49 years old and prostate cancer screening including digital rectal exam (DRE) and PSA testing for all men 50 or older [44], two examples of recommendations that are yet to be supported by solid evidence. In addition, a key driving force in health technology assessments in the United States has been the climate of medical malpractice litigation, which leads the medical profession to consider sensitivity of screening tests as a more important parameter than specificity given the potential legal costs of false-negative results.

Summary and Conclusions

Progress in our understanding of the natural history of cancer and in developments in testing technology and epidemiologic methods have led to an increased reliance on intermediate endpoints as outcomes in screening and primary prevention studies (see also Chapters 4 and 23). However, empirical demonstration that preventive strategies have an impact on the detection of (in the case of screening) or on the incidence of (in the case of chemoprevention) cancer precursors does not equate with proof of benefit from a public heath standpoint. The standard of proof for practice guidelines is more restrictive; preventive strategies must produce a reduction in mortality or at least in cancer incidence to be deemed worthy of adoption on a populations basis. Nevertheless, screening and prevention studies using precursor cancer endpoints play a valuable role in providing the necessary proof of principle to justify the considerable costs and resources required for investigations of cancer incidence or mortality endpoints.

The practice by many health technology assessment groups of conducting rigorous systematic reviews of primary and secondary strategies for cancer have greatly contributed to the establishment of scientifically sound practice guidelines. As reviewed in this chapter, the conclusions by these systematic reviews of evidence indicate that many screening and preventive strategies fall short of their expected or promised impact.

Most successful secondary prevention (screening) strategies for cancer are based on the detection and effective treatment of cancer precursors, leading to a reduction in the incidence of and mortality from invasive cancer. With the exception of the Pap test in cervical cancer, which was proven largely successful on the basis of systematic epidemiologic observations, the other success stories, namely, mammography in breast cancer screening and FOB in colorectal cancer, underwent verification by a higher standard of proof: the RCT paradigm. Also with noted exceptions (chest X-ray and sputum cytology in lung cancer and urinary metabolites in neuroblastoma), lack of evidence of benefit for other screening approaches does not indicate that the benefit may not exist, but rather, that current technology and lack of availability of well-designed studies are hampering our understanding of a possible public health impact of these screening strategies.

Primary prevention approaches are all based on the premise that the natural history of cancer must be arrested in its very early phases (by blocking exposure to carcinogens before it leads to the onset of precursor lesions) or reversed soon after appearance of precursor lesions. Except for a few approaches involving chemoprevention and dietary modification, maneuvers whose efficacy in cancer prevention have been scrutinized by RCTs, the expected benefit for most other primary prevention strategies discussed in this chapter is backed up by the lesser standard of proof of observational epidemiologic studies, albeit with substantial consistency across studies. Consistency in epidemiologic findings for a particular cancer risk association forms the rationale for testing the putative preventive strategy in RCTs. The fact that this has led to an occasional paradoxical result—for example β-carotene in lung cancer prevention among smokers—does not indicate that epidemiologic studies were pointing to the wrong opportunity for intervention, but rather, that the putative maneuver was an oversimplification of the role of dietary fruits and vegetables in cancer causation.

Systematic reviews of published results of evidence in cancer screening and prevention do not necessarily form the only knowledge base that health care agencies and medical professional societies use when formulating practice guidelines. A variety of factors influence the adoption of recommendations, including the system of healthcare delivery in a given country or region, pressure from unconvinced health professionals and patient groups, and fear of medical malpractice litigation. As health and legal professionals and the public become more aware of the value of scientific evidence for or against preventive interventions, the latter situation may change, and such comprehensive reviews may eventually become the main criterion to influence changes in healthcare practices. However, evidence-based medicine is far from being an exact science. No matter how much of the evidence may come from RCTs, a healthy dose of skepticism will always exist when it comes to making sense of information on cancer control and prevention.

References

1. Kramer BS. NCI State-of-the-art statements on cancer screening. In: Greenwald P, Kramer BS, Weed DL (eds) *Cancer prevention and control.* New York: Marcel Dekker, 1995, p. 721.

2. Screening for Cancer (PDQ) Screening/Detection—Health Professionals. Available at URL: *http://cancernet.nci.nih.gov/pdq/pdq_screening.shtml.*

3. Baines CJ, Miller AB. Mammography versus clinical examination of the breasts. *J Natl Cancer Inst Monogr* 1997; 22:125–9.

4. La Vecchia C, Franceschi S, Decarli A, et al. "Pap" smear and the risk of cervical neoplasia: quantitative estimates from a case-control study. *Lancet* 1984; 2:779–82.

5. Herrero R, Brinton LA, Reeves WC, et al. Screening for cervical cancer in Latin America: a case-control study. *Int J Epidemiol* 1992; 21: 1050–6.

6. Laara E, Day NE, Hakama M. Trends in mortality from cervical cancer in the Nordic countries: association with organised screening programmes. *Lancet* 1987; 1:1247–9.

7. Benedet JL, Anderson MB, Matisic JP. A comprehensive program for cervical cancer detection and management. *Am J Obstet Gynecol* 1992; 166:1254–9.

8. Kronborg O, Fenger C, Olsen J, et al. Randomised study of screening for colorectal cancer with faecal-occult-blood test. *Lancet* 1996; 348: 1467–71.

9. Hardcastle JD, Chamberlain JO, Robinson MH, et al. Randomised controlled trial of faecal-occult-blood screening for colorectal cancer. *Lancet* 1996; 348:1472–7.

10. Winawer SJ, Flehinger BJ, Schottenfeld D, et al. Screening for colorectal cancer with fecal occult blood testing and sigmoidoscopy. *J Natl Cancer Inst* 1993; 85:1311–18.

11. Mandel JS, Church TR, Ederer F, et al. Colorectal cancer mortality: effectiveness of biennial screening for fecal occult blood. *J Natl Cancer Inst* 1999; 91:434–7.

12. Winawer SJ, Fletcher RH, Miller L, et al. Colorectal cancer screening: clinical guidelines and rationale. *Gastroenterology* 1997; 112:594–642.

13. Winawer SJ, Zauber AG, Ho MN, et al. Prevention of colorectal cancer by colonoscopic polypectomy: the National Polyp Study Workgroup. *N Engl J Med* 1993; 329:1977–81.

14. Rembacken BJ, Fujii T, Cairns A, et al. Flat and depressed colonic neoplasms: a prospective study of 1,000 colonoscopies in the UK. *Lancet* 2000; 355:1211–14.

15. Gohagan JK, Prorok PC, Kramer BS, et al. Prostate cancer screening in the prostate, lung, colorectal and ovarian cancer screening of the National Cancer Institute. *J Urol* 1994; 152: 1905–9.

16. Henschke CI, McCauley DI, Yankelevitz DF, et al. Early Lung Cancer Action Project: overall design and findings from baseline screening. *Lancet* 1999; 354:99–105.

17. Nanda K, McCrory DC, Myers ER, et al. Accuracy of the Papanicolaou test in screening for and follow-up of cervical cytologic abnormalities: a systematic review. *Ann Intern Med* 2000; 132:810–19.

18. Cuzick J, Sasieni P, Davies P, et al. A systematic review of the role of human papilloma virus (HPV) testing within a cervical screening programme: summary and conclusions. *Br J Cancer* 2000; 83:561–5.

19. Marcus PM, Bergstralh EJ, Fagerstrom RM, et al. Lung cancer mortality in the Mayo Lung Project: impact of extended follow-up. *J Natl Cancer Inst* 2000; 92:1308–16.

20. U.S. Preventive Services Task Force. *Guide to Clinical Preventive Services*, 2nd ed. Washington, DC: U.S. Department of Health and Human Services, 1996.

21. Canadian Task Force on the Periodic Health Examination. *The Canadian guide to clinical preventive health care*. Ottawa: Health Canada, 1994.

22. National Institutes of Health Consensus Development Conference Statement: Breast Cancer Screening for Women Ages 40–49, January 21–23, 1997. National Institutes of Health Consensus Development Panel. *J Natl Cancer Inst* 1997; 89:1015–26.

23. Chalmers I. The Cochrane Collaboration: preparing, maintaining and disseminating systematic reviews of the effects of health care. *Ann NY Acad Sci* 1993; 703:156–63.

24. Abstracts of Cochrane Reviews. The Cochrane Library Issue 4, 2000. Available at URL: http://hiru.mcmaster.ca/cochrane/cochrane/revabstr/mainindex.htm or URL: *http://www.update-software.com/cochrane/cochrane-frame.html.*

25. Towler BP, Irwig L, Glasziou P, et al. Screening for colorectal cancer using the faecal occult blood test, Hemoccult (Cochrane Review). In: The Cochrane Library, Issue 4. Oxford: Update Software; 2000.

26. Martin-Hirsch PL, Paraskevaidis E, Kitchener H. Surgery for cervical intraepithelial neoplasia (Cochrane Review). In: The Cochrane Library, Issue 3. Oxford: Update Software; 2000.

27. Martin-Hirsch P, Jarvis G, Kitchener H, et al. Collection devices for obtaining cervical cytology samples (Cochrane Review). In: The Cochrane Library, Issue 4. Oxford: Update Software; 2000.

28. McCrory DC, Matchar DB, Bastian L, et al. *Evaluation of Cervical Cytology.* Evidence Report/Technology Assessment No. 5. AHCPR Publication No. 99–E010. Agency for Health Care Policy and Research. Rockville, MD: U.S. Department of Health and Human Services; 1999.

29. Agency for Health Care Policy and Research. *Colorectal Cancer Screening.* Technical Review 1. AHCPR Publication No. 98-0033. Rockville, MD: U.S. Department of Health and Human Services; 1998.

30. Noorani HZ, Arratoon C, Hall A. *Assessment of techniques for cervical cancer screening.* Ottawa: Canadian Coordinating Office for Health Technology Assessment; 1997.

31. Cuzick J, Sasieni P, Davies P, et al. A systematic review of the role of human papillomavirus testing within a cervical screening programme. *Health Technol Assess* 1999; 3:1–199.

32. Payne N, Chilcott J, McGoogan E. Liquid-based cytology in cervical screening: a rapid and systematic review. *Health Technol Assess* 2000; 4:1–73.

33. Hubbard SM, Shields VT, Thurn AL. Information Systems in Oncology. In: Devita VT, Hellman S, Rosenberg SA (eds) *Cancer: principles and practice of oncology,* 5th ed. Philadelphia: Lippincott-Raven, 1997, pp. 2983–91.

34. National Cancer Institute. CancerNet PDQ Cancer Information Summaries: Prevention. Available at URL: *http://cancernet.nci.nih.gov/pdq/pdq_prevention.shtml.*

35. Gail MH, Costantino JP, Bryant J, et al. Weighing the risks and benefits of tamoxifen treatment for preventing breast cancer. *J Natl Cancer Inst* 1999; 91:1829–46.

36. Sandler RS. Aspirin and other nonsteroidal anti-inflammatory agents in the prevention of colorectal cancer. *Cancer Principles Pract Oncol Updates* 1997; 11:1–14.

37. The Writing Group for the PEPI trial. Effects of hormone replacement therapy on endometrial histology in postmenopausal women: the Postmenopausal Estrogen/Progestin Interventions (PEPI) Trial. *J Am Med Assoc* 1996; 275: 370–5.

38. The Alpha-Tocopherol, Beta Carotene Cancer Prevention Study Group: the effect of vitamin E and beta carotene on the incidence of lung cancer and other cancers in male smokers. *N Engl J Med* 1994; 330:1029–35.

39. Omenn GS, Goodman GE, Thornquist MD, et al. Effects of a combination of beta carotene and vitamin A on lung cancer and cardiovascular disease. *N Engl J Med* 1996; 334:1150–5.

40. Cochrane Tobacco Addiction Group. Abstracts of Cochrane Reviews. The Cochrane Library, Issue 4, 2000. Available at URL: *http://www.update-software.com/abstracts/g160index.htm.*

41. Cochrane Gynaecological Cancer Group. Abstracts of Cochrane Reviews. The Cochrane Library, Issue 4, 2000. URL: *www.update-software.com/abstracts/ab001035.htm.*

42. Franco EL. Epidemiology in the study of cancer. In: Bertino JR (ed.) *Encyclopedia of Cancer,* Vol. 1. San Diego: Academic Press, 1997, pp. 621–641.

43. Taubes G. NCI reverses one expert panel, sides with another. *Science* 1997; 276:27–8.

44. Fink DJ. Chapter 12: Cancer detection: The cancer-related checkup guidelines. In: Holleb AI, Fink DJ, Murphy GP (eds) *American Cancer Society textbook of clinical oncology.* Atlanta American Cancer Society, 1991, pp. 153–76 (website updated guidelines available at URL: *www2.cancer.org/SiteSearch/www3/SiteCenter.cfm?scDoc=41255*).

Part V
Conclusion

Prospects

Thomas E. Rohan and Eduardo L. Franco

As is made evident in this book, the past few years have witnessed tremendous progress in our understanding of cancer precursors. Nevertheless, many questions remain with respect to precursors, not only (for precursors at some anatomical sites) with respect to their definition, but also with respect to their etiology, detection, and prevention. Although predicting future developments can be a somewhat hazardous undertaking, certain trends and opportunities are discernible with respect to the study of cancer precursors.

It is obvious that pathology has played a major role in the development of cancer epidemiology, given that the current classification of cancers and their precursors is (and has been for some time) based upon histomorphologic criteria [1,2]. Recently, however, the first tentative steps have been taken towards the creation of molecular classifications of cancers based on gene expression patterns [3], and we envisage that similar classifications of cancer precursors will emerge in time, spurred perhaps by recent technological developments such as laser capture microdissection, which can provide access to homogeneous samples of relevant tissue [4]. Advances in the application of molecular methods and new cell sampling techniques to the analysis of human tissue are allowing what are potentially the earliest molecular changes leading to carcinogenesis to be identified. For example, recent observations at some anatomical sites (e.g., the breast and the upper respiratory tract) suggest that molecular changes may precede histological changes [5,6].

Currently, however, it is not clear whether tissue displaying these changes should be considered to be premalignant. Resolution of this question will require follow-up studies in which cancer incidence, or perhaps the incidence of cancer precursors, is compared in individuals with and without molecular changes in normal tissue, and possibly studies in which the prevalence of molecular changes in histologically normal tissue is compared with that in adjacent tissue showing cancer precursors and invasive cancer. Molecular studies of this kind might lead us to revisit our current approaches to the classification of cancer or cancer-predisposing lesions. Indeed, given the increasingly molecular nature of pathological classification, it appears conceivable that in time we will move away from terms such as "cancer precursor" and "invasive cancer" and move towards a system wherein lesions are classified on the basis of the genetic changes that they exhibit as "early" or "late" cancer, without further specification. Existing morphology-based definitions will continue to be used for the foreseeable future, however, given that they form the cornerstone of current approaches to the treatment of cancer.

It is conceivable that molecular approaches to the classification of early lesions (or cancer precursors) will result in changes in our understanding of the etiology of such lesions (and their associated cancers). At the very least, the emerging era of molecular classification will spawn a new round of etiological studies using these classification systems for case definition.

These studies might change our understanding of the etiology of some conditions, and might provide us with new opportunities to begin to understand the etiology of others.

Molecular analysis of cancer precursor lesions might assist with the identification of those lesions which are at particular risk of progression to invasive cancer. This will have implications for the management of individuals harboring such lesions, and might result in increased surveillance or early intervention. Studies designed to identify markers of risk will require well-characterized cohorts, and we anticipate that studies of this kind, which have begun to be reported recently [7,8], will increase in number considerably. Existing biorepositories of tumor tissue with associated epidemiological information might represent a convenient starting point for such studies.

Advances in approaches to the molecular characterization of tumors and their precursor lesions, with the resultant possibility of identifying early lesions on molecular grounds, leads inevitably to the possibility of molecular screening for such lesions, an approach to tumor detection which is already under investigation for invasive cancers [9]. If implemented, these developments will have clinical and ethical implications, because practitioners will be confronted with an expanded array of lesions, the malignant potential and appropriate management of at least some of which may not be clear. For example, with respect to management, adoption of molecular approaches to lesion detection will raise questions as to the appropriate margins for the excision of lesions given that similar molecular changes might be observed in adjacent, morphologically normal tissue [5,6]. Nevertheless, before molecular assays are incorporated into clinical practice, it will be necessary to validate them, to demonstrate that they are superior to current approaches to tumor detection, and to develop and refine the requisite high throughput automation of the assays [9].

Prevention of true cancer precursors will necessarily result in a reduction in the subsequent incidence of the associated cancer at the same anatomical site. As such, cancer precursors serve dual roles as potential targets for preventive agents and as intermediate endpoints for trials testing agents and interventions designed to prevent cancer occurrence. Therefore, approaches to the primary prevention of cancer precursors hold much promise for the prevention of cancer. To date, however, there are relatively few data on the prevention of cancer precursors. For some sites at least, this may reflect a somewhat limited understanding of the etiology and natural history of cancer and its precursors. However, given the current movement towards the use of intermediate endpoints in trials of preventive agents, it is anticipated that there will be a burgeoning of data on the prevention of cancer precursors. This will be the case especially in the area of chemoprevention [10]. Mathematical models of the development of precursor lesions may assist in the development of optimal prevention (and screening strategies) by predicting the effect of an intervention given its proposed mechanism of action [11]. Models for adenoma development [11] and the natural history of human papillomavirus infection [12] have been developed recently, and we anticipate that similar efforts will be made for precursor lesions at other sites, given the increasing interest in prevention.

From an epidemiologic perspective, it is clear that researchers will have to contend with increasingly complex etiologic models when designing observational studies and intervention trials. The use of "softer" endpoints, situated upstream from the earliest morphological changes observable in the natural history of cancer, will pose new challenges to molecular epidemiologists in terms of the safeguards that they will need to employ to avoid the biasing effects of error in the measurement of molecular markers. Although the importance of using accurate and reproducible assays is well recognized, the literature on cancer precursors is not without examples of incoherent results due to misclassification of intermediate endpoints [13,14]. Increasing reliance on prospective studies, with repeated measurements of intermediate endpoints, will help to assuage some of the concerns about misclassification bias. Statistical methods for the analysis of longitudinal data generated in such investigations are a relatively recent addition to the armamentarium of cancer epidemiologists, and they are yet to be fully appreciated as research tools. Use of these methods and judicious use of mediation analysis [15,16] in studies of intermediate endpoints will play a valuable role in helping epidemiologists to decipher the sequence of events and associated molecular changes leading to cancer development.

From the foregoing discussion it should be evident that many disciplines can contribute to the goal of understanding cancer precursors (from many different perspectives). For example, despite the reservations of occasional commentators [17,18], to some extent the blossoming field of molecular epidemiology, entailing incorporation of biologic measurements into epidemiologic research, points the way towards realization of this goal and attests to the power and benefits of a multidisciplinary approach. However, other, perhaps more novel collaborations might be mutually beneficial. For example, transgenic mice (i.e., mice with foreign DNA incorporated into their genome [19]) with specific genetic lesions can develop histological lesions similar to those which precede cancer development in humans [20], and therefore provide insight into the molecular basis of carcinogenesis [19]. Clues as to the appropriate transgenic mouse models that molecular biologists might develop for this purpose might come, in part, from epidemiological studies of the molecular pathogenesis of cancer. This is but one of many possible examples, and we end this book with a plea for novel cross-disciplinary approaches to investigations designed to enhance our knowledge of cancer precursors.

References

1. Saxen E. Histopathology in cancer epidemiology. In: Sommers SC, Rosen PR (eds) *Pathology Annual*, Pt. 1. New York: Appleton, Century and Crofts, 1979, pp. 203–17.

2. Eustis SL. The sequential development of cancer: a morphological perspective. *Toxicol Lett* 1989; 49:267–81.

3. Perou CM, Sørlie T, Eisen MB, et al. Molecular portraits of human breast tumors. *Nature* 2000; 406:747–57.

4. Fend F, Raffeld M. Laser capture microdissection in pathology. *J Clin Pathol* 2000; 53:666–72.

5. Kandel R, Li SQ, Ozcelik H, et al. p53 protein accumulation and mutations in normal and benign breast tissue. *Int J Cancer* 2000; 87:73–8.

6. Westra WH, Sidransky D. Phenotypic and genotypic disparity in premalignant lesions: of calm water and crocodiles. *J Natl Cancer Inst* 1998; 90:1500–1.

7. Rohan TE, Hartwick W, Miller AB, et al. Immunohistochemical detection of c-erbB-2 and p53 in benign breast disease and breast cancer risk. *J Natl Cancer Inst* 1998; 90:1262–9.

8. Gobbi H, Dupoint WD, Simpson JF, et al. Transforming growth factor-β and breast cancer risk in women with mammary epithelial hyperplasia. *J Natl Cancer Inst* 1999; 91:2096–101.

9. Ahrendt SA, Sidransky D. The potential of molecular screening. *Surg Oncol Clin N Am* 1999; 8:641–56.

10. Lippman SM, Lee JJ, Sabichi AL. Cancer chemoprevention: progress and promise. *J Natl Cancer Inst* 1998; 90:1514–28.

11. Pinsky PF. A multi-stage model of adenoma development. *J Theor Biol* 2000; 207:129–43.

12. Myers ER, McCrory DC, Nanda K, et al. Mathematical model for the natural history of human papillomavirus infection and cervical carcinogenesis. *Am J Epidemiol* 2000; 151:1158–71.

13. Franco EL. The sexually-transmitted disease model for cervical cancer: Incoherent epidemiologic findings and the role of misclassification of human papillomavirus infection. *Epidemiology* 1991; 2:98–106.

14. Makni H, Franco E, Kaiano J, et al. *P53* polymorphism in codon 72 and risk of HPV-induced cervical cancer: effect of inter-laboratory variation. *Int J Cancer* 2000; 87:528–33.

15. Freedman LS, Graubard BI, Schatzkin A. Statistical validation of intermediate endpoints for chronic diseases. *Stat Med* 1992; 11:167–78.

16. Buyse M, Molenberghs G. Criteria for the validation of surrogate endpoints in randomized experiments. *Biometrics* 1998; 54:1014–29.

17. McMichael AJ. Invited commentary—"Molecular epidemiology": new pathway or new traveling companion? *Am J Epidemiol* 1994; 140:1–11.

18. Zur Hausen H. Cervical carcinoma and human papillomavirus: On the road to preventing a major human cancer. *J Natl Cancer Inst* 2001; 93:252–3.

19. Guha U, Hulit J, Pestell RG. Transgenic mice in cancer research. In: Bertino J (ed) *Encyclopedia of cancer*, 2nd ed. New York: Academic Press, 2001, (in press).

20. Wang TC, Cardiff RD, Zukerberg L, et al. Mammary hyperplasia and carcinoma in *MMTV*-cyclin D1 transgenic mice. *Nature* 1994; 369:669–71.

Index